FUNDAMENTALS OF **Gynecology and Obstetrics**

DALE RUSSELL DUNNIHOO, M.D., PH.D.

Professor and Vice-Chairman
Department of Obstetrics and Gynecology
Professor of Family Medicine and Comprehensive Care
Louisiana State University School of Medicine
Shreveport, Louisiana

Illustrations by Daniel Clement, M.D.

J. B. Lippincott Company Philadelphia
Grand Rapids   New York   St. Louis   San Francisco
London   Sydney   Tokyo

FUNDAMENTALS OF

Gynecology and Obstetrics

Acquisitions Editor: Lisa McAllister
Compositor: Achorn Graphic Services, Inc.
Printer/Binder: R. R. Donnelley and Sons
Production: P. M. Gordon Associates

1 3 5 6 4 2

Library of Congress Cataloging-in-Publication Data

Dunnihoo, Dale Russell.
    Fundamentals of gynecology and obstetrics/Dale Russell Dunnihoo;
    illustrations by Daniel Clement.
        p.   cm.
    Includes index.
    ISBN 0-397-50964-2
    1. Gynecology.   2. Obstetrics.   I. Title.
    [DNLM: 1. Gynecology.   2. Obstetrics.   WQ 100 D924f]
RG101.D89   1990
618—dc20
DNLM/DLC
for Library of Congress   89-8231
                                                                  CIP

The author and publisher have exerted every effort to ensure that drug selection
and dosage set forth in this text are in accord with current recommendations and
practice at the time of publication. However, in view of ongoing research, changes
in government regulations, and the constant flow of information relating to drug
therapy and drug reactions, the reader is urged to check the package insert for
each drug for any change in indications and dosage and for added warnings and
precautions. This is particularly important when the recommended agent is a new
or infrequently employed drug.

To my wife, Betty

Hippocratic Oath

*I swear by Apollo the physician, and Aesculapius, and Hygeia, and
Panacea, and all the gods and goddesses, that, according to my ability
and judgement, I will keep this Oath and this stipulation—to reckon
him who taught me this art equally dear to me as parents, to share my
substance with him, and relieve his necessities if required; to look upon his
offspring in the same footing as my own brothers, and to teach them this
art, if they shall wish to learn it, without fee or stipulation, and that by
precept, lecture, and every other mode of instruction, I will impart a
knowledge of the art to my own sons, and those of my teachers, and to
disciples bound by a stipulation and oath according to the law of
medicine, but to none others. I will follow that system of regimen which,
according to my ability and judgement, I consider for the benefit of my
patients, and abstain from whatever is deleterious and mischievous. I
will give no deadly medicine to anyone if asked, nor suggest any such
counsel; and in like manner I will not give to a woman a pessary
to produce abortion. With purity and holiness I will pass my life and
practice my art. I will not cut persons labouring under the stone, but will
leave this to be done by men who are practitioners of this work. Into
whatever houses I enter, I will go into them for the benefit of the sick,
and will abstain from every voluntary act of mischief and corruption;
and, further, from the seduction of females or males, of freemen and
slaves. Whatever, in connection with my professional practice, or not in
connection with it, I see or hear, in the life of men, which ought not to be
spoken of abroad, I will not divulge, as reckoning that all such should
be kept secret. While I continue to keep this Oath unviolated, may it be
granted to me to enjoy life and the practice of the art, respected by all
men, in all times! But should I trespass and violate this Oath, may the
reverse be my lot!**

*Reproduced with permission from A. Castiglioni, *A History of Medicine*, ed. and
trans. by E.M. Krumbhaar. New York, N.Y.: Alfred A. Knopf, Inc., Publisher, 1946,
pp. 154–155.

Preface

Educators have known for years that effective education depends in large measure upon their ability to define what it is they wish students to know and be able to do at the end of their formal education. This book is my statement of what medical students, interns, obstetric residents, and family practice residents going through their obstetrics-gynecology rotation must know. I have also attempted to reflect the "Instructional Objectives for a Clinical Curriculum in Obstetrics and Gynecology," developed by an undergraduate medical education committee of the Association of Professors of Gynecology and Obstetrics (APGO) in 1985, and the "Educational Objectives for Residents in Obstetrics and Gynecology," developed by the Council on Resident Education in Obstetrics and Gynecology (CREOG) in 1984. Because it is impossible for students to learn everything, they must exercise a degree of selection and emphasis in their own learning, and educators must assist them in making that selection. My contribution to this effort resides in this book.

I have attempted to present this information according to four basic levels of knowledge: what the student need only be **familiar** with, what to **know** in greater depth, what to **understand** even more thoroughly, and what to know how to **apply**. Typographic evidence of these levels is provided within the text.

Every body of knowledge contains information that has little practical value at the time that one learns it, but which is still an integral part of the basic foundation of that field. The student should at least be **familiar** with that information and be aware of the significance it may have in the future; however, it is not necessary to know it in any great depth. Plain text type will be used throughout the book for this type of information.

Other information requires a greater degree of awareness because it is practical and useful in performing a task. The student should **know** this information in considerable depth. The use of *italics* for words or phrases will alert the student to the fact that this information, and the context in which it is found, should be well known.

An even greater degree of knowledge is necessary if the student is to truly **understand** the interrelationships among the different bits of information that he or she learns, and therefore words or phrases that are in **bold** type should be considered in some depth in relation to the other data.

Finally, the student's ability not only to know and understand the data but also to **apply** those data to the clinical care of the patient is important. The ability to actually apply the knowledge in an accurate and appropriate manner in a clinical situation, which often does not fit the generalized textbook example, is the highest form of knowledge, since it not only requires an extensive database that is thoroughly understood, but also requires that the individual be able to analyze the many variables involved, synthesize such data, and then make the appropriate decisions. Those areas that require the **apply** level of knowledge in a clinical situation will be self-evident and constitute the sum of what I have covered.

I hope that this book will provide a simplified and organized approach to the study of obstetrics and gynecology. Those of my colleagues who are purists will perhaps take me to task for oversimplifying certain aspects of the material. In doing so, my emphasis has been on the practical facts rather than on the absolute data because I feel that the student will benefit more from a straightforward approach early in training and will then learn the exceptions and qualifiers at a later time. I have made no real attempt to be comprehensive, since that type of approach is more properly the goal of a reference textbook to be used by individuals who have already specialized in this field of study. Finally, I hope that my approach will provide direction and point out those salient features of the subject that should be of central concern to the student just entering the field of obstetrics and gynecology.

Acknowledgments

My desire in writing this textbook for medical students, family practitioners, and residents in obstetrics and gynecology was prompted by the recognition that there are few textbooks available that combine the simplicity of knowledge with the practicality of practice. Having been broadly trained myself, it became apparent to me over the years that many textbooks present the material using a general, comprehensive approach rather than teaching some of the specifics of the practice of obstetrics and gynecology. Often, each fact presented is scientifically qualified, with arguments for and against it painstakingly discussed. I decided that a simplified approach to the subject of obstetrics and gynecology was needed in order to highlight new advances in the subject while at the same time presenting the knowledge in such a manner as to make it usable in everyday practice. In addition, a knowledge of some of the historical aspects of medicine seemed to be necessary in order to show the continuity of our profession with medical traditions. To this end, this textbook is dedicated.

No one individual produces a work of this magnitude without the support of many individuals. My wife, **Betty Dunnihoo,** has suffered from the literal absence of her husband during the past four years as I toiled away in what we have euphemistically called my "computer room." The many references that I have reviewed have been supplied in part by **Marianne Jones,** the wife of one of our former family practice residents, who also served as our medical librarian at the E. A. Conway Hospital. **Roy G. Clay, Jr., M.D.,** assistant dean for E. A. Conway Affairs, was very supportive of my efforts. **David Boyle, Ph.D.,** psychologist, reviewed and contributed generously to the chapter on psychosomatic obstetrics and gynecology. **Paul Ware, M.D.,** psychiatrist at the E. A. Conway Hospital, was also of help in putting this chapter into a proper perspective. My eminent colleague **Warren Otterson, M.D.,** chairman of the Department of Obstetrics and Gynecology at the Louisiana State University School of Medicine, Shreveport, assisted me in reworking the section on stress incontinence and the evaluation of the urinary tract in Chapter 12 concerning vaginal disease. In addition, Dr. Otterson assisted me in performing one last review of the oncology portions of the book before it went to press.

Through the years, I have been blessed by having the opportunity of working with some of the leading obstetricians and scientists of our time. Some of these individuals assisted me by critically reviewing the manuscript and encouraging me to persist in my efforts. Others have provided me with the education and the desire to contribute to this great profession that we call medicine. **Kermit Krantz, M.D., Litt. D.,** chairman of Obstetrics and Gynecology at the University of Kansas, Kansas City, Kansas, who is perhaps one of the best known obstetricians of our time, took the time from his busy schedule to evaluate my efforts and to advise me about the contents of the book. Dr. Krantz was also very helpful in assisting me to specifically define the material on stress incontinence and in defining some of the anatomy in Chapter 2. **James Daly, M.D.,** chairman of Obstetrics and Gynecology at the University of Missouri, Columbia, Missouri, an old friend from my days in the United States Air Force, reviewed the oncology portions of the book, along with **John Wheelock, M.D.,** who is currently the director of the Residency Program and chief of the Oncology Division at the Keesler USAF Medical Center in Biloxi, Mississippi. The critical comments of these individuals were invaluable to me in the final editing of the manuscript.

The obstetric portions of the manuscript were reviewed by **William Roberts, M.D.,** chairman of the Department of Obstetrics and Gynecology at the Keesler USAF Medical Center. Dr. Roberts' advice and review were especially helpful and encouraging to me.

The specialized endocrinologic portions of the book were reviewed by **Donald Tredway, M.D., Ph.D.,** chairman of the Department of Obstetrics and Gynecology at the Oral Roberts University, Tulsa, Oklahoma, and **Krishna Singh, M.D.,** director of Endocrinology in the Department of Obstetrics and Gynecology at the Louisiana State University (LSU) School of Medicine, Shreveport, who also provided a final critical evaluation of those sections. **John Mailhes, Ph.D.,** also at the LSU School of Medicine in Shreveport, reviewed the statistical and genetic aspects of the book and was helpful in placing this area in perspective.

I would also like to take this opportunity to especially thank **William Bennett Bean, M.D.,** who edited the delightful book by Robert Bennett Bean, *Sir William Osler: Aphorisms from His Bedside Teachings and Writings,* for allowing me to include some of these aphorisms in my book. I heartily recommend this book, which is published by Charles C Thomas of Springfield, Illinois, to all of my readers. The wisdom espoused by this famous physician is still very apropos today.

Harvey Huddleston, M.D., my associate at the E. A. Conway Hospital, was kind enough to review the entire book, and he has added his helpful comments and suggestions to the manuscript.

Daniel Clement, M.D., my illustrator, has provided the continuity of appearance throughout the book with his fine illustrations. The combination of one author and one illustrator has made this book somewhat unique, and I hope that it will be appealing and educational to the students who read it.

In spite of the concerted efforts of my colleagues in trying to assist me in this endeavor, I must state that any mistakes or errors in this manuscript are entirely my responsibility. I have tried to make this text as error-free as possible, but the writing "gremlins" will probably always have their way, I suspect. Hopefully, there are no major errors or misstatements present in the final version of the book.

And finally, I would like to thank my editors, Lisa Biello, Lisa McAllister, Paula Callaghan, and Betsy Keefer. Their constant support and encouragement was very helpful. Their helpful comments and suggestions made the task so much easier.

Contents

PART I

General considerations

CHAPTER 1

The philosophy of practice

The critical sense and skeptical attitude of the Hippocratic school laid the foundation of modern medicine on broad lines, and we owe to it: first, the emancipation of medicine from the shackles of priestcraft and of caste; secondly, the conception of medicine as an art based on accurate observation, and as a science, an integral part of the science of man and of nature; thirdly, the high moral ideals expressed in that most memorable of human documents, the Hippocratic oath; and fourthly, the conception and realization of medicine as a profession of a cultivated gentleman.

—*Sir William Osler**

1. Our heritage

Aesculapius was a Greek physician who, according to Homer, served in the Trojan wars about 1250 B.C. and was later deified and placed in the pantheon of Greek gods as the god of medicine. As a god, he was considered to be the son of the god Apollo and the goddess Coronis. He was raised by the centaur Chiron, who taught him how to cure all diseases. The virgin sister of Apollo, Artemis, who later killed Coronis because of her unfaithfulness, is remembered as the goddess of women and the protectoress of the young girls of Athens. The daughters of Aesculapius were named **Hygeia** and **Panaceia. The main Aesculapiad Schools of Medicine were located at Cos, Cnidus, and Rhodes.**

Hippocrates the Great (460 B.C.–370 B.C.), the son of Heraclides, was born on the island of Cos. Hippocrates was a legend in his own time and has subsequently been considered the father of modern medicine. He had a long and productive career, much of it as an itinerant physician, and he died at the age of 90 in Thessaly.

The fame of Hippocrates eventually made the school at Cos the best known. Hippocrates studied first under his father, an Aesculapiad physician, and then later under Herodicus, one of the head physicians of the Aesculapiad school on the Asiatic peninsula of Cnidus. More than 60 books have come down to us as the work of Hippocrates; however, it is thought that only a very few of them were actually written by Hippocrates himself. This **Corpus Hippocraticum** (i.e., the Hippocratic Collection) has been variously listed as having between 53 and 72 books covering almost every aspect of medicine.

In his treatise **"Airs, Waters, and Places,"** Hippocrates discussed climatic conditions in relation to health. He emphasized the need for the young physician to observe his surroundings and to evaluate the hygienic and sanitary conditions of a community.

In his work **"Prognostics"** he stated: *"It appears to me a most excellent thing for the physician to cultivate prognosis; for by foreseeing and foretelling, in the presence of the sick, the present, the past, and the future, and explaining the omissions which patients have been guilty of, he will be the more readily believed to be acquainted with the circumstances of the sick; so that men will have confidence to entrust themselves to such a physician."*[1]

---

*Reprinted with permission from Robert Bennett Bean, *Sir William Osler: Aphorisms from His Bedside Teachings and Writings,* William Bennett Bean, ed. Springfield, Ill.: Charles C Thomas, Publisher, 1968, p. 118.

[1] Reprinted by permission from Encyclopaedia Britannica, Inc., *Great Books of the Western World,* vol. 10, "Hippocrates and Galen," Robert Maynard Hutchins, ed. Chicago: William Benton, Publisher, 1952, p. 19.

In **"Of the Epidemics"** the student is instructed that *upon entering the patient's sickroom he should have an authoritative demeanor and be properly dressed; he should speak briefly, have perfect composure, and pay assiduous attention. He should reply to objections, show calm self-control in managing the troubles that may occur, and rebuke those who create a disturbance. He should make frequent visits and be certain to examine the patient carefully so that he will know the case and be more at ease with it, and he must have the will to do what has to be done.*

From the **"Law"** treatise comes the discussion of the qualities that a young man must have if he wishes to become a physician. *Hippocrates commented that whoever wishes to study medicine should possess a natural ability. He should receive instruction in a favorable place. He should be able to pay the tuition. He should love to work and should be willing to spend the time to learn. The student should have a natural ability for medicine, since if he does not, then his efforts will be in vain. The student should acquire the knowledge and reflect on it in a favorable place for study. Finally, he should study for a long time so that his knowledge will eventually bear fruit.* The instructions continue and include the admonition that *the physician must look healthy and must be very clean, decently dressed, and anointed with sweet-smelling unguents. He should be silent, lead a morally irreproachable life, be grave and kind to all, and be serious without being harsh. He should be fair in every respect, and never lose his self-control. The physician must always remain bodily and spiritually clean.*

Hippocrates became very famous in his own time and was considered an authority on medical subjects for many centuries. His treatment of the sick, and his loyalty to the people of Athens, earned him fame and fortune. He was given a coveted Athenian citizenship award and was financially supported for the rest of his life by the people of Athens. Even the children of the Coans were allowed to have an "ephebe's training" in Athens (i.e., one year of army training and one additional year of garrison duty), with the same "rights and privileges as the Athenian children," because their homeland had produced such a great man as Hippocrates.

The Hippocratic Oath begins: "I swear by Apollo the physician, and Aesculapius, and Hygeia, and Panaceia, and all the gods and goddesses, that, according to my ability and judgement, I will keep this Oath

and this stipulation. . . ." The modern physician may still learn from the great physicians of our past.

2. The philosophy of practice

As a physician, you have the unique opportunity of being allowed a glimpse into the intimate details of the lives of the people you serve. In addition, your duties require you to bypass all sense of modesty or privacy, in both yourself and your patient, as you probe and poke into the hidden areas and recesses of the human body. Finally, a patient's answers to your persistent questions frequently reveal your patient's innermost thoughts and feelings and may lay bare basic fears and fantasies. **None of this could happen without your patient's trust in your integrity.** This type of trust has deep roots in the traditions of medicine, roots that predate even the time of Hippocrates.

While there has been a tendency in recent times to consider the practice of medicine to be merely a type of "business," you should bear in mind that the trust the patient places in you as a physician far transcends that accorded to a business person. **Faith that you will place the patient's interests above your own is what gives you the authority to be a physician.** As a consequence, you should treat your patients as you would want your own loved ones to be treated. If, upon objective reasoning, you would not wish your mother, wife, or daughter in the same situation, to receive a certain form of therapy, then you should not subject your patient to it. On the other hand, however, you should not become too emotionally involved in the care of your patients. If you feel very close to your patient emotionally and psychologically, then you might omit certain necessary procedures because of your desire not to "hurt" her. This situation can be very dangerous; one of the reasons physicians traditionally have not treated their own family members is that their judgment may be clouded by their emotional involvement with the person. You should maintain a gentle, caring, and sincere concern for your patients and their problems; however, you should always attempt to **remain objective** in all of your dealings with them. This approach constitutes **a philosophy of practice** that, in my opinion, you should strive to follow throughout your medical career.

3. Responsibilities

There are four major groups to which you, as a physician, owe responsibility: (1) your **family,** (2) your **patients,** (3) your fellow **colleagues,** and (4) your **community.**

a. Family responsibilities

From the moment you begin training, you will realize that you have a conflict between your medical education, with its long hours and intense intellectual focus, and your family life. Ruined marriages and destroyed careers often result when priorities are not set. You owe it to yourself and to your family to work out compromises that will satisfy, to some extent, both your professional life and your home life. You should be aware of the fact that your family will suffer in many areas because of your profession. It requires a truly exceptional person to be the spouse of a physician. Often it is not the amount of time that you spend with your family, but the quality of these relationships that counts.

b. Patient responsibilities

The responsibilities that you have to your patients are both ethical and legal ones. Since the term **"doctor"** means "to teach," one of your tasks is to teach your patient either how to cure her illness or, if incurable, then how to learn to live with it. This rule should be extended one step further in modern medicine to include teaching patients aspects of *preventive medicine.* Having to treat patients who have already developed a disease and have suffered some or all of the ravages of that disease constitutes a *crises type of medicine.* It makes far more sense to teach your patient how to avoid medical problems in the first place than to treat her after she has already developed the medical condition. Encouraging a patient to change her life-style by eliminating smoking, alcohol, and drug abuse is one example of such an approach. Teaching the patient how to handle the stresses in her life may be one of the most valuable services that you may be able to provide. *The preconceptional counseling* of a woman who is contemplating becoming pregnant is another example of modern preventive medicine. Teaching your patient that medicines, or surgical procedures, carry *risks* as well as *benefits* is also important. Educating your patient about the health hazards in her workplace or in her home may prevent future medical problems.

You should always keep in mind *the expenses of medical therapy* and attempt to teach your patient the best way to obtain quality care for the cheapest price. The overuse of emergency rooms for minor illnesses that could have been managed during office hours is one example of inefficient and costly medical care. Furthermore, in treating your patients, you should always go from the *simple to the complex* in ordering tests or performing procedures. Often, a simple inexpensive test may confirm your diagnosis. Ordering a battery of expensive tests is not cost-effective medical care. The *safety of the patient* should always be uppermost in your thoughts whenever you order invasive procedures.

You should try to develop a true rapport with your patient by treating her with respect and courtesy. Never be abrupt, rude, or insensitive to her needs or fears. She has trusted you enough to let you see her emotions and experience her fears, so it becomes your responsibility to never ridicule her or cause her to lose her pride.

Finally, **you owe it to your patient as well as to yourself to maintain and improve your medical skills throughout your career.** *As little as one hour of study each day, if carried out faithfully, will maintain your knowledge base. A little more study, plus your frequent attendance at medical seminars and postgraduate courses, will assist you in improving your skills.*

c. Responsibility to your colleagues

The responsibilities that you have to your fellow physicians are unique. There is an unseen bond between you and every other physician who has ever lived, including those with whom you practice every day. **You should treat your colleagues with respect and honor, and you should never criticize another physician.** This rule does not mean that an *impaired physician* should be allowed to continue in practice, but it does mean that such individuals should be treated with compassion and should be assisted in their efforts to conquer their afflictions, and if at all possible, they should be returned to active practice.

In some instances, you may be asked to testify for or against one of your colleagues in a malpractice action. Since, in a larger sense, you have a responsibility to the patient as well as to your colleague, you should testify about the truth as you see it and let the jury decide the verdict.

d. Community responsibilities

Community responsibilities usually involve *public health concerns,* such as the risks of birth control pills, the problems of teenage pregnancy, or perhaps the medical aspects of proposed laws involving the use of automobile seat belts for pregnant women. Occasionally, you will be asked to talk to high school or church groups on medical subjects, and as such you should always remember that you are **an advocate for your patients.** Their health, and the community conditions that may affect that health, should be uppermost in your mind as you contribute your time and knowledge to community health efforts. All of these activities can be personally satisfying to you and can also be of great benefit to the community.

Community responsibilities involve not only the immediate locality in which you live and practice, but also the larger community of your state as well as the national scene. You should utilize your expertise for the betterment of your patients' health by contributing your time and energies to **state and national medical societies.** This participation may place you in a position in which you may be able to influence the health care of patients throughout the country. As a patients' advocate, you can perhaps rectify those aspects of health care that are inefficient, expensive, and ineffective. Furthermore, you may be able to establish new and innovative approaches to medical care that may benefit large numbers of women. Many lives may be saved by your unselfish sharing of your medical and administrative talents.

A further responsibility that you have to the community concerns medical research. Although it is generally believed by many physicians that medical research is the responsibility of the academician, there are many instances in private practice where important information may be uncovered that would be of benefit to many patients if it were disseminated to the medical profession as a whole. It is therefore important for you to acquire, during your medical training,

those observational and writing skills necessary to record such scientific information for publication in medical journals.

4. An approach to patient care

a. Office procedures

1) Patient responsibilities

You should attempt to teach your patients that they have responsibilities to you, just as you have responsibilities to them. The patient owes you the courtesy of keeping you informed as to her response, or lack of response, to your treatment. You should subtly instruct her in doing this until it becomes second nature for her to do so. **Keeping appointments on time** is also an important point for you to teach your patients, as is the proper way to **break an appointment** in sufficient time for another patient to utilize that time period. Remember that, as a physician, you are the only one who can teach your patients how to properly utilize medical facilities. In doing so, you provide them with far better care for their medical dollar, and in addition, help them become much more knowledgeable about health-care problems. Furthermore, such patients will come to appreciate the demands and pressures of your job and will respect your needs to spend time with your family. Patients who have been well trained by their physicians do not call their physicians in the middle of the night about trivial matters.

2) Appointments

In the management of your practice, you should evaluate your office procedures and routines to determine whether there are **any factors that may be irritating or inconvenient** to your patients. When the patient arrives at your office, her initial contact with your office staff should be pleasurable, reassuring, and comforting. The receptionist should be tactful and cheerful, and she should let the patient know whether you are on schedule and how long she might have to wait before being seen. If you are running late and the patient's medical problem is not critical, then she should be allowed the option of making another appointment, as her busy schedule may be too tight to accommodate the delay. **It is therefore very important for you to make every possible effort to**

remain on schedule in seeing your patients. It is rude and inconsiderate for you to repeatedly run behind schedule and keep your patients waiting for long periods of time. Patients do not appreciate having to plan their schedules around an appointment time, and then being forced to wait inordinate amounts of time to be seen by the doctor. If such delays occur too frequently, many patients will seek care elsewhere or will become hypercritical of your medical efforts.

3) Waiting room

Your waiting room should be spacious, comfortable, and tastefully furnished. There should be adequate reading materials available with good lighting. Remember that your waiting room is a reflection of you as a physician and as a person. If it is shoddy and threadbare, the patient may assume that you have only a few patients or that you are not a successful practitioner. On the other hand, an ostentatious waiting room may make a patient feel that your fees are too high.

4) Office staff

You should choose the personnel that you hire to work in your office very carefully. Every office employee should be cheerful, caring, and industrious. **It is important that your staff like people and that they be willing to show extra compassion for patients who are ill.** An office employee's tactfulness in dealing with an ill patient, who may not be up to observing the amenities of normal contacts with people, will be greatly appreciated by your patient when she regains her health. **Insensitive employees,** or those who talk about confidential matters that they have heard in the office, are to be avoided, not only because they are insensitive to the needs of the patients but also because they may cause legal trouble for you by violating the confidentiality of the physician-patient relationship.

5) The interview setting

When the patient is ushered into your office by the chaperone, you should greet her in a cheerful manner and invite her to sit in a comfortable chair. Some physicians will sit behind a desk, but this **barrier effect** may make the patient feel that you are aloof and unapproachable, unless you have a particularly warm personality. Other physicians may place their desks against a wall and sit next to the patient. This arrangement may convey a feeling of equality that may be effective in dealing with some patients; for shy patients, however, the closeness engendered by the proximity of the chairs may be uncomfortable.

b. The interview technique
1) Structure

The interview is the first contact between you and the patient. It serves not only as a means of obtaining the patient's history but also serves as an introduction to the physician-patient relationship. **This first encounter will set the stage for the development of rapport between you and the patient—a relationship that may last for many years.** You should be careful not to address the patient by her first name or to assume familiarity above and beyond the relationship you have established with her. The patient will generally appreciate an attitude that is courteous and slightly formal in a kindly manner. You should not be frivolous or superficial in your demeanor, but rather, you should **just relax and be yourself.** In treating the patient in a relaxed manner, you put the patient at ease and remove some of the apprehensions she may have concerning her relationship with a "new" doctor.

In taking the history, it is important for you to **structure the interview** to some extent in order to prevent the patient from rambling and wasting time discussing insignificant events. It has been my practice to tell the patient that "I wish to ask a few **background** questions first," after which I would like for her to tell me about any problems she is having (see Chapter 4). This procedure allows me to obtain some basic information as to her chief complaint (in one brief sentence), the menstrual history, possible bleeding problems, and her contraceptive practices. With this minimal database, I can then have the patient give a chronological account of her problem(s), and I am then able to compare it with this baseline information. For example, if the patient's primary complaint is abdominal pain, the previous notation of her last menstrual period, her intermenstrual spotting, and her contraceptive practices may assist me in directing some of my questions toward determining whether a diagnosis of an ectopic pregnancy is in order. Thus, by starting the interview in this fashion, I will have set the structure of the interview and obtained a minimal database that will allow me to place her subsequent problems in a proper perspective. The patient should be allowed to tell her story at this point, with only an occasional interruption to clarify a fact, ask further questions, or fill in a gap in her story. You should write a succinct account in the chart as the patient is telling you of her problems. **This procedure has the effect of reinforcing the fact for the patient that what she tells you is important enough for you to write it down.** If, however, the patient relates intimate or sexual matters to you, then you should stop writing, so as to indicate to the patient that such information will not be recorded in the chart, where it might be seen by office personnel or others. **In addition, it is often advisable to tell the patient that you are omitting such information from the record so that she may be reassured that her privacy will not be violated.**

2) Role of the physician

You may assume one of three basic roles as you interview the patient. You may be: (1) **a dictatorial-authoritative figure,** with the patient being completely passive, or (2) **a cooperative-authoritative figure,** with the patient having almost equal input into her care, or you may establish (3) **a patient-controlled relationship,** in which the patient may at times completely control the situation and have a great deal to say about her care.

a) Dictatorial-authoritative figure approach

In the past, many physicians assumed the dictatorial-authoritative approach to patient care and would brook no interference on the part of the patient in determining the management of the case. This approach placed the patient in the position of a "child" being told what to do by the "severe patronizing parent." With increasing sophistication and maturity on the part of patients today, this type of management has become inappropriate, except in emergency situations where prompt decisions need to be made on the basis of medical necessities.

b) Cooperative-authoritative figure approach

The cooperative-authoritative approach is perhaps the best one for you to use in managing your patient. It allows you to continue to be the authoritative figure but gives the patient maximum input into her medical management. This approach assumes that the patient is an adult who is capable of assuming responsibility for her own health care under the guidance of your professional expertise. The patient thus becomes an active participant in her medical management, and in making decisions concerning her health care, she chooses from among the various options that you present. In presenting the options, you have both the moral and the legal obligation to present all of the facts to the patient in an unbiased manner so that the patient can make an informed decision. Those patients who are not capable initially of assuming complete participation in their health care should be gradually educated by the physician until they do have sufficient knowledge to become an active partner.

c) A patient-controlled approach

In recent times, there has been a tendency on the part of some physicians to allow the patient to almost completely dictate their medical care, even when such a course of action is inconsistent with the patient's safety (e.g., home deliveries). This approach can be dangerous if the proper safeguards are not kept in mind. While a patient may have some strong beliefs concerning her health care, you have an equal or greater responsibility to protect the patient from herself. The patient may not be aware of the dangers of certain courses of action, and it is your duty to inform her of the various risks and alternative approaches to therapy that are available. If the patient still refuses to listen to medical reason, then you should consider referring the patient to another physician who may be willing to follow the patient's dictates, rather than doing something that is medically or personally unacceptable to you.

3) The physician's personality

It is necessary for you to gain insight into your own personality if you wish to be a successful physician. You should be comfortable with your failings, as well as with your virtues, and you should **like** yourself. **The better you know yourself, the better you will recognize problems in your patients.** You will learn that all human beings, while being unique, are also very much alike. Analyze your past experiences and the lessons you have learned in life, since these experiences are the sum total of what you bring to the forefront when attempting to assist your patients. You should be aware of the fact, however, that you have your own personal biases that may not be of much help to your patients. You may need to modify your thinking to fit your patients' circumstances and needs rather than your own. You should mentally put yourself in the patient's position, and then ask yourself, "What is the best approach to this problem that will be of most benefit to the patient?"

4) Nonverbal communication

a) Physician

You should dress appropriate to your role as a physician. Whether you like it or not, your patient will view you as an authoritative figure and will expect you to live up to that role. When you step out of that preconceived image, you lose an important element in the treatment of your patient: **her faith in someone that she looks up to as an authority.** Dress neatly and avoid obnoxious habits, such as smoking and chewing, maintain good dental hygiene and a sweet breath, and conduct yourself in a professional and reserved manner. Do not eat or drink around your patients. Such activity is not only discourteous, but it is nonhygienic as well.

You should be cautious that you do not invade the patient's **"space"** too abruptly or without her permission. **Each individual has a zone about her body that is a "private space."** While you will let loved ones enter this space at will, you will not allow strangers to do so with comfort. By necessity, the physician must enter the patient's "space" to carry out the physical examination. Much of the patient's embarrassment and nervousness concerning the physical and pelvic examination may be related to this concept. **You should also be aware of the fact that when a patient adamantly refuses to have a pelvic examination, or when the patient is very uncooperative during a pelvic examination, the reason may be that she has had a traumatic invasion of her "space" in the past (e.g., sexual abuse, rape).**

Outside of the examination room, you should be careful to avoid close physical contact with your patient. It may take many visits, and a ripening of the professional relationship, before such contact will be considered acceptable by the patient. The astute physician will "sense" what is and is not appropriate in working with the patient. You should pay attention to the patient's nonverbal communication, and when it seems natural and appropriate to place your hand on her arm or shoulder, do so in a gentle and sympathetic manner.

b) Patient

Often the patient's nonverbal communication may tell you far more than her verbal comments, if you are perceptive enough to notice them. You should be able to determine what the patient's mood is on the basis of her posture, her tone of voice, or her facial expression. Patients who are depressed may slump, appear listless, move slowly, talk with a flat, lifeless monotone with many pauses and sighs, and show little interest in their surroundings. Patients who are in pain may walk and sit in a gingerly fashion, often placing a hand on the offending parts of the body, all the while grimacing and frowning with every motion. Their voices may be strained or their speech interspersed with grimaces as the pain strikes them. Brief staccato speech, finger tapping, and the crossing and uncrossing of the legs might signify impatience or anger, depending upon the patient's facial expression. Behavior such as looking off to the side or at the ceiling, giving minimal verbal responses, and fidgeting with or straightening one's clothes may be seen in young girls who are brought to your office by their mother; these actions generally indicate the girl's feigned disinterest in the proceedings. Mixed responses may result from either fear or psychiatric disorders. If the patient smiles with tears in her eyes and tells you of a lump that she has found in her breast through trembling lips, you can be certain that she is frightened that she may have cancer. When a patient calmly smiles at you and tells you about the severe pain that she is having in her abdomen, you should consider this an inappropriate response that may have a deeper psychiatric significance. Finally, you should be aware of the fleeting look that crosses the patient's features when a sensitive subject is broached, or the flickering of an eyebrow when certain things are said. In summary, you should pay attention to all of the patient's nonverbal signals if you wish to "read" your patient appropriately and correctly.

Often, you may find that the patient's basic problem is something entirely different from her presenting complaint. Remember that a patient must have a complaint, a **"ticket of admission,"** in order to see you as a patient. In actual fact, however, the problem that she may be really concerned about could be something quite different. You will have been of little help to her if you do not detect the subtle clues concerning this hidden agenda and allow the patient the opportunity to discuss her real problem openly with you.

c) Telephone calls

It is important that you **do not allow nonemergent telephone calls** to interrupt you while you are with a patient. If you do, the patient you are with receives a clear message that, in the future, she can talk to you more easily by telephone than by coming to your office. During your busy schedule in the office each day, you should allow for a couple of time periods when you can return your patients' calls without interfering with appointments, perhaps while you are having your morning or afternoon coffee break in between patient visits. **You should always make a time-dated note in the patient's chart when you talk to her on the telephone. You should briefly list the patient's problem and your disposition of it as you are talking to the patient in order to document the telephone call.**

d) The examination technique

Your patient should be escorted to the examining room by your chaperone, who should assist her in undressing and being draped in preparation for you to perform the examination. **The chaperone should always remain in the room** throughout the examination so that a charge can never be made that you have acted in an improper manner toward your patient. **It is often helpful to tell the patient, before you actually start, what you plan to do during the examination.** Many women are quite modest, and you should be sensitive to their needs in such an intimate examination. Keep your patient draped as much as possible, except for the area that you are examining, so as to protect her modesty. The patient will recognize other minor courtesies as genuine attempts on your part to make her feel comfortable in a potentially embarrassing situation.

In rare instances, a patient may be outwardly seductive and will invite you to cross the bounds of propriety. It is best to ignore these advances, as if you are unaware of the sexual content involved, since if you openly recognize

them, the patient may feel rebuffed and your professional relationship may suffer. Some things are better left unrecognized, and this is one of them. Consequently, there will be no embarrassment for either party. Should the patient actually verbally proposition you, it is best to assume that she is "kidding" around with you and treat it lightly, and then immediately change the subject. She will get the message that the office environment and the physician-patient relationship are not to be violated.

e) The summing up

Following the examination, the patient should get dressed and return to the office for the final summing up of your findings and the outline of your plan of management. **It is always a good idea to take the patient into your confidence and let her see how you intellectually work your way through her medical problems. This approach not only allows the patient to learn what the possible diagnosis might be, but also allows her to participate in her own care.** When you have thoroughly discussed your findings and the proposed management plan with the patient, you should then ask her if she understands what you are attempting to do in the management of her problem. If you have established a good rapport, the patient will feel free to ask you questions at this point. You should try to teach your patient as much as possible and explain the diagnosis and what you plan to do about it. Invite her comments in an effort to elicit her concerns and fears about her condition and about the treatment plan. Try to answer her questions in simple terms, and avoid scientific medical terminology as much as possible. Occasionally, it may be valuable for you to draw pictures of your physical findings (e.g., an ovarian mass), and explain the factors involved with regard to both the diagnosis and the treatment of her condition.

c. The approach to interim care

Perhaps the area of practice neglected most by physicians is the **disposition** of the patient. **This disposition should cover the interim between the time of the patient's discharge and the time when you will see her again.** Whether you discharge a patient from your office or from the hospital, it is essential for you to record four aspects of the patient's care: **(1) the tests, consultations, or procedures you have ordered, (2) the medications you are** prescribing, with the dosage regimens, (3) the precautions or instructions you have given her, and (4) the date of her return appointment.

1) Tests, consultations, and procedures

If you have ordered laboratory tests on your patient, you should explain their purpose in detail and the necessity for having them done. Most laboratory tests are quite expensive, and the patient deserves to know what she is paying for and whether the tests will truly help in her diagnosis. If there is any risk to the procedures you are requesting (e.g., an intravenous pyelogram), then you should go over the risks and the possible complications involved and explain why these risks are worth taking in her case. If you are referring the patient to another physician or a health-care worker for consultation, you should explain the reasons why you feel this step will be helpful.

You should keep in mind the **three types of consultation requests:** (1) the **total referral** of the patient to another specialist where you expect that physician to **diagnose and treat** the patient without further contact with you (e.g., a fractured finger in a pregnant patient), (2) the **partial referral** of the patient to another specialist for **one-time advice** as to how to proceed with the patient's care (e.g., an anesthesia consultation for the management of a complicated obstetric patient), and (3) the **cooperative referral** of the patient to another specialist where you wish that specialist to **medically follow along with you** over a long period of time (e.g., a pregnant cardiac patient). *The ethics of the second and third forms of consultation are that the specialist should discuss the findings and the recommendations with the referring physician first, and only after the referring physician concurs should the patient be informed of the recommendations.* The consultant should place a note in the patient's chart with his advice and recommendations; however, the referring physician has no real obligation to follow the consultant's advice. Indeed, further consultation from yet another specialist may sometimes be sought by the primary physician.

2) Medications

You should discuss at length with the patient the risks and benefits of any medications you prescribe. Specific precautions concerning adverse reactions are essential if she is to be an active participant in her care. **You should always leave the patient with the impression that she can always call you day or night if she has problems with her medications.** The degree of reassurance that this approach provides the patient is almost a guarantee that she will not call you for minor or superfluous reasons but instead will keep you appropriately informed of any major adverse reactions. It is a good idea for you not to prescribe narcotics or tranquilizers outside of the hospital, in light of the current problems with substance abuse in our society. Rarely will these drugs be needed in the obstetric or gynecologic patient on an outpatient basis.

3) Instructions and precautions

It is essential that you instruct the patient as to what her activities should be in the intervening period between visits and why you feel that she should follow your advice in these matters. For example, following delivery, intercourse and douching should be avoided for a few weeks in order to decrease the risk of a possible pelvic infection. Further, after a period of rest, the gradual resumption of household activities should be discussed. If the patient is breast-feeding, then the care of the breasts and nipples becomes an important topic to talk over with the patient prior to her discharge. **You should outline for your patient all of the instructions and precautions that are necessary to "protect" her until you will see her again.** She should be warned about specific problems pertinent to her case, such as how to recognize undue bleeding, or the subtle signs of infection, and what you want her to do about such eventualities. Your efforts to teach your patient the possible complications that she might encounter during this period, and what she should do about them should they occur, will prevent any undue delay in treatment and will protect the patient's health.

4) The return appointment

The timing for the return appointment conveys to the patient your degree of concern for her welfare. Return appointments should be "tailored" to the patient's needs. If she comes in with a complaint of pelvic pain, and you give her a return appointment in three months, it tells her that you are insensitive to the fact that she is in pain. Such patients should be seen on a more frequent basis until you are able to define the diagnosis and institute appropriate therapy. During these visits, you might develop considerable insight into the patient's problems, and your frequent examinations might define initially unrecognized pelvic pathology as the cause of her complaint. Similarly, a patient who comes in with symptoms of an ectopic pregnancy should not have a battery of tests run and then told to return in one month. Such a recommendation could be quite dangerous; if the patient actually does have an ectopic pregnancy, it could rupture and she could get into serious trouble before she could seek help again.

In selecting the time for your patient's next visit, you should convey to your patient the urgency, or lack thereof, of your concern in her case. Furthermore, you should not dismiss a patient from your care until you have done as much as possible to solve the patient's medical problem. If you fail to arrive at a diagnosis and the patient continues to have problems, then you should seek consultation from other physicians. If you are certain that the patient does not need to be seen again in the near future (e.g., after a routine annual checkup), then the return appointment should be scheduled to take place in no longer than one year. It is better to see a patient more often than necessary than to make the appointments at longer intervals that may be dangerous to the patient's health.

d. The physician's influence

Many of us fail to take into account the role that we play in our patients' lives. What we say is repeated many times over to the patient's friends and relatives. Our opinions are sometimes elevated to heights that would surprise even us if we were to hear them restated by the patient. What we do and what we say to our patients and their families should be approached with a great deal of consideration for the truth. **You should never exceed the boundaries of the scientific data available to you and should never tell your patients inaccurate stories or use allegories to explain their diseases or conditions.** These tales have a way of becoming garbled to the point of unintelligibility and end up being told at a later time to your colleagues, who cannot believe that you would tell your patient such a fanciful tale. **The best policy is always to be honest with the patient. It is also a good policy for you to not be too optimistic about the outcome of any aspect of the patient's care.** All too often, the uncomplicated patient has a tendency to suddenly develop "every complication in the book," at which point the patient and the family members remember with great clarity that you told them "everything was alright." **Never exceed your prognostic capabilities, and always "hedge your bet" by leaving an "out" for yourself if things should take a turn for the worse.** Remember that the patient and her family view medicine as a "black-and-white" situation, and that they generally do not understand that you cannot control every aspect of the patient's care. It is not fair to the patient or to her loved ones to lead them astray by stating that all is well when the patient's condition has not been completely resolved. In addition, in today's litigious society, when things do not turn out perfectly the patient and her family often feel that it must be somebody's fault, and an error on the part of the physician is often suspected, even when everything possible was done to prevent such an occurrence.

CHAPTER 2

Basic pelvic anatomy

Anatomy brought life and liberty to the art of healing, and for three centuries the great names in medicine were those of the great anatomists.

—*Sir William Osler**

1. An overview of practical pelvic anatomy

The astute clinician recognizes the fact that anatomy and physiology form the basis of all clinical diagnoses. Anatomy is perhaps most important in understanding the pathologic lesions of the organism, whereas a knowledge of physiologic principles is necessary to unravel the metabolic derangements of the body. If you wish to practice obstetrics and gynecology, you must have a working knowledge of both of these subjects. The management of pathologic lesions and the surgical procedures necessary to treat them require a thorough knowledge of pelvic anatomy. You should attempt to develop a mental *three-dimensional concept* in your thinking about anatomy and try to visualize the pelvic contents in such a manner that you are able to see the interplay of the muscles and the fascial planes, with their accompanying vascular, lymphatic, and nervous structures, surrounding the pelvic organs as they carry out their functions.

The primary supportive structures of the pel-

vis consist of the musculature and the fascial planes. In order to contain the contents of the peritoneal cavity when the female is in the upright posture, *the pelvic musculature forms a sling-like structure.* The fascial sheaths of these pelvic muscles are also combined and intertwined so as to provide a set of endopelvic fascial planes, or a **skeleton-like fascial framework,** which supports the internal female organs in the center of the pelvis and allows them to maintain their relationship with each other.

During pregnancy, the pelvic structures are greatly distorted by the enlarging uterus. In addition, the abdominal pressure that occurs secondary to the pregnant uterus is directed toward the muscular pelvic sling, which must absorb this pressure and keep the internal genital organs from prolapsing out through the vagina. Furthermore, since the bowel manifests peristaltic action, and the urinary bladder distends with urine, a certain amount of freedom of action is essential in order for these processes to occur without permanently damaging the anatomy of the adjacent organs. **The fascial planes allow the pelvic organs the freedom to distend, move, and change their positions in an independent manner without appreciably affecting the adjacent organs.** The blood vessels, lymphatics, and nerves are found only in these fascial planes, which would seem to be a sensible arrangement given the fact that these structures, in turn, may proliferate or otherwise change position in support of the organs they serve.

It is important for you to consider gynecologic pelvic problems (e.g., pelvic relaxation, stress incontinence, pregnancy, delivery, etc.) from an anatomic point of view. The dynamic status of the pelvic structures and the condition of their fascial planes are the basis for almost all of the abnormalities of pelvic re-

---

*Reprinted with permission from Robert Bennett Bean, *Sir William Osler: Aphorisms from His Bedside Teachings and Writings,* William Bennett Bean, ed. Springfield, Ill.: Charles C Thomas, Publisher, 1968, p. 82.

laxation that we see in clinical practice. An understanding of these anatomical and functional arrangements will often provide you with a much clearer picture of the abnormality and will also assist you in the surgical correction of such problems. The following anatomical discussions are designed to acquaint you with some of these anatomical arrangements. If you plan to perform gynecologic surgery or obstetric deliveries, then it is essential for you to know this information.

2. The bony pelvis

The pelvis is a ring-shaped series of bones that form the pelvic girdle. This girdle supports the person in the upright position and distributes the weight of the body between the two femoral heads. It is subject to disease (e.g., rickets) and traumatic fractures, which can distort its shape. In addition, the pelvis has a different configuration according to the sex of the individual. **The pelvis consists of two innominate bones and the sacrum** (Fig. 2-1). The innominate bones consist of the ilium, the ischium, and the pubic bones on each side. There are *three joints,* including the **symphysis pubis** anteriorly, and the **two sacroiliac joints** posteriorly, which are joined together by strong ligaments (Figs. 2-2 and 2-3). In addition, laterally there is the hip joint, a ball-and-socket type of joint (i.e., the acetabulum) that receives the head of the femur. Strong ligaments surround all of these joints. Above the pelvic brim, which is the division between the true pelvis below and the false pelvis above, are the flaring iliac crests. The true pelvis (i.e., below the iliopectineal line) is of concern from an obstetric viewpoint. The two pubic bones join anteriorly, with the ischiopubic rami extending posteriorly from the pubis to the **ischial tuberosities.** The anterior ischiopubic rami constitute the curve of the obstetric forepelvis. As the rami extend posteriorly and superiorly, the ischial spine juts into the true pelvis. The **greater sciatic notch, or ischiadic foramen,** is superior to the ischial spine and is the portion of the ilium adjacent to the sacrum. The **sacrospinous ligament** extends from the ischial spine to the sacrum. The **sacrum,** composed of five fused vertebrae that taper to the coccyx, articulates with the ilia on each side at the sacroiliac joints and is generally slightly curved and directed somewhat posteriorly.

3. The perineum

You should have a thorough understanding of the anatomical relationship between the various internal pelvic structures and those of the external genitalia. The external genital structures and the vagina function primarily as organs for copulation, whereas the internal organs of the generative system are primarily involved in fetal development and growth. The two systems are then brought together as a functional unit during parturition.

a. Mons veneris

The *mons veneris* is a fatty pad overlying the pubic bone that is generally covered with short curly hair that is called the *escutcheon.* In the female, this escutcheon appears as an inverted triangle, whereas in the male the hair pattern is more of a diamond shape, with the superior point extending upward in the midline toward the umbilicus.

b. Vulva

The vulva consists of two sets of lips, the **labia majora** and the **labia minora,** which cover the **introitus,** or the vaginal opening (Fig. 2-4). The labia majora are somewhat thicker than the labia minora, due to fat deposition, and are usually covered with hair, whereas the labia minora are without hair. The labia minora are usually thin and appear to be covered with a surface epithelium that is more like a mucous membrane than like skin, especially in the nulliparous female. The labia minora fuse in the midline posteriorly to form the **fourchette** (i.e., near the fusion of the labia majora at the posterior commissure).

c. Clitoris

The **clitoris** lies superiorly beneath the prepuce, which is formed from the juncture of the upper lamellae (i.e., small folds) of the labia minora. The lower lamellae form the frenulum of the clitoris. The clitoris has a 2 cm shaft (cylindrical body) surmounted by a 0.5 cm glans that is much like the head of the male penis. The two crura of the corpora cavernosa arise along the ascending pubic rami and unite to form the body of the clitoris, which terminates in the glans. This tissue is erectile and contains a rich vascular

Text continues on p. 18

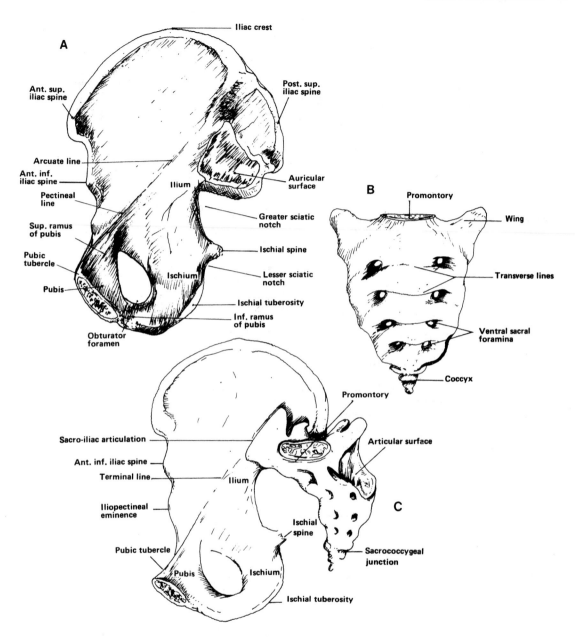

FIGURE 2-1. (A) Medial aspect of the coxal bone. (B) Anterior aspect of the sacrum. (C) Articulated right coxal bone with the sacrum and the coccyx.

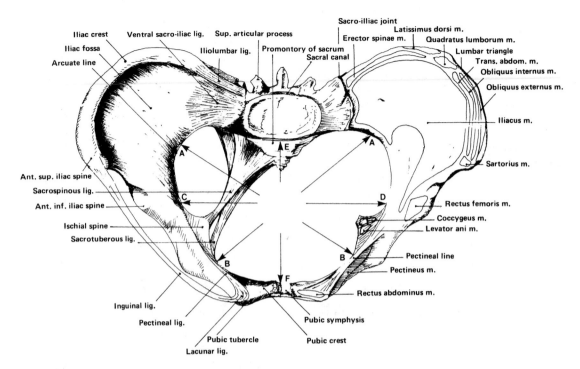

FIGURE 2-2. The female bony pelvis, with the origins and insertions of the muscles indicated on the right and the ligaments shown on the left of the drawing. (A) Sacroiliac joint. (B) Iliopubic symphysis. (C) and (D) Midpelvic brim. (E) Sacral promontory. (F) Pubic symphysis. The ischial spine projects into the pelvic space bilaterally. The greater sciatic (ischiadic) notch lies between (A) and (C) above the sacrospinous ligament. The area between (B) (F) (B) represents the obstetric forepelvis.

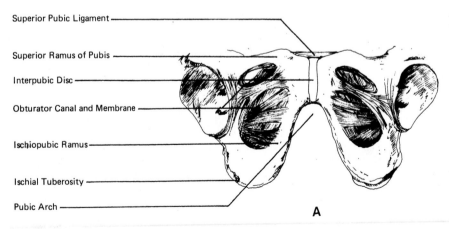

FIGURE 2-3. Anatomy of pelvic joints and ligaments. (A) Subpubic arch view. (B) Inlet view. (C) Posterior view of the sacroiliac joints.

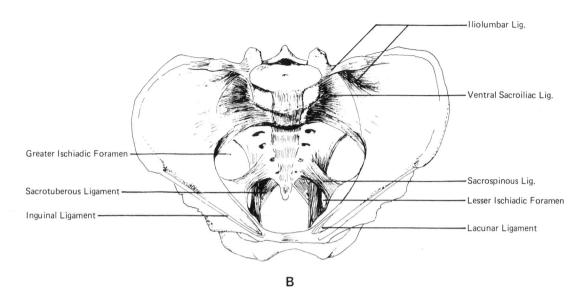

Iliolumbar Lig.

Ventral Sacroiliac Lig.

Greater Ischiadic Foramen

Sacrotuberous Ligament

Inguinal Ligament

Sacrospinous Lig.

Lesser Ischiadic Foramen

Lacunar Ligament

B

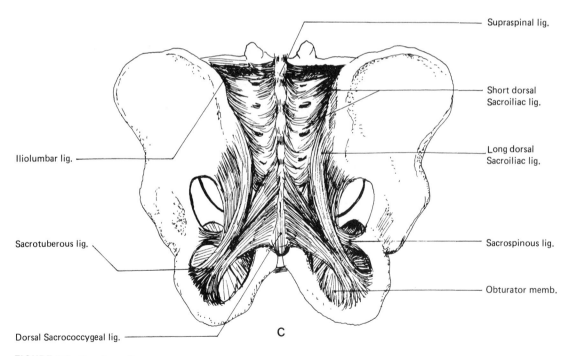

Supraspinal lig.

Short dorsal Sacroiliac lig.

Long dorsal Sacroiliac lig.

Iliolumbar lig.

Sacrotuberous lig.

Sacrospinous lig.

Obturator memb.

Dorsal Sacrococcygeal lig.

C

FIGURE 2-3. *(continued)*

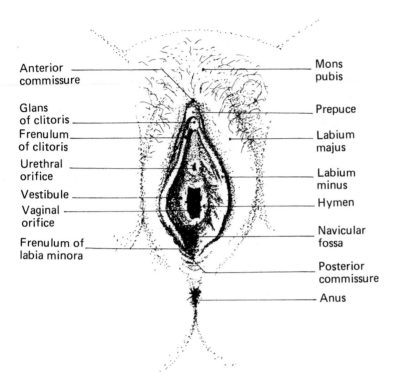

Anterior commissure

Glans of clitoris

Frenulum of clitoris

Urethral orifice

Vestibule

Vaginal orifice

Frenulum of labia minora

Mons pubis

Prepuce

Labium majus

Labium minus

Hymen

Navicular fossa

Posterior commissure

Anus

FIGURE 2-4. Surface view of the perineum and vulva.

supply that is similar to that of the penis in the male. It is also highly sensitive due to the many nerve endings that are present.

d. The vestibule

The **vestibule** is the area enclosed by the labia at the mouth of the vagina. A number of openings enter into it, such as the urethra, the vagina, *the ducts of the Bartholin glands* (vestibular glands), and *the ducts of the Skene glands* (paraurethral glands). There are extensive venous plexuses in the vestibular area, which are liable to injury during childbirth.

e. Hymen

The vaginal orifice in a virginal woman may have an overlying membraneous septum (*hymen*), which may nearly obliterate the vaginal opening. The hymen may have a pinhole-sized opening, or it may have an opening that is large enough to admit one or two fingers. This tissue may easily tear in a radial fashion during first coitus, or as the result of injury, to form a series of small lumps of scarred tissue (i.e., carunculae myrtiformes) that occur at intervals around the introitus.

f. Vagina

The **vagina** is a flattened "H-shaped" muscular tube that extends about 10 cm from the introitus to the juncture with the cervical portio vaginalis, or vaginal fornices, which encircle the cervix like a ring. **It is lined by squamous epithelium arranged in folds called rugae, which are directly affected by the amount of estrogen present.** There are no glands in the vagina. **The vagina is normally moistened by cervical secretions; however, during sexual excitement these secretions are further supplemented by a transudate of fluid which percolates through the vaginal walls from the surrounding vaginal venous and lymphatic plexuses.**

The vaginal wall is composed of three layers of smooth muscle: an outer longitudinal layer, an inner circular layer, and an inner poorly differentiated longitudinal layer. Fibrous endopelvic fascial tissues surround these muscular coats, and it is in these tissues that the blood vessels, lymphatics, and nerves may be found. In contrast, the pelvic spaces (i.e., the paravesical and the pararectal spaces) are relatively free of important structures and are filled wtih loose areolar fatty tissue. The main blood supply to the anterior wall of the vagina is by way of the vaginal branches of the uterine artery, which forms the coronary artery of the cervix and then becomes the midline anterior azygos artery with branches to supply the anterior vaginal wall. The posterior azygos artery is also derived from the coronary artery of the cervix and anastomoses with branches from the middle hemorrhoidal and the internal pudendal arteries to supply the posterior vaginal wall.

4. The perineal body

The **perineal body** lies on a line between the ischial tuberosities in the midline between the vagina and the anus. This fibromuscular structure is the insertion point for the superficial transverse perineal muscles, the bulbocavernosus muscles, the external sphincter of the anus, and some fibers from the anterior and medial divisions of the levator ani muscles. **During delivery, an episiotomy may be performed by incising the perineal body in either a midline approach or a mediolateral one** (see Chapter 26).

5. The pelvic and urogenital diaphragm

a. Pelvic diaphragm

The support of the perineum is dependent upon the pelvic and urogenital diaphragms. The **pelvic diaphragm** contains the levator ani and coccygeus muscles, which form a broad sling within the pelvis that swings forward at the pelvic outlet to surround the vagina and the rectum as a form of sphincter. It inserts into the median raphe in the midline between the rectum and the vagina (Fig. 2-5).

b. Urogenital diaphragm

The **urogenital diaphragm** is a triangular area between the ischial tuberosities and the symphysis pubis that contains the urethral striated sphincter muscles, the urogenital trigone fascia, and the inferior urogenital trigone fascia. This area provides support for the lower urethra and the anterior wall of the vaginal barrel (Fig. 2-6). The vagina, the urethra, the artery of the bulb, the dorsal nerve of the clitoris, and the internal pudendal vessels all penetrate this diaphragm. External to this diaphragm are the superficial transverse

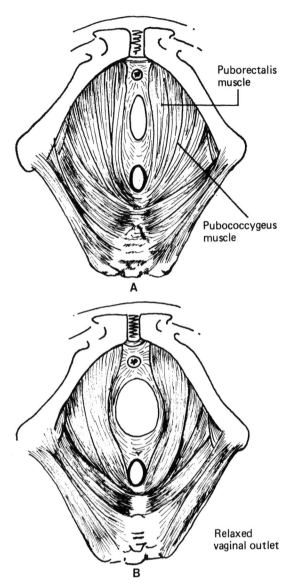

FIGURE 2-5. (A) Perineal view of the levator ani muscle, showing the central hiatus in the pelvic floor produced by the penetration of the urethra, vagina, and rectum. Note the decussations of the levator fibers that pass between the rectum and vagina and support the hiatus. (B) Schematic illustration of a widened hiatus showing separation of the decussating fibers of the levator ani from the perineal body and the margins of the pelvic portal and shortening of the levator plate between the rectum and coccyx. (Redrawn with permission from R. F. Mattingly, and J. D. Thompson, *Te Linde's Operative Gynecology,* 6th ed. Philadelphia: J. B. Lippincott Company, 1985, p. 572.)

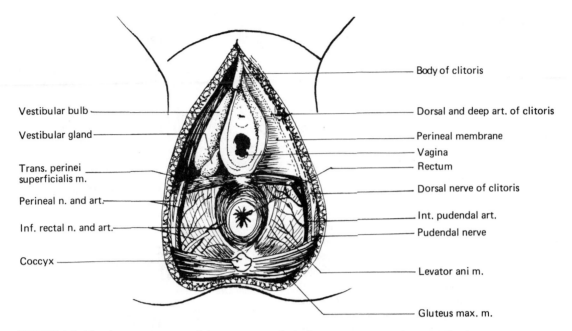

Body of clitoris

Vestibular bulb

Vestibular gland

Trans. perinei superficialis m.

Perineal n. and art.

Inf. rectal n. and art.

Coccyx

Dorsal and deep art. of clitoris

Perineal membrane

Vagina

Rectum

Dorsal nerve of clitoris

Int. pudendal art.

Pudendal nerve

Levator ani m.

Gluteus max. m.

FIGURE 2-6. The deeper structures of the perineum. The bulbospongiosus muscle has been removed on the patient's right side to reveal the vestibular bulb and the vestibular gland. On the patient's left side the contents of the superficial space have been removed to show the inferior layer of the urogenital diaphragm, the internal pudendal artery, and the pudendal nerve.

perineal muscles, the bulbospongiosus muscles on each side of the vagina, and the ischiocavernosus muscles, which arise from the inner surface of the ischial tuberosities and end on the under surface of the crus clitoridis.

6. The pelvic blood supply

It is essential for you to know the details of the blood supply to the pelvic structures. Not only will you encounter these vessels in surgical procedures, but they also form landmarks for the identification of other structures, such as the ureter.

The abdominal aorta at the level of the promontory of the sacrum divides into the common iliac artery, which after a short run again divides into the external and the internal iliac branches. The blood supply of the pelvic genital structures is derived in large part from the internal iliac artery (hypogastric artery) and its

branches. The *external iliac artery* traverses the lateral side of the pelvis and gives off the deep circumflex iliac artery and the inferior epigastric artery just before entering the femoral canal to emerge in the leg as the femoral artery. The **internal iliac artery, or the hypogastric artery,** turns medially and inferiorly at the brim of the pelvis, where it drops down into the true pelvis to supply the uterus and the other pelvic structures. The **ureter** crosses the common iliac artery just superior to its bifurcation into the external and internal iliac arteries.

a. The branches of the hypogastric artery

The hypogastric artery divides almost immediately into its anterior and posterior divisions (Fig. 2-7). The **posterior division** includes three branches, namely: (1) the iliolumbar, (2) the lateral sacral, and (3) the superior gluteal arteries. The **anterior division** gives off the remaining 7–8 branches, which are (4) the obliterated umbilical

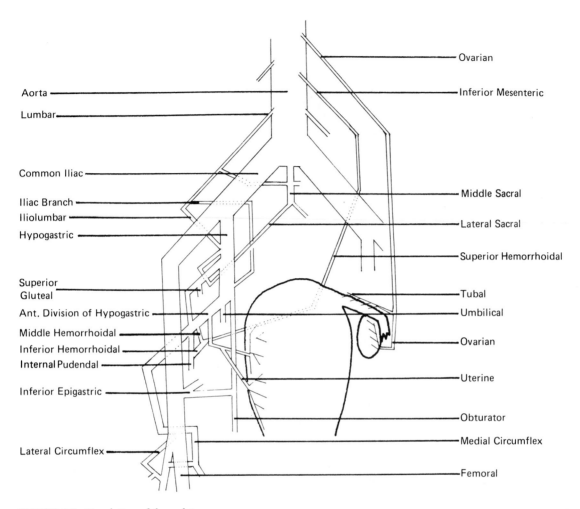

FIGURE 2-7. Circulation of the pelvis.

(and/or superior vesical), (5) the obturator, (6) the uterine, (7) the middle hemorrhoidal, (8) the inferior vesical, (9) the inferior gluteal, and the (10) internal pudendal arteries.

7. The pelvic nerve supply

a. Sympathetic nerve supply

The pelvic structures receive both sympathetic and parasympathetic nerves of the autonomic nervous system. The **sympathetic nerves** enter the pelvis by several routes: (1) by the abdominal sympathetic trunk, (2) in conjunction with the superior hemorrhoidal vessels, (3) by further connections with the ovarian plexus, and (4) via the most prominent para-aortic plexus, which upon entering the pelvis becomes the **hypogastric, or presacral plexus (L1–L4). The presacral plexus** divides into the left and right branches, which descend further into the pelvis to become part of the **deep pelvic plexus** (Fig. 2-8). **The pelvic plexus divides into the anterior and posterior divisions. The anterior division of the pelvic plexus innervates the bladder and the urethra, whereas the posterior division goes to the uterus, cervix, vagina, the rectosigmoid colon, and the anal region.**

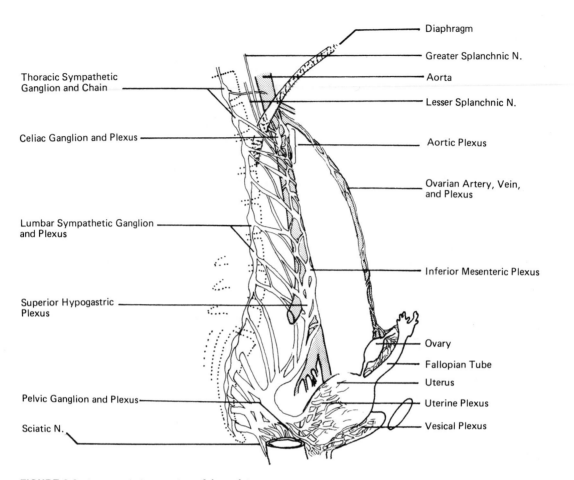

FIGURE 2-8. Autonomic innervation of the pelvis.

b. Parasympathetic nerve supply

The parasympathetic nerves are derived from S2, S3, and S4, and their preganglionic fibers run through the pelvic plexus and thence to the broad ligaments and uterosacral ligaments to supply the uterus and the adjacent pelvic organs.

c. Sensory nerves

The sensory nerves from the uterus run with the sympathetic nerve plexus to L2 and L4 of the spinal cord, whereas the sensory nerves from the cervix generally are transmitted through the uterosacral ligaments and go to S2, S3, and S4. As a consequence, pain from the uterus is generally referred to the lower abdomen. In contrast, pain from the cervix is reflected to the lumbrosacral region.

d. Motor nerves

The motor nerve to the adductor magnus, brevis, and longus and to the gracilis muscles of the thigh is the **obturator nerve, which arises from the anterior divisions of the lumbar plexus (L2, L3, and L4).** It traverses the brim of the pelvis beneath the common iliac vessel to emerge beneath the bifurcation of the common iliac vessel into the external and internal iliac vessels, near where the ureter crosses above the bifurcation. It then descends through the pelvis to the obturator foramen along with the obturator vessels.

The **pudendal plexus** is derived from the anterior divisions of S2, S3, and S4, while the **sacral plexus,** in

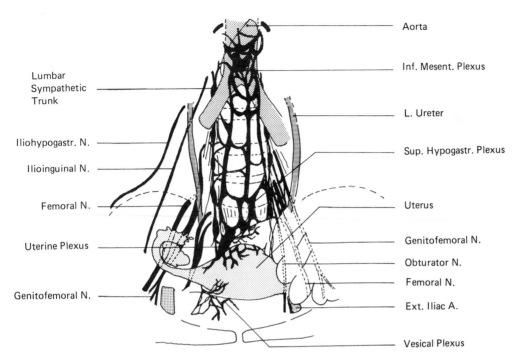

Lumbar
Sympathetic
Trunk

Iliohypogastr. N.

Ilioinguinal N.

Femoral N.

Uterine Plexus

Genitofemoral N.

Aorta

Inf. Mesent. Plexus

L. Ureter

Sup. Hypogastr. Plexus

Uterus

Genitofemoral N.

Obturator N.

Femoral N.

Ext. Iliac A.

Vesical Plexus

FIGURE 2-9. Innervation of the pelvic organs.

addition to the coccygeal nerves, comes from part of S4 and all of S5. The sympathetic and parasympathetic visceral branches of the pudendal plexus enter the pelvic plexus. **The internal pudendal nerve (S2, S3) traverses the sciatic foramen and then extends back through the lesser sciatic foramen into the ischiorectal fossa (Alcock's canal), where it emerges medial to the ischial tuberosities and swings superiorly to supply the muscles of the perineum and vulva. The nerves to the external genitalia** include the iliohypogastric nerve (T12–L1), the genitofemoral nerve (L1–L2), the ilioinguinal nerve (L1), and the pudendal nerve (S2, S3, S4) (Fig. 2-9).

8. The pelvic lymphatics

a. Drainage of the vulva, vagina, and rectum

The lymphatic drainage of the vulva, vagina, and rectum follows three somewhat separate routes (Figs. 2-10 and 2-11). The **lower vagina, vulva, and perineal areas** drain to the superficial inguinal nodes, except for the clitoris and the labia minora, which drain to the deep inguinal nodes. The clitoris may also drain directly to the internal iliac nodes. The lymphatics of the **middle part of the vagina and rectum** drain to the internal iliac lymph nodes. **The upper vagina and the adjacent rectum** drain to the internal and external iliac nodes.

b. Drainage of the cervix, uterus, tubes, and ovaries

The superficial and deep lymphatics of the uterus and cervix drain (1) laterally to the external iliac nodes, (2) posterolaterally to the internal iliac nodes, and (3) posteriorly to the rectal and sacral nodes. These lymphatics follow the endopelvic fascial planes of the pelvis. Some of the cervical lymphatics also drain laterally to the **obturator node,** which is one of the outlying iliac nodes that lies in the obturator canal. The **upper uterine** and the **ovarian lymphatics** follow the ovarian vessels in the infundibulopelvic ligament to the aortic and preaortic nodes. The superficial inguinal nodes drain the area at the juncture of the round ligament and the fallopian tube.

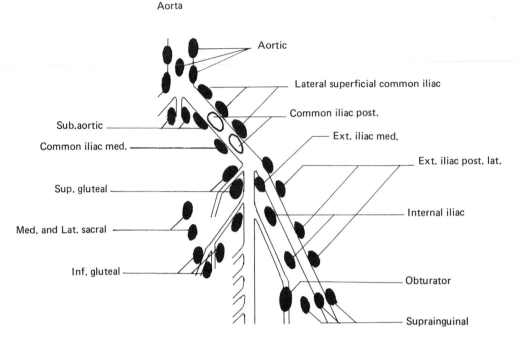

FIGURE 2-10. The lymphatic drainage of the pelvis.

c. Iliac nodes

The internal iliac nodal chain follows the internal iliac vessels and receives drainage from the lower pelvis, perineum, and buttock muscles. **The external iliac nodal chain,** which consists of about 8 to 10 nodes that are located anteriorly, medially, and laterally, follows the external iliac vessel up to the bifurcation of the common iliac vessel and drains the inguinal nodes, the clitoris, the cervix, the upper vagina, the urethra, and the fundus of the bladder. The four to six **common iliac lymph nodes** along the common iliac artery drain the internal and external iliac nodal chains and then connect to the lateral aortic nodes that surround the aorta to form the lumbar trunks on each side, which end in the cisterna chyli.

9. The pelvic fascial planes and spaces

a. Endopelvic fascia

The pelvic organs (i.e., the rectum, the vagina, the bladder, and the urethra) are supported by interlacing condensations of connective tissue that have been referred to as the **endopelvic fascia.** These tissues are somewhat dense in some areas and almost nonexistent in others. These condensations of connective tissue, or pelvic "ligaments," play an important part in separating and supporting the pelvic structures, and in addition, they provide a framework that allows each of these organ systems to function independently of each other. In effect, this fascial tissue forms an "internal skeleton" or framework for all of the pelvic structures.

1) Fascial planes

The fascial planes provide a natural framework for the accompanying blood vessels, nerves, and lymph ducts and nodes that supply the pelvic structures. Because these planes separate the pelvis into separate sections and spaces, they also form barriers to the spread of infections and hematomas. **On the other hand, because these planes contain the vascular and lymphatic structures, they also direct the spread of cancer along the lines of the fascial partitions, or septa, and therefore they form the natural routes of spread for neoplastic disease.**

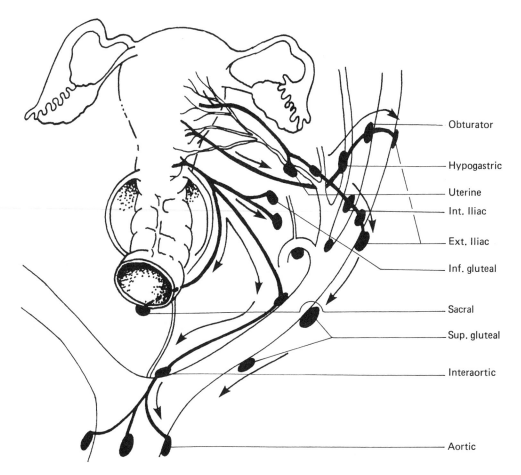

FIGURE 2-11. The lymphatic drainage of the cervix.

These tissue planes and spaces may be illustrated by a frontal cross section taken at the level of the cervix (Fig. 2-12).

2) Spaces

The spaces between the septa contain loose areolar tissue and fat and are essentially free of blood vessels and lymphatics. These areas can be entered surgically with impunity and the fascial septa may be palpated for evidence of an infiltrative carcinomatous process. In the course of performing a hysterectomy, these spaces can be entered to expose the adjacent vascular structures (i.e., to skeletonize the uterine vessels) for easy visual clamping, cutting, and ligation. A thorough knowledge of these connective tissue fascial planes

(septa, partitions), and of the potential spaces between the planes, is absolutely essential for the pelvic surgeon and is necessary for an understanding of the supporting ligamentous structures of the female generative tract.

b. The anterior pelvic planes and spaces

1) Prevesical space

Immediately behind the pubic bone is the *prevesical space of Retzius,* which extends from the pubis superiorly to the umbilicus in a triangular manner. It is bounded on the sides of the triangle by the terminal ends of the hypogastric arteries (*i.e., the obliterated*

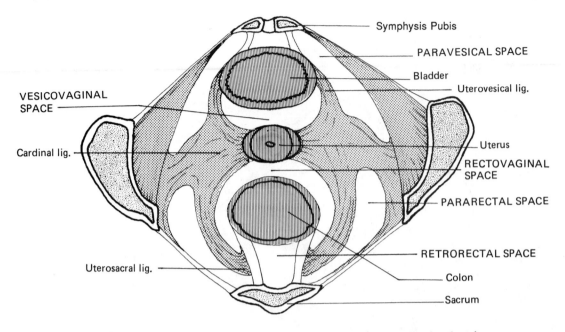

FIGURE 2-12. Cross section of the pelvis at the level of the cervix showing the endopelvic fascial planes and spaces. The cardinal ligament extends to the lateral pelvic wall where it fans out for its attachment. The lymphatics that drain the cervix are contained within this ligament. The paravesical and pararectal spaces contain loose areolar tissue.

umbilical arteries) and contains the *urachus* in the midline, which extends to the umbilicus from the dome of the bladder. The *transversalis fascia* extends from the bladder to the pubis for the full length of the triangle (i.e., from the pubis to the umbilicus).

The *ascending bladder septa* spring from the cardinal ligaments on each side of the cervix and separate the space immediately between the cervix/vagina and urethra/bladder (i.e., the midline vesicovaginal space) from the lateral paravesical spaces. As these septa ascend beyond the bladder to the pubis, they also partition the prevesical space between the bladder and the pubis from the lateral paravesical spaces. The terminal portion of the ureter travels in the lower part of the ascending bladder septum prior to its anterior flexion and entry into the bladder. A portion of each ascending bladder septum at the level of the cervix forms into well-defined bilateral condensations of connective tissue that have been termed the **vesicouterine ligaments,** or the **bladder pillars.** As a consequence, the ureter can be demonstrated on a vaginal hysterectomy by palpating the area just lat-

eral to the bladder pillars after the anterior vaginal cuff has been opened up. Above this level there are a number of blood vessels, such as the inferior vesical artery and the vesical plexus of veins.

2) Paravesical spaces

The **paravesical spaces** lie on each side of the partitioned-off central organs and spaces in the midline and are bounded by the lateral pelvic wall, the cardinal ligament, the internal obturator muscle, the levator ani muscle, and the ascending bladder septum. The two lateral paravesical spaces are filled with fatty areolar tissue. Because they are an area of easy access above the cardinal ligament, they provide a convenient place for the surgeon to digitally palpate the anterior portion of the cardinal ligament on each side of the cervix and out laterally to the pelvic wall for tumor extension. You can palpate the length and breadth of both sides of the cardinal ligament by placing your thumb in the paravesical space and one finger in the pararectal space.

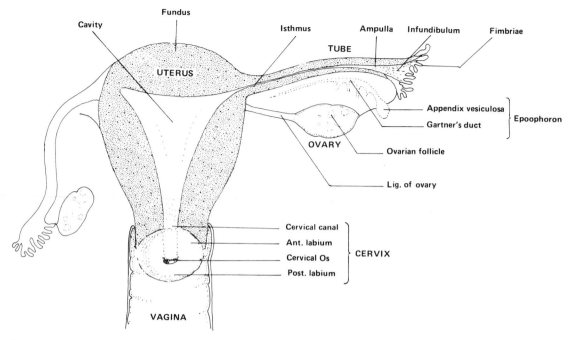

FIGURE 2-13. Schematic section of the internal female organs, anterior view.

c. The posterior pelvic planes and spaces

1) Cardinal ligaments

The cardinal ligament, or Mackenrodt's ligament, separates the anterior and posterior portions of the pelvis. This ligament, a strong condensation of areolar connective tissue (40%) and longitudinal smooth muscle tissue from the vagina and uterus (60%), extends from around the cervix and the vaginal fornices laterally to the pelvic side walls, where it fans out for a broad attachment to the fascia overlying the obturator and levator ani muscles. The **broad ligament** is a large fold of the peritoneum that fans out anteriorly and superiorly above the cardinal ligament and contains the ovarian arteries and veins and the fallopian tubes. **The cardinal ligaments fix the pelvic organs in the middle of the pelvis and provide considerable support for the uterus and bladder.**

2) Uterosacral ligaments

The descending rectal septa descend from the lower border of the cardinal ligament and the cervix to the rectum and then extend beyond to the sacrum. The space between the rectum and the vagina is the **rectovaginal space,** which the descending rectal septa separate from the lateral **pararectal spaces.** Posterior to the rectum is the **retrorectal space.** Bilateral condensations of connective tissue and the peritoneal folds of the descending rectal septa at the level of the cervix constitute the **uterosacral ligaments,** which contain some blood vessels, lymphatics, and the fibers of the parasympathetic and sympathetic nerves.

3) Pararectal spaces

The **pararectal spaces** extend out posterolaterally from the central organ structures. These spaces are bounded by the uterosacral ligaments medially, the cardinal ligament superiorly, and the levator ani muscles of the pelvic floor inferiorly.

10. The pelvic structures

a. The uterus

The uterine cervix inserts into the vagina at the level of the cardinal ligament attachment (Fig. 2-13). **The**

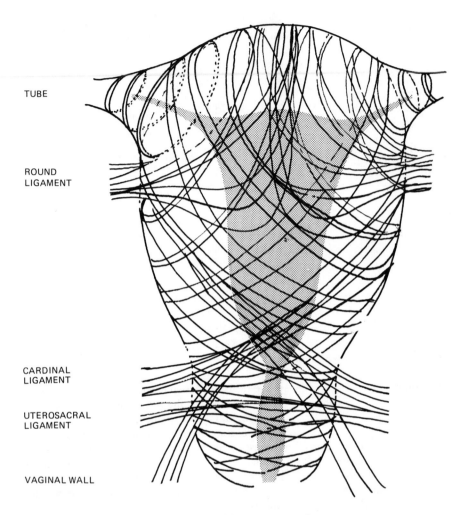

TUBE

ROUND
LIGAMENT

CARDINAL
LIGAMENT

UTEROSACRAL
LIGAMENT

VAGINAL WALL

FIGURE 2-14. Schematic representation of the uterine muscles.

uterus in the mature woman is a pear-shaped organ that is 7.5 cm long, 5 cm wide, and 2.5 cm thick and weighs about 40 grams. The cervical portion is about 2–3 cm in length. The portion that blends with the squamous epithelium of the vagina is called the portio vaginalis, or the **ectocervix,** whereas the portion of the cervix that is usually within the endocervical canal and is covered by columnar epithelium is called the **endocervix.** If the columnar epithelium extends out onto the external surface of the cervix, it is usually covered over with squamous epithelium (i.e., squamous metaplasia) after the onset of puberty.

The uterus has three layers of tissue: serous,

muscular, and mucous. The serous layer consists of the abdominal peritoneal covering, which is tightly bound to the underlying muscular tissue. The smooth muscle of the uterus extends to the fallopian tubes, the ovarian and round ligaments, the vagina, and bilaterally into the cardinal ligaments. The outer layer of the muscular layer is made up of longitudinal fibers, while the inner layer is composed of interlacing spiral fibers with many blood vessels (Fig. 2-14). The cervix normally does not have any appreciable amount of smooth muscle tissue present beyond the internal os distally. The inner mucous lining of the uterus is composed of the **endometrium,** which consists of stromal and glandular tissue that may vary between 2 and 10 mm in thickness as it responds to the steroid hormonal levels that are present. The endometrial lining consists of a basal layer, a spongiosa layer, and a compacta layer. During menstruation, the spongiosa and compacta layers are sloughed, leaving the basal layer. *The outer two layers are then regenerated from the basal layer during the succeeding menstrual cycle under the influence of estrogen and progesterone.*

The blood supply of the uterus is primarily by means of the **uterine artery,** which is a branch of the anterior division of the hypogastric artery. The uterine artery enters the uterus at about the level of the internal os of the cervix and sends a descending branch to the vagina (which forms the coronary artery of the cervix) and an ascending branch up along the border of the uterus (with many penetrating branches to the uterus and fallopian tube). It then extends out along the fallopian tube, where it joins with the ovarian artery, which descends in the fold of peritoneum that is called the **infundibulopelvic ligament.**

The uterus is supported in its midposition in the pelvis by the cardinal ligaments, the round ligaments, the bladder pillars, and the uterosacral ligaments. The round ligaments are fibromuscular bundles of connective tissue that extend from the anterolateral surface of the uterus near the fallopian tube through the internal inguinal rings and the inguinal canals to insert into the labia majora. These ligaments contain blood vessels, lymphatics, and nerves. The round ligaments are quite easily stretched, especially during pregnancy, and therefore they act primarily as "guy wires" in supporting the uterus in the midline of the pelvis.

b. The fallopian tubes

The bilateral **fallopian tubes** are derived embryologically from the paramesonephric (müllerian) ducts. *They are usually about 10–12 cm long and about 1 cm in diameter.* The distal end of the fallopian tube is flared to form a trumpet-shaped area (*infundibulum*) with a series of fine, finger-like projections, or *fimbria.* One of these, the **fimbria ovarica,** is longer than the rest and extends over the surface of the ovary. Owing to the muscular elements in this special fimbria, the tube is kept in close proximity to the ovary during ovulation. The next portion of the tube, called the *ampulla,* progressively narrows down to the segment of the next portion of the tube closest to the uterus, which is called the *isthmus,* just before it

enters the uterus. The part of the tube within the cornual portion of the uterus is referred to as the *interstitial,* or *intramural,* portion of the fallopian tube. Unlike the uterus, the fallopian tubes have four coats: (1) serous or peritoneal, (2) subserous, (3) smooth muscle, and (4) a mucous layer. The peritoneum is not as tightly bound to the tube as it is to the uterus. The blood vessels and nerves are found in the subserous layer. The muscular tissue of the tube is composed of two layers: an outer longitudinal layer and an inner circular layer. The internal lumen of the tube is thrown into a series of folds, or plica, which are covered with a mucosa composed of ciliated columnar epithelium.

c. The ovaries

The ovaries consist of paired structures that measure 3–5 cm long, 1.5–3.0 cm wide, and 1.0–1.5 cm thick and weigh about 3–8 grams. They have a pinkish-white appearance and usually have multiple small cystic structures (a pebbly appearance) beneath their surface. The ovary is supported by ligaments at each pole: the suspensory ligament (i.e., infundibulopelvic ligament), attached to the posterior wall of the broad ligament, and the **utero-ovarian ligament,** attached medially to the uterus. The blood supply is by way of the ovarian arteries, which arise from the aorta just below the renal arteries and traverse the infundibulopelvic ligament to the ovarian hilum. An ovarian venous plexus drains the blood via the ovarian vein in the infundibulopelvic ligament to enter the inferior vena cava on the right side and *the left renal vein on the left side.* Fibers of the sympathetic nervous system from the 10th thoracic segment, and from the aortic, renal, and celiac plexuses, traverse this ligament as well. Remnants of the embryologic mesonephric tubules (*wolffian ducts*) may appear within the broad ligament (the epoophoron and the paroophoron) or in the cervix and upper vagina (Gartner's duct cyst).

d. The ureters

The **ureters** are tubular structures that extend from the renal pelves to the bladder. They are about 25–30 cm in length and cross the brim of the pelvis at about the bifurcation of the common iliac vessels into the external and internal iliac (i.e., hypogastric) arteries. The ureter then drops into the true pelvis near the

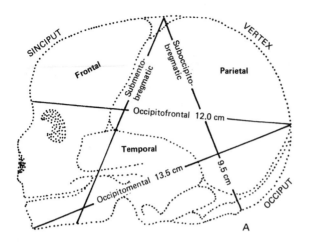

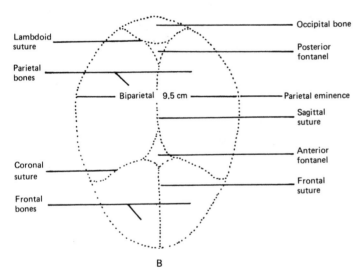

FIGURE 2-15. Bones of the fetal head. (A) Lateral view. (B) Superior view.

lateral borders of the uterosacral ligaments and proceeds down along the uterine cervix to the point where the uterine artery enters the uterus at the level of the internal os. At this juncture, the ureter passes beneath the uterine artery and then immediately swings anteriorly and superiorly to join with the bladder, which lies above the uterus. When the ureter is touched, a peristaltic wave will usually occur. If the ureter is rolled between the thumb and the forefinger, it has a "rubber-like" consistency. On occasion, when it is impossible to visually identify the ureter, this palpable finding may assist you in identifying its location.

11. The fetal head

In obstetrics it will be necessary for you to know the basic landmarks of the fetal skull, since you will have to evaluate these anatomic features in the management of labor.

a. Landmarks

The fetal skull is somewhat unyielding in its passage through the birth canal and thus it constitutes the "measure of the pelvis," whereas the breech is a smaller and more compressible part of the fetus. The base of the head is surmounted by the vault of the skull. The bones of the base of the skull are usually ossified and therefore not compressible, whereas those of the vault (i.e., cranium) are thinner, less ossified, and can be easily compressed to produce overlapping of the skull plates (i.e., molding).

Anatomically, from the **superior view,** the posterior portion of the fetal skull consists of the posterior occipital bone, which is joined to the two lateral parietal skull plates by the membraneous **lambdoid suture** (Fig. 2-15). This juncture of the three bony plates forms a Y-shaped **posterior fontanel** (lambda) with the lambdoid and the long **sagittal suture.** The **biparietal diameter (9.5 cm)** extends across the largest transverse diameter of the skull, which is somewhat posterior to the mid-skull position because of the more posterior swelling of the parietal eminences. The average term circumference of the fetal skull in the occipitofrontal diameter is about 34.5 cm.

The anterior portion of the fetal skull consists of the junction of the two lateral parietal skull plates, which are separated by the sagittal suture with the two frontal bony plates to form the coronal suture and the frontal suture, which thus produces a larger diamond-shaped **anterior fontanel** (bregma). One or both of the anterior and posterior fontanels are utilized during the vaginal examination during labor to determine the position of the fetal head. This information, when supplemented by Leopold's maneuvers, can accurately define the fetal position.

b. Diameters

When viewing the fetal skull from the **lateral position,** it is important to note the brow area (the **sinciput**), the posterior portion of the top of the skull between the fontanels (the **vertex**), and the extreme posterior portion of the skull (the **occiput**), since these are also important landmarks in labor. The **sub-occipitobregmatic diameter (9.5 cm)** measures the well-flexed fetal head in the usual position for labor. The **submentobregmatic diameter (9.5 cm)** measures the face presentation, extending from the anterior fontanel to the neck and jaw region. Since this diameter is the same as the usual suboccipitobregmatic presentation, the infant will have little difficulty in delivering if the chin is anterior. When the chin is posterior, however, the fetal head is already greatly hyperextended, thus preventing it from extending any further for delivery.

The **occipitofrontal diameter (12 cm)** measures the deflexed head (e.g., military attitude, occipitoposterior position) and extends from the elevated area between the orbital ridges (glabella) and the external occipital protuberance. This larger presenting diameter will frequently slow the progression of labor and, in such cases, delivery of the fetus may require either a forceps rotation or a cesarean section. The **occipitomental diameter (13.5 cm),** the longest diameter of the fetal head, measures the fetal head with a brow presentation. Due to the large presenting diameter, a persistent brow presentation has a poor prognosis for vaginal delivery.

CHAPTER 3

Basic neuroendocrinology

Science since Darwin is fact upon fact, instance upon instance, experiment upon experiment, principle upon principle, which fitly joined together by some master mind may establish some great truth.

—*Sir William Osler**

1. Introduction

In order to understand the reproductive endocrine functions of the female patient, it is necessary for you to develop an appreciation of the sequence of actions of the various transmitters that orchestrate the cycle of menstruation. The central nervous system, especially the hypothalamus, utilizes neurotransmitters and neurohormones for internal communication and stimulation of the pituitary gland, which in turn secretes gonadotropic hormones to regulate and stimulate the follicles and the stroma of the ovaries. By means of both positive and negative feedback mechanisms, the ovarian hormones modulate the timing and the secretion of these neurohormones and gonadotropic hormones so as to produce a finely tuned, smooth, and coordinated ovarian function, which is then reflected in the normal menstrual cycle by the periodic stimulation and shedding of the uterine endometrium.

---

*Reprinted with permission from Robert Bennett Bean, *Sir William Osler: Aphorisms from His Bedside Teachings and Writings,* William Bennett Bean, ed. Springfield, Ill.: Charles C Thomas, Publisher, 1968, p. 63.

a. Hypothalamic neurohormone secretion

1) Gonadotropin releasing hormone (GnRH)

The release of gonadotropic hormones by the anterior pituitary gland is controlled by **gonadotropin releasing hormone (GnRH). This decapeptide neurohormone is produced in the peptidergic neural cells in the arcuate nucleus of the hypothalamus in the floor of the third ventricle of the brain.** These cells are responsive to the hormones produced by the target organ endocrine gland cells as well as to other neurotransmitters produced within the brain, such as dopamine, norepinephrine, serotonin, melatonin, and endorphins.

After it is produced in the hypothalamus, GnRH is released in a pulsatile fashion into the axonal tuberoinfundibular tract to the portal vessels and is then transmitted via the hypothalamic hypophyseal portal circulation to the anterior pituitary gland, where it stimulates the secretion of the gonadotropic hormones, which include the **follicle-stimulating hormone (FSH)** and the **luteinizing hormone (LH).** The secretion of these gonadotropins is also pulsatile, and they in turn stimulate the ovary to produce estrogens, progesterone, and androgens. **The half-life of the GnRH is only a few minutes,** and therefore its effects upon the menstrual cycle must depend upon repeated complex feedback mechanisms from the other neurotransmitters, the gonadotropic hormones, and the steroid hormones that are produced in the target organs. These mechanisms provide for an almost constantly modulated release of the GnRH at a specific pulse frequency. **The pulse frequency of the GnRH secretion is apparently important,** since optimal GnRH secretion, at least in the monkey, requires that there be one pulse per hour, consisting of 1 μg GnRH per minute for six minutes. One group of chemicals, the catecholamines (e.g., epinephrine, norepinephrine, and dopamine), are thought to help regulate the pulse frequency of the GnRH secretion. Another regulator involves the **catecholestrogens,** which are produced in the hypothalamus by the enzymatic conversion of estrogens to form a compound that has both an estrogen side and a catecholamine side. These compounds may interact with the catecholamines to affect the secretion of GnRH. **Norepinephrine,** a neurotransmitter produced in the mesencephalon and in the lower brainstem, is thought to **stimulate GnRH secretion. Dopamine** is produced in the arcuate and paraventricular nuclei of the hypothalamus, where it acts to **inhibit the secretion of GnRH. Serotonin may also be inhibitory to GnRH secretion;** however, its exact role is unknown at the present time. These biogenic amines are also involved with the emotional and behavioral aspects of the individual and thus play an important role in pyschosomatic problems (see Chapter 5).

2) Other releasing factors

Other releasing factors present in the central nervous system control the secretion of other agents. Dopamine is the neurohormone that most likely controls the release of prolactin. While most of the neurohormones are releasing hormones, dopamine is the **prolactin inhibiting factor (PIF).** Bromocriptine, a derivative of ergot, has been used clinically to treat hyperprolactinemia. This drug probably exerts its effect by stimulating the dopaminergic system, which in turn produces dopamine to inhibit the secretion of prolactin. **Thyrotopin releasing hormone (TRH)** is present in many areas of the brain and effects the release of thyroid-stimulating hormone (TSH), which in turn effects the secretion of the thyroid hormones. The thyrotropin releasing hormone also has an antidepressant effect.

3) Other neurotransmitters

A number of other peptides have been found in the central nervous system. These include: (1) the substance P (a transmitter of pain), (2) neurotensin (which regulates changes in body temperature and pituitary hormone levels), (3) somatostatin (which inhibits the release of prolactin, growth hormone, and TSH, and may be a pain transmitter), and (4) the endorphins.

a) Endorphins

This latter group of peptides, the **endorphins,** are derived from **β-lipotropin,** which along with adrenocorticotropic hormone (ACTH), share a common precursor, **pro-opiomelanocortin** (see Chapter 42). The β-lipotropin has no morphine-like activity, but when it is further degraded, it results in enkephalin, beta-melanocyte-stimulating hormone (β-MSH), and α-, γ-, and β-endorphins. Alpha (α) and gamma (γ) endorphins and enkephalin have opioid properties similar to those of morphine, whereas β-endorphin is five to ten times more powerful than morphine.

There are opioid receptors present in the limbic system (the site of euphoric emotions) and throughout the brain and spinal cord, as well as in the sensory nerve endings. **These opioids are capable of stimulating the release of growth hormone, ACTH, and prolactin. They also inhibit TSH, LH, and FSH.** These endogenous opiates **inhibit the production of GnRH** in the arcuate nucleus area of the hypothalamus. They also **inhibit dopamine release,** with a resultant increase in prolactin levels. Since patients with *menstrual disturbances associated with stress and exercise* have been found to have low gonadotropins and elevated prolactin levels, it is thought that these menstrual disturbances may be due to these mechanisms. The administration of either endorphins or morphine to an individual will produce identical findings, indicating that both compounds have a similar effect. If an opiate antagonist, such as naloxone hydrochloride (Narcan), is administered, then the levels of FSH and LH will increase and the prolactin level will decrease.

There may be two main endorphin systems present—one in the hypothalamus and the other in the pituitary. While each of these systems may have their own control feedback systems, this theory is currently a controversial subject. The pituitary endorphin system seems to be mainly affected by stress stimuli, whereas the ovarian steroids may perhaps modulate the hypothalamic beta-endorphin system.

The endorphins apparently modulate the frequency of GnRH release and decrease the frequency of the LH pulse. Interestingly, although LH pulses have been associated with postmenopausal hot flashes, naloxone hydrochloride does not modify the characteristics of the LH pulse in this situation. In some individuals, a chronically elevated or depressed level of opioid activity may interfere with normal menstruation.

Opiates and the opioid peptides are also thought to have an effect on the *appetite.* Beta-endorphin, when injected into the brain of a rat, will increase the amount of food intake. The cyclic nature of endorphin levels has been implicated as a cause of depression, fatigue, and irritability in the premenstrual syndrome (PMS). One postulated etiology of PMS is that a temporary addiction to the rising opiate levels may occur during the luteal phase of the menstrual cycle, and with the abrupt decrease in the levels of these compounds at the time of menstruation, the patient experiences a withdrawal reaction with the excessive release of catecholamines, which produces some of the symptoms of PMS (see Chapter 42).

4) Tropic hormones, action, and regulation

The releasing hormones and the anterior pituitary hormones are examples of tropic hormones, which perform their functions by uniting with specific cellular receptors on the cell membranes of the target tissue. When this union occurs, the **adenylate cyclase system is activated** in the membrane wall, which causes the conversion of adenosine triphosphate (ATP) to **cyclic adenosine 3′, 5′-monophosphate (cyclic AMP).** This cAMP-receptor protein complex activates the protein kinase, which contains two regulatory subunits and two catalytic subunits, the latter of which are released to catalyze the phosphorylation of the cellular proteins to produce the physiologic events specific to the hormone's function. This immediate response of increased steroidogenesis is by phosphorylation, rather than by means of gene transcription.

The modulation of specific cellular receptors for hormones in either a positive or negative manner has been termed "up or down regulation." Some hormones have the ability to stimulate an increase in the numbers of their own cellular receptors (i.e., up regulation). The down regulation for polypeptide hormones apparently occurs as a process in which there is an *internalization* of the receptors into the cell, which then limits the number of receptors available and thus the amount of hormonal activity that can occur. An excess in the concentration of certain hormones (e.g., GnRH, LH) will instigate the process of internalization. The modulation of the activity of the adenyl cyclase system may occur in the presence of nucleotide *stimulatory* regulatory units and *inhibitory* regulatory units.

Recently, some of the intraovarian nongonadotropic regulators have been classified as being either **paracrine** or **autocrine.** While the **endocrine** regulators of folliculogenesis are blood borne, cells that have **paracrine** communication include those in which the diffusion of the regulator is locally to a different type of cell. The cells that produce regulators that act upon their own surface receptors have been classified as having **autocrine** communication.

b. Pituitary hormones

1) Anterior pituitary hormones

A number of hormones are secreted from the anterior pituitary gland. These are: (1) the adrenocorticotropic hormone (ACTH), (2) the thyroid-stimulating hormone (TSH), (3) the follicle-stimulating hormone (FSH), (4) the luteinizing hormone (LH), (5) the growth hormone (GH), and (6) prolactin. The secretion patterns of some of these hormones are regulated by their specific hypothalamic releasing factors or, in the case of prolactin, by an inhibitory regulator, and by the feedback mechanisms from the target organs.

2) Posterior pituitary hormones

The posterior pituitary hormones are oxytocin and arginine vasopressin. Neurosecretory cells in both the supraoptic and the paraventricular nuclei of the hypothalamus produce these polypeptide hormones and transport them by means of the transport peptides called neurophysins. **Neurophysin I is an estrogen-stimulated transport peptide that accompanies the release of oxytocin, whereas neurophysin II is a nicotine-stimulated peptide associated with the release of vasopressin.** The presence of increased levels of vasopressin may also be related to increased learning and memory capabilities, since the administration of vasopressin has been associated with improved memory in brain-damaged individuals.

Oxytocin may be released by the manipulation of the cervix and the uterus, or by coitus (i.e., the Ferguson reflex). This is an important point to remember in dealing with patients who have premature labor, since premature contractions may be stimulated by the oxytocin release that occurs with sexual activity. In addition, a number of prostaglandins are present in the semen, which might also stimulate uterine contractions. Oxytocin is released with neurophysin I at the time of the LH surge during the menstrual cycle. Oxytocin is also released with suckling, or with the manual stimulation of the breasts and nipples. This response has recently been utilized as a "stress test" during the third trimester to determine the status of the infant. The afterpains that many multiparous patients experience during the postpartum period, especially during nursing, are due to the release of oxytocin, which stimulates uterine contractions.

Oxytocin is present in large amounts in the meconium and in fetal urine and may be responsible for the "precipitate labor" sometimes seen in association with fetal distress. Maternal oxytocin levels increase during the *second stage of labor;* however, there is no evidence that oxytocin itself initiates the labor process. Interestingly, the levels of fetal oxytocin are elevated during the *first stage of labor,* and this oxytocin may cross into the maternal compartment.

Osmoreceptors present in the hypothalamus are responsible for the regulation of blood volume. In addition, there are volume receptors (i.e., stretch receptors) present in the left and right atria, the aortic arch, and the carotid sinus. The regulation of the blood volume appears to be determined by the myocardial receptors that are located in and around the atria and the great vessels and are most prominent in the low pressure system (i.e., the right atrium). These receptors are primarily concerned with the regulation of the antidiuretic hormone (i.e., vasopressin) and aldosterone. In conditions of prolonged bedrest or weightless conditions, such as in water submersion or travel in outer space, an overfilling of the right atrium occurs due to the effect of the loss of gravity on the column of blood in the inferior vena cava. These receptors sense this increased venous return to the right atrium as being representative of hypervolemia, which triggers a loss of water and sodium in the urine, which in turn results in a decrease in the intravascular volume. This hypovolemia may then result in dizziness and syncope when the individual again resumes the upright position under normal gravity conditions.

The atrial natriuretic factor (ANF), a hormone produced in the atrial epicardial myocardium and released whenever the atrium is stretched, causes a profound natriuresis and diuresis. This factor is the first endogenous agonist that utilizes the cyclic guanosine monophosphate (cGMP) membrane-bound mediator in effecting its action on the cell. ANF is stimulated by: (1) increased vascular volume, (2) increased atrial pressure, (3) hyperosmolarity, (4) hypoxia, and (5) an increased heart rate. Increased plasma levels of ANF cause: (1) a decrease in arginine vasopressin (i.e., ADH), (2) arterial vasodilatation, (3) a decrease in arterial pressure, and (4) an increased heart rate. On the venous side of the vascular system, ANF causes: (1) vasoconstriction, (2) increased capillary pressure, (3) decreased blood volume, (4) decreased venous return, and (5) a decreased cardiac output. ANF causes a decrease in aldosterone release. In the kidney, ANF causes: (1) a decreased renin release, (2) decreased angiotensin II levels, (3) an increased urine flow, and (4) an increased excretion of sodium, potassium, chloride, and calcium. ANF apparently influences blood pressure and blood volume regulation in the fetus as well.

c. Ovarian hormones

1) Estrogen

In 1923, Edgar Allen and Edward Doisy were the first to demonstrate the presence of estrogenic substances in the ovarian follicle. By 1929, Doisy and a German investigator, A. Butenandt, were able to crystallize estrone from the urine. In 1930, J. S. L. Browne was able to isolate estriol from placental tissue. Finally, in 1936, D. W. MacCorquodale and associates were able to isolate the principle estrogen, estradiol-17β.

The ovary produces three main estrogens: estradiol-17β, estrone, and estriol (Fig. 3-1, Fig. 3-2). Estrone is produced by the aromatization of androstenedione. A further degradation of estrone results in the production of estriol, the weakest of the estrogens. Estradiol-17β results from the aromatization of testosterone. Almost all of the estrogen that is produced comes from the ovary. The excretion of estrogens is generally accomplished by the liver, which

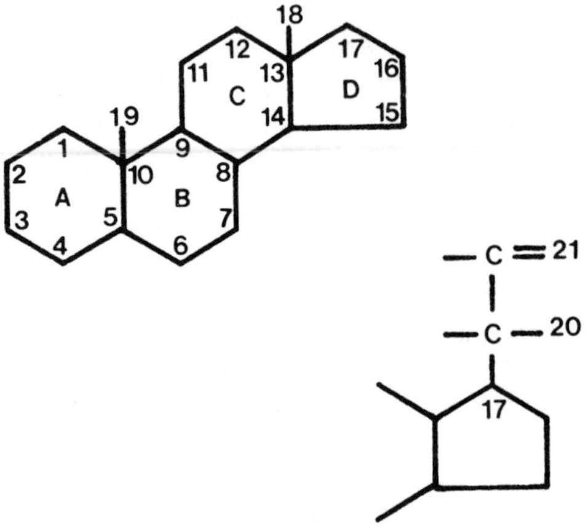

FIGURE 3-1. Basic steroid formula structure, with the cyclopentanophenanthrene ring system. Each ring is identified by a letter from A to D. Carbon atoms are numbered in the sequence shown.

conjugates these hormones with a glucuronide or a sulfate for excretion in the urine and bile.

Estrogens are growth-stimulating agents that specifically affect their target tissues (i.e., breasts, bladder, urethra, and the genital system). Estrogen decreases both FSH and LH secretion, although the latter may be stimulated at the point of ovulation during the normal menstrual cycle by a positive feedback mechanism. In the presence of elevated estrogen levels, there is an increase in the levels of a number of the blood components, such as the **sex hormone–binding globulin (SHBG)**, fibrinogen, and some of the lipoprotein complexes. The development of the secondary sexual characteristics is due to the secretion of adequate amounts of estrogens during puberty.

2) Progesterone

In 1928, **George Corner** and **Willard Allen** were able to isolate a new hormone (progesterone) from sow's ovaries, which they initially named "progestin." Over the next couple of years they were able to crystallize and characterize it, as did another investigator, **Butenandt,** who in 1930 was also able to characterize the new hormone as a steroid (Fig. 3-3). This new hormone was then given the name **progesterone** by both groups of investigators. By 1937, E. H. Venning was able to determine that the excretion of preg-

nanediol in the urine correlated with the secretion of progesterone and was indeed a metabolite of progesterone.

Progesterone is secreted primarily by the corpus luteum of the ovary, or by the placenta if a pregnancy should occur. The continued support of the LH secretion stimulates the secretion of progesterone during the secretory portion of the menstrual cycle after ovulation has occurred. Progesterone has a maturational effect on the estrogen-prepared target tissues and effectively inhibits the growth-stimulating effect that occurs with estrogen stimulation. The secretion of progesterone increases the body temperature by about 0.4–1.0°F, and basal body temperature charts provide a marker for determining ovulation in patients concerned about possible infertility.

3) Androgens

The stroma of the ovary is capable of producing androgens under the influence of LH stimulation during the menstrual cycle. The theca cells, when stimulated by LH, produce androstenedione and testosterone, which are aromatized to produce estrogens in the granulosa cells of the corpus luteum (Fig. 3-4).

4) Steroid hormone action

The mechanism of steroid action on cellular receptors is poorly understood. It has been thought that steroid hormones (e.g., estrogens, progesterone, androgens, mineralocorticoids, and glucocorticoids) exerted their action by diffusing across the cell membranes of the target tissue cells where they would bind with cytoplasmic receptor proteins (ligands), which would then transport them to the nuclei. This hormone-receptor complex is then transformed or activated and bound to the nuclear DNA, where the messenger RNA (mRNA) is synthesized and transported to ribosomes in the cytoplasm to produce specific proteins. While the main action of the steroid hormones is the regulation of the intracellular synthesis of proteins, the mechanism, as outlined above, has come under increasing scrutiny and doubt. The "heat-shock proteins" have apparently been identified as being the same as the 90,000 molecular–weight steroid-receptor components, but their functions are unknown. They may be important in regulating cellular pro-

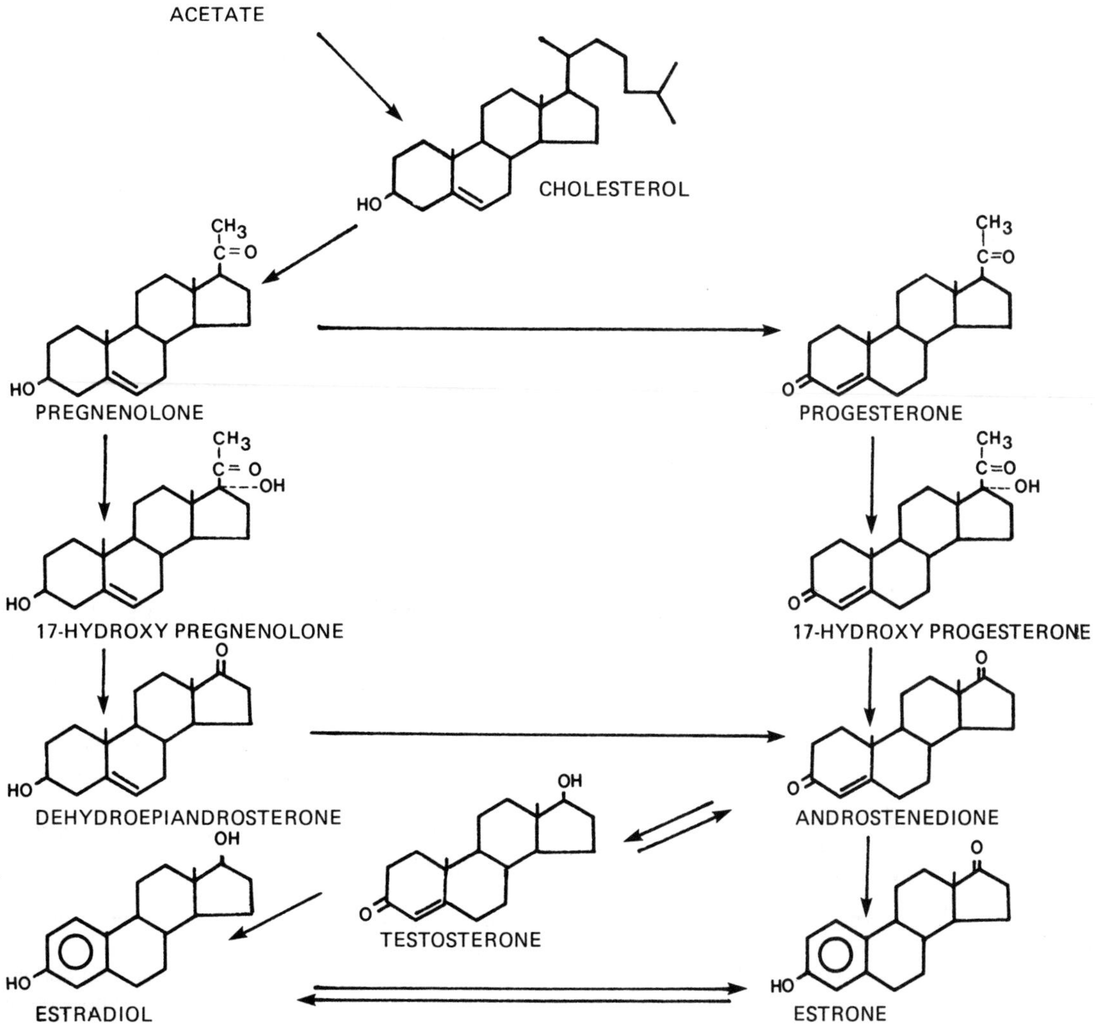

FIGURE 3-2. Pathways for the synthesis of ovarian hormones.

cesses; however, more studies in this area will be necessary before their exact function can be defined.

2. The onset of puberty

The specific event that initiates the onset of puberty is unknown. At about 6–8 years of age, the follicle-stimulating hormone (FSH) and the dehydroisoandrosterone (DHA) levels begin to rise; however, it is not until about 10–12 years of age that the luteinizing

hormone (LH) and the estrogen values begin to increase. **The onset of puberty is associated with pulsatile secretion of LH that occurs during sleep.** This pattern of LH release apparently does not occur either before or after puberty, but only at its onset, and it is thought to represent the early maturational changes in the hypothalamus.

Gonadotropin releasing hormone (GnRH) is produced in a pulsatile fashion and serves to stimulate both the development and the release of the gonadotropins. The gonadotropins (FSH, LH), in turn, stimu-

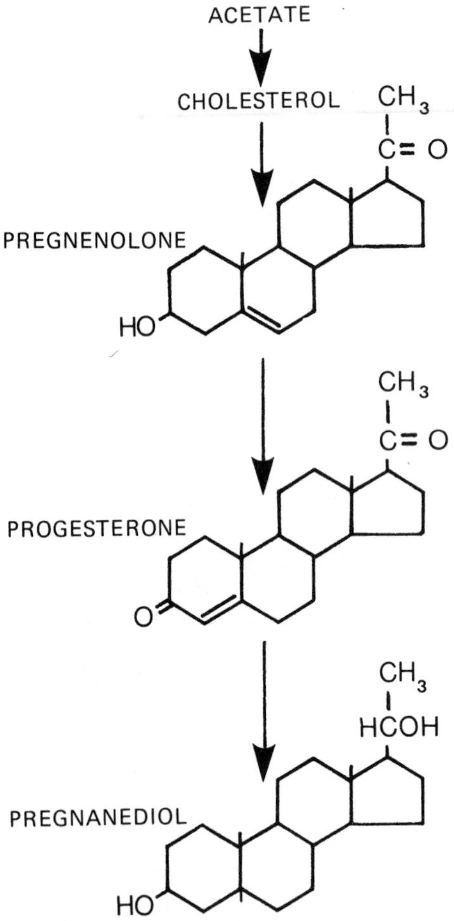

ACETATE

CHOLESTEROL

PREGNENOLONE

PROGESTERONE

PREGNANEDIOL

FIGURE 3-3. The synthesis of progesterone.

late the ovary to produce the sex steroid (estradiol), which by midpuberty begins to provide a feedback mechanism that assists in the control of the menstrual cycle. GnRH secretion is independent of this steroid feedback mechanism until just prior to menarche.

As puberty takes place, the hypothalamus becomes increasingly less sensitive to the negative estrogen feedback mechanism. The hypothalamic release of GnRH increases in response to this perceived "lack of estrogen production," which results in an even greater production of the gonadotropins and estradiol. At the same time, the "hormonal gonadostat" becomes reset at an increasingly higher level of function until the adult level is reached.

a. Weight/fat theory

It has been suggested that puberty may be triggered by the individual's attainment of a specific body weight or body fat content. **A body weight of 48 kg, or a body fat content in excess of 17%, has been considered to be the "critical weight/fat content" necessary to provide a metabolism capable of initiating the menstruation process.** In support of this concept, it has been noted that obese girls (i.e., 20–30% over normal weight) experience an earlier menarche than do thinner girls. Also, in girls who are underweight, or in those who have less than normal amounts of body fat, the menarche may be delayed. During the past 100 years, the age of onset of puberty seems to have gradually declined; this earlier onset of puberty has most likely been due to the fact that the girls of today have better nutrition and reach the critical weight/fat content at an earlier age than in previous generations.

b. Sequence of menarcheal events

The usual sequence of events at the time of puberty is as follows: (1) thelarche (breast development) at 9.8 years, (2) adrenarche (pubic and axillary hair development) at 10.5 years, (3) a maximal growth spurt at 11.4 years, and finally (4) menarche (the onset of menses) at 12.8 years. The entire process extends over about a two- to four-year period.

Breast development and the growth of **pubic and the axillary hair** have been adequately described by Tanner's classification system (Fig. 3-5). Each stage of the development encompasses about 1 year, with the final adult stage being reached at about the age of 14.

The growth spurt begins at about the age of 10 and extends through ages 15–16, with a peak at about 11.4 years. The height increase is of the order of 6–11 cm (2–4 inches) during the first year, with a reduction to about 6 cm (2.5 inches) after menstruation begins.

The onset of menarche in girls in the United States occurs at an average age of 12.8 years, with a range of 9.1 to 17.7 years. During the first few years following menarche, the hypothalamic-pituitary axis gradually matures as the setpoint of adult hormonal functioning of the menstrual cycle becomes steady and reliable. Until this maturation process takes place, however, it is to be expected that the incidence of anovulation will be high and that the initial men-

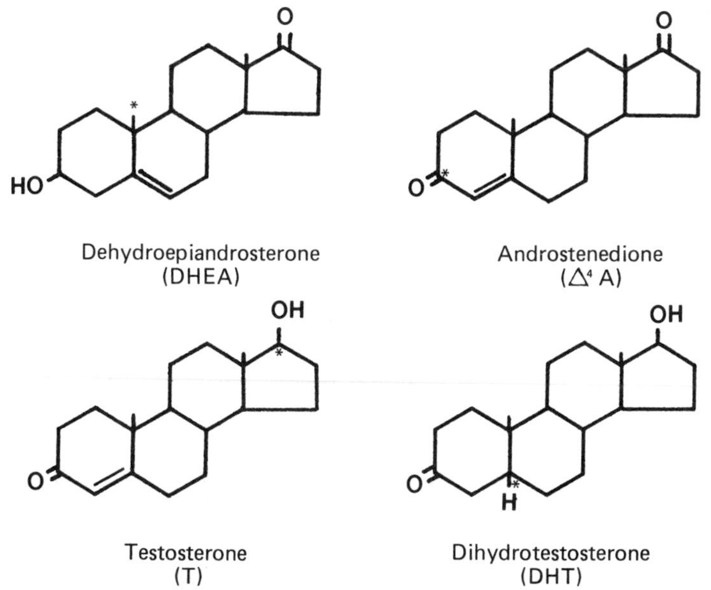

Dehydroepiandrosterone
(DHEA)

Androstenedione
(Δ^4 A)

Testosterone
(T)

Dihydrotestosterone
(DHT)

FIGURE 3-4. Major serum androgens. Asterisk indicates sites affecting androgen potency. (Redrawn with permission from D. N. Danforth and J. R. Scott, eds., *Obstetrics and Gynecology,* 5th ed., Philadelphia: J. B. Lippincott Company, 1986, p. 897.)

strual cycles may be irregular and variable in interval, duration, and flow.

3. Precocious puberty

a. True puberty

Puberty in the United States is considered to be precocious if it occurs prior to the age of eight years. The sequence of menarcheal events, however, may be confused in precocious puberty, in that the growth spurt may occur initially; the menarche may be the first event to occur; or the onset of adrenarche, thelarche, and the growth spurt may all occur simultaneously. **True sexual precocity (i.e., constitutional, idiopathic) is probably the most common form of precocity, since it is the cause in about 54% of the reported cases.** This condition may occur in families in which there is a history of early onset of puberty in other family members (i.e., constitutional). In others, it may occur much earlier than eight years of age, and in these instances it has been thought to be due to the early maturation of the hypothalamic-pituitary-ovarian axis under a normal higher cortical brain control, as electroencephalographic tracings in these patients have revealed a high frequency of abnormalities.

b. Historical findings

The patient's *growth history* should receive special attention. The progression of menarcheal events in precocious puberty may be confused and often may be slower than normal. You should evaluate the patient's height, since these girls are initially tall for their age; however, owing to the fact that they have a premature closure of their epiphyses, their eventual height may be much shorter. Nearly one-half of these patients will end up being less than 5 feet tall (the range is from 4 feet 5 inches to 5 feet 8 inches). *The onset of the patient's dental eruption is more closely allied to the chronological age than to the skeletal age.* **A left hand-wrist film will usually define the skeletal age.**

A history of encephalitis, meningitis, hydrocephalus, von Recklinghausen's disease, cranial trauma, or the ingestion of certain drugs can be important factors in such cases. The presence of a *foreign body* in the vagina of a young girl may be the cause of genital bleeding. If the patient has ingested exogenous estrogenic medications, such as diethylstilbestrol, a darker pigmentation of the areola and of the nipples may occur.

c. Other diagnostic possibilities

About 5% of the cases of sexual precocity are due to abnormalities of the central nervous sys-

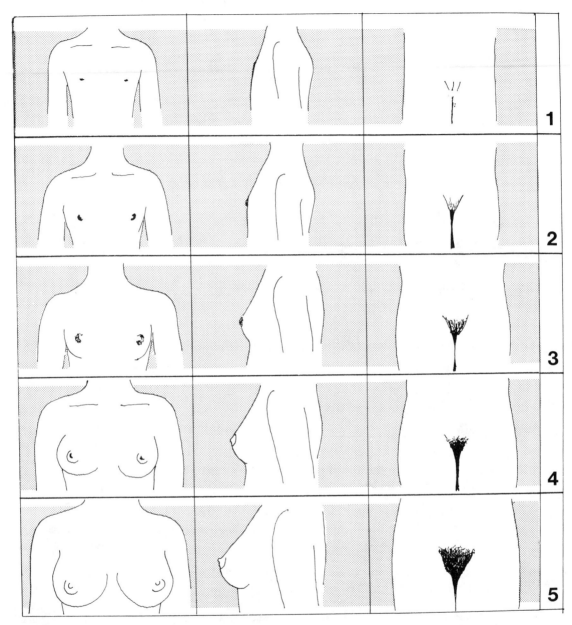

FIGURE 3-5. Tanner's classification of breast development: (1) Stage I—Preadolescent with elevation of papilla only; areola not pigmented. (2) Stage II—Breast-bud stage with elevation of breast mound; increased diameter of areola. (3) Stage III—Increased breast mount with no separation of areola contour. (4) Stage IV—Elevation of papilla and areola to form secondary mound above breast level. (5) Stage V—Only papilla is elevated; areola recessed to general contour of breast.

Tanner's classification of pubic hair development: (1) Stage I—Preadolescent with no pubic hair. (2) Stage II—Sparse growth of downy hair along labia. (3) Stage III—Sparse growth of dark coarse hair over pubis. (4) Stage IV—Adult hair spread over a smaller area with no spread to medial thighs. (5) Stage V—Normal adult female hair pattern with spread to medial thighs.

tem. Precocious puberty may occur in the presence of central nervous system tumors, such as a craniopharyngioma, a hamartoma, a suprasellar cyst or teratoma, or an optic nerve glioma. However, the exact mechanism involved is unknown. Skull films may be of value in making the diagnosis in these cases.

1) McCune-Albright syndrome

The McCune-Albright syndrome (i.e., polyostotic fibrous dysplasia) consists of "cafe-au-lait" skin spots, multiple disseminated cystic bone lesions, and precocious puberty. A history of bone fractures and precocious puberty should alert you to this diagnosis. The McCune-Albright syndrome is seen in about 4% of patients with precocious puberty. Giantism, hyperthyroidism, and Cushing's disease have also been associated with this syndrome, leading some authors to suggest that it may be a multiple-endocrine-adenoma syndrome.

2) Primary hypothyroidism

Primary hypothyroidism may be associated with precocious puberty, and these patients may also have *galactorrhea*. In such cases, the thyrotropin-releasing hormone (TRH) is elevated, which in turn elevates the thyroid-stimulating hormone (TSH), the follicle-stimulating hormone (FSH), and the luteinizing hormone (LH). Treatment of the hypothyroidism will usually reverse the sexual precocity. The thyroid function should always be assessed in patients with precocious puberty.

3) Ectopic gonadotropin production

Ectopic gonadotropin production occurs in less than 0.5% of cases of precocious puberty. Tumors that have been implicated in ectopic gonadotropin production are dysgerminomas and chorioepitheliomas of the ovary and hepatomas of the liver. The presence of abdominal tumors, or ascites, should alert you to the possibility of this diagnosis.

4) Tumors

An increased level of sex steroid production can be a cause for precocious puberty and may be associated with ovarian tumors in about 8%, with adrenal tumors in 1% and with congenital adrenal hyper- *plasia in 28% of cases.* **The most common ovarian tumors that produce estrogens are the granulosa-thecal cell tumors, teratomas, gonadoblastomas, lipoid cell tumors, cystadenomas, and ovarian carcinomas.** Estrogen production produces breast growth and vaginal bleeding, along with skeletal maturation. *About 80% of these tumors are palpable on abdominal or pelvic examination.* A **luteoma,** a small tumor that produces both estrogen and progesterone, may produce a pseudosexual precocity. Follicular and luteal cysts may cause a waxing and waning of the sexual precocity symptoms as the cysts come and go. **Adrenal tumors are not common;** however, an adrenal carcinoma may secrete estrogen and may be the cause of precocious puberty.

5) Premature thelarche

Premature thelarche (i.e., breast development prior to eight years of age) is a relatively common phenomenon. It is probably secondary to an abnormal sensitivity of the end-organ to low levels of estrogen.

6) Premature adrenarche

Premature adrenarche is probably secondary to the secretion of weak androgens, since the blood dehydroisoandrosterone sulfate (DHAS) and the 24-hour 17-ketosteroid urinary excretion are only slightly elevated in these cases. It has been noted that girls with scoliosis have a higher incidence of premature adrenarche.

d. Treatment

The treatment goal in true precocious puberty is to stop the growth process so that the patient's ultimate height will be protected. The administration of 400 mg of medroxyprogesterone acetate (Depo-Provera) intramuscularly every three months will inhibit gonadotropin production: However, it will not delay the closure of the epiphyses. This therapy is no longer used to treat precocious puberty. Currently, the use of GnRH in a continuous rather than a pulsatile fashion has been successfully used in the treatment of precocious puberty patients. This treatment eliminates the menstrual periods, delays the closure of the epiphyses, and inhibits the development of the secondary sexual characteristics. You should also provide psychological support for the patient and for her family.

4. Delayed puberty

Probably less than 1% of girls in the United States fail to enter menarche by the age of 18. These patients should be considered as cases of primary amenorrhea and should be evaluated as such. A few patients may have a simple constitutional delay of menarche. Others may have disorders of gonadal failure, of steroid synthesis, or of the hypothalamic-pituitary axis, or they may have a chronic nonendocrine disease. The bone age should be determined by hand-wrist X-ray films. FSH and LH levels, growth hormone (GH) levels, thyroid studies, skull films, and a karyotype of the leukocytes should also be obtained in these patients.

a. Gonadal failure

In those patients with **gonadal failure,** treatment with conjugated estrogen (Premarin, 1.25 mg/day from day 1 to day 25 each month, and progesterone (Provera), 10 mg/day from day 13 to day 25 each month, will allow the bone age to catch up to the chronologic age and will promote normal maturation with appropriate epiphyseal closure. **In patients below the age of 12 who are predicted to achieve a height of more than 6 feet by the Bayley-Pinneau tables, and who do not wish to attain this height, it is possible to enhance the closure of the epiphyses by administering higher doses of estrogen (e.g., Premarin, 10 mg/day from day 1 to day 25, in association with Provera, 10 mg/day from day 13 to day 25).** Hand-wrist films should be obtained every six months to assess bone growth until the epiphyses have closed.

5. Normal menstruation

a. Menstrual cycle

Menstruation (L. *menstrudare,* to discharge the menses) is the orderly, periodic (monthly) sloughing of the outer two-thirds of the endometrial lining of the uterus in response to the cyclic interplay between the hormones of the hypothalamus, the pituitary, and the ovaries. **The events of the menstrual cycle may be divided into: (1) the follicular phase, (2) ovulation, and (3) the luteal phase.**

1) Follicular phase

The follicular phase of the menstrual pattern encompasses the first 10–14 days of a 28-day menstrual cycle, counting from the first day of menstruation, although this phase is somewhat variable in length. During this period, multiple primordial follicles in the ovary begin to grow and mature in anticipation of ovulation. One of these follicles will be singled out to be the one follicle that ovulates. Recently, it has become evident that there may be a number of different **regulators** of the events of folliculogenesis. To be effective, these agents should be produced locally, manifest their activity locally (i.e., paracrine and autocrine function), and should be necessary for proper ovarian function. Some of these factors may include the epidermal growth factor (EGF), transforming growth factors (TGFα, TGFβ), insulin-like growth factors (Sm-C/IGF-1), and the fibroblast growth factor (FGF). These regulators work in cooperation with luteinizing hormone (LH) and follicle-stimulating hormone (FSH) in aiding the ovarian follicular granulosa cell differentiation and replication.

By the time of puberty, there are only about 300,000 to 500,000 germ cells remaining in the ovary. This reduction of the ovocytes occurs by means of a recurrent ripening and atresia that continues not only throughout the intrauterine life, but also throughout the reproductive life of the woman. **During approximately 40 years of reproductive life, a maximum of about 400–500 ovocytes can be ovulated, if ovulation occurs each and every month.** In actual fact, however, some of the time ovulation does not occur. **Thus, for every ovocyte that is ovulated (or even without ovulation), there are another 1,000 or more that will be lost by atresia each month; by the time of menopause, almost all of the ovocytes will have been exhausted.**

a) Primordial follicle

The primordial follicle consists of an ovocyte that was arrested in the diplotene stage of prophase during meiosis at about 7 months of intrauterine gestation. It is surrounded by a single layer of granulosa cells.

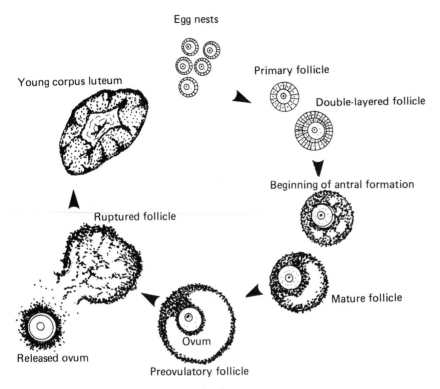

Egg nests

Young corpus luteum

Primary follicle

Double-layered follicle

Beginning of antral formation

Ruptured follicle

Mature follicle

Released ovum

Ovum

Preovulatory follicle

FIGURE 3-6. Sequence of events in follicular maturation.

b) Preantral follicle

After the onset of puberty, the preantral follicle of the ovary begins to develop as the primordial follicle enlarges and develops a *zona pellucida,* along with several more layers of granulosa cells. The zona pellucida surrounds the egg. The granulosa cells primarily manufacture estrogen; however, they are also capable of producing androgens and progesterone. The FSH receptors on the granulosa cell, in the presence of FSH, cause the aromatization of androgens into estrogens. Continued follicular growth is dependent upon the production of increased amounts of estrogen. The combination of FSH and estrogen stimulates the proliferation of granulosa cells and causes an increase in the amount of FSH receptors. **The greater the number of FSH receptors, the greater the conversion of the androgens into estrogens by aromatization.** The androgen level in the preantral follicle becomes important, because at lower concentrations, the androgens fuel the conversion process to

produce more estrogens, whereas higher concentrations may exceed the ability of the aromatization conversion mechanism to process the androgens and thus result in atresia of the follicle.

c) Antral follicle

The antral follicle differs from the preantral follicular phase by the formation of a cavity between the granulosa cells. This cavity is filled with follicular fluid so that the ovocyte, with its zona pellucida and its own layers of granulosa cells, is nearly surrounded by the cavity. Increased levels of FSH and estrogen are then necessary to produce follicular fluid and to sustain the growth of the follicle (Fig. 3-6). The granulosa cells are encompassed by a basement membrane, outside of which are connective tissue cells organized into two layers: the theca interna and the theca externa (G. *theka,* a box or sheath). **The explanation of how steroid hormones are synthe-**

sized within the follicle has been referred to as the "two-cell theory," since it posits that the cooperation of both the granulosa cells and the theca cells is required to develop the follicle to the point of ovulation. The granulosa cells contain the FSH receptors, while the theca cells contain the LH receptors. **The theca cells produce androgens under the influence of LH. The granulosa cells, under the influence of FSH, convert these androgens into estrogens by the aromatization process.** The antral follicular fluid contains a high concentration of estrogen, which is necessary for the continued growth and development of the follicle. **The follicle selected for ovulation** becomes *the most estrogen-dominant follicle* in the midst of all other follicles, which have much less estrogen. The predominant follicle eventually grows to about 25 mm in diameter. **As the estrogen concentration of the dominant follicle continues to increase, the negative feedback mechanism that it generates tends to suppress the hypothalamic-pituitary FSH secretion, and in so doing deprives the other lesser follicles of their FSH support.** With the loss of this support, there is less estrogen produced in the lesser follicles. They then develop an androgen dominance, which leads to *follicular atresia*. As the midcycle approaches, FSH, in conjunction with the high estrogen environment, stimulates the granulosa cells of the follicle to produce LH receptors in preparation for ovulation and the development of the subsequent corpus luteum.

d) Preovulatory follicle

The preovulatory ovarian follicle produces increasing amounts of estrogens, reaching a peak about 24–36 hours prior to ovulation. LH increases gradually and then at midcycle shows a sudden positive estrogen feedback surge (as the result of the increasing plasma estradiol levels) that reaches a peak about 10–12 hours prior to ovulation (Fig. 3-7). LH induces luteinization in the granulosa cells, which results in the initiation of progesterone production. Due to LH stimulation of the theca tissue of the ovary, there is a 15% increase in the androstenedione values and a 20% increase in the testosterone levels in the peripheral plasma. This androgen release serves to hasten the process of follicular atresia in the lesser follicles and also stimulates the libido of the woman. This increased libido may be important from a teleologic viewpoint, in that it encourages sexual intercourse at a time when pregnancy is most likely to occur.

2) Ovulation

Ovulation occurs about 10–12 hours after the midcycle LH peak, on about day 14 of the menstrual cycle. The increasing progesterone levels, by a negative feedback mechanism, may perhaps assist in terminating the LH surge. The LH surge initiates the luteinization of the granulosa cells, increases the synthesis of prostaglandin, increases histamine release, and increases the local concentration of proteases (which weaken the follicular wall). Within several minutes to an hour, the follicular wall will rupture with the release of the ovum, probably as a result of the proteolytic degeneration of the collagenous connective tissue of the follicular wall. The prostaglandins also increase in the follicular fluid and reach a peak at the time of ovulation. **The presence of prostaglandins appears to be essential for this rupture to occur, and perhaps is also necessary for the extrusion of the ovocyte-cumulus mass.** It has been noted that smooth muscle is present in the ovary.

It must be remembered that at birth the primary ovocyte was arrested in the prophase of the first meiotic division. **At the onset of the LH surge, the ovocyte resumes its reductional division (i.e., meiosis)** with the formation of the first polar body and a secondary ovocyte, which has 23 chromosomes in 2 monads. **Before the male and female pronuclei unite at the point of fertilization, a further division occurs to form one monad with 23 single chromosomes (22 + X) and a second polar body.**

3) Luteal phase

The luteal phase of the menstrual cycle begins with ovulation and ends with the onset of menstruation. It encompasses about 14 days, plus or minus 2 days, and this length of time appears to be much more constant than the length of the follicular phase. Following ovulation, the granulosa cells grow larger, become vacuolated, and begin to accumulate a yellow pigment called *lutein*. The extent of the luteinization is probably dependent upon the number of LH receptors present on the granulosa cells. The capillaries penetrate the layer of granulosa cells to reach the central cavity, where blood may accumulate (hemorrhagic corpus

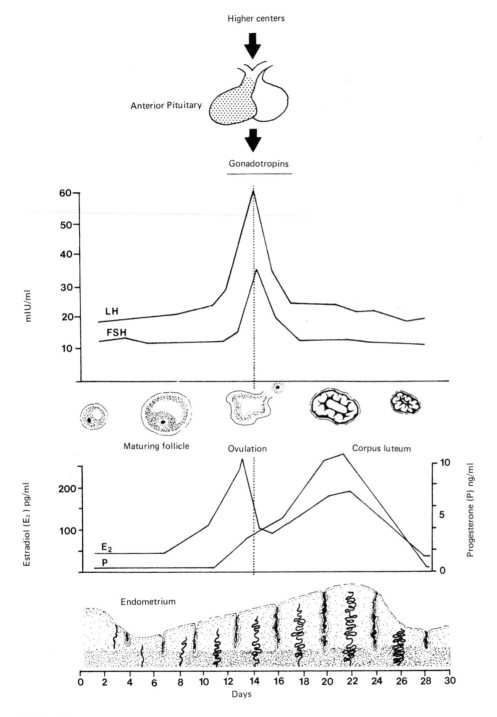

FIGURE 3-7. Diagrammatic representation of the events that occur throughout the menstrual cycle. The estradiol (E_2) level peaks at about day 12, the FSH and LH levels peak at about day 13, and ovulation occurs on day 14.

luteum). *This vascularization is complete by day 22–23.* The life span and the capability of the corpus luteum to produce progesterone is dependent upon the continued support of LH, which begins to decline by about day 23–25 of the menstrual cycle so that menstruation may occur at about day 28, unless the corpus luteum is "rescued" by the developing placenta of a pregnancy.

b. Menstruation

During the menstrual cycle, estrogen stimulates the proliferation of the endometrium. With ovulation and the development of the corpus luteum, progesterone counteracts these effects and allows the endometrium to mature. If pregnancy does not take place, the **withdrawal of the progesterone results in tonic contractions of the spiral arterioles.** This loss of blood flow to the superficial endometrial layers causes shrinkage of the tissues, **ischemia,** and stasis of blood flow. The endometrium then releases **prostaglandins,** which cause contractions of the uterine muscle, which in turn cause disruption of the endometrial arteries, leading to hemorrhage and lysis of the superficial two layers of the endometrium (the spongiosa and compacta) with desquamation and sloughing. This discharge of endometrium and blood constitutes the menstrual flow.

CHAPTER 4

Gynecologic and obstetric history and physical examination

The best Physician is also a Philosopher.
—*Galen (ca. A.D. 131–210)**

1. Taking the medical history

a. Listening

There are certain basic data about the patient's history that you must obtain during your evaluation of her. It has been truly stated that you should **"listen to the patient Doctor, and she will tell you the diagnosis."** Certainly, many of us do not really listen to what people are saying to us. We are either thinking ahead about what we want to say or listening only to refute whatever it is the other person is saying. If you truly devote all of your attention not only to the words but also to the inflections and the overall attitude and composure of the patient (i.e., nonverbal communication), you will receive a number of messages aside from the patient's actual words. A degree of **empathy** develops that allows you to "sense the undercurrents" and the "behind-the-scenes reasons" for the patient's problems. During the interview, you should become very sensitive to the subtle changes in the patient's composure and be aware of her emotional and psychological responses to your questions. An experienced physician can usually develop a fairly accurate

evaluation of the patient's general approach to life and her orientation to her socioeconomic and physical environment within the first five minutes of the interview.

b. Gynecologic history

The traditional obstetric-gynecologic interview includes a complete evaluation of all aspects of the patient's medical and surgical history (Table 4-1). This type of survey should be obtained on a patient at periodic intervals and should be accompanied by a thorough comprehensive physical examination. If you have never seen the patient before, then it is a good idea to perform a *complete history and physical examination* initially and then annually on the patient. If there are significant changes in the patient's health status, these steps may need to be performed more often, depending upon the circumstances. In practice, most patients do not receive a complete examination on each and every office visit. Not only would this procedure be too time consuming for the physician, but it would be of little benefit to the patient. Instead of obtaining such a complete compilation of data, a **brief evaluation** may better serve the patient, especially if it covers the pertinent obstetric-gynecologic data needed by the practicing physician. This abbreviated entry in the medical record is a summary of the basic gynecologic history that you should take from your patients (Table 4-2). Its brevity belies the importance of the information that it contains. This summary lists all of the basic data that you should obtain during your outpatient clinical evaluation and forms the basis for determining your initial diagnosis and plan of treatment. Some of this data may be detailed as follows.

---

*Reprinted with permission from Encyclopaedia Britannica, Inc., *Great Books of the Western World,* vol. 10, "Hippocrates and Galen," Robert Maynard Hutchins, ed. Chicago: William Benton, Publisher, 1952, p. 163.

TABLE 4-1. Obstetric and gynecologic history

  I. Demographic data: age, parity, and race.
 II. Chief complaint: major symptoms.
III. Menstrual history:
   A. Menarche: usual interval, duration, flow, presence of cramps.
   B. Last menstrual period (LMP): date and character of flow.
   C. Previous menstrual period (PMP): date and character of flow.
   D. Intermenstrual bleeding (IMB): date and character of flow.
   E. Postcoital bleeding (PCB): date and character of flow.
   F. Premenstrual symptoms (PMS): type, intensity, duration.
   G. Perimenopausal symptoms: type, intensity, and duration.
   H. Vaginal itching, irritation, discharge.
   I. Hygiene: douching, bowel care, powders.
   J. Birth control method that is practiced: satisfaction, duration.
 IV. Present illness: A narrative account of the patient's problems with a pertinent review-of-systems (ROS).
  V. Obstetric history:
   A. Dates and details of past pregnancies and deliveries.
   B. Weight, sex, and outcome of infants.
   C. Complications, surgical procedures, and abortions.
 VI. Sexual history:
   A. Frequency, satisfaction, orientation, and types of sexual activity.
   B. Frequency of orgasm and female initiation of the sex act.
   C. Dyspareunia or other sexual problems.
   D. The patient's sexual concerns.
VII. Work history:
   A. Place of employment, home, workplace.
   B. Job description, exercise level.
   C. Exposure to industrial or home drugs, abusive habits, chemicals, toxins, radiation, or other hazardous conditions, such as extreme temperatures, loud noises, or infective agents from household pets.
   D. Tolerance of patient to home and work environment.
VIII. Medical history:
   A. A complete review of systems.
 IX. Surgical history:
   A. The surgical procedure, date, doctor, hospital, diagnosis, and complications.
  X. Allergic history: Drugs, pollens, other agents.
 XI. Transfusion history: Number of units, reactions, when administered.
XII. Accident history: when, where, frequency.
XIII. Stress history: on the job, in the home, with relatives.

1) Age

The patient's age is one of the most important pieces of information you will obtain because it will, to some extent, determine the types of illnesses that you should consider in the face of certain complaints. For example, in a *premenarcheal girl,* vaginal bleeding is usually due to a foreign body in the vagina; however, it may also mean that the child has ingested some of her mother's birth control pills. Vaginal bleeding may also be due to ovarian tumors or precocious puberty (see Chapter 3). The *teenage girl* who is not pregnant will almost always have dysfunctional bleeding due to anovulation. Vaginal bleeding in the *woman of reproductive age* should always suggest pregnancy first, with all of its complications, such as a threatened abortion, an ectopic pregnancy, or a hydatidiform mole. Other considerations include endometrial polyps, cervical carcinoma, and leiomyomata. In the *perimenopausal woman,* vaginal bleeding should suggest endometrial

TABLE 4-2. Brief obstetric and gynecologic history (y.o. = years old; G = gravida; P = para; W = white; F = female; 12 × 28 × 5 N = menarche age 12, interval 28 days, duration of flow 5 days, normal flow; LMP = last menstrual period; PMP = previous menstrual period; PCB = postcoital bleeding; IMB = intermenstrual bleeding; BCP = birth control pills; PMS = premenstrual syndrome; No. Douche = number of douches per week)

THE GYNECOLOGIC HISTORY AND PHYSICAL EXAMINATION

This 24 y.o. G_2P_{2-2002} W/F comes in with:

Chief Complaint: Pelvic Pain
                   6 months duration

Present Illness: 12 × 28 × 5 (N) - mild cramps
                   LMP: June 2 (N)   No PCB or IMB   On BCP (Type)   PMS
                   PMP: May 2 (L)   No Vag. Disch. No. Douche

Narrative of Present Illness

Obstetric History
Sexual History
Work History

Physical Examination: Breasts:
                        Abdomen:
                        Pelvis:
                            External Genitalia
                            Vagina
                            Cervix
                            Fundus
                            Adnexa
                            Rectal

Impression: 1) (Differential Diagnoses)
              2)

Disposition: 1) Tests, Consultations, and Procedures
              2) Medications and Dosage
              3) Instructions and Precautions
              4) Return Appointment

              _____
                        Signature/Date

carcinoma, although dysfunctional uterine bleeding is also common in this age group. Bleeding in the *postmenopausal patient* has to be strongly considered to be due to carcinoma of the endometrium, and these patients must be evaluated by a fractional D&C of the uterus.

2) Reproductive history

You also need to know about the woman's reproductive performance, including her gravidity, parity, and previous pregnancy outcomes. A **nulligravida** is a woman who has never been pregnant. A **primigravida** is a woman who is pregnant for the first time, whereas a **multigravida** is one who has previously been pregnant. **Parity** refers to whether an infant has previously been delivered. A **nullipara** is a woman who has never carried a pregnancy beyond 20 weeks' gestation. A **primipara** is one who has delivered one infant, either alive or dead, who weighed greater than 500 grams, or who was beyond 20 weeks' gestation at the time of delivery. A **multipara** is one who has delivered more than one infant. A **grand multipara** is a woman who has given birth to six or more infants of 500 grams or more. **The pregnancy outcome** is usually recorded as the number of full-**T**erm infants, **P**remature infants, **A**bortions (i.e., a fetal weight of less than 500 grams, or a gestational age of less than 20 weeks), and **L**iving infants. *The gravidity and parity with the fetal outcome* may be briefly expressed in a shorthand listing as follows: **G-P-T-P-A-L.** For example, if the woman tells you that she has been pregnant three times, has two living daughters, one of which was premature, and that she had one miscarriage, then you would note that she is a G3P2-1112 on her chart. Some physicians will leave off the parity category and record the notation as G3-1112. Either of these brief notations will provide you with the required information as to the patient's reproductive history in a very small amount of space. Another method of notation indicates the gravidity, the parity, the number of abortions, and the number of ectopic pregnancies (e.g., G3P1A1E1). If the patient is currently pregnant, then the current pregnancy should be included in the above coding systems. Finally, another method records only the parity and is written as para 1112 (full-term, premature, abortions, and living children). During labor, the patient should be referred to as a **parturient,** whereas following delivery, she should be considered a **puerpera** until six weeks postpartum.

3) Menarcheal history

Your patient's menarcheal history is very important. The *age* when menstruation began, the *usual interval* between her periods, and the average *duration* and *amount* of menstrual flow should be recorded. These data establish the woman's menstrual history, against which her current menstrual periods may be compared. You should enter on the woman's chart the onset and character of the **last menstrual period (LMP)** and the **previous menstrual period (PMP)** as a minimum database. In some instances, you may need to inquire about even earlier menstrual periods as well (e.g., P^2MP, P^3MP).

You should always find out whether the patient has experienced any abnormal uterine bleeding. In cases involving **intermenstrual bleeding (IMB),** or **postcoital bleeding (PCB),** the character of the bleeding and its time of onset during the menstrual cycle may be important factors in arriving at a correct diagnosis. For example, spotting just prior to the menstrual period associated with a prolongation of the period may indicate the presence of irregular shedding of the endometrium (i.e., irregular maturation) due to a hormonal imbalance. Spotting on and off during the cycle may indicate the presence of endometrial polyps. Spotting or bleeding after coitus may frequently be due to a cervical erosion or an endocervical polyp.

As you listen to your patient's responses to your questions about her menstrual periods, keep in mind that the normal range of the menstrual interval is 21 to 35 days, with the usual or average interval being about **28 days.** The usual **duration of flow is about 3–5 days,** while the normal range may be between one and nine days. **The amount of flow is usually 25–60 ml of blood loss during each period.** The hemoglobin level will begin to fall if the patient loses 60–80 ml of blood or more per month. The most consistent pathologic cause of menorrhagia is the presence of uterine leiomyomas, and von Willebrand's disease is the most common hereditary disorder that has been associated with menorrhagia. If your patient tells you that she fully soaks more than five pads per day for more than three days during her period, then she can be considered to be a heavy bleeder. The gradual development of anemia, with a hemoglobin level of less than 10 g/dl and a hematocrit of less than 30%, will confirm this finding. The iron loss during menstruation, when averaged over 365 days, is about 0.5 mg per day; however, the actual loss with each period may be of the order of 4–50 mg. **Any variations in the menstrual flow should be compared to the patient's normal range of menstrual values over most of her life, and especially during the previous few months, to determine whether there have been any recent changes.** Keep in mind that the patient's evaluation of blood loss may be highly subjective, and that it may be either greatly understated or grossly exaggerated.

A recent history of abrupt changes in the menstrual flow, however, may be significant.

With this basic information, it becomes possible for you to determine whether the patient has had any heavy or prolonged bleeding, or **hypermenorrhea.** This type of menstrual bleeding may be further classified as being **menorrhagia** (heavy bleeding), **polymenorrhea** (frequent periods), or **metrorrhagia** (bleeding in between periods). **Hypomenorrhea** (scanty periods) has also been classified as **oligomenorrhea** (infrequent periods) or **amenorrhea** (absent periods).

4) Cramps/pelvic pain

You should ask the patient whether she has cramps with her periods, since mild to moderate cramps with the menses are often present in the patient who is ovulating. In teenagers and in women beyond 40 years of age, however, the incidence of ovulation is much less than during the reproductive years. **The patient may provide you with other evidence that she is ovulating by reporting mid-cycle lower abdominal pains (mittelschmerz), which are associated with two or three days of pelvic pressure and an increased amount of clear, mucoid vaginal discharge.** Severe menstrual cramps should alert you to the possibility that the patient may have some other pelvic pathology, such as endometriosis or pelvic inflammatory disease. Many patients may report having experienced severe cramps with periods prior to their first pregnancy, after which the cramps disappeared. This type of cramping is usually due to the presence of a slightly stenotic cervix that was corrected by the cervical dilatation during labor and delivery.

If pelvic pain is a prominent complaint, you should ask your patient to fully describe the pain. The pain may be **constant or intermittent, sharp or dull,** or **diffuse or localized.** You should also ask whether the pain radiates to another part of the body. You should determine whether the pain occurs during or after intercourse **(dyspareunia),** or whether it is associated with her menses **(dysmenorrhea)** (see Chapter 42). Sometimes the pain may be relieved by a change in body position or by a particular medication, but occasionally the pain may be resistant to all treatment. You may obtain a sense of the **severity of the pain** by asking the patient whether it keeps her awake at night. Severe pain will prevent the patient from sleeping, whereas mild to moderate pain may allow the patient to at least doze. You should ask the patient if there are certain specific **precipitating factors that seem to cause the onset of the pain, or whether there may be factors that aggravate the pain once it occurs. Psychological factors and the sociologic environment may play a major role in patients who experience chronic pelvic pain, since the somatization of many social, sexual, and psychological problems may tend to localize pain in the pelvis** (see Chapters 5 and 14).

5) Contraceptive practices

The contraceptive practices of the individual assume a place of considerable importance in the patient evaluation. **Pregnancy is always a consideration in any patient who is of reproductive age.** Furthermore, if oral contraceptives or intrauterine devices are being used, any bleeding problems could be secondary to the use of these agents. Other symptoms, such as weight gain, edema, or cramping, may also be related to certain forms of contraception (see Chapter 45).

6) Vaginitis

In obtaining the baseline historical data on your patient, you should ask about the presence of any vaginal discharge or irritation. First, though, you should make a distinction between **leukorrhea** and **vaginitis.** A **leukorrhea** is a nonirritating, clear, mucoid vaginal discharge that is not abnormal and that often occurs in women who are under stress or who douche repeatedly. **Vaginitis, on the other hand, is usually accompanied by itching, irritation, and a foul-smelling discharge. There are three common organisms that may cause vaginitis: (1) Trichomonas, (2) Candida, and (3) Gardnerella.** There are specific treatments for each of these organisms, and therefore the organism should be positively identified by using a wet saline smear (see Chapter 12).

7) Premenstrual syndrome

You will also want to ask your patient whether she has experienced any symptoms of the **premenstrual syndrome (PMS).** These symptoms generally consist of bloating, nervousness, headache, irritability, and depression, as well as a variety of other symptoms, during the 7–10 days prior to the menstrual period. While almost all women experience some of these symptoms to a mild degree, it is important to determine whether your patient's symptoms are sufficient to warrant therapy (see Chapter 42).

8) Sexual history

You should always take a simple sexual history from your patient. The information that you obtain is frequently important in your overall evaluation of the patient, and at times, such data may constitute the basis for the patient's symptomatology. There may be many stressful problems in your patient's life, some of which might involve the complex sexual relationships between her and her consort. Sexual questions should be asked in a matter-of-fact, routine manner, and the tone used should be indistinguishable from that of questions concerning the cardiac or gastrointestinal systems. **If you act embarrassed or appear to be reticent about discussing sexual matters, the patient will sense this and will not confide in you.** When the patient does confide in you, do not be judgmental, and never register surprise or shock at what the patient tells you, nor at the language she may use to describe her problem. On the other hand, you should not revert to the "language of the streets" in discussing her problem but should gently use more simple scientific terms (with appropriate explanations) to assist her in talking about the problem. Do not belittle her or make her feel as if she is talking about something that is not quite "nice." Be honest with her, and remember that, in general, most types of sexual activity are medically permissible as long as both parties agree to it, and as long as no one individual is being exploited.

It is important also to recognize that your patients will have different sexual life-styles. While teleologically speaking, a heterosexual relationship is essential for the propagation of the species, this fact does not preclude other loving relationships. There is nothing wrong with people "loving one another," although some parts of our society have difficulty with the sexual expression of this "love" (i.e., heterosexuality, bisexuality, homosexuality). Indeed, many homosexuals are very intelligent and talented individuals who are quite mature and gentle people. **Lesbian patients constitute about 4% of the patient population, and they will have a completely different orientation toward sexual matters than heterosexual patients. To fail to recognize that these patients have a right to their own sexual expression is to deny reality.** Whether you approve of such sexual preferences or not as a person has little to do with your function as a physician. It is important, however, for you to be aware of the different approaches to such matters that your patients may have so that you do not alienate them by asking inappropriate questions and thus failing to be sensitive to their needs. **Your job as a physician is not to pass moral judgment on your patient's religion, lifestyle, or sexual preference, but to treat her impartially and fairly, according to accepted medical standards.**

Simple questions will usually elicit some aspects of the sexual history and open the door for the patient to discuss her sexual life with you if she so desires. **Your questions may include: "Do you have a current sexual partner?" "How often do you have sex?" "How often do you have a climax?" "Do you have any problems in your sex life?"** One or more of these questions may reveal the patient's sexual preference. Once you have an indication of whether the patient is heterosexual, bisexual, or homosexual, then you may want to explore these sexual approaches in a little more depth if there seem to be any problems involved or if the patient has questions or concerns.

Bisexual and homosexual patients may have questions concerning some of the venereal diseases, especially AIDS, and their risks in contracting such diseases. If these individuals keep their sexual contacts down to a very few trusted individuals, or preferably to only one carefully chosen individual, then the risk of contracting a sexually transmitted disease is minimal. Since venereal diseases are infections, individuals who have had many sexual contacts with other people (who in turn are also having many contacts with other people) are at the highest risk.

Keep in mind that bisexual and homosexual couples have difficulty in solving the same sexual and nonsexual problems that heterosexual couples have trouble with (see Chapter 17).

9) Work history

The high-technology world that we live in exposes us all to an increasing variety of hazardous chemicals, toxins, and irradiation in our homes and in the workplace. **Questions about your patient's work envi-**

ronment, as well as her home situation, may provide valuable information about her well-being and her possible exposure to hazardous agents. It is important to have some knowledge of the different types of industry in your community and the possible hazardous conditions that may be present in the workplace. For example, if your patient works in a battery factory, this should alert you to the possibility that she may develop lead poisoning.

Pregnant patients often request a leave of absence from their jobs during pregnancy because of work problems or problems with the pregnancy. It is your responsibility to investigate the type of job that your patient performs and understand the hazards she might be exposed to in her place of work. The patient can tell you just what her job entails and can often name the types of chemicals or other hazardous substances that she may be exposed to in her job. If she is unable to do so, however, the industrial health nurse at the workplace, or an occupational physician in the factory, can often supply you with information as to the risks of the different work situations in a particular industry (see Chapters 23 and 28). Regional Occupational Safety and Health Agency (OSHA) consultants may also be helpful. Do not allow the employer, the insurance company, or the patient to deter you from making medically sound recommendations.

10) Presenting complaint

Finally, you will need to explore the reasons for your patient's visit. You should ask for specific information about her complaint in order to define the problem and provide a set of working diagnoses. Do not be dismayed if you cannot give the patient a specific diagnosis on her first visit. In many instances, it will require several visits before the diagnosis may become evident. The hardest words that a young physician may utter are **"I don't know."** If you are honest with the patient, however, and tell her that you will make every effort to find out what the problem is, almost all patients will have respect for you and your honesty and will stay with you until the diagnosis is clarified. Whatever you do, be certain that you do not jump to a **premature conclusion** and tell the patient a diagnosis that is not based on the facts. When the true diagnosis is later revealed, it is difficult to explain to the patient how you could have been so wrong in your initial assessment. Similarly, you should never imply that the patient's problem "is

all in her head" (i.e., a psychological problem). If you do, you will incur the patient's undying enmity and she will probably never return to you for medical care. Patients who do have psychological problems as a cause of medical difficulties should be taught how to handle the stress in their lives. It may take a number of visits before the patient may accept such an evaluation; however, if the baseline laboratory data are negative and no pathology can be found to explain her symptoms, then the patient may be more amenable to this approach. She should be made aware of the fact that she herself can affect her health in a positive manner and that the maladaptation syndrome is common to all people in one form or another (see Chapter 5).

c. Obstetric history

In addition to the gynecologic history, you should collect information about your patient's obstetric experiences, with an emphasis on the present pregnancy, if one exists. If the patient herself does not suspect that she is pregnant, you may be alerted to this possibility by her reports of amenorrhea or irregular bleeding. This suspicion may lead to the identification of such common symptoms of pregnancy as undue fatigue, nausea and vomiting, breast swelling and tenderness, and an increased frequency of urination. If the patient presents with a history of irregular bleeding instead of the classic amenorrhea of pregnancy, then you should consider other diagnostic possibilities, such as an ectopic pregnancy, a threatened or inevitable abortion, a molar pregnancy, a ruptured corpus luteum cyst, or dysfunctional uterine bleeding.

You should follow up on all other positive historical findings with an in-depth analysis of the symptoms using the traditional review-of-systems (ROS) approach.

2. Hospital progress notes

In the management of both obstetric and gynecologic patients in the hospital, the initial history and physical examination is followed by writing the daily progress notes. These may be organized in a problem-oriented manner by using the SOAP format, in which the patient data is recorded daily as follows: (1) the **S**ubjective patient complaints, (2) the **O**bjective physician findings, (3) the **A**ssessment of both the subjective and objective data, and (4) your **P**lan of management for the patient. Outpatient records, however, do not lend themselves to this type of format, and the abbreviated gynecologic history, as outlined above, provides a much more thorough evaluation of the patient on each office visit and allows the physician to rapidly identify almost all of the common gynecologic problems that may occur. The use of a continuing "problem list" is also often useful in the management of the outpatient.

3. Gynecologic examination

a. Initial examination

Historically, the introduction of the pelvic examination was not without its problems. The patient's modesty was considered to be of prime importance. The pelvic examination in the early nineteenth century was performed under sheets or under the patient's skirts and precluded the actual visual examination of the genitalia. **James Young Simpson** was perhaps the first physician to stress the importance of the bimanual examination in 1850. **Charles D. Meigs,** a Philadelphia physician who had previously spoken out against the concept of puerperal sepsis and anesthesia, also opposed the vaginal speculum as an instrument of indecency. In 1850, **James P. White** of Buffalo, New York, was chastised for performing a delivery in the presence of students. The profession considered a physician to be incompetent if he could not conduct labor by touch alone. As time progressed, the lax attitude that had allowed the physician to examine an unclothed prostitute finally prevailed to include the lady of good breeding.

After taking a complete medical history and a general as well as a specific complaint-oriented review of systems (ROS), you will have identified certain areas on which you will want to focus attention in the physical examination in order to explain the patient's symptomatology. Always keep in mind, however, that some other pathology may be present that has not yet produced sufficient symptoms to alarm the patient. Thus, it becomes essential that you do not gloss over any aspect of the examination in your pursuit of the obvious pathology. Both gynecologic and obstetric patients should receive **a complete and thorough initial physical examination.** The primary areas of emphasis, however, do differ somewhat for the two types of patients. In the obstetric patient, you should be interested in those areas of the examination that pertain to the successful outcome of a pregnancy, whereas in the gynecologic patient, you should pay more attention to any complaints the patient may have.

b. Follow-up examinations

After completing the initial physical examination, most physicians tend to believe that the data will almost never change over a short period of time. As a consequence, the subsequent medical treatment may be based entirely upon this *one examination,* with no further attempt being made to reconfirm the physical findings as the treatment regimen proceeds. Not infrequently, what you may find on an examination on one day may change or completely disappear on subsequent examinations a day or two later. It is a good rule to repeat the general physical or pelvic examination every few days while the patient is under treatment, or on each and every outpatient visit. Often, in the hospital, the patient's course of therapy may not progress as well as you might like. In such cases, it has been well stated that *"when all else fails, go back and examine the patient."* Not infrequently, you may find some new pathology that may completely change the diagnosis and the course of therapy.

c. Adolescent examination

The examination of the adolescent is rather special, and it may be quite difficult to perform unless you take the necessary time to educate the teenager as to how it is to be accomplished and why it is being done. The preparation of the adolescent begins during the initial interview. The patient should be aware of the fact that *she* is your patient and that what she tells you will not be divulged to her parents without her permission, except in an emergency life-threatening situation or if surgery is indicated. This *assurance of privacy* is essential if you expect the teenager to reveal to you any intimate facts about her life.

Prior to performing the physical examination, it is important that you carefully explain what you are going to do and why each part of the examination is important. Keeping up a constant "patter" of explanations as you progress through the examination will serve as a distracter while at the same time it will reassure the girl about what you are doing. It is not advisable to go into any great scientific detail in these explanations, and in fact, the use of technical terms may actually "turn off" the patient from what you are saying and defeat the purpose of the explanation. A brief explanation in a quiet, professional tone of voice is often sufficient to allay the patient's fears. Your constant coaching, reassurance, and explanatory comments will keep the patient's mind off what you are doing, and will not allow time for her to formulate her fears and concerns. Before she knows it, the examination will be over, and she will then realize that it wasn't as bad as she had expected. How you conduct this first examination will set the stage for the girl's subsequent pelvic examinations in the future, and *a gentle, caring physician who takes the additional few minutes to teach the adolescent patient how to relax so that her first pelvic examination is not uncomfortable will be remembered fondly by the patient for the rest of her life.*

d. Physical examination

The routine annual cancer-screening examinations should consist of the following (as a minimum): (1) the breasts, (2) the abdomen, (3) the pelvis, and (4) a Papanicolaou smear.

1) Breast examination

The inspection and palpation of the breasts are the mainstays of the breast examination. With the patient assuming various positions, you should inspect the breasts for dimpling, skin retraction, abnormal contour or depressions, or any deviation of the nipples from their normal position (Fig. 4-1). The **first position** consists of having the patient sit quietly with her arms at her sides. Usually one breast (often the left one) is larger than the other. The nipples will normally show a slightly outward deviation bilaterally. In the **second position,** you should have the patient raise her arms high over her head while the same inspection is carried out. The **third position** involves having the patient place her hands on her hips and stretching her elbows backwards so as to tighten the muscles across the chest. In the **fourth position** the patient stretches her arms out in front of her and leans forward so that the breasts may be inspected in the dependent position. The **fifth position** consists of having the patient lie supine on the examining table while you examine

the breast in a systematic fashion. **The breast should be palpated in each of the four quadrants, and then beneath the nipple, using the "flats of the fingers."** Any significant lumps will become apparent in most instances. The patient then returns to her resting upright position and *the axillae are thoroughly palpated for lymph nodes.* In addition, the *supraclavicular* areas should be thoroughly palpated to detect the presence of any enlarged lymph nodes. An attempt should be made to express secretion from each nipple, and if any is obtained, a *cytologic smear* should be performed. The patient should be instructed as to these basic positions and should be taught how to examine her own breasts in front of a mirror and while lying supine in bed. This breast self-examination should be carried out by the patient in the first half of the menstrual cycle each month (see Chapter 16).

Transillumination, thermography, and mammography have all been utilized in the diagnosis of breast masses. Cystic masses may be needled and the liquid contents sent for cytologic diagnosis (see Chapter 16).

2) Abdominal examination

You should examine the abdomen of the patient in the supine position. It should first be observed for the presence of any scars or other surface landmarks and for its general configuration. This observation should be followed by the palpation and percussion of the underlying organs, such as the liver, the kidneys, and the spleen. You should determine the presence of bowel sounds and their character, the presence of tenderness or rebound, and the presence of any abdominal masses. **Any masses noted should be described in terms of their shape and consistency, their location and mobility, and their size in centimeters. You should ask your patient to point to any area of pain with specifically one finger.** This procedure will often localize the primary area of concern much more precisely than if you assume that the pain is generalized. The area where the pain is located should be palpated only after all of the other areas have been examined, so as to avoid any unnecessary voluntary guarding. The palpation of the inguinal area for a hernia with the patient in a standing position and after a Valsalva's maneuver or a cough should also be carried out. You should also seek the presence of costovertebral angle (CVA) tenderness over the kidneys bilaterally.

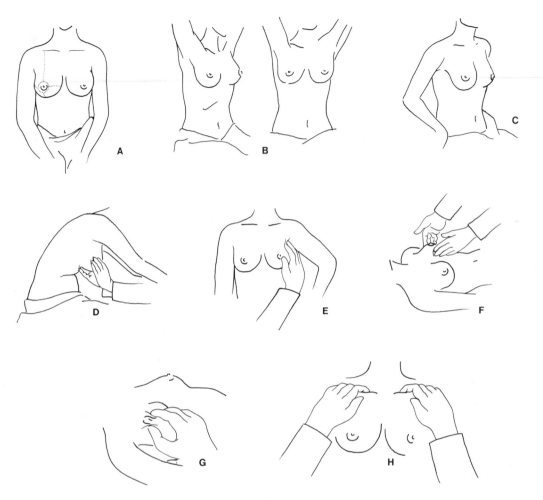

FIGURE 4-1. Breast examination. (A) First position with the patient sitting quietly with her arms to her side. (B) Second position with the patient's arms raised high as the physician carries out the inspection. (C) Third position with the patient stretching her elbows backward and tightening the muscles of her chest. (D) Fourth position with the patient leaning forward. (E) With the physician palpating each axilla. (F) Fifth position with the patient lying supine as the breast is palpated in a systematic fashion. (G) An attempt should be made to express any material from the nipple. (H) Palpation of the lymph nodes in the supraclavicular areas of the neck.

3) Pelvic examination

You should carry out the pelvic examination in a systematic manner in order to avoid missing important information. The patient should be instructed to empty her bladder prior to the examination. She then should be placed in a comfortable lithotomy position on the examination table with her legs in the stirrups and her buttocks slightly overhanging the end of the

table. *She should be instructed to remain relaxed and to keep her legs widely separated in order to facilitate the examination.*

You, as the examiner, should take a seat on a stool placed between the patient's legs, and a light should be positioned so as to obtain maximal illumination of the perineum. *It is reassuring to the patient when you inform her as to what you wish to do during the examination, before actually doing it.* The palpation of the inguinal lymph nodes, as the first skin contact, will tend to "break the ice" and allow the patient to relax for the remainder of the examination.

a) External genitalia

You should thoroughly inspect the external genitalia for lesions, masses, inflammation, or other pathology (see Chapter 11). The labia should be palpated for cysts or lumps, and the clitoris should be inspected for size (normal size is about 2.0 by 0.5 cm). The labial folds should then be spread widely and the urethral and vaginal orifices inspected. The placement of a finger beneath the urethra along the anterior vaginal wall will sometimes identify the presence of a urethral diverticulum or express any material that might be present in the Skene's glands. The palpation of the vaginal introitus at the five and seven o'clock positions with the thumb and forefinger will detect the presence of a Bartholin's duct cyst. The fourchette and the perineal body should be inspected for old obstetric scars or for a loss of tissue due to poor healing. In a virgin, the presence of a tight hymenal ring instead of carunculae myrtiformes may preclude a vaginal examination; however, much can be learned from a bimanual rectal examination.

b) Vaginal examination

You should place two fingers in the parous vagina and exert pressure posteriorly to visualize the lower vaginal canal. The patient should then be instructed to bear down, in order to detect any relaxation of the vaginal walls. If the anterior vaginal wall balloons downward, then a **cystocele** (or a cystourethrocele) is present. In the presence of a **rectocele,** the posterior vaginal wall will balloon downward toward the introitus on a Valsalva's maneuver. If the uterine cervix descends to the level of the introitus, then a **first-degree uterine prolapse** is present. A descent of the uterus through the introitus is indicative of a **second-degree prolapse.** When the entire uterus prolapses out of the vagina, then a **third-degree prolapse** is present. When a posterior vaginal ballooning mass appears to originate high in the vagina between the uterosacral ligaments, then an **enterocele** is present. Any or all of the above conditions have been termed **pelvic relaxation.** Such relaxation is indicative of lacerations or destruction of the endopelvic fascial support of the pelvic structures. This loss of pelvic support may distort the relationships between

the bladder and the urethra, which may result in a loss of urine when coughing or straining. Such a condition has been termed **stress incontinence** (see Chapter 12).

A clean, warm speculum should be placed in the introitus after spreading the labia with the fingers of one hand in order to avoid pinching or dragging the labia into the introitus when the speculum is inserted. The speculum is directed somewhat posteriorly until it is fully inserted, at which time it is gently opened and brought back to the horizontal position as the cervix comes into view. The presence of an ectropion, erosion, or other lesions of the cervix, or lesions of the vaginal walls (fornices) surrounding the cervix, should be noted (see Chapter 13). *Do not use lubricant jelly on the speculum, as it will interfere with the reading of a Papanicolaou smear.* Water can be used if a lubricant is necessary. A Papanicolaou smear of the vaginal, cervical, and endocervical areas, obtained by using a wooden spatula or a cotton-tipped swab, is then smeared on a microscopic slide and immediately placed in a 95% alcohol-ether solution before it can dry out.

If the woman has had no previous pregnancies, the external cervical os will usually be small and round. In a parous woman, the os will usually be gaping with stellate scarring that was secondary to the birth trauma. During the slow removal of the speculum, the vaginal mucosa from the cervix to the introitus should be inspected for the presence of any lesions. The presence of **rugae** (mucosal folds) is indicative of a good estrogen effect, as is the thickness of the vaginal mucosa. **In a postmenopausal woman who is not on estrogens, the mucosa will be thin, atrophic, and without rugae.** If the patient has complained of vaginal irritation or discharge, a cotton-tipped swab of the secretions should be obtained and placed on one slide with a drop of saline (i.e., a wet smear), and on a second slide with a drop of a 10% solution of potassium hydroxide (i.e., KOH smear) for later examination under a microscope for vaginal pathogens (e.g., Trichomonas, Candida, Gardnerella). If gonorrhea is suspected, a Gram-stained smear and a culture using Thayer-Martin agar can be obtained. If Chlamydia trachomatis is suspected, a special culture media or enzyme testing may be used (see Chapter 12).

c) Bimanual examination

The bimanual examination consists of using both of your hands, with one inside the vagina or rectum and

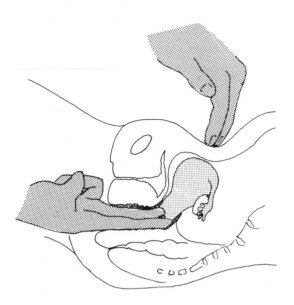

FIGURE 4-2. Bimanual palpation of the uterus by ballottement technique.

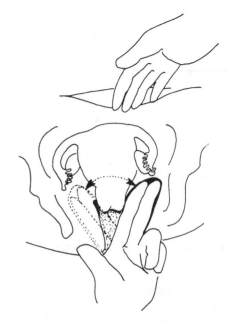

FIGURE 4-3. Bimanual palpation of the adnexa by ballottement technique.

the other on the abdominal wall, to palpate the pelvic and abdominal structures. It is very important for the patient to completely relax during this procedure, since voluntary guarding of the abdominal musculature will effectively prevent an evaluation of the pelvic organs. The use of force to overcome the patient's guarding will only cause pain for the patient and will not produce any worthwhile information. You should place two fingers in the vagina, one on each side of the cervix initially, and then on further examination the fingers should be placed in each adnexa. By **gentle ballottement** of the pelvic structures with the hand on the abdominal wall, their location can be easily determined (Fig. 4-2). The fingers positioned in the vagina provide orientation for where the pelvic organs are located in relation to the cervix and uterine body, while the ballottement defines their size and position without undue pain to the patient (Fig. 4-3). **Any pelvic mass that is detected in the bimanual examination should be defined as to its position, mobility, consistency, and size in centimeters** (Fig. 4-4). *The position of the uterus should be noted as anteflexed, retroflexed, anteverted, or retroverted, along with its size and consistency* (Fig. 4-5). The uterus is shaped like a slightly rounded pear, and in pregnancy its superior-inferior diameter in centimeters roughly corresponds to the number of

weeks of gestation; in later pregnancy, from 16 to 34 weeks, the fundal measurement is equivalent to the weeks of gestation. Therefore, the superior-inferior dimension of a uterus during the 12th week of gestation will measure about 12 cm (Fig. 4-6).

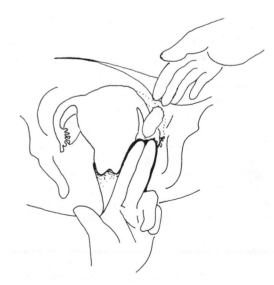

FIGURE 4-4. Bimanual palpation of the ovary by ballottement technique.

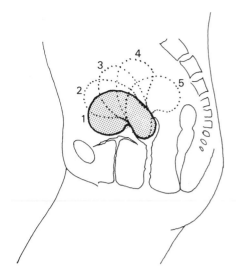

FIGURE 4-5. Positions of the uterus. The sequence of positions that are shown are (from front to back): (1) anteflexion, (2) anteversion, the normal position, (3) mid-position, (4) retroversion, and (5) retroflexion. If both the cervix and the uterine body have moved backward toward the sacrum with a retroversion, then the term "retrocession" is used. In such cases, the uterine body may line up with the vaginal canal and function as a piston whenever there is an increase in the intra-abdominal pressure. This condition may cause a prolapse of the uterus, if the uterine supports are weak.

The adnexal structures should also be carefully evaluated. **The ovaries should not be palpable in the premenarcheal girl or in the postmenopausal woman; if the ovary can be palpated in such patients, it should be considered abnormal and should be investigated. The normal ovary may measure as large as 5.0 by 3.0 by 1.5 cm in size.** It is essential to properly describe the ovarian size in centimeters in order to determine whether you have detected a true ovarian enlargement (see Chapter 15).

It is very important to perform a **rectal examination** on every patient. Not only will this examination allow you to detect rectal pathology, but it will also allow you to obtain a much better bimanual pelvic examination. In many cases, palpating the posterior portion of the uterus and determining the relationships of the adnexal structures to the posterior cul-de-sac may be very valuable in detecting pelvic disease.

4. Obstetric examination

You should not only assess the general physical condition of your patient but also her capability to carry a pregnancy safely to a successful conclusion. The anticipation of potential problems and the prevention of them should be satisfying to you as a professional and should assure that your patient will have a safe delivery of a quality infant. The main areas of concern in the obstetric physical examination are the abdominal and pelvic findings.

a. Abdominal findings

1) Fundal measurement

In performing your abdominal examination, you should specifically evaluate the uterus and its contents. The height of the fundus in centimeters is measured from the top of the fundus to the top of the symphysis pubis. This measurement should be made in a straight line rather than over the bulge of the uterine fundus (Fig. 4-7). The measurement in centimeters should equal the number of weeks of gestation from about 16 to 34 weeks, after which the measurements and the weeks of gestation will no longer correspond. Thus, the fundus during the 26th week of gestation should have a measurement of 26 cm.

2) Leopold's maneuvers

The classic Leopold's maneuvers should be carried out during each office visit in the third trimester to determine the lie of the fetus (Fig. 4-8, Fig. 4-9, Fig. 4-10, Fig. 4-11). With a little practice, you will be able to identify the fetal lie easily. Such information is quite valuable during the course of labor. You should be able to define the fetal poles (i.e., the head and buttocks) and the position of the fetal back and small parts. If the fetal back is closer to the umbilicus than are the small parts, then the fetal back is anterior. If the small parts are closer to the umbilicus than is the back, then the fetal back is down, or posterior (Fig. 4-12). Determining the exact position of the fetus is frequently helpful in assessing labor problems. The **fetal presentation** refers to the part of the fetus that overlies the pelvic inlet (cephalic or breech). The **fetal lie** refers to the relationship of the fetal long axis to the long axis of the mother (longitudinal, oblique, or transverse). The **fetal position** re-

Text continues on p. 62

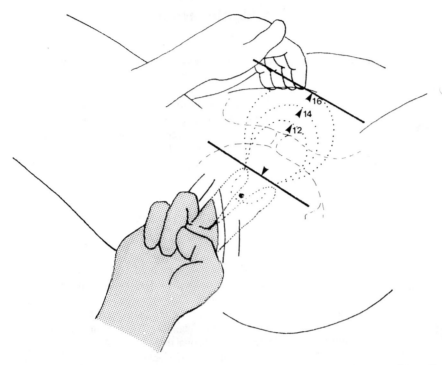

FIGURE 4-6. Measurement of a 12-, 14-, or 16-week gestation uterine superior-inferior diameter on bimanual pelvic examination. Beyond 8 weeks, the superior-inferior measurement in centimeters should equal the number of weeks of gestation.

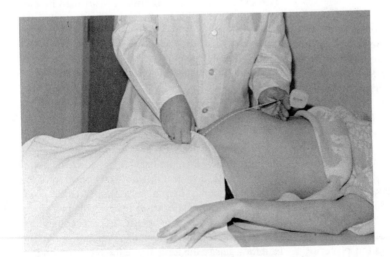

FIGURE 4-7. The proper way to measure the fundal height. The measurement should be taken from the top of the syphysis pubis in a straight line to the top of the fundus, rather than "over-the-hump" of the fundus.

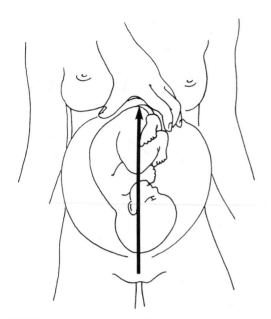

FIGURE 4-8. The first Leopold's maneuver to locate the fetal part in the fundus of the uterus.

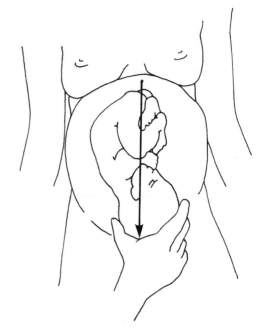

FIGURE 4-10. The third Leopold's maneuver to locate which pole of the fetus is presenting in the inlet.

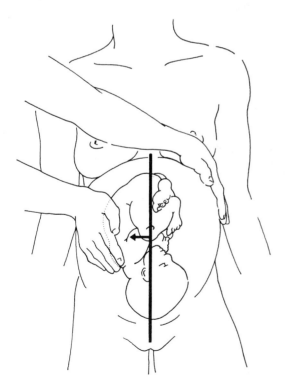

FIGURE 4-9. The second Leopold's maneuver to locate the fetal back.

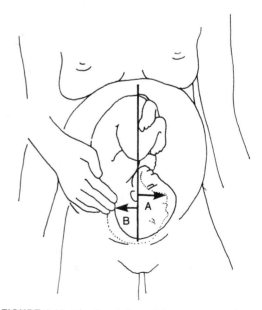

FIGURE 4-11. The fourth Leopold's maneuver to locate the side of the cephalic prominence. (A) If the head is flexed, the prominence will be on the side of the fetal small parts. (B) If the fetal head is extended, the prominence will be on the side of the back.

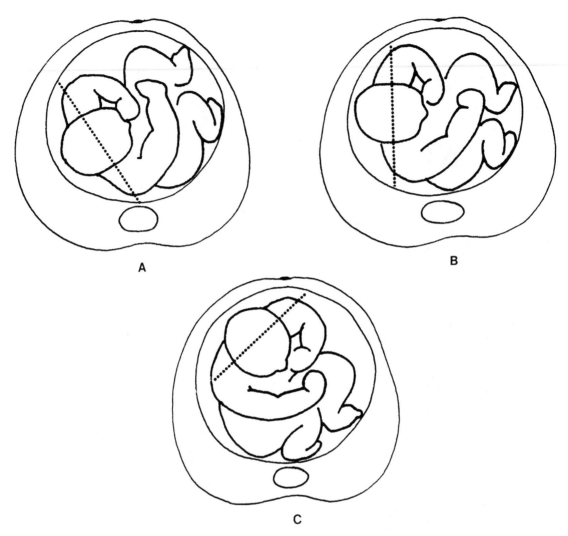

FIGURE 4-12. Cross section view of the fetus in relation to the umbilicus. (A) Posterior position. (B) Transverse position. (C) Anterior position.

fers to the relation of the presenting part to the maternal pelvis, either left or right (left occiput anterior, right occiput posterior, left sacrum posterior, etc.). The **fetal attitude** is the position of the fetal parts to one another, such as the head in relation to the shoulders (i.e., flexion, extension).

3) Fetal movements

Usually, the fetal movements (i.e., **quickening**) will be detected by the "aware" patient by 17–19 weeks of gestation. You should instruct the patient to watch for this finding to make it more accurate. The fetal heart tones can be detected very early in pregnancy with a Doppler ultrasound (i.e., at about 12 weeks' gestation); however, with the use of the **DeLee-Hillis stethoscope,** the fetal heart tones may not be heard until about 18–20 weeks' gestation. Retrospectively, if the fetal heart tones (by the DeLee-Hillis stethoscope) and the quickening have been present for at least 21–22 weeks, then the patient will quite likely be at term.

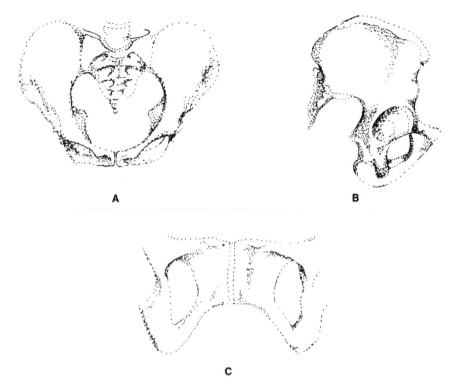

A

B

C

FIGURE 4-13. Gynecoid pelvis. (A) Inlet view. This view shows that the inlet is nearly round. (B) Lateral view. On the this view it is noted that the sacrosciatic notch is average and the sacrum has a normal inclination. (C) Subpubic arch view. In this view the arch has an angle greater than 90 degrees, and the side walls are straight.

4) Estimated date of confinement

In order to arrive at the **estimated date of confinement (EDC),** it is necessary to subtract three months and add seven days to the first day of the last menstrual period **(Nägele's rule).** Since this method is often inaccurate, with an error rate of ($\pm$) three weeks, in determining the estimated date of confinement, the fetal heart tones and quickening observations become more helpful in the final assessment of the gestational age of the pregnancy.

b. Pelvic findings

1) Observation of the patient

The pelvic examination of the pregnant patient is carried out in the same manner as for the gynecologic patient, except that the obstetric bimanual examina-

tion includes the basic pelvic measuration. **Prior to the bimanual examination, it is important to observe the patient in an upright anteroposterior view and in a lateral view. Furthermore, it is essential to observe the patient as she walks in order to detect the presence of a limp or a gait abnormality that might indicate a pelvic girdle problem.** If you keep in mind the classic features of **the Caldwell-Moloy pelvic classifications (i.e., gynecoid, anthropoid, platypelloid, and android types of pelves),** it will be quite easy for you to tentatively identify the basic pelvic type from these observations. The woman who has the usual feminine curves to her hips and buttocks will almost always have a *gynecoid pelvis* (Fig. 4-13). If she has broad hips from the anteroposterior view but has a narrow silhouette with flattened buttocks from the lateral view, then you should suspect a *platypelloid pelvis*

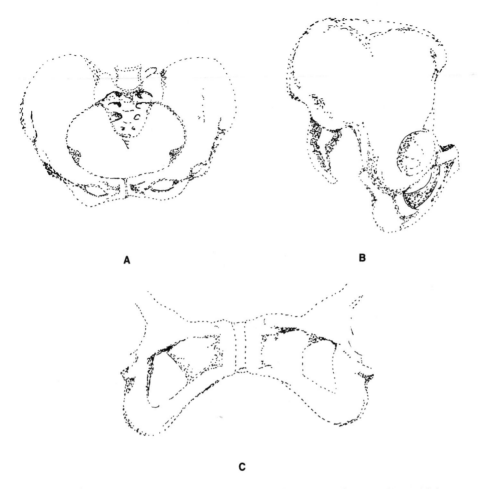

A

B

C

FIGURE 4-14. Platypelloid pelvis. (A) Inlet view. The inlet is wider than it is deep, and the forepelvis is fattened. (B) Sacrosciatic notch appears narrow, but due to the flattening of the pelvis it is actually wide. (C) Subpubic arch view. The arch is wider and may be 100 degrees or more.

(Fig. 4-14). The woman who has a "box-like" pelvis, which is both deep and wide, has an *anthropoid pelvis* (Fig. 4-15). Finally, the woman who has no feminine curves at all but has a hip structure like that of a boy is said to have an *android pelvis* (Fig. 4-16).

2) Clinical pelvimetry

Once you have tentatively identified the type of pelvis that the patient has by observing her in the walking and standing positions, you should perform the pelvic examination to confirm your impression. Some sim-

ple practical pelvic measurements that may be of assistance in this regard are: (1) the biischial diameter (8.5–10 cm), (2) the angle of the subpubic arch (greater than 90–100 degrees), (3) the curvature of the forepelvis, (4) the diagonal conjugate (more than 11.5 cm), (5) the placement and shape of the sacrum and coccyx, and (6) the ischial spines (Table 4-3).

a) Pelvic measurements

1. The biischial diameter. This diameter measures the distance between the ischial tuberosities and

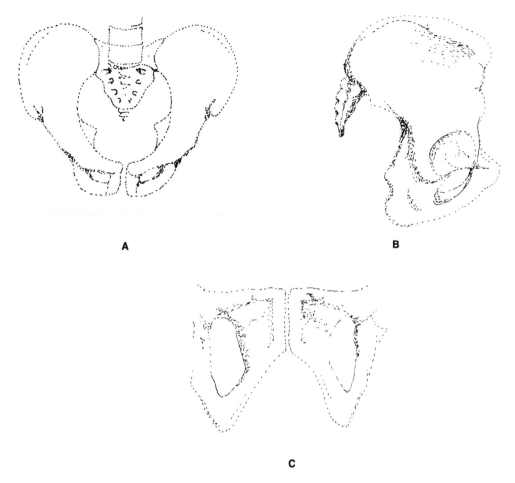

A

B

C

FIGURE 4-15. Anthropoid pelvis. (A) Inlet view. The inlet is deeper than it is wide. The forepelvis is narrowed, but not as much as in the android pelvis. (B) Lateral view. The sacrosciatic notch is wide with a normal inclination of the sacrum. (C) Subpubic arch view. The arch may be slightly narrowed, but it is still within the normal range of 90 to 100 degrees.

is easily determined by measuring the distance with your closed fist. You should know the width in centimeters of your fist, which is placed between the ischial tuberosities to obtain a rough measurement. Any value of more than 8.5 cm indicates that the outlet is normal and that an android pelvis is not present (Fig. 4-17). The value of the biischial diameter plus the posterior sagittal measurement (7.5 cm) should exceed 15 cm in an adequate outlet. The **posterior sagittal diameter** measures from a line between the ischial tuberosities (i.e., at the fourchette of the vagina) to the tip of the coccyx.

2. The angle of the pubic arch. This angle is easily observed by placing your thumbs on each tuberosity and then aligning your first fingers with the pubic rami. The angle thus formed should be *at least 90 to 100 degrees*. If the angle is less than 90 degrees, then an android pelvis is present (Fig. 4-18).

3. The curvature of the forepelvis. This curvature may be assessed by placing two fingers in the vagina up behind the symphysis pubis and sweeping them back and forth to determine the shape of the forepelvis. In the gynecoid pelvis, this is a nice smooth curve. In the platypelloid pelvis, there is almost no

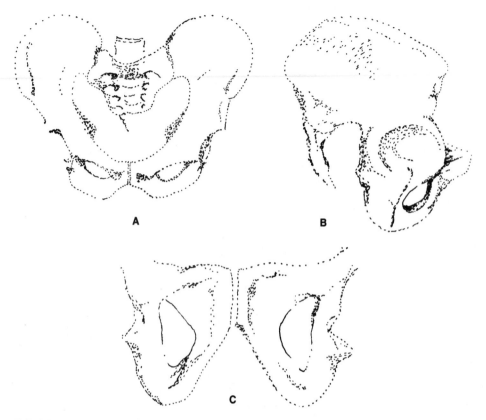

FIGURE 4-16. Android pelvis. (A) Inlet view. The inlet is more triangular than round with a more acute angle to the forepelvis. (B) Lateral view. The sacrosciatic arch is narrowed with the sacrum inclined anteriorly. (C) Subpubic arch view. The arch is narrowed to 90 degrees or less and the side walls converge. The pelvis tends to funnel from the inlet to the outlet.

TABLE 4-3. Characteristics of four basic types of pelves of average size

	Type of pelvis			
Characteristic	Gynecoid	Android	Anthropoid	Platypelloid
Anteroposterior diameter of inlet	11 cm	11 cm	12+ cm	10 cm
Widest transverse diameter of inlet	12 cm	12 cm	<12 cm	12 cm
Forepelvis	Wide	Narrow	Narrow	Wide
Sidewalls	Straight	Convergent	Divergent	Straight
Ischial spines	Not prominent	Prominent	Not prominent	Not prominent
Sacrosciatic notch	Medium	Narrow	Wide	Narrow
Inclination of sacrum	Medium	Forward (lower third)	Backward	Forward
Subpubic arch	Wide	Narrow	Medium	Wide
Transverse diameter of outlet	10 cm	<10 cm	10 cm	10 cm
Bone structure	Medium	Heavy	Medium	Medium

Source: Reprinted with permission from D. N. Danforth and J. R. Scott, eds., *Obstetrics and Gynecology,* 5th ed. Philadelphia: J. B. Lippincott Company, 1986, p. 634.

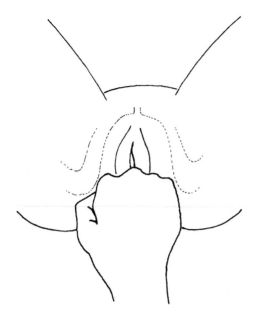

FIGURE 4-17. Estimation of the biischial diameter.

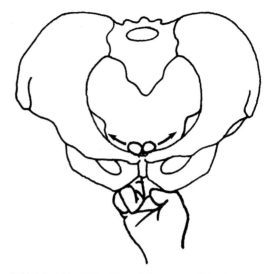

FIGURE 4-19. Estimation of the curve of the fore-pelvis.

curve at all, since it is flattened out. In the android pelvis, the curve is almost acute and is easily recognized in relation to the other measurements. In the anthropoid pelvis, the curve is similar to that of the android pelvis but is wider (Fig. 4-19).

4. The diagonal conjugate. This diagonal measures the depth of the pelvis from the inferior border of the symphysis pubis to the top of the sacral promontory. This value is normally of the order of *12.5 cm or more.* Each examiner should measure his or her own reach by measuring the distance from the base of the thumb to the tip of the second finger (Fig. 4-20); the result should then be recorded as 12.5 cm (or whatever your measurement is) "R" (reached), or "NR" (not reached). Usually, only the platypelloid and the android pelves will have a reduced diagonal conjugate measurement. To approximate the actual measurement between the pubis and the sacral prom-

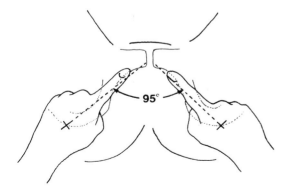

FIGURE 4-18. Estimation of the angle of the pubic arch.

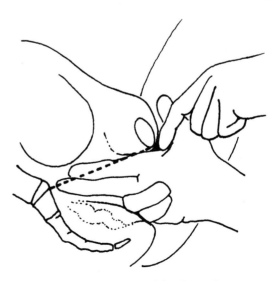

FIGURE 4-20. Measurement of the diagonal conjugate.

ontory, you should subtract 1.5–2.0 cm from the diagonal conjugate, which is called the *obstetric conjugate.*

5. The sidewalls of the pelvis. These are usually straight in the gynecoid and platypelloid pelves and are slightly divergent in the anthropoid pelvis. The android pelvis is conspicuous by its converging sidewalls, which give it a "funneling" effect from the pelvic inlet to the pelvic outlet.

6. The shape of the sacrum and the coccyx. These shapes should be ascertained by palpation. The sacrum may be directed anteriorly or posteriorly, and it may be flattened or curved. In a platypelloid pelvis, a flattened and anteriorly directed sacrum may encroach significantly into the mid-pelvis. The coccyx may also be directed anteriorly or posteriorly, and may be fixed or mobile. If it is hooked anteriorly and is immobile, you may have to fracture it during labor in order to deliver the infant.

7. The ischial spines. The ischial spines represent the mid-pelvis (or the zero station, when the leading edge of the fetal head is at this level), and the distance between them is not clinically measurable. In the android pelvis, the spines are blunt and thick and encroach into the mid-pelvic space. The sacrosciatic notch flares to each side above the ischial spines, and it is narrowed only in the android pelvis. The sacrospinous ligament forms the lower border of the notch and extends from the ischial spine to the lateral margins of the sacrum. It is usually 2.5 cm in length in the normal gynecoid pelvis.

b) The significance of the pelvic findings

Having taken these measurements of the pelvis, what then can be said as to their value in the management of the patient? The finding of a gynecoid pelvis is reassuring, in that it indicates that the size of the patient's pelvis should be adequate for delivery, unless she has: (1) a fetal malpresentation or (2) a large baby or (3) she is less than 5 feet tall. In any of these instances, the pelvis may prove to be inadequate. The common practice of assuming that because a woman has delivered a previous infant of a certain weight proves that she has an adequate pelvis for another baby of that size is incorrect, since even a malpositioned baby of a lesser size may not deliver easily or at all (see Chapter 38).

If an **android pelvis** is found, it is almost a foregone conclusion that the patient will have some difficulty in her labor and may end up having a cesarean section owing to a *deep occiput transverse arrest.* Foreknowledge of this type of pelvis is of value in preventing any undue delay in recognizing the problem during labor.

In the **platypelloid pelvis,** a *deep transverse arrest* is not uncommon. Since the fetal head normally enters the inlet of the pelvis in an occiput transverse position or an oblique position, there must be enough room in the mid-pelvis to allow it to convert to an occiput anterior position. If the sacrum is flattened and anterior, then such is not possible and a cesarean section will be necessary. If the sacrum is directed posteriorly, however, then the labor and descent of the fetal head may continue to progress, with the rotation of the head from the occiput transverse position to the occiput anterior position when it reaches the perineum. In such a situation, you may usually anticipate a vaginal delivery.

In the **anthropoid pelvis,** the great depth of the pelvis becomes the problem. The fetal head may internally rotate in either direction, and an occiput anterior or an occiput posterior position may occur with almost equal ease. As a result, the *occiput posterior* presentation may occur more frequently in this type of pelvis than is normally the case. This is particularly true if the fetal lie is on the right side, since the fetus tends to lie more posteriorly on its back in the right paracolic gutter.

5. Diagnosis, management, and disposition

a. Diagnosis

After you have obtained a complete history and have thoroughly examined the obstetric or gynecologic patient, it is then possible for you to arrive at a working diagnosis, or an **impression.** Since there are only so many ways that the human body can manifest disease by symptomatology, and since there are many diseases that produce similar symptoms, it becomes evident that in most instances you must determine the actual diagnosis from a list of possibilities (i.e., **the differential diagnosis list**). This list indicates the possible disease processes that would perhaps explain the findings. The various possibilities are usually listed from the most likely to the least likely diagnoses.

b. Management

You should investigate the possible diagnoses that might explain the patient's symptoms by utilizing various laboratory procedures and tests, or by repeating the physical examination, which may either alter the position of these diagnostic possibilities or eliminate some of them entirely from the list. It is important that any laboratory studies you obtain be necessary, either to confirm your diagnosis or to rule out other diagnoses on the differential list. **It is axiomatic that you must obtain the results of any laboratory examination that you order and that you make a determination as to whether the result is normal or abnormal.** It is always a good practice to list each laboratory request in the test/consultation section of your disposition section, and then to use this list to remind yourself to find out the results of these tests.

c. Disposition

Once the diagnostic possibilities have been defined and a plan of investigation outlined, it becomes essential to **define the patient's care in the interim period between her outpatient visits.** The disposition consists of four major areas: (1) the tests, consultations, and procedures ordered, (2) the medications and dosage, (3) the instructions and precautions, and (4) the return appointment (see Chapter 1).

CHAPTER 5

Psychosomatic obstetrics and gynecology

A third noteworthy feature in modern treatment has been the return to psychical methods of cure, in which faith in something is suggested to the patient. After all, faith is the great lever of life.

—Sir William Osler*

1. General considerations

The term "psychosomatic" refers to the relationship that exists between the mind and the body that results in physical or mental symptomatology. According to this definition, changes in the emotional and psychological states of the mind may affect the individual's physical body. In addition, changes in the physical state of the body may affect the individual's mental and emotional states. The causes of psychosomatic problems are many and varied. Most psychologists and psychiatrists agree that the etiology is two-fold: The first is that most patients learn faulty methods of dealing with stress and problems as children; the second is that most patients allow themselves to become their own worst enemies in the present by creating many of their own problems. The status of the patient's health is largely dependent upon her peception of her environment and her reaction to it based upon her systems of ethics, beliefs, and values. The astute physician will consider the patient and her illness in relationship to not only her environment, but also in regards to her psychological devel-

opment and beliefs, when attempting to carry out therapy.

a. Historical aspects

Stress has been recognized as a psychophysiological problem since the time of Socrates (470–399 B.C.). The French physiologist **Claude Bernard** (1813–1878) was recognized for his discussions of the **milieu interieur,** or the internal environment of the body. **H. Selye** (1936) was the first to describe a syndrome, later called the **general adaptation syndrome (GAS) or the biologic stress syndrome,** that can be produced by a number of different types of situations. This was also referred to as the **alarm reaction** because it seemed to call up the body's defensive mechanisms. In 1939, W. B. Cannon espoused his theory of **homeostasis,** in which the body's physiologic processes attempt to maintain a steady state. He emphasized that emergency situations, such as pain and rage, stimulate the sympathetic nervous system to prepare the individual for either **fight or flight.**

b. Stages of the adaptation syndrome

The first stage of the adaptation syndrome, or the initial response to stress, is the **alarm reaction.** If the individual survives the initial environmental stress or threat, then a second stage occurs in which the individual begins to develop a **resistance** to the stress. If the stress is overly prolonged or very severe, then a stage of **exhaustion** will finally develop in which the individual can no longer cope at all. While recovery can occur from the stage of exhaustion with rest and recuperation, some degree of **wear and tear** on the individual's body will eventually result if there are repeated episodes of stress.

---

*Reprinted with permission from Robert Bennett Bean, *Sir William Osler: Aphorisms from His Bedside Teachings and Writings,* William Bennett Bean, ed. Springfield, Ill.: Charles C Thomas, Publisher, 1968, p. 102.

1) The alarm reaction

"Stress" should be defined both in reference to: (1) the person, and (2) the environment. The response then involves both: (1) the individual's **appraisal** (perception) of the environmental threat, and (2) the individual's response in managing (coping with) the stress experience. **The individual's appraisal consists of her assessment of the environmental situation in terms of its "meaning to herself"; the amount of jeopardy perceived to be present is highly subjective.** After the individual judges and analyzes the amount of threat or harm that may result from the situation, the response becomes one of "What am I going to do about it?"

Some individuals repeatedly create what has been termed **novel stress,** which provides a way of testing one's personal control over a given situation. In such individuals, the climbing of a mountain, the flying of a plane, or the driving of a race car provides a self-initiated, measurable risk that is controllable and conquerable. Mastering repeated stresses like these can increase a person's self-confidence and reduce fear and anxiety. This type of stress is healthy and enhances the individual's personal growth. Thus, one's perceived ability to control the stress situation removes the harmful aspects of the stress.

The appraisal stage brings together the sum total of the individual's (1) past experiences, (2) previous methods of coping, (3) basic personality traits, and (4) current "load" of other stresses (i.e., coping reserve). One of the biggest misconceptions about stress is the irrational belief that most of it is caused by the environment. **The fact is that it is usually the individual's appraisal or perception of the environment that causes most stress.** For example, if two people are walking through the woods and come upon a harmless snake, each individual may have a different reaction. One could run away in fear, while the other, who recognized that the snake was harmless, could look at it with curiosity and show no signs of fear. Thus, the same environmental stimulus will have provoked two separate reactions that are based upon different appraisals of the danger involved, based on different belief systems.

One approach to this concept is the **A-B-C model.** The "A" represents the *action* or event that occurs. The "B" is our *belief system* concerning that action or event, and the "C" is our reaction (behavior) or method of *coping* based upon our belief system. The most important part of this model is the **belief sys-tem,** which explains why the two individuals in the example reacted differently to the same environmental stimulus.

The individual's appraisal of the environmental situation may elicit one of six basic feelings—love, sexual feelings, joy, anger, sadness, and fear—which sets in motion the physiologic responses of the alarm reaction. Trauma, hemorrhage, or other life-threatening injuries may also elicit this response. The intensity of the response, however, is based upon many factors.

The **suppression or blocking** of one of the six basic feelings may lead to physiologic changes that may cause physical damage to the individual. The emotion of **love** is elicited in situations in which a loving or caring feeling is engendered, whereas **sexual feelings** occur whenever the proper chemistry or emotion between two people causes sexual arousal. **Joy** occurs whenever an experience produces good feelings, and **anger** often occurs when someone does not do what we wish them to do. **Fear** obviously will occur whenever we become afraid or apprehensive about some perceived danger, and **sadness** develops whenever we sustain a loss or become disappointed in someone or something. **If for some reason we block these emotions, then we may develop a psychosomatic illness.**

Normally, most well-adjusted individuals are aware of their feelings in a given situation. They allow themselves to experience this emotion and follow through with an appropriate expression of the feeling so that the feeling is resolved. **In contrast, the patient who develops a psychosomatic illness has usually blocked or suppressed an emotion or feeling.** For example, it is not considered socially acceptable for an employee to become angry when her supervisor makes unreasonable demands upon her time and energies. Since she cannot show her anger without endangering her employment, she may suppress or block her feelings of anger and substitute another emotion, such as depression. This response may lower the individual's resistance and make her more susceptible to infection or to the development of neoplastic disease. This substitution of one emotion or feeling for another may have cultural or regional patterns as well. One Southern practitioner has observed that some Southern men substitute anger in situations in which they experience fear or sadness. In addition, some Southern women will substitute sadness whenever they have problems with sex or anger.

2) Stage of resistance

In the second stage, after the initial alarm reaction, the individual develops a degree of resistance. This type of response allows the individual time to mobilize her resources in an attempt to manage the problem. Depending upon the duration and intensity of the stimulus and the individual's "coping reserve," this process may continue for quite a long period of time. Eventually, however, the individual's resources may begin to fail.

3) Stage of exhaustion

The third stage begins when the individual's coping capabilities fail. For example, one can imagine the extreme stress that a soldier might face over days or weeks on the front line of combat. The stress of the constant threat of death or mutilation, the persistent fire-fights with the enemy, and the loss of companions and friends could produce a degree of strain that could literally attack an individual's sanity. Eventually, the human psyche in such a situation will "give up" and succumb to the ravages of the environmental threat. In most civilian situations, death or injury is not part of the threat; however, an equally dangerous and mutilating danger to the psyche may be present if a humiliating or ego-damaging event is involved. **The individual may pay a physiological price for these environmental insults that may translate into problems with physical health.**

c. Physiological response to stress

Any disturbance of the physiologic steady state (i.e., homeostasis) of the body, be it an internal stimulus (e.g., illness) or an external stimulus (e.g., a threatening environmental situation), may elicit the alarm reaction. It has been postulated that some sort of central mediator, such as the endorphins, may stimulate the release of adrenocorticotropic hormone (ACTH). This hormone then triggers the release of cortisol from the adrenal gland in order to suppress the individual's immune system and inflammatory responses. Catecholamines are also released to further activate the body's adaptive mechanisms.

1) Emotional states

The emotional states generated by the alarm reaction tend to release certain biogenic amines that may have a profound effect upon the organism. The brain's catecholamines, such as epinephrine, norepinephine, and dopamine, are chemical modulators of neuroendocrinologic functions (see Chapter 3). These neurotransmitters also apparently affect the mood and the behavior of the individual. It has been shown, for instance, that a decrease in these biogenic amines may be associated with depression.

The catecholamines regulate the pulsatile release of gonadotropin releasing hormone (GnRH). This regulation is modified by the gonadal steroids and the endorphins. Through their effect on GnRH, the menses may cease or become disordered (i.e., dysfunctional uterine bleeding). Dopamine may suppress the production of GnRH activity in the arcuate nucleus. **Norepinephrine stimulates GnRH release.** Opioid compounds stimulate growth hormone, prolactin, and ACTH, and inhibit gonadotropins (FSH, LH) and thyroid-stimulating hormone (TSH). The effects of the releasing factors on the other systems may also be interrupted. Prolactin secretion may be influenced by the level of dopamine (which is probably the prolactin inhibiting factor). Thyrotropin-releasing hormone (TRH) may also be effected, which in turn may effect the release of TSH. **All of these effects may be related to emotions such as anger, fear, and the other strong feelings that tend to trigger the fight-or-flight mechanism.** Serotonin and monoamine oxidase production may be related to depression and, in turn, the monoamine oxidase levels may be influenced by the estrogen levels. **It is obvious that there is a considerable amount of interplay between these various biogenic amines, the pituitary hormones, the feedback hormones of their target organs, and the behavioral aspects of the individual, much of which is still unknown.**

2) Systemic effects

With the release of systemic epinephrine, there is an increase in the blood pressure, in the strength of the myocardial contractions, in the cardiac output, in generalized vasoconstriction, and in the coronary blood flow. In addition, the effects on the central nervous system result in an increase in the individual's alertness and may produce restlessness, tremor, headaches, and apprehension. The effect of epinephrine on the metabolism causes

hyperglycemia and a release of fatty acids. Stress also causes the release of ACTH, cortisol, and androgens. The individual's response to pain may be diminished, however, through the release of **beta-endorphins.**

All of these responses would be of benefit to the organism if a fight-or-flight situation did in fact exist. For example, if an individual was walking in the woods and suddenly was confronted by a large ferocious brown bear, the alarm reaction would be of great benefit to the individual as she turned and took flight. The outpouring of epinephrine would stimulate the heart and produce a greater cardiac output in order to support the exertions. The hyperglycemia would supply the actively working leg muscles with fuel. The release of endorphins would dull the sense of fatigue and pain due to the exertions. Unfortunately, though, **repeated** episodes of the **release of epinephrine have been found to produce ischemic damage to the myocardium and to the arterial walls, leading to necrosis;** it is obvious that this survival response may become damaging to the individual if it is repeated too often or is too prolonged.

The stress-related increase in corticosteroids and catecholamines have been shown to inhibit both cell-mediated and humoral immunity. This transient **immunodeficiency syndrome** makes these individuals more susceptible to infections and to the growth of neoplasms. The hypothalamic nervous control of the thymus and spleen may also play a role in this response.

It has only been within the past few years that we have recognized that neurotransmitters and hormones are capable of effecting such changes. Furthermore, it has become increasingly apparent that many diseases and conditions may be secondary to imbalances in these reciprocal control systems. **We might refer to a normally functioning system as an "adapted" system, in that it is functioning as it was designed to function and is self-regulating. When it stops functioning in an appropriate manner—and when the control systems fail and disease results—then it becomes "maladapted."**

3) The maladaptation syndrome

The breakdown in adaptive behavior has been the subject of research for the past 30 years. Extreme situations exposing individuals to maximum stress (e.g., concentration camps, combat, severe traumatic injuries) have provided evidence of how coping mechanisms may fail. Some investigators have attempted to find stress determinants within the experience itself; however, there has not been a good correlation between the objective experience and the coping response. **Instead, there seems to be a closer relationship between: (1) how the individual perceives (appraises) the environmental situation in the light of past experiences, and (2) how the person copes with the situation.** Thus, a specific environmental threat may elicit little or no response from one individual (who does not perceive the problem to be personally very threatening), whereas another person (who perceives the environment to be very threatening) may show a maximal response. We may perceive our environment in a number of ways, but all of these perspectives are based upon our past experiences. These "belief systems," which are also called **"self-talk,"** may include the following concerns: "I must please everyone"; "I must be loved by everyone to be a worthwhile person"; "I need my family's and friends' approval to feel good"; "If I'm not worrying, then I am not showing love and concern"; and many more too numerous to review.

If we invoke these types of responses inappropriately, such as: (1) in a nonthreatening situation, (2) in an exaggerated manner, or (3) in a manner in which the response is prolonged beyond the point of danger, then we release all of the physical and emotional mechanisms for the fight-or-flight response inappropriately. The term **maladaptation syndrome** has been coined to describe these inappropriate adaptation responses. By maladaptation, I mean that the individual has a form of **adjustment disorder** that results in a physiologic response that may be prolonged enough or repeated often enough to eventually cause physical damage to the person's organs and tissues. Thus, when the individual persists in reacting in a maladaptive manner over time, disease may result.

The arousal responses that an individual develops to both the external environment and the internal environment are mainly learned in childhood. If the responses are appropriate and of the right intensity, then the person will not usually be subject to psychosomatic diseases. **If the individual learns at an early age to respond to the environment in an**

inappropriate manner, however, then that person may continue these maladaptive responses into adulthood. An inappropriate response is one in which there is a suppression or blockage of one of the six basic feelings (i.e., love, sexual feelings, joy, anger, sadness, or fear) rather than the expression of such feelings in an appropriate manner. The question as to what constitutes "stress" thus may be different for each individual and is dependent upon the person's earlier learned responses to the environment. For example, if the child is stressed by an approaching test in school and responds by becoming ill (illness being acceptable in our society, whereas the inability to cope is frowned upon), the child may learn that this type of coping response brings rewards (the child doesn't have to go to school and take the test); illness may then become a perpetuating inappropriate response in similar situations at a later time. When the child becomes an adult, however, this avoidance behavior may not be as effective in coping with life's situations as when she was a child. Another example might be as follows. Suppose you are treating a pregnant patient who is showing signs of clinical depression. At first you may assume that this depression is caused by the pregnancy, when in reality the patient is very happy about her pregnancy. Rather, the patient may be depressed because she is trying to continually please and obtain approval from an overprotective mother who is constantly trying to run her life now that she is pregnant. Her attempt to please her mother is inappropriate as a married woman and results in depression.

a) Psychosomatic vs. psychiatric problems

Psychosomatic problems tend to involve only one organ system, which might be considered to be the individual's "shock" organ. Thus, stress may cause cardiovascular system problems (e.g., hypertension) in some people, gastrointestinal disease (e.g., duodenal ulcers) in others, or musculoskeletal problems (e.g., tension headaches) in still others. Since there may be a genetic predisposition in the development of duodenal ulcers, the **maladaptation syndrome** may occur either as a response to a genetic predisposition or in response to an environmental stress.

It is essential that you separate those diseases that are **psychiatric** from those that are **psychosomatic (psychophysiologic).** Diseases that are psychiatric in origin arise in the mind and are not necessarily reflected in the bodily functions. Some examples of such psychiatric diseases would be schizophrenia or manic depressive disease. Those diseases that are psychophysiologic may arise either in the mind or in the body, but in contrast to psychiatric problems, they have a direct effect upon bodily functions. Repeated or prolonged psychophysiologic responses may ultimately cause the physical breakdown of specific organs or tissues, which then results in disease (e.g., peptic ulcer, hypertension).

There are two types of patients who have an excessive preoccupation with their body: patients who are depressed (a psychosomatic disorder), and patients with Briquet's syndrome (a psychiatric disease). About 1% of psychiatric patients convert their feelings into physical symptoms and claim to have symptoms that have no clear organic explanation. **This somatization syndrome (i.e., Briquet's syndrome) is really a psychological, psychiatric disorder.** The disorder is said to be present when the patient reports having 12–60 symptoms from at least 9–10 symptom groups without any apparent physical cause. The multisystemic symptomatology usually begins prior to the age of 30. **These patients do not eventually develop the physical diseases, as do the stress-maladapted patients.** Indeed, these patients end up suffering from iatrogenic problems, usually having three times the number of operations for their symptoms than the normal patient. Thus, the main hazard for these individuals is not the symptoms themselves, but rather, the aggressive physician who wishes to operate in order to be certain that the patient does not have a serious disease. This diagnosis should be considered in patients who have gynecologic abdominal pain or irritable bowel syndrome. *The contract between the physician and the patient in these cases should not be a "dramatic cure," but should include a realistic acknowledgment of the problem on the part of the patient and a "negotiated" plan as to what progress can be expected over time.* Unfortunately, the presence of somatization syndrome is no guarantee that the patient will not develop a "real" organic disease while under observation. These patients need to have a long-term relationship with their physician.

One way to determine whether your patient has a real organic problem or a psychosomatic one is to explore the past 2–3 years with the patient. Many times these patients have what has been termed a **bottled hurt.** This term refers to significant events in the patient's life with which she has not dealt effectively. **In effect, the individual blocks the expression of her feelings, which then causes a physiologic reaction.** An example might be the recent death of a loved one, a divorce, an alcoholic spouse, or financial setbacks. A recent case involved a 40-year-old patient who came in for a routine checkup and had a complaint of migraine headaches. As the discussion proceeded, it was noted that her father had died suddenly two years before; however, she had remained "strong" at the funeral and did not cry. Furthermore, she had not visited the cemetery since the day he was buried. It was obvious that she was suffering from "bottled hurt." She was counseled to go to the cemetery with some flowers. There, she finally allowed herself to say "I love you, Dad" and was then able to cry. Following this, the migraine headaches disappeared.

d. Stress reduction (coping) mechanisms

1) Self-effectance

The ability of an individual to cope effectively with her environment is dependent upon the person's range of resources and past experiences. The individual's **self-esteem,** understanding of the problem, plans for the management of the problem, ability to see herself as being capable of producing a positive outcome, ability to imitate others who have been successful in similar situations, ability to control her emotions, and the kind and amount of support and assistance that is available from loved ones are all important. The coping mechanism is a dynamic process, and not a static mechanism. The individual's ability to develop these coping mechanisms has been termed **self-effectance** by some authors.

2) Inappropriate coping mechanisms

The immediate alarm reaction response to an environmental stress may be elicited **inappropriately.** When this occurs, the organism pays a price by developing symptoms of illness, and eventually, by actually causing physical damage of the organs involved. This repeated failure to cope results in an uncontrolled alarm reaction physiologic response (i.e., hypertension, vasospasm, tachycardia, cortisol release, etc.) and will eventually result in sustained hypertension,

coronary artery disease, and perhaps a loss of host resistance to infections or cancer. This type of inappropriate (i.e., maladapted) response is based upon a faulty belief system that we have learned in childhood. **In effect, we are our own worst enemy.** As you gain clinical experience through the years, you will become more impressed with the truth of this statement.

2. Patient evaluation

You should attempt to determine: (1) the emotional, (2) the socioeconomic, and (3) the physical status of your patient. Every individual will have certain events in her life that may be interpreted as being stressful. Problems with one's spouse or children, difficulties with relatives or coworkers, worries about money and bills, and fatigue due to long working hours or lack of sleep may weaken the patient's coping mechanisms and produce physical symptoms. The real challenge to the physician is to learn how to sort out the real physical problems from the psychosomatic ones and to realize that at times they may be interrelated. By definition, a psychosomatic illness is one in which an emotional or psychological state results in a physical effect that disrupts the patient's well-being. *To be more specific, psychosomatic illness may affect one's life in any of the following ways: (1) a change in sleeping patterns, (2) a change in eating patterns, (3) a change in interpersonal relationships, (4) a change in emotional feelings or psychological states, or (5) a change in the individual's ability to cope with everyday stress.*

a. Emotional evaluation

The patient's life-style should be briefly reviewed to determine whether any changes have taken place in the way that she approaches life. You should ask questions such as: *(1) "How have you been sleeping lately?" "Are you waking up at night after going to sleep, and then having a hard time getting back to sleep?" "Are you tired most of the time?" "More tired than you should be for what you are doing?" (2) "How have you been getting along with your husband or boyfriend?" "How are you getting along with your parents?" "How are you getting along with your children?" "Do you feel that you can talk to your husband and parents and do you feel that they listen to you when you need to share your feelings?" (3) "How has your appetite been lately?" "Do you eat more when you are nervous or upset?" "Are you eating less than usual?" (4) "Have you or others noticed that you have had a change of temperament lately?" "Do you lose your temper more easily than before?" "Do you have as much patience with people?" "Do you find yourself avoiding people and wanting to be alone more than usual?" (5) "Do things get on your nerves more easily lately?" "How well do you handle day-to-day-stress?"* If these questions are asked in a gentle and kindly manner, few if any patients will be offended by them.

Usually, one or more of these questions will cause the patient to open up and confide in you. It is important that you not be judgmental in obtaining this information. In addition, you should not belittle the patient's concerns or be tempted to immediately give advice without thinking about the problem. Remember that it is not the environment per se that is important, but the patient's appraisal of that environment that creates the stress. After you have evaluated the patient completely and have performed a thorough physical examination, you may wish to provide simple straightforward suggestions (i.e., directive therapy) if it appears that the problem is not particularly complicated with other underlying psychological problems. If such suggestions prove to be inadequate in solving the patient's problem, then consideration should be given to referring the patient to a professional psychological counselor or psychiatrist.

b. Socioeconomic evaluation

It is also worthwhile to evaluate your patient's socioeconomic status. There are many people in our society who do not have even the basic essentials to maintain a proper existence. Hunger, filth, poor housing, and disease seem to be the lot of far too many people. Many of these people have entered the poverty class after losing their jobs. After a lifetime of supporting their families, these individuals may be reduced to relying upon charity hospital care, food stamps, and welfare checks. Not only have they had a shock to their ego in losing their chance to support themselves, but they are further humiliated by the loss of control over their lives. Other people have been chronically poor throughout their lifetimes, and due to a lack of marketable skills, they have skirted the financial edge of an independent existence for years. Such a constant struggle to maintain one's life may lead to crime, drug abuse, and alcoholism as the only escape from the terrible reality that these people experience in their everyday lives.

You should question your patient as to her source of income and the type of job (if any) that she or her husband has. Her place of residence in your community may alert you to her financial status. Sometimes, large debts and other bills may be an all-consuming worry to the patient. You might ask questions such as: "If you had one wish for material things, what would you wish for?" "If you could have all of the money you needed, what luxury would you like to have the most?" Often the patient's choice may be very revealing, not only as to aspirations for a better life, but also as to her greatest concerns at the present time. Most people can resist the ravages of stress for a period of time (i.e., stage of resistance); however, a limit is eventually reached. In these patients, the crushing situation of poverty may be so severe over a period of time that it finally overwhelms her coping responses to the point where she develops physical symptoms (i.e., stage of exhaustion).

c. Physical evaluation

The patient who has manifested recurrent or persistent symptoms secondary to her failure to cope with stress may eventually develop other damaging physical changes in her body that are due to these ineffective coping mechanisms. For example, the nervous, chronically anxious individual may utilize a variety of stress reducers that are medically unacceptable. The use of cigarettes will reduce nervous tension but will also cause long-term damage to the pulmonary and cardiovascular systems. The use of alcohol may result in the well-known damage to the liver and brain. **Overeating is a common device to reduce tension in the American population, and the secondary problems of obesity include hypertension and diabetes mellitus.** Many diseases may be due to the individual's inability to cope with the stresses of modern-day life. Chronic or repetitive stresses combined with a high cholesterol diet, lack of exercise, and smoking is more than likely the basis for coronary artery disease and myocardial infarction.

Your examination of the patient may uncover a number of such habits that are hazardous to the patient's health. Educating the patient as to the proper manner of maintaining her health may be very beneficial; however, it should be recognized that advice alone will not correct the problem. The patient must first be motivated to change her life-style, and the threat of future death may not be a persuasive argument. Acceptable alternative stress-reducing techniques must be offered to the patient if success is to be achieved.

3. Treatment of maladaptive behavior

In the treatment of specific diseases during the past few years, attempts have been made to modify the individual's "appraisal" processes in transactions with the environment. Biofeedback techniques have had some success in the treatment of specific problems, such as headaches; however, such voluntary control of the emotions for one specific problem has not always corrected the individual's responses to other stress-related conditions.

The use of a more generalized approach, in which there is an effort to teach the person how to identify those patterns of thinking or behavior that tend to precipitate maladaptive responses, and then to intervene in the process so as to substitute a more benign coping response **(i.e., cognitive-behavior intervention),** is perhaps a better method of reducing these damaging and repetitive physiological changes. This method would allow the individual to alleviate fear, anger, and other emotions that cause the alarm reaction and the resulting bodily illnesses and to substitute a more relaxed and effective response to a stressful stimulus. Such stress-reducing (or anxiety-reducing) activities as alcoholism, drug abuse, smoking, and other inappropriate and dangerous behavioral traits would no longer be needed to enable the person to withstand the rigors of everyday living in a stressful environment. Your recommendation that the patient take up a hobby, enter an exercise program, or engage in other sports activities may provide your patient with a more healthy method of reducing stress.

You have a responsibility to attempt to teach your patients how to cure their illnesses. The basic premise that you should teach is that **"You are as healthy as you think you are,"** and as such, it is within the patient's power to help herself. Your encouragement and efforts to teach patients that they can indeed effect a positive outcome of their diseases, including infections, hypertension, and other illnesses, will go a long way toward improving their chances of a cure. Furthermore, disease may often be *prevented* by the patient's *positive approach to health.* You might ask the patient a simple question: "On an average day, how much time do you spend in processing **negative thoughts,** or in other words, what percentage of every day do you spend thinking negative thoughts about yourself or about your situation?" Negative thoughts are destructive to one's health and should be replaced by **positive thoughts. It is truly healthful to "count your many blessings." While initially this approach may not be easy, in time it will become second nature to the patient and will provide a shield against illness.**

a. Crisis medicine vs. preventive medicine

Medicine as it is practiced today is primarily "crisis" medicine rather than "preventive" medicine; we treat the patient after the disease has occurred instead of preventing it from occurring in the first place. The greater the cost of medical care to society, the greater the push will be in the future toward preventing disease. Self-destructive life-styles (e.g., alcoholism, drug abuse, smoking, and perhaps eventually maladaptive behavior!) may no longer be covered by health insurance in the future. **People may be required to be responsible for their health and may also be required to learn how to better adapt to their environment.** The basic reason for the success of our species on this planet has been our overall ability to adapt to the physical environment; however, we have had considerable difficulty in adapting to "ourselves" and to our fellow humans. It is time that we concentrated our efforts toward teaching our fellow humans to adapt to their human environment. Individual and global violence, destructive life-styles, and *unrestrained greed and the seeking of power* must be curbed if humankind is to continue to survive and prosper on this earth.

CHAPTER 6

Sexual assault

There is no more difficult art to acquire than the art of observation, and for some men it is quite as difficult to record an observation in brief and plain language.

—*Sir William Osler**

1. Definitions

The term "rape" is a non-medical word (L. *ra-pere*) meaning "to take by force" or "to snatch." Legally, a forcible rape is considered a crime of violence rather than just sex and is in the same category as assault and other aggressive crimes up to and including murder.

In the past, there has been a great tendency on the part of the general public to place at least a part of the blame for rape on the victim herself. Perhaps the reasoning behind this concept was that this act is, on the surface at least, a "sexual" act, and therefore the woman must have enticed or otherwise aroused the male into committing it. It has become increasingly clear, however, that such is not the case and that the woman does not usually "invite the assault." There are a number of reasons why rapists commit these crimes of violence, only some of which are related to sex per se. The very young, the very old, and the mentally incompetent are the most susceptible to being raped. More rapes occur in the warmer months of the year than in the cooler ones, most commonly in August.

Many rapes occur between 10 P.M. on Saturday and 2 A.M. on Sunday. About 80% of the victims are single, divorced, or separated. Rapes are intraracial rather than interracial in 90% of the cases. Studies have shown that between 70–100% of victims are threatened with bodily harm and that 30–40% of the women are threatened with a weapon. In 10–46% of the victims, there will be evidence of violence in the form of bruises, lacerations, minor fractures, or other physical damage.

Statutory rape is said to have occurred when the sexual act (i.e., carnal knowledge, or vaginal penetration of the female by means of force) is performed upon a girl who is legally under the age of consent (usually 18 years old), which may be different for each state. Also, the exact definition of **rape** may vary from state to state and often only requires a degree of carnal knowledge (e.g., sodomy, fellatio). In some instances, this sort of sexual activity is referred to as a **deviant sexual assault** (i.e., contact between the sexual organs and the other individual's mouth or anus without consent). **Sexual molestation** is the term used when there is noncoital sexual contact without consent. In some jurisdictions, the term **sexual battery** is utilized to include any forceful sexual activity. In a few states, **marital rape** has been recognized. Although the victims of rape have generally been female, there is a growing awareness that men are sometimes raped as well; it would appear that male-to-male rape in penal institutions, for example, is a major problem.

The incidence of rape is about 30:100,000 females in rural areas and about 85:100,000 to 100:100,000 females in the large cities of the United States, and these numbers seem to be increasing every year. Perhaps as few as 10–20% of rapes are reported to the police. About one-third of

---

*Reprinted with permission from Robert Bennett Bean, *Sir William Osler: Aphorisms from His Bedside Teachings and Writings,* William Bennett Bean, ed. Springfield, Ill.: Charles C Thomas, Publisher, 1968, p. 59.

all rapes are done by repeat offenders. About 25–50% of rape victims are adolescents. Unfortunately, less than 1% of all offenders are prosecuted and sentenced to go to jail.

2. The rapist

The crime of rape is one of violence and aggression. The majority of rapists are from the lower socioeconomic levels of society, but they occasionally come from the higher levels of society as well. **The rapist is frequently less than 30–35 years of age, and often knows the victim.** The rapist plans his crime and continually repeats it using the same approach each time. It has been estimated that by the time the rapist is caught, he may have committed as many as 14 rapes. The reasons behind the act of rape vary somewhat from one rapist to another but may often be related to feelings of sexual inadequacy or to a poor family-life environment while growing up.

3. Types of rape

Rape usually involves an expression of force and hostility. The types of rape may be categorized as: (1) the power rape, (2) the anger rape, and (3) the sadistic rape.

a. The power rape

The **power rape** is thought to be one of the most common of all rapes and usually involves a teenage boy who has concerns about his virility. He fantasizes about his victim and plans out his attack ahead of time. While he may use force to control the situation, his main purpose is sexual intercourse, not injury. The victim often knows the rapist and may even date him. After an evening on the town, the girl may allow the initial sexual advances of her date but then changes her mind. The rapist persists, and then the rape occurs. He may not derive any particular sexual gratification from the rape. Many of these **date rapes** are never reported because the victim feels that perhaps she may have led the attacker on and that she herself may be to blame for the rape. Her emotional attachment to the rapist makes the rape even more confusing to her.

b. The anger rape

The **anger rape,** the next most common type of rape, is usually **an impulsive act.** The intent of the rapist is to degrade, humiliate, and injure his victim, often in response to a stressful situation in his life that causes him to feel helpless and wronged by others. The man therefore takes out his anger on the nearest woman available. Due to the intent to injure, there is more danger to the victim in this form of rape.

c. The sadistic rape

The **sadistic rape** occurs in about 5% of cases, and constitutes the most violent and dangerous type of rape. These cases involve ritualistic sexual deviation and sexual trauma that often leads to rape-homicide. The rapist is a sadistic individual who has a long history of abusive behavior in his family, at work, or in other areas of his life. Although some of these offenders are "closet sadists" and may put on a face of gentleness to the world, they commonly abuse their wives and children at home. These rapes are premeditated and are designed to destroy the individual victim—if not in actuality, at least symbolically. The degree of violence and the magnitude of mutilation and torture frequently produce long-lasting psychological scars in the victim, if she survives.

4. The medical evaluation of the rape victim

a. Initial contact with the patient

Initially, you should make every attempt to establish rapport with the patient and offer psychological support. The rape victim will usually experience an immediate acute emotional and behavioral reaction to the act of rape. **The rape experience constitutes a violation of the patient's beliefs as to the safety of her environment and attacks her concepts of trust, self-confidence, and self-esteem.** Shock, and a disbelief that the rape has occurred, may be combined with an inability to concentrate or to make decisions. These feelings are further confused by the psychological revulsion and the remembrance of her fear during the encounter. The aches and pains associated with the actual physical assault further add to her trauma.

Two phases to the "rape trauma syndrome" have been identified: the acute, or disorganized, phase and the reorganization phase. During the **acute, or disorganized, phase** the patient may be in psychological shock and may not be able to control her behavior. Her defense mechanisms will be lost and she may be unable to cope with her own feelings as well as the demands of her environment. She will usually be fearful, confused, and humiliated and will have feelings of anger, guilt, and embarrassment. She may experience sleep disturbances, eating difficulties, and an inability to concentrate on her normal day-to-day activities. Her mood may swing considerably as she reviews the assault in her mind in anger, frustration, fear, and guilt. Irritability and psychosomatic complaints will usually be present. The acute phase may last for days or weeks before the patient appears to begin to **reorganize** her life. At this point, she will begin to emotionally move away from the psychological aspects of the sexual assault. During this time, however, she may go through the stage of an **outwardly satisfactory adjustment,** followed by another period in which there is a **resurgence of the rape trauma** in the form of nightmares and daytime recollections of the event. During this time, the patient should talk out her feelings and be allowed to express her anger about the rape. Having a sympathetic person to talk to during this period is quite helpful. Most women will eventually reorganize their lives and heal their psychological wounds. Some women, however, will have long-term sequelae from the event and may ultimately require psychiatric assistance to overcome the emotional and mental scarring. This phase is often dependent upon the previous history of the patient, the current support from her friends, and ultimately, upon her inner strengths. Economic stress, prior victimization, loss of self-esteem, and maladaptive stress mechanisms, however, may all retard the patient's recovery.

b. The interview

An understanding, compassionate, empathetic, non-judgmental, and caring approach should be utilized by the physician in the management of the patient who has been raped. The initial history and physical examination should be carried out in a quiet, private room located apart from the open emergency room area. The date, time, and circumstances of the sexual assault should be obained. **The term "rape" should not be used, since it is not a medical, but a legal term. The time that has elapsed since the alleged assault is important, because the patient's complaint that the sexual assault occurred against her will, will be based upon a prompt reporting of the event (i.e., the so-called "hue-and-cry" rule).** The patient's clothes should be preserved for the police. *The place that the assault occurred* is also of paramount importance, since grass stains or other environmental material may be present on her clothes. *Evidence of resistance on the part of the patient* (i.e., scratches, torn clothing, bruises, and other wounds of the body or genital areas) may support the patient's claim that the assault was against her will. The use of a weapon by the assailant is usually the factor that causes women to press charges. Photographs of any bruises or lacerations may need to be obtained by the police photographer. The type of violence, the language, and the threats that were used should also be recorded. Did the patient know the attacker? What were the circumstances of the encounter? How many people were involved? The classic "who, why, where, when, and what" type of interviewing approach should be used. **You should quote the patient as often as possible to illustrate the salient features of the history.** *A statement as to the patient's state of orientation and emotional condition should be made.* The time when the patient last had intercourse and when she last douched or bathed should also be recorded. An accurate menstrual history is important, as is the method of contraception that is being used, since pregnancy may occur as a result of the rape.

5. Physical examination and gathering evidence

a. The rape kit

The forensic aspects of a rape case places the physician in a position of being an expert for the court in the legal sense. You should try to uncover as much information as possible in your evaluation of the rape victim. Many hospitals now have a special **rape kit** that contains all of the necessary medical and legal forms as well as proper materials for the collection of the specimens.

b. Bodily injuries

All of the bodily injuries of the patient should be carefully noted and described. You should look for *finger-shaped bruises* on the body. Bite marks, signs that the victim was choked, and other evidence of struggling or scratching, should be photographed with the patient's *written permission*. The time that has elapsed since the event should be kept in mind, since initial reddened areas may become purplish bruises a few hours later. *Material under the fingernails should be collected* with a sharp wooden fingernail file and placed in a specially labeled glassine bag. Foreign matter that you find on the patient's clothes, on her body, or in her vagina may help to verify the location of the assault. Since there is usually close pubic contact at the time of coitus, *the patient's pubic hair should be combed and any foreign loose hair collected in a glassine bag.* Samples of the patient's pubic and scalp hair should be collected, labeled, and placed in other glassine bags.

Lacerations in the genital area are quite significant and you should be very careful to describe, measure, and perhaps photograph such injuries. Small surface lacerations may be emphasized by placing a 1% aqueous solution of toluidine blue stain over the area and then swabbing it off with a cotton-tipped applicator containing lubricating jelly. The lacerations will retain the stain and stand out from the remaining areas of the skin.

c. Laboratory specimens

You should obtain a *blood specimen* from the patient to determine her blood type and Rh. *Since about 80–85% of the population are secreters (i.e., they secrete blood antigens in their saliva and body fluids), a sample of the liquid material in the vagina should be collected to determine if the semen of the assailant may contain a blood group different from that of the patient.* The patient's saliva may be tested by having her chew a cotton pledget, which is then allowed to dry (without being touched) and placed into a glassine bag. You should prepare wet vaginal smears by aspirating material from both the vaginal pool as well as from the cervical canal, which are then immediately placed on glass slides with a drop of saline and observed under the microscope to detect *the presence of sperm.* **If motile sperm are present in the vagina, it usually means that they were ejaculated there**

no longer than 8–12 hours previously. If there are nonmotile sperm present, then no prediction can be made as to when they were deposited, since they may have either died within the past 30 minutes, if there is a hostile cervical mucus, or may have been there for several days. **Within the cervix, sperm may remain motile for as long as seven days, and they may be present for an additional length of time beyond the loss of motility.** Permanent slides should be prepared of the vaginal and cervical smears. In addition, air-dried swabs of vaginal secretions should be placed in a container to detect the presence of an elevated level of *acid phosphatase* (>20 King-Armstrong units), which is considered to provide positive evidence for the presence of semen even if there is no sperm present (e.g., in men who have had a vasectomy or who are azospermic). This procedure is also done to determine the presence of choline, prostatic antigen, blood group antigens, and proteins. Additional samples of semen may be obtained from the ejaculate deposited onto the external genitalia or other areas of the body (i.e., pharynx, anal area, skin). You can collect this material by swabbing the area with a saline-soaked swab, which is then air dried and placed in a container.

d. Chain of evidence

The proper handling of the materials collected in a rape case is very important. Legally, there must be no chance that the **chain of evidence** can be broken. You must hand-carry the material to the necessary support personnel (laboratory) or police technicians and sign off the transfer of the material on a receipt. If this procedure is not followed, the legal case for the prosecution may be lost on a technicality, since the question could be raised by the defense as to the true origin of the specimens.

If you should be asked to testify, you must realize that you are appearing as an expert and that you should be neutral in your testimony. Just tell the truth as to what you did and what you saw. Use the record freely to refresh your memory. Always be courteous and answer each question carefully and truthfully. **Any physician competent to perform a physical examination and gather the evidence is considered to be qualified to serve as an expert witness in a rape case, so the fact that you may be an intern or a resident has little bearing on** your capabilities in this area as far as the court is concerned.

6. Treatment

Always remember that while you may be involved in a legal situation for the society in which you live, you still have a physician's obligation to treat the patient in an appropriate manner according to the standards of medical care.

a. Sexually transmitted diseases

You should consider the possibility of gonorrhea, syphilis, or chlamydial infection in every rape patient. It has been estimated that the risk of acquiring a gonorrheal infection from a rape is 1:30, while the risk of contracting syphilis is about 1:1,000; consequently, a gonorrheal culture and a serological test for syphilis must be obtained in these cases. Another serological test for syphilis must be repeated six weeks later if the first test is negative. Prophylaxis for the possible presence of gonorrhea may be given, which consists of 4.8 million units of aqueous procaine penicillin I.M. after orally receiving 1.0 gram of probenecid. The oral administration of 500 mg q6h of tetracycline for 14 days will also treat a chlamydial infection if it is present (see Chapter 12).

b. Pregnancy

Depending upon the method of birth control that the patient has been using, you may need to administer medication in an attempt to prevent conception in the rape patient (see Chapter 45). Some of the drugs that have been used are: (1) ethinyl estradiol, 5 mg p.o. for 5 days; (2) Premarin, 25–50 mg I.V. per day × 5 days, (3) Ovral, tabs 2 stat and tabs 2 in 12 hours, or (4) diethylstilbestrol, 25 mg b.i.d. for 5 days. **A beta human chorionic gonadotropin (β-hCG) pregnancy test should be obtained before such treatment is instituted, especially if there is a question about the presence of a pregnancy that antedates the sexual assault.**

c. Psychological care

The long-term psychological aspects of the patient's care should be considered carefully, **since often the most significant injury that the patient experiences is in this area.** Many communities have rape crisis centers with qualified counselors who are available to offer emotional and psychological assistance to the rape victim over the ensuing months. In severe cases, the patient may need psychiatric counseling. Keep in mind that the husband or "significant other" involved with the patient will also have to adjust to the experience.

7. The sexually abused child

a. Child abuse

Any child with a sexually transmitted disease, a genital laceration, or a strong history of suspected sexual abuse should be reported to the child protective services. Usually the child appears to be normal and without objective evidence of trauma but is brought in by the parents because the child related that someone fondled her or made other improper advances. Occasionally, the child molester will be a stranger who makes only one attempt to sexually molest the child. These instances are usually quickly reported to the parents and to the police. Often, however, the assailant is a neighbor or relative who tells the child that they are playing a game and thus lures her into the sexual play. In many instances, the abuser will simulate intercourse by rubbing his penis between the labia or the buttocks of the child. This type of abuse is usually kept a secret for some time, so that there may have been sexual abuse of a long-standing nature by the time the child is brought in for examination. In cases involving boys, masturbation and oral sex may be involved in the molestation episodes. Not all sex offenders fit the typical stereotype of "dirty old men." Many offenders are adolescents who were abused sexually themselves as younger children. It is thought that these adolescent offenders may be more amenable to treatment than adult sex offenders.

b. Incest

Incest perhaps occurs more often than has been previously suspected, with the father of the victim being the abuser in 75% of the cases and a close family member being involved in the other 25%. Generally, the sexual abuse will have been going on for a considerable period of time before it is brought to light. The child frequently develops a poor self-image and a weak ego structure. The families of these children often have other problems as well, including alcoholism, domestic violence, and mental illness. Because of this poor family example, girls raised in these types of families will often seek out a similar family situation when they leave the home and will marry men who will reproduce the same kind of chaotic family situation. The child who has been the victim of an incestuous relationship at home may become a behavioral problem in school. Delinquency, lying, stealing, and running away from home are a few of the manifestations of these disturbed children. While rapists are generally less than 35 years of age, the child molester may be of any age and may include much older men. If force is used, then the assailant is called a **child rapist.**

A complete examination of the child is necessary in order to decrease the emphasis on the genital region. A gentle pelvic speculum examination should be done, if possible, using a nasal or virginal speculum. If the hymen is intact, a urethral and rectal swab for gonorrheal cultures should be carried out.

8. The battered wife, child, or elderly person

The battered-wife syndrome has only recently received the attention that it deserves. While perhaps as many as 25% of women who are seen in the emergency room are there because of domestic violence, only about 3% will be identified as such by their treating physicians. Some of this perhaps stems from the physician's unwillingness to "get involved" in the domestic affairs of the family; however, it should be recognized that such abuse may not be limited to just the **wife** but may also include the **children** (battered-child syndrome), and the **elderly** (elderly abuse) who live in the home. There are between 500,000 and 2.5 million cases of elderly abuse in the United States each year. **Moreover, these domestic "spats" may eventually lead to severe injuries or to the murder of one or more people if they are not curbed at an earlier stage.** Battered-women shelters, safe houses, and other protective services are available in many communities, and you should utilize them to the fullest extent in stopping this unnecessary violence. Temporary restraining orders, criminal complaints, legal separation with child custody and support, or divorce are all options that the patient may want to pursue. You should attempt to assist your patient in utilizing those options and any other community resources that are available.

CHAPTER 7

Death and dying

. . . .

He should observe thus in acute disease: first, the countenance of the patient, if it be like those of persons in health, and more so, if like itself, for this is the best of all; whereas the most opposite to it is the worst, such as the following: a sharp nose, hollow eyes, collapsed temples; the ears cold, contracted, and their lobes turned out; the skin about the forehead being rough, distended, and parched; the color of the whole face being green, black, livid, or lead-colored.

—*Hippocrates (460–370 B.C.)**

. . . .

1. The physician's role

It has been said that physicians have a four-fold greater fear of death than most people, and that this may be one of the reasons they initially enter the field of medicine. Perhaps our subconscious thinking said, "I will study medicine in an effort to learn more about death, so that I may understand my own death better." **Whatever the reason for entering the field, it does seem that some physicians view the death of a patient as a failure on their part to conquer the disease and to thwart the ultimate ending of physical existence.** This issue may be especially difficult for physicians who specialize in obstetrics and gynecology, since obstetricians have a strong desire to alleviate pain and suffering and to bring life into the world.

---

*Reprinted with permission from Encyclopaedia Britannica, Inc., *Great Books of the Western World.* vol. 10, "Hippocrates and Galen," Robert Maynard Hutchins, ed. Chicago: William Benton, Publisher, 1952, p. 19.

a. Continuing care

Often when a cure has not been effected, the physician may feel that his role has ended and that there is little more he can do for his patient. This denial of the death process may stem from his own fear of dying. The compassionate physician, however, will not abandon his patient, nor will he feel guilty for his failure. *Indeed, our role is to teach the patient how to cure her ailment, or if incurable, then to teach her how to live with it; it is also our role to aid the dying patient with sensitivity and compassion.* The terminal process is a special area of health care that gives the physician an opportunity to experience much personal growth. The nobility of the human spirit surfaces in times of adversity, and what greater adversity exists than that of approaching death?

2. Patient communication

The first problem that faces the physician is how to tell the patient that she is dying. This initial communication is never easy, and sometimes we feel so sad for our patients (and for our own wounded ego for failing) that we paint a bleaker picture than we should. There have been many patients in the past who were given the "death sentence" by their physicians only to outlive their doctor by many years. Attempting to prognosticate and pinpoint the patient's actual life span is unscientific; there are apparently patients on record who have been diagnosed as having cancer but who conquered their disease without treatment and were found at autopsy years later to be totally free of the disease. By the same token, the patient should not be misled into believing that she has a minor illness that will "go away" in time. **The physician who has had the foresight to "educate" the patient right from the start of the diagnostic workup and treatment regimen has an edge on the one who does not.** Making the patient your partner in the management of her condition helps both of you adjust to the changing health problems, be they mild or serious. You should inform the patient appropriately of her condition in general terms and explain what she might expect in the future. In addition, you should encourage hope, and you should dispel any doubts that the patient may have about your continued support and your desire to keep her as comfortable as possible and free of pain.

3. Stages of dying

The dying patient will generally pass through the various stages of grief that Elizabeth Kübler-Ross has described. **The patient's behavior may range through the stages of: (1) denial and isolation, (2) anger, (3) bargaining, (4) depression, and finally, (5) acceptance.** Although many patients may pass through all of these stages, some may stop at one stage, which will then become that individual's method of coping with the threat of death.

In the **first stage, of denial and isolation,** the patient "cannot believe that it is happening to her." She is in a state of shock. The patient feels that it just cannot be true that she has a terminal illness, and that "a mistake must have been made." She may think that there must have been a mixup in the laboratory pathologic reports. The patient may "doctor shop" to obtain a different opinion that will contradict what she thinks is an erroneous diagnosis. This denial acts as a buffer so that the individual can gradually adjust to the implications of impending death. The family and the medical health-care team may tend to avoid the patient, which leads to further isolation and loneliness. The patient may withdraw within herself and avoid normal contacts with others.

The **second stage, of anger,** eventually replaces denial and the patient reasserts herself. "Why me?" becomes the question. The patient's anger may be directed toward the physician, and she may complain bitterly that the physician is no good and "doesn't know anything." In addition, she might complain that "The doctors are rude and uncaring in their treatment of the patients," and that "the nurses also do not care; they make you wait for your medications and they just don't seem to understand what you need." The patient becomes more demanding of the nurses and the doctors as her anger increases.

During the **third stage, that of bargaining,** the patient may attempt to "make a deal with God." The patient hopes that God will cure her if she agrees to be "good" in the future. She promises to "dedicate her life to God" if He will only spare her, or if He will at least give her some additional time—anything at all to postpone death.

The **fourth stage, of depression,** occurs as the patient realizes that there is no help. God has not heard her plea. She is dependent upon the doctors, the nurses, and the family, and none of these people truly understand the amount of pain and suffering that she is going through. The bills are piling up, and there may be financial burdens placed upon the patient and her family. This depression about the impending future losses is necessary and serves to prepare the patient to finally come to grips with the reality of her death and to "accept" the inevitable.

In the **fifth stage, of acceptance,** the patient finally comes to grips with the situation and develops a quiet acceptance of her impending death. The patient will be at peace with herself and will be in a state of void, or emotional exhaustion. She may only want to be left alone to "die in peace." The patient may become withdrawn and lose interest in her surroundings and even in her loved ones during this time. Some patients will seem to almost will themselves to die and, not infrequently, they may actually do so. The patient may maintain a faint flicker of hope throughout all of these stages, feeling that there is always the remote chance that a miracle could happen. The patient may maintain this hope for long periods, or one day she may just "give up" and die within a few days.

4. The prognosis and new advances

It is important that the patient be kept aware of any new scientific therapeutic approaches that might apply to her condition, and she should also be aware of the fact that you are continually evaluating such information for possible application in her case. The numerous pseudo-scientific cures that are promulgated in the press and through the advertising media should be rationally and factually explained to the patient. You will also need to educate the family in order to prevent them from placing unfounded hope in special "fad cures" and unorthodox methods of therapy. The patient may naturally reach out for any charlatan treatment regimen in the remote hope of a cure. Many of these "supposed cures" become very expensive, and their perpetrators hawk their wares under the guise that "orthodox medicine knows that they are effective and is suppressing such cures because of financial considerations."

5. The day-to-day management of the dying patient

a. Attitudes

Unfortunately, when people have incurable illnesses, those around them, including their physicians, begin to treat them differently. The family and the children no longer discuss their usual mundane activities and the humorous events that occur in the family circle in the patient's presence, perhaps because of a feeling that such matters are too insignificant to bother a dying person with them. However, quite the reverse is true. *These patients will undoubtedly be depressed and grieving, but the usual everyday events of their families will often pull them out of such depression and reestablish a balance in their lives.* The family members should be encouraged to share their activities with the patient. **They also should be encouraged to speak about the cancer (or other illness) to the patient in an encouraging and positive manner.**

b. Family counseling

Keep in mind that the family members may also have **guilt feelings** of their own concerning their previous relationships with the patient. Some may even blame themselves for the patient's condition. You will need to bring these feelings out into the open during your conferences with the family members, where you can assist them in understanding their feelings and discuss how they can assist the dying patient as well as themselves. **In many respects, when your patient is dying, you become the physician and counselor for the whole family.**

6. Goals in the management of the dying patient

a. Comfort

The main goal in the management of the dying patient is to provide the most comfortable and effective existence possible consistent with the patient's personal desires. Many patients seem to be shut out of the decision-making process, and often everyone except the patient seems to be making the decisions. **The patient's desires should be foremost and should be honored whenever possible. Death with dignity has rightfully become an important concept in recent years.**

b. Living will

In some states, a patient may make out a **living will** requesting that the physician not use extraordinary means to maintain life. While the terms euthanasia (G. "easy death") and "mercy killing" have bad connotations, the patient's right of determination as a partner in the decision-making aspects of her care would seem to make such living wills a valid concept. Such wills allow the patient to truly die with dignity. It is obvious that such considerations require a great deal of mature judgment on the part of the patient, and each situation must be evaluated on its own merits. In those cases in which the physician and the patient are partners in health care, and when the patient has a sense of control over her fate, then there is actually a greater desire on the part of the patient to maintain her life as long as possible.

c. Terminal care

Another goal in the management of the dying patient is to allow the patient to remain at home for as long as possible and perhaps to die at home as well. While this approach may create problems for the rest of the family, the cost of terminal hospitalization may otherwise be prohibitive. The family members will usually do much better in caring for the patient if you provide adequate information to them as to what they should do in any medical eventuality. If you do not adequately prepare them for the patient's death, and the patient should die at home, then you may increase their guilt feelings of having done too little for the patient during the terminal event. Of more importance, by keeping the patient near the people, the environment, and the material things that she is familiar with, she will usually do much better and will maintain her physical and mental capabilities for a longer period of time than she would have done had she remained in an impersonal hospital with its sterile, alien environment.

d. Pain control

Adequate pain medication should be made available to allow the patient to be comfortable during the dying process. Even if addiction were to be a concern, which it is not, these patients do not usually become addicted. Often when the patient is pain-free, she will take more interest in her environment and may be more capable of providing for herself. Pain is a very crippling symptom that can occupy almost all of the patient's attention and thus should be alleviated whenever possible. Indeed, the patient should be catered to in all of her desires; if she wishes to have alcoholic beverages or tranquilizers in order to cope with the affliction, then these agents should not be denied. The same rule applies to any supportive medication that will make the quality of the patient's life better.

7. The death of the patient and the survivors

The death of the patient sets up a series of problems for the survivors. Even though the patient may not have died suddenly, but only after a long illness, the relatives still may feel that they (or you) did not do enough for the patient while she was alive. **Mixed emotions, consisting of a sense of relief at the death of the patient along with a sense of failure about not expressing love for the deceased during life may produce guilt in some of the relatives.** Those relatives who do not mourn sufficiently at the time of the death are much more prone to develop psychological and physical symptoms at a later time. Your counseling role does not stop with the death of the patient but should extend into the post-death period. Encouraging the relatives to express their feelings in a one-to-one relationship with you may be beneficial. It has been said that the normal grieving response usually takes about one year for survivors to complete.

8. Fetal death

The obstetrician is often faced with the management of the patient who has lost her baby, either by stillbirth or by a neonatal death shortly after delivery. *The manner in which the patient copes with a fetal death is based upon many factors,* including: (1) the patient's physical and psychological health at the time, (2) the degree of her foreknowledge that the death might occur, (3) the degree of her desire to have the baby in the first place, and (4) the nature and number of previous losses and her ability to cope with those situations. Other familial, cultural, and social factors may also be involved, as well as the degree of marital harmony that may be present.

a. The patient's response

The patient may develop a number of emotional symptoms and behavioral patterns in response to her grief. She may have feelings of guilt; she may magnify her failure to do certain things during her pregnancy; and she may blame herself as being the cause of the baby's death. She may become hostile to the physician and nurses, or to her husband. She may become withdrawn and preoccupied with thoughts of the baby and the loss of her future plans for it. Finally, she may develop physical symptoms that cause her to choke up or have nervous tension or pain. **A breakdown in the normal patterns of behavior may occur and inappropriate responses may be elicited.**

The patient who delivers a "normal" baby also has to adjust at the time of birth from the *idealized concept* of the baby to the *actual appearance* of the baby. This adjustment involves grief over the loss of the idealized child, as opposed to the real child. If the baby is normal, then this adjustment phase is usually of no consequence and the transition is relatively easy. If the infant is abnormal, however, then the transition may be quite difficult. Furthermore, if the child is born dead, then she may suffer even more intense grief over the loss of what the idealized baby might have been. In the process, she may go through the five stages of grief; namely, (1) denial, (2) anger, (3) bargaining, (4) depression, and (5) acceptance. The grieving process may last for over a year and will dominate the patient's thoughts during this time as she gradually accepts the loss and moves on with her life. A **shadow reaction,** or **anniversary reaction,** involving a flare-up of the grief reaction, may occur on the baby's birth or death dates.

b. The physician's response

The physician's response to a grieving patient and the stillbirth or neonatal death will also vary, depending upon the physician's background and training. **At one and the same time, the physician is cast in the role of being somehow responsible for the fetal loss and also being the counselor for the patient.** As a physician, your ego may be involved in this perceived inadequacy, helplessness, and failure to prevent the catastrophe, and yet you must aid and comfort the patient as you struggle with your own fallen image of yourself. **In effect, both the patient and the physician are undergoing the grieving process to some degree.** Dealing with death on a personal level with the patient is often difficult for the physician, since it strikes at the physician's own basic fear of death. This fear may cause you to reject the tragedy or to gloss over it when talking with the patient. It may cause the physician to make such inappropriate statements as "you can always have another baby," or "you should put this behind you and forget it." It takes a great deal of maturity and confidence in one's abilities to be able to lay aside your own personal feelings and concentrate on the patient's problem. It is helpful to encourage the patient to express her feelings and to let her know that her responses are shared by many women in similar straits. In addition, remember that the father will be going through the grieving process as well and that you should assist him in expressing his feelings and facing the loss of his idealized child.

c. The management of the stillborn infant

It is important for the mother and father to see their stillborn infant in order for them to verify that the child is truly dead. They may need to touch or hold the infant. Furthermore, they should partake in naming the child, preparing the birth certificate, and making funeral arrangements. Each of these actions allow the couple to accept the fact of death and to emotionally move beyond it. Naming the baby provides a definite identity for the baby and allows the parents to remove the baby from the "it" category to that of a real person even though the baby is dead. A lock of the baby's hair, a handprint or footprint, the ID bracelet, and other momentos may be treasured later by the couple.

The physician can play an important role in helping the patient throughout the mourning process and can monitor her response as well as her husband's response to the fact of death. Recognizing that parental guilt may play a large role in the grieving process, you should make every attempt to **obtain an autopsy** and to find out whether the condition could be repeated in future pregnancies. Sometimes, determining what went wrong can mitigate the bereavement considerably. This is especially true if a rare, nonrepeating congenital anomaly is found that would have precluded the survival of the child under any circumstances (e.g., renal agenesis).

Telling the parents initially of the baby's death, or impending death, should be carried out in a quiet place with the father, the mother, and perhaps also the other close relatives present. The fact of death should be communicated in a clear and a concise manner, without any assumption of guilt for the death, and without stating any hasty conclusions as to the cause of death. Even though you may feel that somehow you have failed the patient, you should not convey this to the patient or to her family. You should manifest the concern that you feel at the turn of events, even to the point of tears, if you feel that moved by the baby's death. **Do not be dismayed, however, if the patient or her family attempts to place the blame for the baby's death on you.** If asked, you should calmly explain your management in a nondefensive manner and reassure the patient that you will be happy to go into the management of her case in greater detail in a few days when the shock of the baby's death has dissipated somewhat, particularly if an autopsy is to be performed. The use of kindly gestures and of touching the patient in a comforting manner will often convey your sincerity more than your words.

You should attempt to subtly define the **family dynamics** that may be going on as you convey the bad news to them. Separate sessions with some of the family members may be necessary to answer their questions and to allow you to make them "part of the team" in providing support for the grieving parents.

CHAPTER 8

Wound healing

Halsted's fundamental surgical principles: (1) Every operation whether unusual or commonplace must be performed with the utmost care; (2) tissues must be handled with the greatest gentleness; (3) the field of operation should be unstained with blood; (4) a step must never be taken blindly; and (5) the time required to complete the operation is subordinate to accurate and thorough performance.

—*Samuel James Crowe, M.D.**

*Reprinted with permission from Samuel James Crowe, *Halsted of Johns Hopkins: The Man and His Men.* Springfield, Ill.: Charles C Thomas, Publisher, 1957, p. 93.

1. Wounds

a. Types

Wounds have been classified as being clean (Type 1), clean-contaminated (Type 2), contaminated (Type 3), and dirty and infected (Type 4).

1. **Clean wounds** are atraumatic operative wounds that do not involve the respiratory tract, the alimentary tract, the genitourinary tract, or the oropharyngeal cavity. In these wounds, there has been no break in aseptic technique, no infection is present, and no drains have been left in place. The incidence of infection in this type of wound is 1–5% in obstetric and gynecologic incisions.
2. **Clean-contaminated wounds** are operative wounds that may enter the respiratory tract, the alimentary tract, the genitourinary tract, or the oropharyngeal cavity. Minor breaks in aseptic technique may have occurred. The incidence of infection in this type of wound is 3–11%.
3. **Contaminated wounds** are ones in which there are soft tissue lacerations or other traumatic injuries. When there has been a major break in aseptic technique, a major gastrointestinal spillage, or entry into the genitourinary tract (or other systems) in the presence of infection, then the wound is classified as being contaminated. The incidence of infection in this type of wound is 10–17%.
4. **Dirty and infected wounds** are those that are obviously heavily infected prior to surgery, and they may contain foreign bodies or necrotic tissue. The incidence of infection in this type of wound is over 27%.

2. Wound healing

a. Factors that affect wound healing

If the wound is closed with an *undue amount of tension* on the suture line, the initial edema that develops will strangulate the blood supply and will thus delay or prevent adequate healing. On the other hand, if the wound closure is unduly loose without regard for the *closing of the dead spaces deep within* the wound, then these spaces will fill up with serum or blood, which will lead to the development of a seroma or hematoma and the subsequent dehiscence of the wound. Poor general nutrition, deficient hydration, anemia, or necrotic tissue or foreign bodies in the wound may adversely affect healing. In addition, if the patient has had previous irradiation, has a current infection, or has been treated recently with corticosteroids, collagen formation in the wound may be inhibited. The practice of shaving the operative site is to be discouraged unless the hair growth will interfere with the closing of the wound edges. If this is the case, then the shaving should be accomplished utilizing sterile clippers in the operating room just prior to the surgery.

b. First intention

When an operative wound is closed in an aseptic manner with the proper approximation of the tissue, the wound should heal promptly with minimal scarring (i.e., by first intention). **There are three phases of primary wound healing: (1) inflammatory response, (2) fibroplasia, and (3) maturation.**

The **inflammatory response phase** occurs during the **first five days.** The immediate response of the tissue involves the vasoconstriction of the small blood vessels; however, this stage does not last for more than about 5–10 minutes, after which it is followed by vasodilatation with a leakage of plasma into the area. A scab begins to form so as to seal off the surface and prevent further contamination. The leukocytes begin to adhere to the endothelium of the venules so that they are densely covered in 30–60 minutes. The leukocytes (i.e., predominantly polymorphonuclear leukocytes initially and then mononuclear leukocytes later) migrate through the vessel walls by diapedesis, and the red cells make a rouleaux formation and tend to temporarily plug the capillaries.

The degree of localization of the inflammation and the amount of pus developed is determined by the extent of the tissue injury, the degree of the cellular reaction, and the amount of polymorphonuclear leukocytes that accumulate. The amount of circulation present and the extent of the lymphatic drainage of the area are also important factors in the development of pus collection. Vasodilatation **(redness),** plasma leakage into the tissues **(swelling),** and **increased heat** in the area of injury are accompanied by increased tissue pressure and the presence of other tissue products, which produce **pain.** These are the **four classic cardinal signs of inflammation** that were first described by Celsus in the first century A.D.—"rubor et tumor cum calor et dolor" (i.e., redness and tumor with increased heat and pain).[1]

One of the substances that may accumulate at the injury site is **fibronectin,** an insoluble glycoprotein with a high molecular weight that plays a role in adhesion formation and in the localizing process during the first 24–48 hours. This substance finally disappears when the fibrous protein synthesis period predominates in the fibroplasia phase.

The mast cells contain granules that consist of 5-hydroxytryptamine **(serotonin), heparin, and histamine.** Early in the course of injury, these cells lose their granules. **Both serotonin and histamine cause an increase in the vascular permeability.** Other chemical subtances are also released in the injured tissue, such as **proteolytic enzymes,** which may be capable of activating the kallikreins. **Kallikrein** may also be activated by the Hageman factor (i.e., Factor XII). The plasma enzyme kallikrein releases bradykinin and kallidin from the alpha-2-globulin kininogen. These kinins apparently then act upon the microvasculature in a manner similar to that of serotonin and histamine to increase the vascular permeability at the injury site.

Injury is thought to activate the phospholipase of the cellular membranes to release arachidonic acid. **The arachidonic acid is converted into the various prostaglandins by the enzyme prostaglandin synthetase.** The prostaglandins E_1 and E_2 may play a role in wound healing. During the initial cellular phase of the injury response, the neutrophilic granulocytes are the first cells to enter the area of injury. As the pH of the injury site is lowered, the lysosomal enzymes of these cells are released. These neutrophils apparently aid in the clearing of any infection present in the area, allowing for the subsequent healing of the wound. The macrophages then enter the wound and clean up the cellular debris and remove any foreign bodies and necrotic material. This stage is usually completed by the fifth day.

After the blood clots and debris have been removed, the second phase of healing occurs. **This fibroplasia phase extends from about the fifth to the fourteenth to twentieth day.** The fibroblasts begin to move into the area and to utilize the fibrin and fibronectin strands as a framework for the orientation of the proliferating fibroblasts. As the new collagen is deposited, these strands gradually disappear. New capillaries migrate into the area along with the fibroblasts. Endothelial budding of these capillaries is a classic finding and lends a pinkish-red color to the

---

[1]Albert S. Lyons and R. Joseph Petrocelli, II, *Medicine: An Illustrated History.* New York: Harry N. Abrams, Inc., Publishers, 1978, p. 248.

tissues. By the 21st day, the wound will have regained about 30% of its previous tensile strength.

From two weeks up to a year or two, the wound undergoes the final healing phase—that of reorganization, or the maturation phase. After the collagen deposition has repaired the injury site, there is a gradual *remodeling or maturation* of the area as the new capillaries regress and the amount of glycoprotein and mucopolysaccharide in the wound decreases. Collagen synthesis also gradually decreases as the maturation phase is completed. The skin scar will change from a pinkish-red color to a silvery grey color after a year as the new capillaries disappear. Fascia will reach 80% of its prior strength in about two years, whereas it will only take about 28 days for the bladder and bowel to attain the same strength. No tissue attains its original strength after injury.

c. Second intention

If an abdominal wound breaks down and dehisces, it may be allowed to heal by second intention if the rectus fascial plane remains intact. The subcutaneous tissues may be packed open to allow the surface to granulate from the base of the wound up to the surface. When a wound closes by second intention, it closes by the contraction of the wound rather than by primary union. Granulation tissue develops on the exposed edges of the incision and the wound slowly heals in from the bottom to the surface, thus creating a widened and somewhat weaker scar. If the surface of the wound closes before the bottom has closed, an abscess cavity will be formed.

d. Third intention

A delayed closure of the wound (i.e., healing by third intention) refers to the secondary closure of the wound about 4–6 days after its initiation. The closure of a wound by this technique is a safer method of closure whenever the wound is contaminated, dirty, or infected. The rectus fascia should be closed at the time of the initial surgery with interrupted, permanent, single-filament sutures and the subcutaneous tissues and skin left open. The wound should be cleaned and debrided of necrotic, or nonviable, tissue and then allowed to remain open for a few days. The granulation tissue that is formed provides an added degree of protection against infection. An accurate approximation of the underlying tissues as well as of the surface at the time of the secondary closure will result in the healing of the wound by third intention.

Recently, a simplified approach to the *clinical management* of wounds using the concept of **color-coding** has been described. A new wound, or a wound that has healthy granulation tissue present, will be **red.** This type of wound will heal well. If infection is present, the wound will be **yellow,** owing to the inflammatory exudate, and healing will be retarded. These wounds will require cleansing, the use of clean, moist dressings, and perhaps topical antimicrobial treatment. If necrosis is present in the wound, these areas will be **black.** Debridement must be performed in these cases before proper healing of the wound can take place.

3. Sutures

A suture is a thread of some sort of material that is used to tie off blood vessels (i.e., ligature) or to sew together two tissue surfaces. Throughout the years, many substances have been used to accomplish these goals, such as silver wire, silk, cotton, linen, horsehair, and the intestinal tissues of different animals. In recent years, new synthetic materials have been developed that are not only stronger and last longer than many of the previous materials but are also less reactive in the tissues. The surgeon should select sutures on the basis of *tensile strength* and should use the *smallest size* consistent with this goal so as to minimize the amount of tissue reaction to the suture material.

In addition to the proper use of suture material, certain **basic principles of surgery** must always be observed by the surgeon. **Gentleness in the handling of tissues is perhaps the first and foremost principle of surgical technique.** The surgery should be **carefully performed** and **without undue haste.** Surgical dissection should almost always be carried out on **tissues that are under tension.** The sutures should not be placed under undue tension, but should be placed so as **to approximate the tissue, not strangulate it. Hemostasis should be meticulous** so that the field of surgery is not obscured. The **thinnest suture possible** commensurate with the task to be performed should be used. Finally, the surgeon should thoroughly **understand the anatomy** of the area in which he is working.

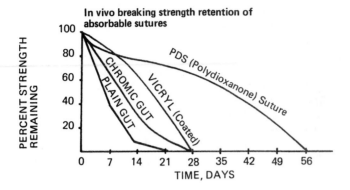

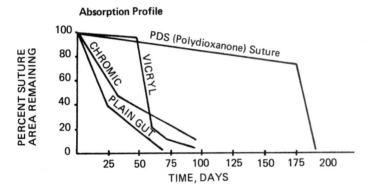

FIGURE 8-1. In vivo breaking strength retention of absorbable sutures. (Redrawn with permission from Ethicon, Inc.: *Wound Closure Manual.* Sommerville, N.J.: Ethicon, Inc., 1985, p. 17.)

4. Suture materials

a. Absorbable sutures

Sutures may be divided into absorbable and nonabsorbable types. Absorbable sutures are slowly digested by the body's enzymes or hydrolyzed by body fluids until they disappear. Some examples of absorbable sutures are: (1) surgical gut, plain catgut, and chromic catgut, all of which are derived from the submucosa of sheep or beef intestine, (2) collagen sutures, either plain or chromic, which are made from the flexor tendons of beef, (3) polyglactin 910 coated or uncoated sutures (Vicryl), which are copolymers of glycolide and lactide with polyglactin 370, and calcium stearate if coated, (4) polyglycolic acid suture, which is a homopolymer of glycolide (Dexon "S"), (5) copolymer of glycolic acid and trimethylene carbonate (Maxon), and (6) polydioxanone (PDS) suture, which is a polyester of poly (p-dioxanone).

The absorbable sutures are classified as to their tensile strength and their absorption rate

(Fig. 8-1). Each of these features is independent of the other, so that even though the absorption is slow, the loss of tensile strength may be rapid. In general, the **tensile strength** decreases to about zero in approximately the following time periods for these absorbable sutures: (1) **plain gut**—21 days; (2) **chromic gut**—28 days; (3) **collagen**—about 10–12 days; (4) coated **Vicryl** (a braided suture)—28 days; and (5) **PDS** (a monofilament suture)—beyond 56 days. The **absorption** of these sutures occurs at about the following rates: (1) **plain gut**—about 70 days; (2) **chromic gut**—more than 90 days; (3) **collagen**—about 56 days; (4) coated **Vicryl**—about 90 days; and (5) **PDS**—at about 180 days.

b. Nonabsorbable sutures

The **nonabsorbable sutures** include three U.S.P. classes of suture: **Class I**—a silk or synthetic fiber of monofilament, braided, or twisted construction; **Class II**—a cotton, linen, or synthetic fiber that is coated;

and **Class III**—a single monofilament or multi-filament wire suture.

Nonabsorbable sutures are neither digested nor destroyed by the body enzymes or fluids. When placed on the skin surface, they must be removed postoperatively; if they are buried in the body, they will become encased in scar tissue. **Nonabsorbable sutures** include: (1) **surgical silk,** raw silk spun by the silkworm, (2) **virgin silk,** which are the natural silk fibers, (3) **dermal silk,** which is silk that has been tanned with a protein coating, (4) **surgical cotton,** from long staple cotton fibers, (5) **linen,** from long staple flax fibers, (6) **stainless steel wire,** which is a specially formulated iron-nickle-chromium alloy, (7) **nylon** (Ethilon, Nurolon, Surgilon, Dermalon), a polyamide polymer, (8) **polyester fiber, uncoated and coated** (Ethibond, Ethiflex, Mersilene, Ti-cron, Dacron), a polymer of polyethylene terephthalate, (9) **polypropylene** (Prolene, Surgilene), a polymer of propylene, and (10) **dacron** (Lutex).

Silk suture loses most of its tensile strength in about one year, and it essentially disappears by the end of two years. **Cotton suture** loses about 50% of its tensile strength in about six months, but only loses an additional 10–20% more over the course of two years. Since the diameter of the strands of linen are difficult to control, and its tensile strength is less than that of other sutures, linen is seldom used today. **Steel suture,** although difficult to handle, has excellent strength and is essentially inert. Since electrolytic problems may occur between other metals and the steel wire sutures, this type of suture should not be used in close proximity to metallic prostheses. **Nylon suture** has a superior tensile strength, is elastic, elicits minimal tissue reaction, and is eventually hydrolyzed in the tissues at a rate of about 15–20% per year.

In general, multifilament sutures tend to tie well with the usual number of square knot throws. In contrast, monofilament sutures tend to have a "memory," and require additional knot throws. Of course, in any situation in which the suture is critical, it is often wise to use additional knot throws. A square knot has the best holding power and should be used with at least two or more throws, depending upon the location and the type of suture material. The square knot may be tied with one hand or with two hands (Fig. 8-2, Fig. 8-3). In some situations the surgeon may prefer to tie the square knot with an instrument (Fig. 8-4). Pro-vided that the square knots are laid appropriately, there is no difference between the one-hand and the two-hand ties.

One additional suturing technique involves the use of metallic or absorbable clips. During the past 30 years, **mechanical stapling devices** have gained some favor in surgery. The modern internal stapling device places B-shaped staples of fine wire-like material or absorbable suture in staggered double rows. The gastrointestinal anastomosis (GIA) stapler is 5 cm long and will place two staggered lines of staples in the intestine, which can then be divided with a scalpel. The thoracoabdominal (TA) stapler places a double row of staples, and then the tissue may be cut with a knife. The end-to-end anastomosis (EEA) stapler will anastomose two purse-stringed bowel segments together in an end-to-end fashion, and a circular knife can then be used to cut the bowel below the double layer of staples. The ligate-and-divide (LDS) stapler may be used to ligate vascular pedicles. Certain devices will also place clips in the fascia and in the skin as well. Some are reloadable and are made of disposable plastic. Although these instruments decrease the amount of time required to do a surgical procedure in some instances, the cost of these instruments is quite high compared to that of the usual suture material.

5. Suture procedures

a. Suture preference

It should be recognized that each surgeon will have his own preferences as to what types of suture material to use at different steps of an operation. These preferences are learned during the physician's training and have a tendency to acquire an "absolute" quality about them as the years progress. As a consequence, they tend to become the "standard" against which all other approaches and new suture materials are measured. To some extent, however, it is not so much the suture material that is important as much as it is the surgeon's ability to use the suture appropriately.

b. Vascular ligatures

Vascular pedicles may be tied off with **ligatures** to accomplish hemostasis. These ties, or ligatures, may

Text continues on p. 99

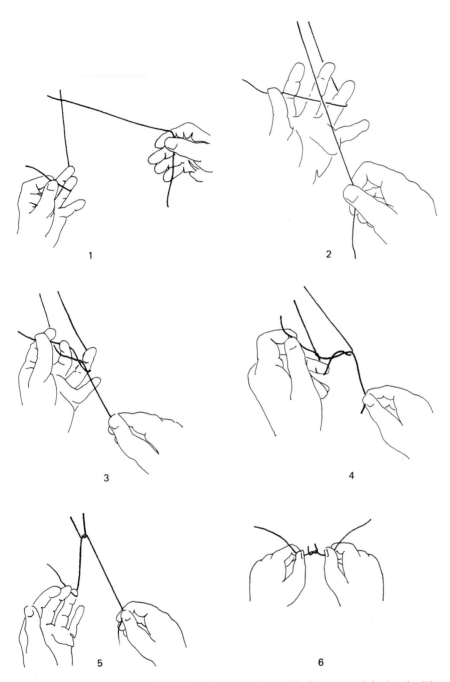

FIGURE 8-2. One-hand tie: (1) holding the suture lines, (2) placement of the hands, (3) starting the first knot, (4) tying first knot, (5) laying the first knot, (6) finishing first tie, (7) starting second knot, (8) position of hands, (9) completing second knot tie, (10) beginning to lay second knot, (11) laying second knot (note the crossing of the hands to produce a square knot), (12) finishing second knot tie.

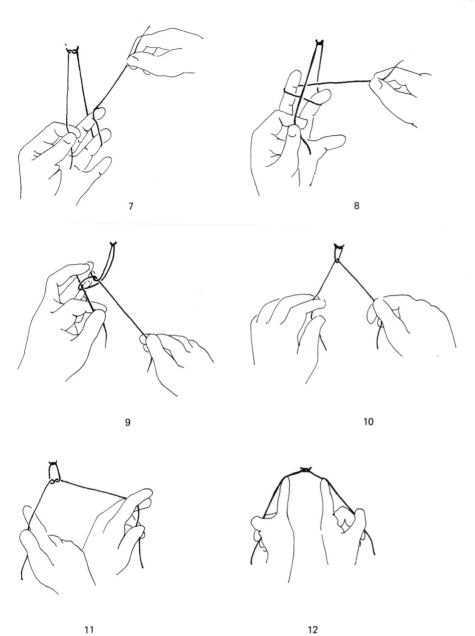

7

8

9

10

11

12

FIGURE 8-2. *(continued)*

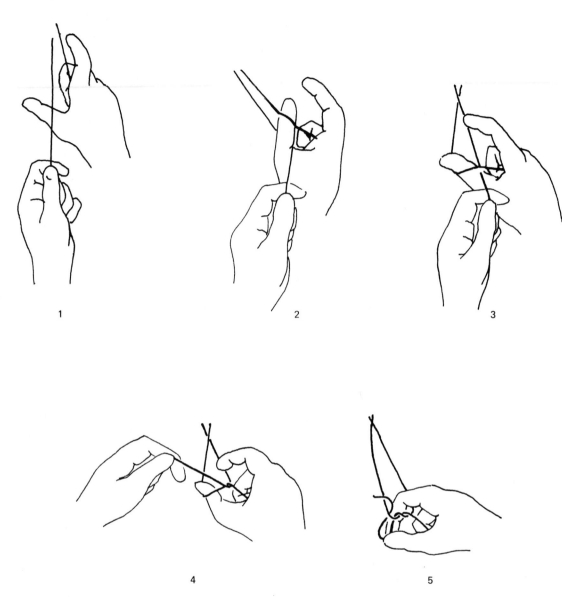

FIGURE 8-3. Two-hand tie: (1) holding suture lines, (2) position of hands for first knot, (3) starting tie, (4) beginning to tie the knot, (5) mid-tie, (6) finishing tie of first knot, (7) positions of hands for second knot, (8) beginning tie, (9) mid-tie, (10) completing tie, (11) laying of second knot.

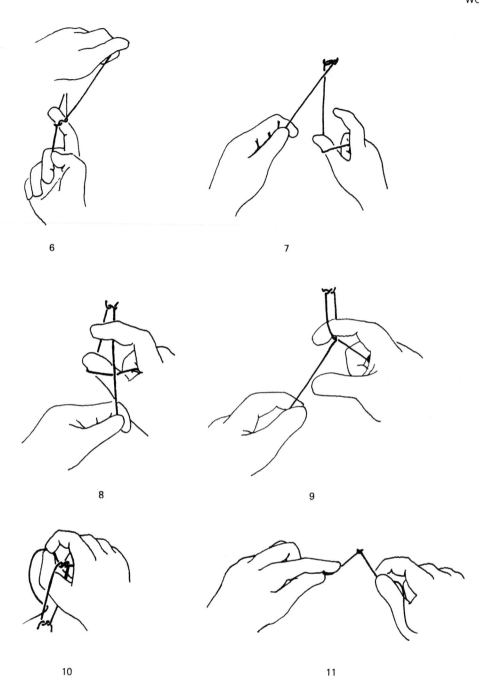

6

7

8

9

10

11

FIGURE 8-3. *(continued)*

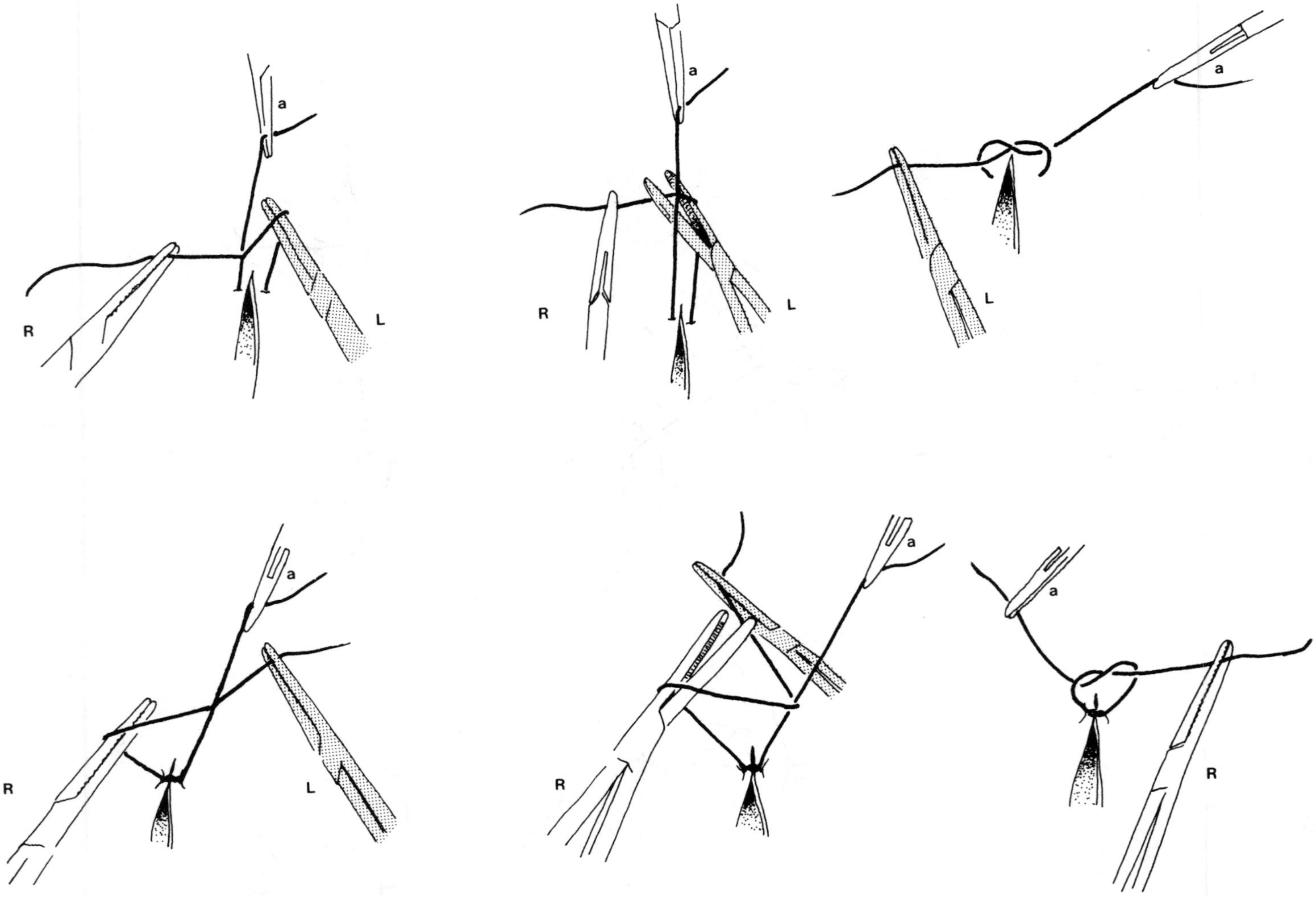

FIGURE 8-4. Instrument tie.

98

be handed to the operator in the following ways: (1) **as a free tie,** which is then manually passed around the tip of the clamp that is holding the end of the vessel, or as a **suture tie** using a needle (Fig. 8-5), (2) **as a banjo string,** in which the suture extends from the end of a straight clamp, which is then passed around the vascular clamp (good for deep pelvic ligatures) (Fig. 8-6), or (3) the suture may be threaded through a curved needle and passed as **a transfixion suture,** in which the suture is sutured to the pedicle (Fig. 8-7). The transfixion suture should not be used on a vascular pedicle unless a free tie or banjo-string tie has been placed more proximal to the transfixion suture first. In obstetrics and gynecology, surgical gut (e.g., 0 to 3-0 chromic catgut), or Vicryl, is commonly used inside the abdomen; however, nonabsorbable sutures may be used as long as they are not placed near the bladder mucosa, the vaginal mucosa, or in the subcutaneous tissues. Permanent sutures have a tendency to migrate to a "surface," and they may work their way through the tissues to the epithelial surface. In infected patients, monofilament sutures should be used instead of the multifilament (braided) sutures, since the latter have a tendency to sequester micro-organisms between the filaments and do not allow the migration of polymorphonuclear cells.

6. Abdominal closure

a. Peritoneum

The posterior parietal peritoneum of the pelvis may be closed with a continuous 2-0 plain, 2-0 chromic catgut, or 2-0 Vicryl suture, which is placed with minimal tension to approximate the peritoneal edges and to eliminate any areas into which the bowel might herniate causing a later postoperative bowel obstruction. Following the pelvic surgery, it is advisable to cover the operative field by placing the sigmoid colon and the omentum over the site. If the anterior peritoneum is closed by sutures, it is important to constantly visualize the placement of the tip of the needle so as to preclude the inclusion of a loop of bowel in the closure. This closure may be made by a running 2-0 absorbable suture with about every third stitch being locked. Some surgeons do not close either the posterior or the anterior peritoneum because of the supposedly increased incidence of peritoneal adhesions and the possibility of subsequent bowel obstruction.

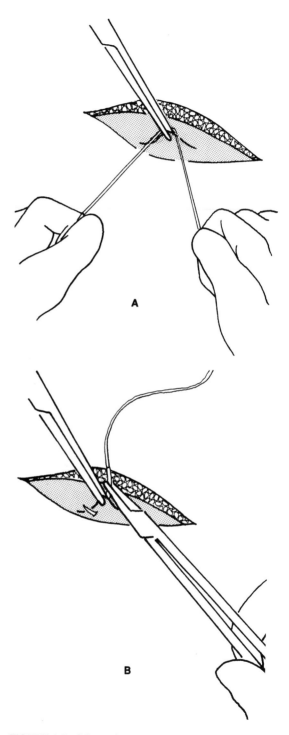

FIGURE 8-5. (A) Single strand ties. (B) Suture ligatures.

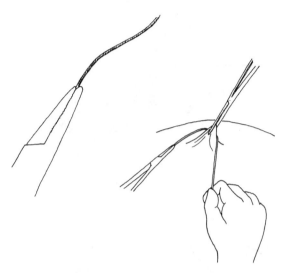

FIGURE 8-6. "Banjo string" tie. This suture provides good control of the ligature in cases in which a deeply placed ligation is to be performed. The suture material should issue from the tip of the forceps. When tying, the tip of the banjo string forceps should be placed on the tip of the vascular clamp and the vascular clamp rotated slightly with the point directed away from the banjo string. This allows the ligature to be easily tied without slipping off of the pedicle.

b. Retention sutures

In patients who are obese, anemic, diabetic, in poor condition, or who have had previous irradiation, it is advisable to place additional supporting **"retention sutures" in the abdominal wall upon closing the abdomen.** These are usually nonabsorbable (e.g., stainless steel, Prolene), widely placed, interrupted sutures placed either above the peritoneum to include the fascia, subcutaneous tissues, and skin, or through-and-through sutures that include the peritoneum and all layers of the abdominal wall. A plastic or rubber bridge is often used to keep the suture material off of the skin incision line. These sutures should be loosely tied to accommodate tissue swelling and may be readjusted at a later time postoperatively. Retention sutures should be removed after about 10–14 days.

c. Fascial sutures

Nonabsorbable sutures should be used in tissues that heal slowly, such as the abdominal wall rectus fascia. A Smead-Jones interrupted nonabsorbable suture may be placed in the fascia to provide for a strong fascial closure (mass closure) (Fig. 8-8). In a midline lower abdominal incision, the rectus fascia should be closed with 2-0 **nonabsorbable, interrupted, figure-of-eight sutures** placed at about 1–2 cm intervals with an adequate amount of fascial edge (1 cm) included in each bite. These sutures should not be tied under undue tension so as to strangulate the tissue, but should be tied with moderate tension to merely approximate the tissue. The muscles usualy do not need to be closed except when they are widely separated. In such a case, a few figure-of-eight or mattress sutures may be placed to approximate the muscles to the midline.

d. Subcutaneous sutures

When the skin incision is initially made, the following principles should be considered. The length of the incision should generally be slightly larger than the

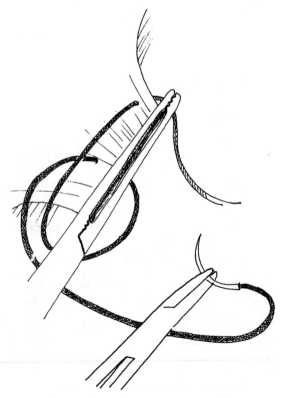

FIGURE 8-7. Transfixion suture.

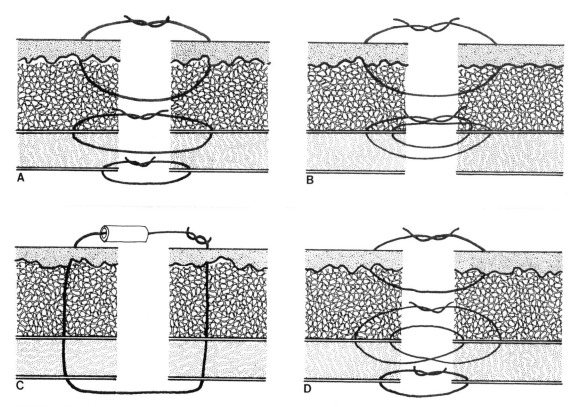

FIGURE 8-8. Abdominal incision closure techniques. (A) Layered. (B) Smead-Jones. (C) Through-and-through. (D) Far-near.

width of the surgeon's hand. The length of the subcutaneous tissue, fascial, and peritoneal incisions should be progressively smaller. You should avoid undercutting the deeper portions of the incision so that the closure will not leave unclosed dead spaces at the apices of the incision. These undercut areas may commonly collect serous effusions and cause seromas or hematomas in the incision. With the closure of the abdominal wall, the subcutaneous tissues should be approximated with interrupted 2-0 or 3-0 absorbable sutures that are placed at about 2–3 cm apart so as to completely obliterate the "dead space." Although some investigators have indicated that there is a higher incidence of wound infections when subcutaneous sutures are placed to obliterate the dead space, this has not been true in my experience.

e. Skin sutures

The skin may be closed in a variety of ways; however, the most cosmetic closure involves the use of the **sub-cuticular suture.** Although mattress sutures and metallic clips take less time to place than do subcuticular sutures, they often leave unsightly small pinpoint scars in the skin after the healing has occurred. In performing the subcuticular closure, it is important to be sure that each succeeding bite is placed at the exit point of the previous suture (Fig. 8-9). Nonabsorbable skin sutures should be removed in about 5–8 days, except for those about the face and neck, which should be removed in 2–5 days to prevent undue scarring.

f. Common types of suture techniques

The **common types of suture techniques** that are used in various surgical procedures include: (1) the vertical and horizontal mattress suture (Fig. 8-10), (2) the locking suture (Fig. 8-11), (3) the figure-of-eight suture (Fig. 8-12), (4) the interrupted and continuous suture (Fig. 8-13), (5) the interrupted Lembert and the continuous Lembert sutures (Fig. 8-14), and (6) the

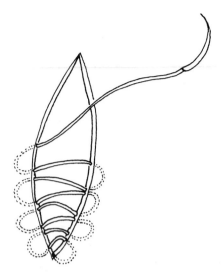

FIGURE 8-9. Subcuticular suture. Note that each bite starts where the previous suture exited. Do not place tension on the suture line.

pursestring suture (Fig. 8-15). Some of these sutures have particular applications, whereas others are used more generally. The vertical and the horizontal mattress sutures are often used in skin closure. The locking suture is often utilized to obtain hemostasis of the vaginal cuff after a hysterectomy. Figure-of-eight sutures are often used in areas where there is persistent bleeding and a specific bleeding vessel cannot be isolated, or in the approximation of friable tissues. Interrupted or continuous sutures are used in many different situations. The interrupted or continuous inverting Lembert suture is often used in the closure of a uterine incision made for a cesarean section. The pursestring suture is used in closing the peritoneum after a vaginal hysterectomy or in the closure of the appendiceal stump after an appendectomy.

7. Needle design

Surgical needles have three basic components: (1) the eye, (2) the body, and (3) the point (Fig. 8-16).

a. The eye

The eye of a surgical needle may be one of three different varieties: (1) swaged on (i.e., eyeless), (2) closed, and (3) the French eye

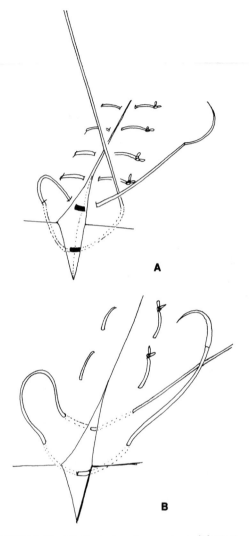

FIGURE 8-10. (A) Vertical mattress suture. (B) Horizontal mattress suture.

(split or spring eye). Approximately 80% of sutures now have the needles swaged on so that the suture is intimately attached to the needle. Such needles minimize tissue trauma, since there is no undue bulging at the point where the suture joins to the needle. In addition, the needle size and shape is appropriately mated to the suture. Controlled-release swaged-on sutures will "pop off" with a sudden tug on the needle. This latter type of needle is ideal for situations in which interrupted sutures are needed, since you can place many sutures rapidly.

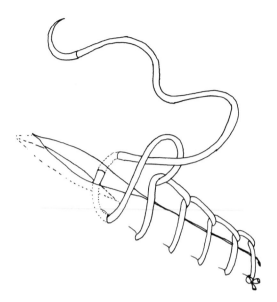

FIGURE 8-11. Locking suture.

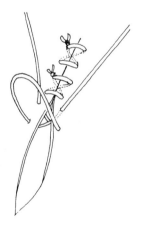

FIGURE 8-12. Figure-of-eight suture.

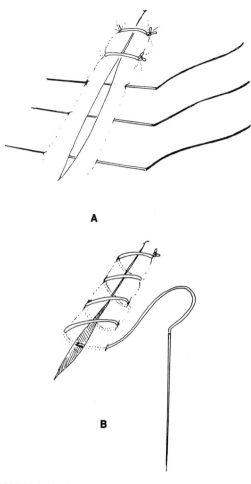

FIGURE 8-13. (A) Interrupted sutures. (B) Continuous suture.

Closed-eye needles have an eye much as an ordinary sewing needle, and therefore must be threaded each time before use. The large size of the eye and the strand of thread that passes through it will cause more tissue damage than the swaged-on type.

The **French eye** is a slit into which a suture may be snapped into place. These are often used with silk sutures to close the fascia, since, like the pop-off sutures, they can be placed rapidly due to the quick release mechanism.

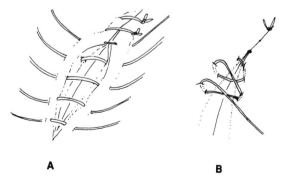

FIGURE 8-14. (A) Interrupted Lembert suture. (B) Continuous Lembert inverting suture.

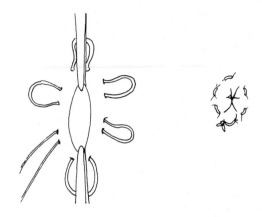

FIGURE 8-15. Pursestring suture.

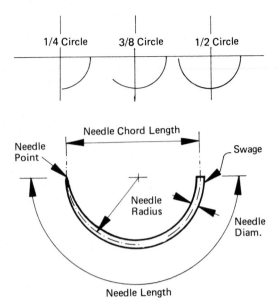

FIGURE 8-16. Anatomy of a surgical needle. (Redrawn with permission from Ethicon, Inc.: *Wound Closure Manual.* Sommerville, N.J.: Ethicon, Inc., 1985, p. 46).

b. The body

The cross-sectional area of a needle's body may be round, flattened, rectangular, triangular, or oval. Longitudinal ribbing may be present to prevent the rotational movement of the needle in the needle holder. The chord length (i.e., the distance from the point to the swage) is also an important feature.

The needle may be straight or curved. Straight needles are used for skin suturing (e.g., Keith needles). Curved needles are the most commonly used type and require that the surgeon rotate his or her wrist in passing the half-circle needle through the tissue.

c. The point

The point of the needle is always designed to penetrate the tissue in a smooth manner. Since the skin is relatively tough, **cutting needles** are preferred when sewing skin. Minimal tissue damage may be expected with **round or tapered needles,** which are used in tissues that are easily penetrated. **The size of the chord of the needle** depends upon where the needle will be utilized. Small-chord needles are more appropriate for small areas in which the "swing" of the needle is limited by the anatomical restrictions. **The shape of the needle** (i.e., the fraction of a circle that is encompassed, either ¼, ⅜, ½, or ⅝) is also important, with the half-circle needle being the one most commonly used in gynecologic surgery.

8. Surgical instruments

All medical students are exposed to the various common surgical instruments during their clinical rota-

tions on a surgical subspecialty service; however, minimal attempts have been made in the past to teach the students the advantages of each of these tools. Perhaps the reason for this has been that physicians have developed their own likes and dislikes regarding surgical instruments. Indeed, a listing of just some of the different hemostatic clamps (e.g., Kelly, Halsted, Mayo, Ochsner) is indicative of the fact that many physicians design their own instruments for specific surgical procedures.

It is worthwhile, however, to at least have an acquaintance with the common surgical instruments. **Hemostatic clamps** come in a variety of sizes in order to accommodate their use in the open abdominal cavity as well as within the small confined spaces of the pelvis. Their tips may be *straight or curved* (e.g., Crile, Kelly, Pean), or they may have a right-angled tip, as is seen in the Mixter hemostatic forceps. The grooves along the clamp surface may be transverse (e.g., Halsted), or longitudinal (e.g., Carmalt). The tip may contain a beak-like projection that inserts into a notch in the other blade of the forceps (e.g., Ochsner), which provides for a better grip on the tissue in order to prevent the tissue from sliding out of the clamp (Fig. 8-17, Fig. 8-18).

A ratchet lock between the finger-hole rings is pro-

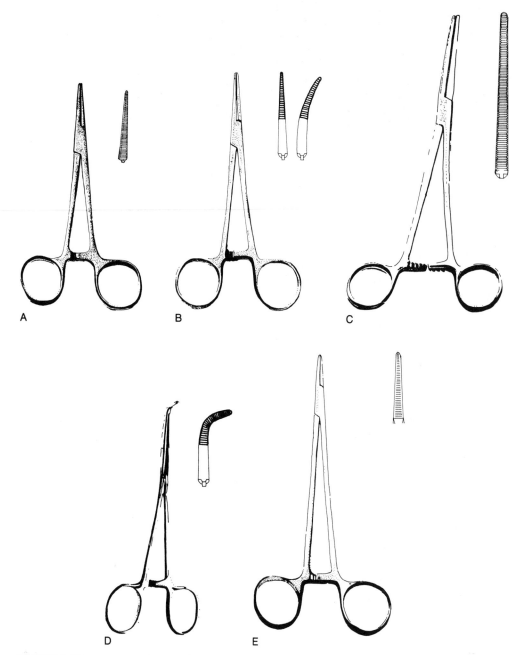

FIGURE 8-17. Hemostatic forceps. (A) Crile forceps. (B) Kelly forceps. (C) Péan forceps. (D) Mixter forceps. (E) Halsted forceps.

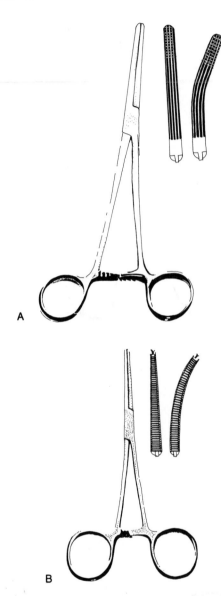

A

B

FIGURE 8-18. Tissue grasping forceps. (A) Carmalt. Note the longitudinal grooves in the blades, which aid in grasping the tissue. (B) Ochsner. Note the tooth at the end of the clamp, which keeps the tissue from slipping out of the clamp.

vided to keep the blades of the clamp closed. When hemostatic clamps are placed, they should always be closed completely so that the vascular pedicle does not slip out of the jaws. Larger forceps (e.g., Pean, Kelly, Heaney, Ochsner, Carmalt) are used to grasp

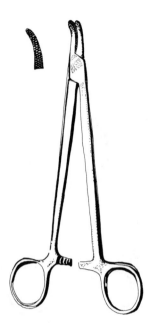

FIGURE 8-19. Heaney needle holder.

large bites of tissue along the side of the uterus or in clamping the infundibulopelvic ligaments during a hysterectomy. Small forceps (e.g., Halsted mosquito) are used to clamp small blood vessels in the subcutaneous tissues and on the surfaces of various organs.

A special clamp is used to hold the needle during the placement of sutures. These clamps are called **needle holders,** and they may be straight or curved (e.g., Heaney) (Fig. 8-19) and may come in several lengths.

The **knife handles** have replaceable blades that may extend in a straight forward fashion or may turn in at a 45-degree angle. The blades come in a variety of sizes, such as 10, 11, 12, 15, 20, 21, 22, and 23, and they may be slightly curved or straight, or wide or narrow (Fig. 8-20). You should hold the knife with your thumb and first two fingers when cutting tissue; to hold the knife as you would a pencil is usually only necessary on very delicate or small incisions.

Surgical **suture scissors** may be straight or curved. You should not cut sutures with **tissue scissors,** which will dull the cutting edge of the operating scissors. The tissue scissors used for cutting fascia (e.g., Mayo) are usually heavier than the usual dissecting

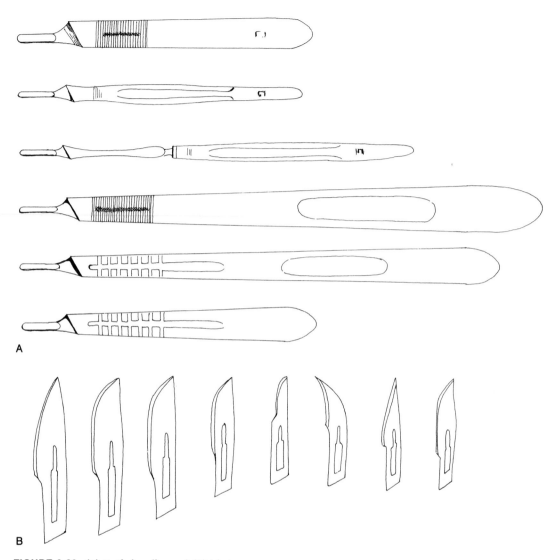

FIGURE 8-20. (A) Knife handles and (B) blades.

scissors (e.g., Metzenbaum), which are slightly more delicate and have longer handles (Fig. 8-21).

There are a variety of tissue **thumb forceps** available. The tips may be *smooth* (with cross striations), *toothed, or broad* (e.g., Russian). The small tissue forceps (e.g., Adson's thumb forceps), are used in the closure of the skin. Long forceps (e.g., dressing forceps, tissue forceps) may be used deep in the pelvis, where there is little room available to maneuver (Fig. 8-22).

Towel clamps assist in maintaining the drapes in position about the area of the surgical incision. A **single-toothed tenaculum** is utilized on the anterior cervix to stabilize the uterus during an endometrial biopsy (Fig. 8-23). A **multi-toothed tenaculum** (e.g., Lahey Goiter vulsellum) is helpful in elevating and placing traction upon the uterine fundus or the cervix during an abdominal or vaginal hysterectomy.

There are a number of special **retractors** that can be used to provide exposure of the operative site,

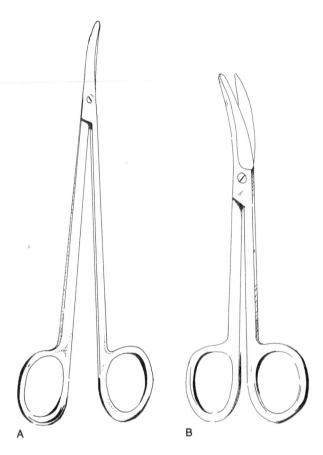

FIGURE 8-21. Operating scissors. (A) Metzenbaum scissors. (B) Mayo scissors.

A   B

such as the **Richardson,** the Richardson-Eastman, the **Deaver,** and the Mayo. In addition, **malleable ribbon retractors** may be shaped to fit into odd-shaped areas to provide exposure (Fig. 8-24). There are more complex **self-retaining retractors,** such as the Balfour and the O'Sullivan/O'Connor (Fig. 8-25).

A **suction tube** may be used to remove large amounts of blood and fluids from the surgical site. Small pledgets of gauze may be folded and placed between the jaws of a **sponge forcep** to hold tissues aside and remove blood staining over a small area. In the performance of a cesarean section, **Pennington clamps** may be used to assist in the closure of the uterine incision and to suppress some of the bleeding from the cut edges of the uterine muscle (Fig. 8-26).

During vaginal surgery, a **weighted speculum** may be placed in the vagina for the exposure of the vaginal vault. The visualization of the lateral or ante-

rior vaginal areas with a **vaginal retractor** blade allows the surgeon to operate within this small space with adequate exposure (Fig. 8-27).

9. Wound dehiscence

Any wound breakdown is referred to as a **wound dehiscence.** The term **evisceration** is often used synonymously when there is total dehiscence of the abdominal wall with the possible exteriorization of the bowel. While this complication is rare (0.3–3%), it may carry a mortality rate as high as 15–20% when it does occur.

Some of the etiologic factors that have been implicated in wound dehiscence are: (1) low vertical abdominal incisions, (2) the types of sutures utilized, (3) the strength of the tissues, (4)

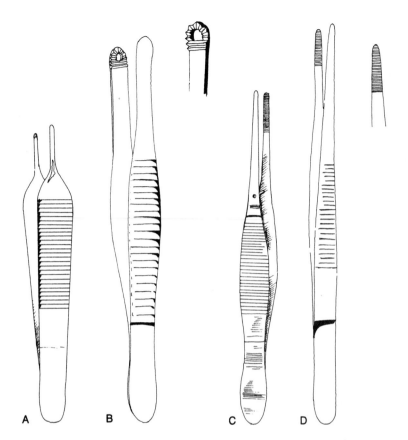

FIGURE 8-22. Grasping forceps. (A) Adson forceps. (B) Russian forceps. (C) Thumb forceps. (D) Dressing forceps.

the mechanical stresses that the wound is exposed to in the postoperative period, and (5) systemic factors.

It has been noted in some studies that there is a greater incidence of wound dehiscence when absorbable suture is used in the closure of the fascia. Low midline verticle incisions have a higher incidence of dehiscence than do transverse incisions. If the sutures are placed too far apart, or if the tissue bites do not include a sufficient amount of fascial tissue, then dehiscence is more likely to occur. *Elderly, obese, diabetic, infected, or protein-deficient patients will also have a higher wound disruption rate than others. Finally, patients who have excessive coughing, vomiting, or abdominal distention postoperatively have a greater risk of wound dehiscence due to the mechanical disruption of the sutures. Dehiscence usually occurs on about the fifth to the eighth postoperative day.*

The treatment of a surgical wound dehiscence, if the fascia has been disrupted, is immediate surgical closure. The wound should be opened, cleaned, debrided, and then closed with through-and-through retention sutures at an interval of about 5–6 cm. These retention sutures should remain in place for 10–14 days. The fascial edges should be closed with interrupted, nonabsorbable, monofilament sutures (e.g., Smead-Jones) to prevent later incisional hernias. Broad-spectrum antibiotics should be utilized in almost all cases, since infection is associated with more than half of all cases of dehiscence.

10. Abdominal drains

Drainage is accomplished by placing one or more drains into a restricted space in the abdomen or

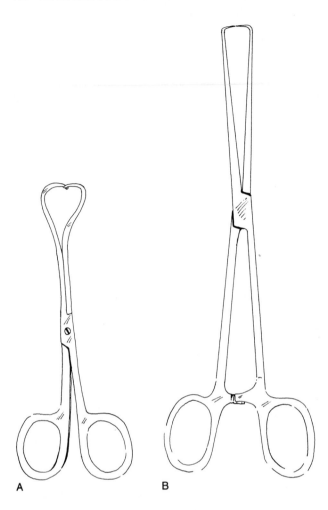

A   B

FIGURE 8-23. (A) Towel clamp. (B) Tenaculum.

within the abdominal wall and leading them to the outer skin surface or into the vagina. **The purpose of a drain is to drain a specific collection of blood, serum, or pus.** This drainage allows the small space to collapse so that a seroma, a hematoma, or an abscess will not develop. Usually, drains are placed to take care of a capillary ooze that cannot be corrected by vascular clamps or hemostatic agents. The drainage of the entire abdomen is not feasible.

a. Drain types

In order to drain a small dead space of fluid material, the drain must be **soft and flexible** so that it may be placed in odd positions within the tissues without

damage to the surrounding organs by erosion. The drain should be able to be easily removed following surgery and should be nonreactive with the tissue. **A passive outflow drain,** such as a simple tube, a corrugated rubber drain, or a Penrose drain, will allow the fluids to migrate through the drain by gravity and tissue pressure. **A closed-suction drain,** such as the Jackson-Pratt and the Hemovac drains, utilizes a negative suction to the drain tube in order to drain areas where gravity will not function. Since these drains will also suction tissue into the drain holes, an open suction or **sump drain** can be used to allow equalization of the pressure in the space. The Davol, Shirley, Saratoga, and Axiom brands are examples of commercial sump drains.

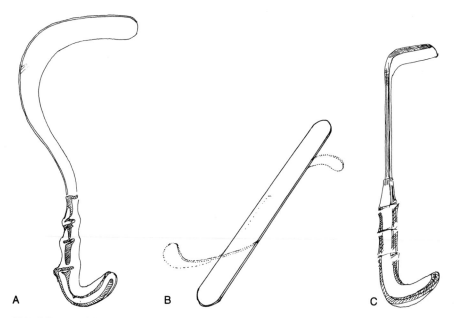

FIGURE 8-24. (A) Deaver retractor. (B) Malleable retractor. (C) Richardson retractor.

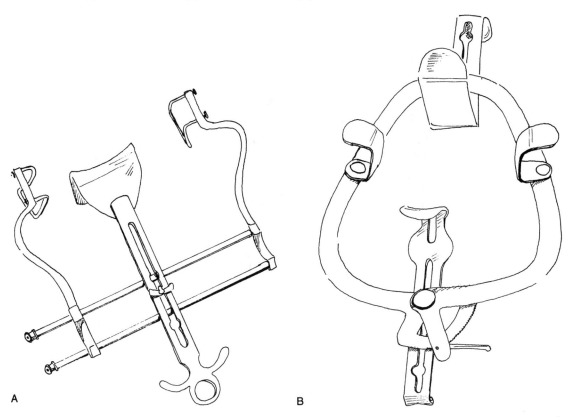

FIGURE 8-25. (A) Balfour self-retaining retractor. (B) O'Sullivan/O'Connor self-retaining retractor.

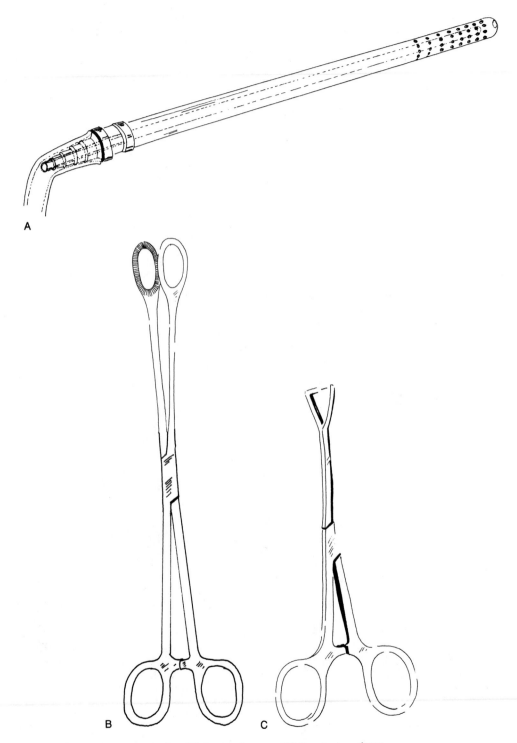

FIGURE 8-26. (A) Suction tube. (B) Sponge forceps. (C) Pennington clamp.

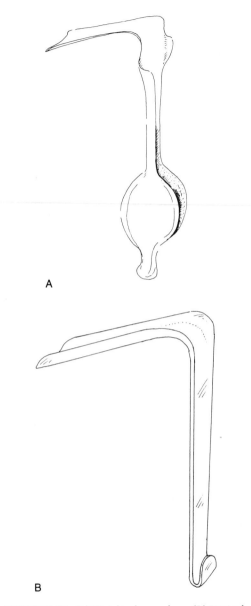

A

B

FIGURE 8-27. (A) Weighted speculum. (B) Vaginal retractor.

b. Complications

Drains that remain in place for longer than 72 hours may cause a secondary infection to develop (1–3%). If the drain exits through the wound itself, the infection rate may be higher (e.g., 4%); thus, a separate stab wound should generally be used. Incisional hernias also seem to be less common when a separate stab wound is utilized. A drain tube might also cause damage to adjacent organs and may erode into blood vessels.

c. Indications for drains

In any traumatized wound, even after debridement, there will be areas of devitalized tissue still remaining that may form the nidus for the development of an abscess. Suction drains in such wounds may decrease this risk by removing fluids. Pelvic abscesses that point into the cul-de-sac of Douglas can frequently be opened by a vaginal colpotomy incision, with the placement of a Malecot drain after the abscess cavity adhesions and loculi have been digitally broken up.

d. Drain management

It is important to know how to properly place the drain within the tissues in a closed space. There should be a *sufficient number of holes present* in the drain to assure that they will not become easily plugged by debris following surgery. The drain should be remote from the suture line but should not be longer than necessary. Following surgery, the drain should be *slowly advanced each day* to allow the bottom of the "dead space" to seal itself and to prevent the development of an abscess cavity. **Usually, when the amount of fluid return greatly diminishes (24–72 hours), the drain may be safely removed.**

CHAPTER 9

Gynecologic and obstetric statistics

• • • • • • • • • • • • • •

Teach him how to observe, give him plenty of facts to observe, and the lessons will come out of the facts themselves.

—*Sir William Osler**

• • • • • • • • • • • • • •

1. Introduction

During your medical career, you should learn to utilize medical statistics that deal with **demographics** (i.e., population statistics) as well as those that deal with **sample studies** (i.e., experimental statistics). Both of these fields are very important in the practice of medicine and will provide you with a coherent view of the medical world. Sample statistics are included in almost every medical journal article that you will read, whereas population statistics will acquaint you with the occurrence rates of various conditions.

Obstetrics is that branch of medicine concerned with the reproductive performance of the female, whereas gynecology consists of the study of diseases and conditions of the female generative tract. The subject of obstetrics has far-reaching significance; it is not an exaggeration to state that it literally involves the fate of the whole human race. The causes and manifestations of congenital anomalies are of supreme importance because the effects of environmental toxins, chemicals, and irradiation on the developing human organism at least have the potential of being truly catastrophic for future generations. Certainly, on a smaller scale, the fate of

countries and empires throughout the centuries have undoubtedly been influenced by the level of competence possessed by their obstetric attendants. For example, in 1817, George IV of England had no sons and only one daughter, Princess Charlotte of Wales. Dr. Richard Croft, who was the son-in-law of Thomas Denman (one of the leading conservative physicians of his day), was her obstetric attendant. Dr. Croft allowed the Princess to labor for more than 50 hours, 24 of which were in the second stage of labor (52 hours after the escape of the liquor amnii). Not only was a stillborn male infant delivered, but the mother died as well. Later, it was felt that the judicious use of forceps to effect the delivery could perhaps have saved both of their lives. The loss of this potential male heir shifted the line of succession to Queen Victoria. Dr. Richard Croft later committed suicide.

The collection of vital statistics in obstetrics allows us to monitor the reproductive parameters of the human race. The term **obstetrics** is derived from the Latin word **obstetrix (midwife),** which may be defined as that branch of medicine that is concerned with the birth process, including those conditions that attend it before and after. The root French word **obstare** (to stand in front of, or to stand in the way) is also often quoted as a possible origin of the word. While the term **midwifery** has been used more commonly in England than in the United States, the term **obstetrics** has become the more popular designation in the past 50 years.

2. Obstetric statistics

a. Basic statistics

It is important for the **vital statistics** of obstetric care to be collected and evaluated on an ongoing basis. It is

---

*Reprinted with permission from Robert Bennett Bean, *Sir William Osler: Aphorisms from His Bedside Teachings and Writings,* William Bennett Bean, ed. Springfield, Ill.: Charles C Thomas, Publisher, 1968, p. 46.

equally important that such data be expressed in a logical and standard manner so that a comparison may be made of the data from different areas of the world.

In 1986, it was estimated that there were 3,371,000 babies born in the United States and that about 2,099,000 people died. The fertility rate was about 64.9 live births per 1,000 women aged 15 to 44 years. The overall mortality rate of the population was 8.7 deaths per 1,000 population. The infant mortality rate was 10.4 per 1,000 live births. It was estimated that 2,400,000 couples were married that year, to give a marriage rate of 10 per 1,000 population.

The following terminology has been generally accepted:

1. **Fertility rate.** The fertility rate is the number of live births per 1,000 women between the ages of 15 and 44 years of age.

2. **Birth.** The complete expulsion of a fetus from the mother is considered to be a birth. If the fetus is born dead, then a distinction must be made between a "birth" and an "abortion." The definition of an **abortion** varies slightly from state to state, but in most states it is defined as the birth of any "dead fetus that weighs less than 500 grams" (in Louisiana it is 350 grams) or, if the weight is unknown, then any "fetus whose gestational age is less than 20 weeks" is considered an abortion.

3. **Live birth.** Any fetus that is born with any signs of life (e.g., breathing, heart beat, voluntary movements, or crying) is considered a live birth regardless of the fetal weight or the gestational age.

4. **Stillbirth.** A stillbirth is the birth of a fetus who shows no signs of life and who weighs more than 500 grams, or who has a gestational age greater than 20 weeks.

5. **Stillbirth rate (Fetal death rate).** The stillbirth rate is the number of stillbirths per 1,000 infants born.

6. **Neonatal death.** The definition of a neonatal death is divided into early and late deaths. An **early neonatal death** is one in which a liveborn infant dies within the first 7 days of life. A **late neonatal death** is one in which the infant dies within the first 28 days of life, excluding the first 7 days. Another evaluation involves the neonatal interval, which may be categorized as: (1) **neonatal period I:** from birth through 23 hours and 59 minutes, (2) **neonatal period II:** 24 hours through 6 days, 23 hours, and 59 minutes, and (3) **neonatal period III:** from 7 through 27 days, 23 hours and 59 minutes. Neonatal deaths are recorded per 1,000 live births.

7. **Neonatal mortality rate.** The neonatal mortality rate is the number of neonatal deaths that occur per 1,000 live births.

8. **Perinatal mortality rate.** The perinatal mortality rate is the number of stillbirths and the number of neonatal deaths per 1,000 live births. The current perinatal mortality rate in the United States is of the order of 15:1,000 live births. Another evaluation involves the perinatal interval, which consists of: (1) **perinatal period I:** 28 weeks of completed gestation through the first 7 days of life, and (2) **perinatal period II:** which extends from 20 weeks' gestation through the first 27 days of life.

9. **Infant death rate.** The infant death rate is the number of infant deaths under 1 year of age per 1,000 live births. In the United States (1983), the infant mortality was 10.9.

10. **Term birth.** A term birth is one in which the infant is delivered between 38 and 42 weeks' gestation.

11. **Premature birth.** A premature birth is one in which the infant is delivered prior to 38 weeks' gestation.

12. **Postmature birth (postterm, postdates).** A postmature birth is one in which the infant is delivered after 42 completed weeks' gestation.

13. **Maternal mortality rate.** The maternal mortality rate is the number of maternal deaths that occur due to the reproductive process per 100,000 live births. Maternal deaths have been subdivided according to the different etiologies as follows:

    a. **Direct maternal death.** A direct maternal death is one that is directly attributable to obstetric causes or the quality of the obstetric care, usually within a time period of 42 days after the pregnancy; however, in some jurisdictions the time limit is 90–120 days.

    b. **Indirect maternal death.** An indirect

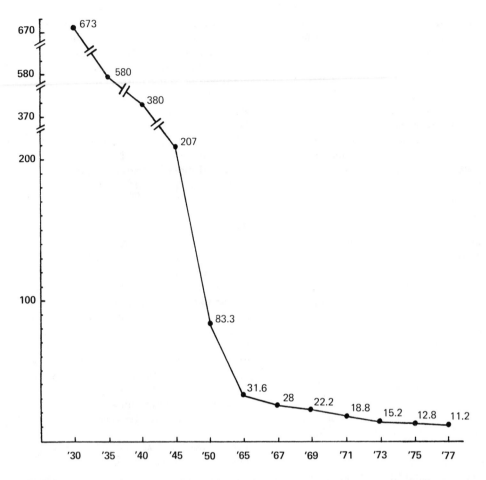

FIGURE 9-1. Maternal deaths per 100,000 live births in the United States from 1930 to 1977. (Adapted from Mortality Statistics, 1977, National Center for Health Statistics HEW, vol. 28, no. 1 (Suppl), May 11, 1979. Redrawn with permission from D. Cavanagh, R. E. Woods, T. C. F. O'Connor, and R. A. Knuppel, *Obstetric Emergencies,* 3rd ed., Philadelphia: Harper & Row, Inc. (J. B. Lippincott Company), 1978, p. 421.)

maternal death is one in which the death is attributable to a concomitant disease or condition that is not directly related to the pregnancy but may have been aggravated by the pregnancy.

   c. Nonmaternal death. A nonmaternal death is any maternal death that occurs by accident or through any other causes not related to the pregnancy.

14. Reproductive mortality. Reproductive mortality consists of those deaths that are either the direct result of pregnancy or of the use of contraceptive techniques per 1,000 women.

b. Causes of maternal deaths

The maternal mortality rate in the United States decreased dramatically between 1930 and 1977 (Fig.

9-1). **The maternal mortality rate in the United States in 1985 was 7.8:100,000 live births with nearly three-fourths of the deaths occurring in blacks.** This disparity between the races is probably due to the generally unfavorable social and economic conditions that are present in the black population, coupled with the fact that black patients tend not to seek appropriate antepartum care as often as white patients. The maternal mortality rate has decreased about 30-fold over the past 40 years; however, it has been estimated that 75% of these deaths are still possibly preventable, which indicates that there is considerable room for improvement in the future. Since patients in the lower socioeconomic groups, especially nonwhite patients, have a higher maternal mortality rate, it would seem that future government expenditures for obstetric health care should be largely directed toward these people.

The triad of hemorrhage (about 13%), pregnancy-induced hypertension (i.e., toxemia) (about 17%), and infection (about 8%) have accounted for about 38% of all obstetric maternal deaths. Embolism as a cause of maternal death has also been more common in recent years and has been reported in some studies to be as high as 20%. *Anesthesia-related deaths occur in about 4% of cases. Cardiac disease has also been listed as a common cause of maternal death, and cerebral vascular accidents account for about 4% of maternal deaths.*

There is generally an increase in the maternal mortality rate in patients who are 35 years of age or older, as compared to those patients who are 20–29 years old. In a recent report prepared by the Centers for Disease Control (CDC), it was noted that women 35 years of age or older have a 4-fold increased incidence of dying in childbirth compared to younger women. The leading causes of death in this older group were obstetric hemorrhage, embolism, and hypertensive conditions, in that order. Interestingly, the maternal mortality rates are highest in the southern United States and lowest in the western portion of the country. It has also been noted that about 27% of the deaths have occurred in unmarried patients.

About 17% of maternal deaths occur in pregnancies that have abortive outcomes, such as ectopic pregnancies, abortions, and cases involving hydatidiform moles (see Chapter 27). **The maternal mortality rate for patients who undergo cesarean sections is less than 1:1,000.**

c. Causes of fetal deaths

The perinatal mortality rate has decreased over 50% during the past quarter-century to a level of about 15:1,000 live births (1985). Usually, stillbirths (7.9:1,000) make up about one-half of the perinatal mortality rate, with the neonatal deaths (7.0:1,000 live births) (1985) accounting for the remainder. Although the perinatal mortality rate is a crude reflection of the quality of overall obstetric practice, fetal morbidity is a much better measure of the level of care. Even this, however, is not an accurate measure of care. Not all of the fetal neurological and intellectual deficits that occur in infants can be explained on the basis of the quality of obstetric care. Many infants who have sustained significant neurological damage have acquired such injuries early in the pregnancy due to uncontrollable factors. The obstetric attendant should not be held responsible by the patient, or by the courts, for an infant who sustains such damage, unless there is clear-cut evidence of a cause-and-effect relationship between inappropriate health care and the damage that is present in the infant.

The most prominent cause of perinatal mortality and morbidity is prematurity, and it is in this group that a large proportion of the neurologically damaged infants may be found. In the past, obstetric management of the labor and delivery process may have played a more important role in fetal damage; however, obstetric care has dramatically improved over the past 35 years, which is reflected in the decrease in the perinatal mortality rate from 39.7:1,000 in 1950 to 15.0:1,000 in 1985. The prenatal recognition of congenital anomalies has also improved. The usual incidence of abnormalities is about 2–3% at birth; however, by the end of the first year, this figure increases to 7.5% as other anomalies are detected.

A number of changes in obstetric management over the past quarter-century have contributed much to the improvement of both maternal and perinatal morbidity and mortality rates. The development of high-quality physician training programs, the availability and proliferation of very potent antibiotics, the expansion of blood-banking capabilities, and the liberalization of the indications for cesarean section have all been important advances. The development of highly sophisticated neonatal intensive care techniques, as well as the advent of the use of ultrasound and electronic fetal monitoring, have also provided the physician with an unparalleled opportunity to salvage infants that only a few years ago could not have been saved.

3. Demographic statistics

a. Introduction

The practicing physician should properly be concerned about population dynamics. **Demography may be defined as the statistical study of the size, density, distribution, and vital statistics of human populations.** Your responsibility as a physician does not stop with the treatment of your patients on a one-to-one basis, but extends to the people in your community, state, country, and even to the rest of the world. The occurrence of a peculiar fetal anomaly would be an unusual event in the busy physician's practice. If several infants with a very rare anomaly were to be delivered within a community, or even in a particular state or group of countries, the conclusion that some toxin or environmental factor might have caused these anomalies becomes inescapable. *Such was the case with the medication thalidomide, which was administered as a sedative to pregnant women throughout Europe in the late 1950s and early 1960s. Nearly 4,000 to 5,000 infants developed phocomelia (seal-limb deformity) before the problem was recognized, and then an additional period of time occurred before it was traced to thalidomide and the drug was taken off the market. By that time, more than 8,000 infants had been affected by phocomelia.*

In order to detect trends in a disease or abnormal condition, data must be collected to identify the normal incidence of the various problems. This may be done by taking a *census* of a group of people or by conducting a *survey* in which a *representative sample of the population* is studied, and then extrapolating the results to apply to the whole group. In most modern societies, many events are now recorded routinely, such as births, deaths, marriages, divorces, and adoptions; however, even 200 years ago, such was not the case. The first U.S. population census was taken in 1790.

b. Terminology

A number of statistics have been used to monitor changes in the population. Some of these parameters

determine the growth or stability of a country's population; others look at the survivals in different age groups; while still others determine the average life span of members of the population.

1. **The crude birth rate (CBR)** is the number of total births per 1,000 total population per year at midyear. The crude birth rate (CBR) may be high (i.e., more than 40) in countries such as Nigeria or Senegal, where there is little or no birth control, or less than 20 in countries like the United States, the Soviet Union, and Italy. In the United States between 1975 and 1980, the crude birth rate was 15.
2. **The crude death rate (CDR)** is the number of deaths per 1,000 total population per year at midyear. The high values (i.e., more than 15) are usually found in underdeveloped countries, while low values (i.e., less than 10) are found in countries with relatively young populations, such as Korea, Brazil, and Colombia. Both the crude birth rate (CBR) and the crude death rate (CDR) are influenced by the age and predominant sex of the population.
3. **The crude rate of natural increase (CRNI)** consists of the crude birth rate (CBR) minus the crude death rate (CDR) per 1,000 population per year. Thus, if there is a larger CBR than CDR, then the population is increasing.
4. **The population growth rate (PGR)** consists of the crude rate of natural increase (CRNI) plus the sum of the migration of people in and out of the population.
5. **The age-specific fertility rate (ASFR)** is the number of live births per 1,000 per year within a specified age group, which has usually been designated as either 15–44 or 15–49, utilizing 5-year groupings within these limits.
6. **The age-specific marital fertility rate (ASMFR)** refers to the number of live births per 1,000 per year among married women within a specific age group. This statistic contrasts with the *general fertility rate (GFR),* which is the number of live births per 1,000 women of reproductive age (i.e., 15–44 or 15–49 years).
7. **The life expectancy (LE)** is the average number of years of life remaining in individuals at a specific age. When this figure is projected from birth, it becomes the life expec-

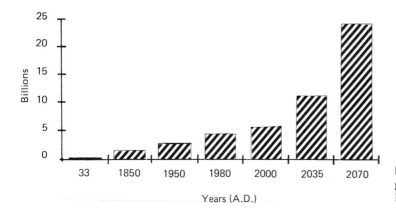

FIGURE 9-2. World population growth with projected population levels.

tancy of the population as a whole. Since women live longer than men, the life expectancy (LE) is usually computed on the basis of sex. The 1985 LE projection at birth for males is 71.2 years, whereas for females it is 78.2 years.

c. Trends

A stable population is the fixed age structure a population attains with a constant level of fertility and mortality and no migration. A stationary population occurs when these statistics are equal and the growth rate is zero. **The world population growth is currently increasing at a rate of about 2% per year. This means that the population will double in 35 years and triple in 55 years.** With the population of the world estimated at 4.4 billion in 1980, it has been projected that the world population in the year 2000 will be about 6.2 billion. About 2 billion of these people will reside in China and India. **To place these statistics in proper perspective, it should be recalled that the world population at the time of Christ was about 250 million people. By 1850, there were nearly 1.2 billion people in the world; the world population increased to 2.5 billion by 1950 and to 4.4 billion by 1980.** If present trends continue, there may be more than **12 billion people in the world by the year 2035,** and more than **24 billion by 2070.** It is obvious that there is an exponential component in these increases that is just beginning to be truly appreciated (Fig. 9-2). The resources of the world may be sorely taxed by such great numbers of people. In animal population

studies, when a certain population density is reached, the number of animals stabilizes to conform to the available food supply. This stabilization is achieved through an increased amount of infertility and stillbirths until births and deaths become essentially equal. In regard to our own species, it remains to be seen what kind of society we will eventually develop. Because of the possibilities of nuclear war, humankind itself may be the "most endangered species" on the planet earth, in that for the first time in history, we now have the capability to destroy all life on the planet. Furthermore, because medical science is conquering disease at an ever-increasing rate, perhaps we will reach our ultimate population level very quickly unless our aggression results in a global war with the elimination of much of the population, or unless the bulk of humankind travels to the stars, the final frontier, and relieves the earth of population overcrowding. Since the most aggressive members of our species are likely to be at the forefront of such a migration into space, the biblical injunction that "the meek shall inherit the earth" (Matthew 5:5) may indeed come true.

4. Sample statistics

One might inquire as to just why a non-research-oriented practicing physician should be interested in such things as a *statistical significance,* the *normal, or Gaussian, distribution,* and the *null hypothesis.* The answer is simple. **Every clinical decision requires the physician to draw on past experience as well as knowledge of current information available**

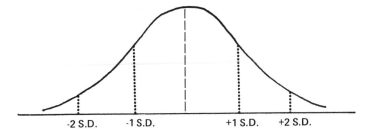

FIGURE 9-3. Normal statistical distribution curve.

in textbooks and scientific journals. In order to properly utilize this information, you must be able to evaluate it in terms of its "significance." To do this requires some degree of appreciation as to just what the statistical data means and whether it is information that might be relied upon to be true.

a. Null hypothesis and significance

One basic assumption usually made in evaluating research data is that **there really is no true difference between the study group and the control group**; in other words, that the difference is due to chance alone. **This assumption is called the null hypothesis.** In order to reject the null hypothesis and accept an alternative one, it is essential to use a level of probability (i.e., significance) that is small enough to remove the possibility of error as much as possible while at the same time being careful not to make this level of probability so strict that it allows the null hypothesis to be falsely rejected. The use of the 5% level (i.e., $P = 0.05$), means that there is a 95% chance that the two groups are really different and that the chance of error is only 5%. Obviously, if you select a level of significance of 1:1,000 (i.e., $P = 0.001$), and the sets of data are different enough to reach this level of significance, then your chance of making an error decreases to 1:1,000. On the other hand, if the selected level of significance is not reached, then you must accept the null hypothesis and accept the fact that the two groups are probably not really different after all. Having said this, however, **it is important that you realize that either accepting or rejecting the null hypothesis does not exclude the possibility that either decision could be wrong.** Other factors, such as sample size, cause-and-effect relationships between data, inappropriate statistical tests, and bias can all affect the data and the final truth or falsity of the decision.

b. Type I error (false rejection of the null hypothesis)

One of the risks in testing for statistical significance is the possibility that you may falsely reject the null hypothesis, and in so doing, accept the study hypothesis as being true when it is not. This has been termed a type I error.

c. Type II error (false acceptance of the null hypothesis)

A type II error is the exact oposite of a type I error. **In this situation, you accept the null hypothesis and falsely reject the study on the assumption that there are no true differences between the two groups when there really are differences.**

Chance plays a big part in both type I and II errors. The sample may be too small in a type II error to show the true differences, or there may have been other confounding factors. The significance level allows you to decrease the risk of these errors ($P = 0.001$), but it does not eliminate the uncertainty entirely. Statistics merely quantify the uncertainty; they do not eliminate it.

d. Normal curve

Any group of normally distributed data values will range from one extreme to the other, with the largest number of values falling somewhere between these extremes. This *normal curve* assumes that 5% of the values will be at the extremes, with 95% residing between them (Fig. 9-3). The concept of "normal" for a sample is based upon the actual value that one might find in the entire population that the sample is derived from.

Often, it is not possible or even feasible to count every case in the total population. As a consequence, a **sample** must be selected as a representation of the

TABLE 9-1. Statistical evaluations

| Test | Gold standard | |
	Diseased	Disease-free
Positive	a = The number of individuals diseased and positive with new test (*true positive*)	b = The number of individuals disease-free and positive with new test (*false positive*)
Negative	c = The number of individuals diseased and negative with new test (*false negative*)	d = The number of individuals disease-free and negative with new test (*true negative*)
	Total diseased	Total nondiseased

Reproduced with permission from R. K. Riegelman, *Studying a Study and Testing a Test.* Boston: Little, Brown and Company, Copyright © 1981, p. 121

population. **The larger the sample, the closer the sample mean value will be to the actual value in the total population.** Such samples have an inherent possibility of error, however, even when they are obtained correctly. In general, it may be assumed that if many random samples of a rate of occurrence of a disease (i.e., 1:100) are obtained, then on the average the sample rates will be the same as for the entire population. If a curve is constructed of these sample rates, a normal statistical curve will result, with some of the rates being equal to the mean value in the population but many of the other rates being higher or lower than this rate.

The statistical test known as the **standard error** attempts to evaluate the size of the error that results from a sampling. The standard error is important because 95% of the time the true population mean will lie within two standard errors of the sample's mean. This range has been called the **95% confidence limit.** For the sampling to be representative of the overall population, however, requires that the sample be randomly obtained and free of major bias.

e. Size of sample

The size of the standard error indicates how well the sample has estimated the true value in the population. The standard error is affected by the size of the sample—the larger the sample, the smaller the standard error.

In reading reports of scientific studies in medical journals, it is important to look at the sizes of the sample populations used. If a study comprises a **small number of observations,** the chance that the sample was not truly representative of the overall population is much greater than when a large number of observations are made. The type of study is also important. In cross-sectional and retrospective studies, the outcome reflects the characteristics of the patients, whereas in experimental and prospective studies, the outcome is related to the disease process.

Keep in mind that a type I error involves showing a statistically significant difference where there is none (i.e., false rejection of the null hypothesis), and a type II error involves failing to show a statistically significant difference where there is one in the overall population (i.e., false acceptance of the null hypothesis), of which the study group is but a small sample.

The incidence of a particular variable in a prospective study is an important factor in defining the size of the sample population. Very rare conditions may not lend themselves to a prospective study at all, because if the study variable is of a very low incidence, sufficient numbers of patients cannot be studied to arrive at significant levels. For example, if the rate of strokes is 1:100,000 in nonusers of birth control pills and is 1:10,000 in pill users, then the difference in the outcome is 0.01 − 0.001%, or 0.009%. In order to demonstrate a statistically significant difference for a study variable incidence this small, the sample sizes might need to be more than 100,000 patients for each group.

f. Diagnostic discrimination

Because of their relative accuracy in separating the normal from the abnormal (the diseased from the

TABLE 9-2. Diagnostic reliability of clinical tests

1. **Total diseased** = (a) True positive + (c) False negative

2. **Total nondiseased** = (b) False positive + (d) True negative

3. **Sensitivity** $= \dfrac{\text{(a) True positive}}{\text{(a) True positive + (c) False negative}} = \dfrac{\text{(a)}}{\text{(a) + (c)}}$

4. **Specificity** $= \dfrac{\text{(d) True negative}}{\text{(b) False positive + (d) True negative}} = \dfrac{\text{(d)}}{\text{(b) + (d)}}$

5. **The predictive value**

   (positive test) $= \dfrac{\text{(a) True positive}}{\text{(a) True positive + (b) False positive}}$

6. **The predictive value**

   (negative test) $= \dfrac{\text{(d) True negative}}{\text{(c) False negative + (d) True negative}}$

7. **Efficiency** $= \dfrac{\text{True positive + True negative}}{\text{True positive + True negative + False positive + False negative}}$

disease-free), some kinds of medical tests constitute a standard against which all new tests are then compared. We can refer to one of these baseline tests as the **Gold Standard** (Table 9-1). For example, if we wish to evaluate the Papanicolaou smear and its effectiveness in detecting the presence of cervical cancer, then we need a positive gold standard reference—such as the pathological examination of the cervices of women undergoing hysterectomies—in order to determine whether the Pap smear actually does detect cancer and in what percentage of cases. A test that can act as a gold standard provides a baseline reference to which other tests may be compared. The **sensitivity** of a test refers to its ability to correctly determine the proportion of **those patients with the disease** (i.e., true positive). The **specificity** of a test refers to its ability to correctly identify the proportion of **those patients who are disease-free** (i.e., true negative) (Table 9-2). The **predictive tests** relate to the matter of false positive tests and false negative tests in estimating the tests' overall effectiveness in predicting the presence or absence of disease. The **efficiency** of a test is the combination of both positive and negative predictive values.

While you may not be interested in calculating the statistics of the scientific data that you may be exposed to during your continuing medical education, you should at least ask yourself some basic questions before you accept the author's findings in a scientific paper.

1. **Study design.** Does the study design enable the appropriate data to be obtained for answering the question(s) proposed? Were the study aims clearly delineated? What kind of study is it (prospective, retrospective, experimental, cross-sectional)?

2. **Sample size.** Is the sample size sufficient to provide statistical significance?

3. **Selection bias.** Was there selection bias in choosing the study and control groups? Were the study and control patients treated in an identical manner? Was it possible for the various parameters to be manipulated in an unequal manner by the treating physicians (e.g., by using yellow medication pills vs. white placebo pills)? Were there significant side effects of the medication that made it obvious which pill was the medication and which was the placebo?

4. **Analysis of the data.** Was the analysis of the data done correctly and compared appropri-

ately with the control group? Was the most appropriate statistical test used?

5. **Significance.** Were the differences in the data statistically significant?

6. **Interpretation.** Did the authors draw a valid interpretation from the comparisons made between the study and the control data?

7. **Limits of the data.** Did the authors extrapolate their data appropriately and not exceed the limits of their data?

8. **Conclusions.** Do the conclusions make sense and agree with other studies, and/or with your own experience? If not what are the possible reasons for the different conclusions?

Exercising critical judgment in your appraisal of the data presented in the journals will not only provide you with a more intelligent clinical perspective in the use of such data but will also allow you to retain such information more easily because you will have scrutinized the paper more thoroughly. This approach will also prevent you from accepting invalid information and applying it to your everyday practice of medicine.

CHAPTER 10

Practice management

. . . .

Believe nothing that you see in the newspapers—they have done more to create dissatisfaction than all other agencies. If you see anything in them that you know to be true, begin to doubt it at once.

—*Sir William Osler**

. . . .

1. Professional liability risk management

a. Introduction

During the past few years, **malpractice** lawsuits have become so prominent and widespread that the problem has reached crisis proportions in some specialties. Some of the largest monetary awards that have ever been awarded have been in the field of obstetrics. As a consequence, the cost of insurance coverage has increased considerably each year, which has directly increased the cost of medical care to the patient. In addition, the newspapers and periodicals have had a "field day" in their coverage of suits against doctors and hospitals. Furthermore, family practice physicians and obstetricians in many areas of the country have stopped practicing obstetrics because of the excessive risk and the cost of malpractice insurance premiums.

Is there actually more malpractice being committed today than ever before? Do we really have such bad physicians that we need to thoroughly clean house and put these physicians out of business? Or is it only

that the public has come to expect such miraculous cures and superior results from modern medicine that when the outcome is less than perfect, the patient suspects that someone must be at fault? A distinction must therefore be made between a bad outcome, or a **medical maloccurrence,** and **medical malpractice.** Although less than optimum results may be obtained in the delivery of a baby, such a result, while tragic, does not necessarily mean that the physician is guilty of malpractice.

The quality of medicine practiced in the United States today is the finest that the world has ever seen. The perinatal mortality rate has decreased dramatically; however, whenever a "bad" baby is delivered, the public looks for a scapegoat to explain why this particular baby is not perfect. **More and more evidence is accumulating to indicate that physicians are not responsible for many of these "damaged" babies, that these infants must have sustained irreparable damage at an earlier period in pregnancy, and furthermore, that the physicians could not have anticipated nor prevented many of these tragic outcomes.**

b. Communication

Effective professional liability risk management begins with good communication and rapport between you and your patient. You should always treat your patient with courtesy, compassion, and understanding. Rudeness, long waiting times in the office, and insensitivity to the patient's needs and concerns are factors that are guaranteed to strain the rapport between you and your patient. *Honesty and candidness with the patient is extremely important.* You should be careful not to make prognostic statements that are not warranted by the facts of the

---

*Reprinted with permission from Robert Bennett Bean, *Sir William Osler: Aphorisms from His Bedside Teachings and Writings,* William Bennett Bean, ed. Springfield, Ill.: Charles C Thomas, Publisher, 1968, p. 64.

case. When you do not know the solutions to the patient's problems, let the patient know of your dilemma. Share the possible approaches to solving the problem with the patient and enlist her aid in making the decisions. Fully inform her of the various alternative medical and surgical approaches, their risks and benefits, and assist her in evaluating each one. *Patients who work as partners with their physicians in making important decisions concerning their health care are not usually prone to bring suit when things do not work out as well as they might have hoped.*

c. Quality of practice

The backbone of professional liability risk management is the quality of the medical practice. You must maintain your skills and your knowledge base sufficiently to provide your patients with the latest techniques of modern medical care. In addition to your own care of the patient, you must be certain that the other members of your health-care team also practice risk management, including your partners, the nurses, and the other office staff personnel, as well as the other consulting physicians who may come into contact with the patient. The words or actions of an uncaring, rude chaperone or an inefficient, arrogant office clerk can sometimes trigger a lawsuit. Your choice of partners or consultants should also be based not only upon their medical expertise, but also upon whether they have any personality traits that might make them a risk for litigation. **Future medical school training will perhaps emphasize more thoroughly the need for physicans to develop communication skills and sensitivity in dealing with their patients and with fellow professionals.**

d. The medical record

The medical record is crucial to the defensibility of your professional care of the patient. The medical record is a chronological account of the patient's visits, telephone calls, laboratory procedures, letters, notes of conversations, diagnoses, and treatment. It presents **your capabilities as a physician** as you obtained the history and performed the physical examination. It indicates the **thoroughness** of your investigations into the patient's medical problems. It also provides a record as to the number of **missed visits** on the part of the patient, and the **de-**

gree of compliance with which the patient carried out your instructions during the course of treatment. The medical record should be written in such a way that the course of events may be easily followed. **The logic of your approach to the patient's medical problems,** your differential diagnosis list, the manner in which you performed your workup so that the patient's safety was always assured as much as possible, your precautions and instructions, the frequency of return visits that indicated your concern about the patient, and the **documentation** that the patient was completely aware of any changes in her condition throughout the course of therapy all provide evidence of the quality of care you provided should the patient bring litigation against you at a later time. The immediacy of the medical record provides a mantle of credibility in litigation proceedings that transcends the remembered accounts by either the patient or the physician at a time remote from when the medical care was delivered. **A loss of even a part of the medical record may seriously jeopardize a physician's defense in a malpractice suit.**

1) Recordkeeping

The medical record indicates the quality of care that the patient has received, and by inference, the capabilities of the physician who rendered that care. If the record is good, it reflects the efforts of a skillful, dedicated, and conscientious physician who gave his patient quality care. If the record is bad, it infers that both the physician and the care were probably substandard. **Never place a note in the record that you do not want to see as the "headlines in tomorrow's newspaper."** Derogatory or belittling statements about the patient are unprofessional and are devastating to the physician's case when read aloud in a court of law. *In addition, you should never make disparaging comments in the record about other professionals.* The medical record is a **legal record,** and one that should contain only facts. Unnecessary speculation as to what you will do in the future is not effective management, as future changes in the patient's condition might alter the situation considerably.

The medical record is also a *communication tool between the medical health-care team members* concerning the various aspects of the patient's care. It forms *a permanent written record of the chronological events of the patient's course,* the types of diagnostic tests utilized, and the facts and reasoning behind the various decisions that were made in the overall care of the patient.

Your concern about producing an accurate, objective, comprehensive, timely, and legible record can only be interpreted by a jury as an extension of your concern for the patient and for all of the aspects of her case. On the other hand, sloppiness, both in the content and in the writing, and a lack of completeness and objectivity in the progress notes, combined with operative dictations that were done days or months after the procedures were performed, all point to a physician that, at the very least, is not very meticulous or concerned about the details of the patient's care. In addition, a physician's failure to correctly and completely fill out the diagnoses and procedures on the hospital face sheet of a hospitalized patient is ample evidence for the opposing lawyer to imply that the physician is sloppy and prone to error, as this information is required upon the discharge of the patient from the hospital. **Such lack of concern and a failure to be meticulous in your chart work could be interpreted by a jury as being sloppy and could be further extrapolated into a conviction that any physician who could be that sloppy could also commit malpractice.**

Any alteration of the medical record should be carried out by making a single line through the error, which is then initialed and dated by the physician. This should be done as infrequently as possible, since it implies that the physician has made an error that he subsequently had to correct. If the physician could make one error, then it is conceivable, in the eyes of the jury, that he could perhaps have committed another error—one that may have led to the current malpractice case. Whatever you do, **DO NOT ALTER a record after receiving a notification from an attorney that you are being sued.** By the time that you are notified, the lawyer has already obtained a certified copy of the record. If there are any changes in the original record on later evaluation, the jury can only conclude that you were attempting to cover up a case of malpractice.

e. Informed consent

The courts have determined that every patient is entitled to an explanation as to: (1) the risks, **(2) the benefits, and (3) the alternative forms of treatment, before undergoing medical or surgical therapy.** The basis for this rule is that the patient must give her **informed consent** to any treatment plan. The operative word in this statement is *informed,* in that the patient must be provided with a sufficient amount of information to enable her to make an intelligent choice as to which, if any, therapy she wishes to accept. The elements involved are the risks or hazards involved in each form of therapy and the potential benefits she may expect to receive from such therapy. *This information should cover not only the alternative approaches to therapy (e.g., medical, surgical), but also the choice of no treatment at all.* There is confusion about this rule because it varies from state to state. Some states utilize the "patient materiality standard" (i.e., the informational needs of the patient), while others use the "professional medical standard" (i.e., what the customary or reasonable physician would have told the patient under similar circumstances).

1) BRAIDED

It has been suggested that the mnemonic acronym **BRAIDED** offers a convenient reminder of what ought to be discussed and documented with any patient who is making a significant medical or surgical decision, especially those who are deciding upon a sterilization procedure. The **B** addresses the **benefits** that the patient should expect to obtain by accepting a particular course of action. The **R** lists the **risks** of the procedure. The **A** involves the **alternative forms of treatment.** The **I** allows the patient to make **inquiries** about things that concern her. The **D** relates not only to the patient's need to make a **decision** but also to her right to change her decision if she so desires. The **E** addresses the **explanations** that you should give to your patient concerning the various approaches or procedures and your answers to the patient's fears and concerns. Finally, the **D** alludes to the **documentation** in the chart and in the operative permit that a discussion of the risks and benefits and the alternative procedures was indeed carried out by you and, in addition, that the patient understood the meaning of her decision to accept or reject a particular course of action. A shorter, and perhaps more easily remembered, version of this mnemonic acronymic device might be **BRAD,** in which the essential elements of **B**enefits, **R**isks, **A**lternative treatments, and **D**ocumentation are considered as the nail (i.e., a brad) that "nails down" the agreement between the patient and the physician.

In order for you to truly obtain an informed consent—one that will probably not be challenged successfully—you should be aware of the fact that a progress note should also be made in the medical chart. You should not only have your hospital's operative permit form appropriately filled out, signed, and witnessed by persons who are not on the operative team and who are not members of the patient's family, but **you should also show evidence in the body of the chart (i.e., a progress note attesting to these facts) that you personally discussed the risks and benefits and alternative forms of treatment** with the patient, and that, having been fully informed, she requested that you proceed with a certain form of therapy. **Drawing pictures of the pathology in your progress note as you talk with the patient, with notations concerning possible major complications such as hemorrhage, infection, etc., may also be of value to indicate that you personally discussed these things with the patient and that the consent was not obtained by a nurse.** Remember that the relatives cannot give informed consent unless they are acting as a legal guardian for a minor or for a mentally incompetent individual.

There are several **exceptions to the rule of informed consent.** These include: (1) an emergency situation where intervention is necessary to prevent the death or injury to the patient, (2) cases where the patient would have agreed to the treatment regardless of the risks involved, (3) cases where the patient waives her right to be informed of the risk, (4) cases in which the disclosure of the risks would be against the best interests of the patient, (5) cases in which the patient is legally incompetent, in which case the legal guardian would then have to be informed and would have to make the decision, (6) cases where the risks involved are commonly known to lay persons, or the patient is already aware of them, and (7) risks that are not normally associated with the procedure when performed appropriately. Whenever possible, you should document any unusual circumstances in the record in such a way that anyone reading the record would understand your actions completely in retrospect.

Should a postoperative or posttherapy complication occur, you should notify the patient immediately and remind her that you had discussed such an eventuality with her prior to the start of treatment. Be sure to document this conversation in the progress notes on the chart.

You should keep abreast of local, state, and federal laws, in addition to any other legislation that may affect your practice of medicine, as well as the policies and guidelines issued by the various specialty societies in their efforts to set standards of care. Finally, it is wise to follow the rules and regulations of your hospital, since it is difficult to legally justify violations of local rules that govern the medical practice in your local hospital situation.

Religious matters have at times placed the physician at odds with the proper care of certain patients. On July 1, 1945, *The Watchtower,* the official publication of the Jehovah's Witnesses, explicitly prohibited the taking of blood into the body on the penalty of the loss of eternal life. While this prohibition involves whole blood, packed red blood cells, plasma, and platelets, it does not prohibit albumin, immune serum globulin, or antihemophilic components. The use of **extracorporeal hemodilution** is acceptable to Jehovah's Witnesses as long as the blood is kept in physical continuity with the individual. The blood loss during a surgical procedure in such a patient contains less red blood cells (due to the hemodilution) and thus the absolute numbers of red blood cells lost is reduced. In any patient in which there is hemodilution, the viscosity decreases as the hematocrit falls, which results in a decreased peripheral vascular resistance and an increased venous return that causes an increase in the cardiac output. If there is a reduction of the hematocrit to 20%, the increase in cardiac output will provide for a cardiac output sufficient to deliver 100% oxygen to the tissues. **A physician who administers blood to an adult who does not consent to the procedure is liable for civil damages.** Under the First Amendment, the freedom to believe in the religion of one's choice is absolute; however, the freedom to act is somewhat modified by the fact that the pregnant patient's decision (to not receive blood) also affects the child, who also has a right to live. In most instances of this type, you should seek the aid of a judge to determine whether the patient should become a ward of the court so that the decision of whether the patient should receive the blood in a critical situation may be made by the judge.

A similar situation may occur when the mother refuses to grant permission to perform a cesarean section in the face of fetal distress. In such a situation, **a judge and the opposing lawyers should be convened immediately at the patient's bedside and the arguments heard.** It has been pointed out, however, that if a good outcome is not obtained by the cesarean section (if approved by the judge), then the physician may still be liable for not protecting the interests of the fetus and providing adequate and timely medical care. Furthermore, the question arises as to the rights of the mother in such a situation.

There are a number of medico-legal problems such as these that you may confront in your practice. Your main concern should be to provide your patient with the best care possible; however, it is the responsibility of society to protect the physician from litigation when he does provide such care.

2. Insurance

a. A tort action (malpractice action)

The failure to exercise due care and to utilize the skills appropriate to your training form the basis of a malpractice action. Such a legal action, called a **tort,** allows a person who has sustained damage to his person or property to recover monetary damages. **In order for a tort action to have merit, however, three conditions must be satisfied: (1) There must be a deviation from the standard of care, (2) the patient must have suffered an injury, and (3) the deviation from standard practice must have been the cause of the patient's injury.** Since there is no firm legal "standard of practice," expert testimony is necessary to determine whether a deviation has taken place.

Some states have set up **medical panels** composed of neutral doctors and lawyers who review each patient's case and make a decision as to whether there is any merit involved. If they find that there is no merit and the case is pursued anyway, then the panel of physicians will testify against the patient. If there is merit, then the panel will testify against the physician. In some other states, physicians have set up a **patient-physician arbitration agreement** that patients sign prior to therapy. This procedure has the effect of screening out the litigious-minded patient. It also may include provisions that the plaintiff's lawyer must disclose his entire case and reveal his expert witnesses to the arbitration panel of neutral physicians in cases involving more than $25,000. In effect, this type of agreement requires that the case be litigated twice, which would discourage the pursuit of nonmeritorious cases by the plaintiff's lawyer. To be effective, the patient should sign the agreement 7–31 days prior to the proposed treatment or surgery.

b. Types of insurance policies

It is important for you to be aware of the types of insurance available to protect you against any legal liability that may arise from your practice of medicine. *In reviewing professional liability insurance, you should be aware of the insurer's obligations concerning: (1) the payment of judgments against you, (2) whether your written consent must be obtained before an out-of-court settlement is made, (3) whether punitive damages will be covered, (4) whether the acts or omissions of your office personnel will be covered, and (5) whether the medical expenses of the patient may be paid without admitting guilt.*

A **claims-made policy** is one that provides you with protection against claims that are made during the life of the policy. In this type of policy, if you discontinue the policy and then are subsequently sued for an event that occurred during the time that the policy was in effect, you are **NOT covered,** unless you have purchased an **additional tail policy** to cover you beyond the termination date of the policy. This additional tail policy may be quite expensive.

An **occurrence policy** is one that provides protection for you against claims that occur during the policy period, regardless of when the suit is filed. In contrast to the claims-made policy, no tail policy is required. This form of insurance is more expensive, and in view of the large numbers of claims in obstetrics, these policies in the future may become either prohibitively expensive or totally unavailable.

3. Common legal terms

1. **Abandonment.** The premature termination of the physician-patient relationship before the patient has had a sufficient amount of time to seek further appropriate care, resulting in some type of damage to the patient.
2. **Assault and battery.** An unlawful, harmful,

or offensive contact with another person's body without his or her consent.

3. **"Captain of the ship" doctrine.** A doctrine that holds the physician responsible for the acts or omissions of other members of the medical health-care team.

4. **Complaint.** The document in which the claimant sets forth the charges against the defendant physician.

5. **Contingency fee.** A lawyer-client arrangement by which the lawyer only recovers his fee if he wins the suit, as opposed to the fee-for-services arrangement. Under the contingency-fee plan, if the case is lost, the lawyer receives nothing.

6. **Court trial.** A trial in which the judge sits in judgment without a jury.

7. **Jury trial.** A trial in which the jury hands down the verdict. A jury trial is constitutionally guaranteed; it may be waived by both parties, but not by only one party.

8. **Deposition.** A question-and-answer period for a witness that is taken under oath by lawyers prior to the trial. It serves as a discovery process and also "freezes" the testimony of the individual for the later trial, in which the person may or may not be called to testify again.

9. **Federal court system.** Another form of court system, similar to the state court system, which only hears certain types of cases, such as those malpractice cases that are brought from out of state.

10. **General damages.** The intangible losses that will occur in the future, such as the loss of future income, expected pain and suffering, loss of the quality of life, and other losses that are claimed by the plaintiff.

11. **Special damages.** Past losses, such as the loss of income or the cost of medical expenses.

12. **Punitive damages.** Damages requested by the plaintiff in an effort to punish the defendant.

13. **Loss of consortium.** A damage claim submitted by a family member for loss of comfort, companionship, or, in the case of the spouse, the loss of sexual relations.

14. **Negligence.** The failure on the part of a physician to diagnose or treat the patient's illness with the same due care that a similarly trained physician would use in the same or a similar circumstance.

15. **Privileged communication.** All of the communication between the patient and her physician, or between a lawyer and client, that cannot be divulged without the individual's oral or written permission. The medical chart is a part of the communication between the patient and the physician and is therefore considered to be privileged information.

16. ***Res ipsa loquitur.*** A Latin phrase meaning that "the thing speaks for itself." This doctrine may be invoked in blatant cases of negligence (e.g., when a sponge is left in the abdomen after surgery).

17. **Standard of practice.** What reasonable and prudent physicians, with comparable training and experience, would do in similar situations. While at times the reference point for this determination is what the physicians in the local community would do (community rule), there is a strong move to make the type of practice that is carried out throughout the United States the reference point (national rule).

18. **Statute of limitations.** A period of time during which a plaintiff may institute a claim. The patient may exceed this limitation in certain instances, if she could not have known of the injury during the allocated time period.

19. **Subpoena.** A court order requiring a person to appear at a legal proceeding to give testimony or produce documents.

20. **Suit.** The filing of the necessary papers with the court by the patient to recover from an alleged malpractice action by a physician.

21. **Tort.** A wrongful act that causes damage to another person, or to that person's property. The perpetrator is called a "tortfeasor."

22. **Summons.** A legal document commanding a person named in a suit to appear and answer the complaints on a certain date and at a specific time and place.

23. **Trial court.** The place where witnesses appear to provide testimony concerning the suit in question.

24. **Vicarious liability.** A physician's liability for the acts or omissions of his office nurses and other personnel.

25. **Alternative liability.** This is not a joint tort, but involves the independent acts of two or more individual tortfeasors, only one of which has injured the patient.

4. Education of the patient

a. The summing-up conference

After you have interviewed the patient and performed the physical examination, you should sum up your findings for her. **Patient education begins with this first summing-up conference.** You have the responsibility to teach your patient as much as possible about her condition, whether it be a normal pregnancy, or a case of uterine cancer. **You should always encourage an atmosphere in which your patient will feel free to ask you any medical question at any time.** During this conference, you should attempt to teach the patient what you have found out about her problem and what significance you place on each of the symptoms and findings. Let the patient mentally "walk through" your diagnostic workup and tentative diagnosis with you so that she will understand your approach to the problem. Reassure her that you will work with her in getting her back to health. **The patient should understand that she is a partner in her health care and that she has the obligation to promptly inform you of any changes in her condition.** In return, you should reassure the patient that you will keep her informed as to any changes in your diagnoses or in your plan of management.

b. Office patient-education techniques

A variety of pamphlets as well as monographs on obstetric and gynecologic matters should be made available to your patients in the waiting room. In addition, patients are a "captive audience" while in your waiting room, and this time offers you a golden opportunity to further educate them by using videotape presentations. There are many **videotape programs** available covering such topics as breastfeeding, oral contraceptives, exercise in pregnancy, the hazards of smoking in pregnancy, and many others that may assist your patients in understanding the various diseases and conditions. It is very difficult for the patient to sit in a waiting room where a video

is playing without looking at the presentation. Videos can also be used in specific situations. In the management of a diabetic woman, for example, a videotape presentation may be invaluable in **teaching the patient** how to self-medicate herself with insulin and how to test blood glucose levels to maintain an adequate control of her disease.

Another use for videotape presentations is that of informing your patient about the risks and benefits of a variety of surgical procedures. Having the patient sign an informed consent and a statement that she has watched such a presentation, and that she has had her questions answered by her physician, may provide a significant defense in a later litigation procedure.

5. Education of the physician

a. Data retrieval

Today we are living in a world in which informational material in all areas of knowledge is increasing very rapidly. In medicine, this *knowledge explosion* is of such proportions that more than a quarter of a million new references are added to the MEDLINE database system alone each year. The **MEDLINE system** is a database that has been developed by the **National Library of Medicine (NLM).** This database is only one of the many databases available from **Medical Literature Analysis and Retrieval System (MEDLARS).** It is essentially a computer compilation of data that may be found in the **Index Medicus,** the **Index to Dental Literature,** and the **International Nursing Index. MEDLINE has about 800,000 references from the biomedical literature published over the previous three-year period from about 3,000 journals in the United States and in foreign countries.** You can also obtain data from previous compilations from 1966 to the present; altogether, this database includes approximately 5 million references. Each month about 20,000 to 25,000 records are added.

The other 15 databases included under **MEDLARS** are the **BIOETHICSLINE** (short form, BIOETHICS), which provides references on the ethics of health care and biomedical research, with more than 13,000 citations being added since 1973, and 1,800 to 2,000 citations now being added each year; **POPLINE** (population information online), with more than 100,000 citations from 1970 to the present, and about 10,000 citations being added each year; the **HEALTH** (Health Planning and Administration), with about 200,000 references on health planning, management, personnel, and related subjects from 1975 to the present, and 2,500 to 3,000 records being added monthly; **TOX-LINE** (toxicology information online), with references from 1965 to the present; **CHEMLINE** (a chemical online dictionary), with more than 650,000 records; **PDQ** (Physician Data Query), an index of more than 1,000 NCI-sponsored active protocols from the CLINPROT file; **CLINPROT** (Clinical Cancer Protocols); **CANCERLIT** (Cancer Literature), with more than 300,000 references and a monthly update of about 5,000 citations; **RTECS** (Registry of Toxic Effects of Chemical Substances), with more than 70,000 potentially toxic chemicals listed; **SERLINE** (serials on-line), with about 40,000 serial titles; **AVLINE** (audio-visuals online), listing about 11,000 audiovisual teaching packages since 1975, and about 100 new records being added each month; **HISTLINE** (history of medicine online), with about 50,000 citations; **CANCERPROJ** (summary of ongoing cancer research projects); **DIRLINE** (Directory of Information Resources), with information on more than 14,000 resource centers; and **CATLINE** (catalog of bibliographic records covering the biomedical sciences), with about 600,000 references.

Overall, MEDLARS contains more than 6 million references to books and journals that have been published in the health sciences since 1966. There are two additional subsidiary online files—the **Name Authority File** (listing about 185,000 personal and corporate names), and the **MeSH Vocabulary File** (which includes about 14,000 Medical Subject Headings and 28,000 chemical substances). All of these reference libraries are accessible by computer. While most of the accessing computers belong to medical libraries at the present time, there is an increasing trend for physician-owned personal home computers to access such databases for literature searches.

b. Personal computers

During the past few years, there has been an increasing use of personal computers among physicians. The availability of relatively inexpensive computers that are simple to learn how to use has opened the door for many people to benefit from the tremendous versatility of such equipment.

1) Practice management

Over the next few years, every physician's office will become computerized in order to manage patients' files and hopefully eliminate many of the difficulties that occur when large amounts of patient data are manually manipulated. Appointments, billing, and other business transactions will be computerized so that you will not have to spend so much of your time being involved in the business aspects of your medical practice. Long-term reviews of the types of diseases being seen in different months, the average load of patients each month, and other patient-related activities might allow you to plan your vacation in a low-volume month, so that your patients are minimally inconvenienced and your income is not adversely affected. It may also provide information as to the beginning of an infectious epidemic, the clustering of congenital anomalies, or the association of certain complications with some of your operative procedures. It may also provide you with data concerning the effectiveness of some of your medications or the incidence of side effects with these drugs.

2) Patient records

The application of data processing techniques to the medical record may improve the quality of care and facilitate cost containment. The medical record could be made much more efficient and complete by the use of a computer. Your ability to look at different aspects of the patient's long-term course in a graphic manner could be important in the management of the case. Sorting the symptoms and their relationship to a database of symptomatology on different related diseases would perhaps improve your diagnostic skills. The ability of the obstetric attendant to retrieve a patient's record on a bedside computer while talking to a patient on the telephone in the middle of the night would eliminate many problems in management.

3) Diagnostic assistance

In the future, physicians may be able to use personal computers to tap into the large mainframe computers that contain enormous amounts of information on the management of almost every medical disease or condition. This development would seem to be the only answer to the information explosion in medicine, since we could utilize the speed and sorting capabilities of the computer to narrow the search for pertinent medical data that are applicable to a specific patient problem. As such, we might expect to submit each of the symptoms and physical findings that have been found in a particular patient to a computer (with proper weighting of the importance of each piece of data), and then proceed through a systematic list of different diagnoses. While the final selection of a diagnosis and the treatment plan would have to remain with the physician, the assistance of a computer could be extremely valuable. The extensive database that would be immediately available to you in your management of any medical problem would be truly astounding. Every patient would be an extensive learning process for you in updating your own experiential database with that of the literature database and the experiences of other physicians throughout the world. Information as to the cures and the results of your treatment of patients would have to be fed back into the computer by your office staff so that there would be a continuous updating of all medical information; however, this would be a small price to pay to be able to obtain up-to-date treatment protocols and prognostic information.

It seems entirely possible that in the near future, physicians who do not become proficient in the use of computer equipment to access the large data banks of the mainframe computers, and who do not become fluent in the extraction of specific informational material from such sources, may be at a severe disadvantage in practicing medicine.

4) Continuing medical education

The large quantity of written material to which physicians are currently exposed in just one week already attests to the increasing impossibility of keeping up with all of this information. In addition, much of the current medical material is not relevant to the physician's day-to-day practice of medicine, but is related to basic research or to extremely rare conditions. Obviously, the "written" medical journals might undergo some significant changes in the future. Instead of receiving a printed magazine journal in the mail, the physician might expect to receive his updated "summary of specific conditions" (i.e., medical journal) in the form of a computer floppy disk, or the physician might connect his computer to a modem (through the telephone) to a medical computer service that would off-load monthly (or weekly or even daily) database

material into the personal computer. Every physician's choice of disease entities to review could be individualized according to what the physician desires. The only remaining "medical journal" tradition that might be retained would be an "editorial section" (on the computer service) to alert physicians as to the general trends in medicine, and to the disease entities that might be on the increase. The computer networks could also provide a forum for physicians to express their opinions about current medical matters. The use of the computer would not eliminate the physician's medical writing skills, but might actually enhance them, since the appropriate patient data entered into the computer for archiving purposes would still have to be filed in an acceptable written format.

Currently, technical bulletins and other educational materials are available to physicians *via computer* through the American College of Obstetricians and Gynecologists (ACOG). In addition, the **ACOG Integrated Academic Information Management System (IAIMS),** which will provide a core knowledge base for the practitioner of obstetrics and gynecology, will probably be in place by 1992. This database will be available on the **ACOG NET,** a computer network that will be available to the practicing physician and accessed by means of a personal computer and a modem. Such a network will allow individual physicians to communicate with one another and to obtain immediate consultations from world-renowned experts on patient problems. It will also allow ACOG committees to meet online and respond quickly to matters that affect health care for women. Messages to other physicians may be left on national or specific clinical-problem bulletin boards. Learning courses may be reviewed (e.g., PROLOG—personal review of learning in obstetrics and gynecology), and interactive clinical situation management programs may be accessed to improve your cognitive skills. **"Shareware" software programs** may be downloaded onto your computer to allow you to improve the various phases of your office management needs (e.g., accounting, communication, and office management). "Shareware" programs are developed by individuals who ask that if you try the program and decide to use it, then you should send a minimal fee to the author.

There will be no limits to the benefits that may accrue from the use of computers, not only to you personally in your practice of medicine, but also to the profession of medicine as a whole. Everything from the compilation of your case lists for the specialty board examinations early in your career to the planning of your retirement accounts at the end of your practice days will be done on computers. It is important, therefore, that you obtain computer skills during your residency training.

6. Financial aspects of practice

Physicians have received payment for their services since the dawn of time. The physicians in ancient Egypt accepted goods and services for their care of patients; however, temple physicians, army doctors, and those who took care of workmen were probably salaried and thus did not charge the patients individually. Physicians also charged for the medicines that they dispensed, since they usually prepared these concoctions themselves. In addition, most physicians were specialized and took care of only one disease or one body part—not too different from modern times.

You should place a price on each of your services that is similar to what other physicians charge who practice in your area. These charges should take into account the amount of skill needed to perform the service, the cost of the equipment involved, the cost of your expenses to provide the service, and the cost of malpractice insurance. In effect, the charge is directly related to your overhead expenses in doing business and making a living. While the practice of medicine is a profession, not a business, your efficiency in keeping your overhead expenses low will be reflected in lower charges for your services to the patient. You should educate the patient as to how these charges are

arrived at, so that she will in turn recognize that when she fails to keep her appointment without notifying you, she eliminates a block of time in which you could have received income by seeing another patient. Less income means a proportionately greater amount of overhead and results in higher fees for all patients. This is also true with regard to those patients who fail to pay their bills.

Patients should be encouraged to pay your charges at the time of the office visit. Major credit cards, checks, and cash should be accepted. Insurance forms should be signed over and the patient should pay the difference that is not covered. If you allow the patient to leave without paying, then the first and second billing notices that are sent to the patient for payment will increase your overhead expenses. While all physicians take care of some patients without charging them, this decision should be your choice, not the patient's. Free care should be extended to the families of your fellow physicians, dentists, nurses, and members of the ministry. Those individuals who are unwilling or unable to pay their bills should be seen in city, county, and charity hospitals that have been set up to provide excellent care without charging the patients any fees—or at least no more than they can easily pay according to their income level. If your practice has an excessive number of patients who do not pay, then you will either suffer in your own income, which affects your wife and family, or you subject your other patients to inordinately high charges in order to make up the difference and stay in practice. In either case, such misplaced altruism becomes unfair to all concerned.

PART II

Gynecology

CHAPTER 11

Vulvar disease

The physician's challenge is the curing of disease, educating the people in the laws of health, and preventing the spread of plagues and pestilences.
—*Sir William Osler**

In this and the next two chapters, some of the sexually transmitted diseases (STD's) will be discussed. These diseases are caused by such organisms as Trichomonas vaginalis (trichomoniasis), Candida albicans (monilial vaginitis), Gardnerella vaginalis (vaginitis), Chlamydia trachomatis (lymphogranuloma inguinale, cervicitis, urethritis, PID), Calymmatobacterium granulomatis (granuloma inguinale), Neisseria gonorrhoeae (gonorrhea, PID), Treponema pallidum (syphilis), the Herpes simplex viruses (herpes), AIDS, the human papilloma viruses (condyloma acuminatum), molluscum contagiosum, Haemophilus ducreyi (chancroid), and hepatitis B (hepatitis). In addition, two parasitic conditions, pediculosis and oxyuriasis, will also be discussed.

1. Infections

a. Pediculosis

An infestation with certain **body lice** is common among the lower socioeconomic groups, who may also have other sexually transmitted diseases. The *Pediculus humanus capitis* (head louse), the *Pediculus humanus corporis* (body louse), the *Phthirus pubis* (pubic or crab louse), and the *Sarcoptes scabiei* (scabies or itch mite) are transmitted from person to person in crowded living conditions, or whenever there is prolonged skin-to-skin contact, rather than by sexual intercourse alone. While the other body lice may be vectors for typhus, trench fever, and relapsing fever, the crab louse and the scabies mite are not known to be vectors for any other diseases.

1) Phthirus pubis (crab louse)

The **Phthirus pubis,** or crab louse, is well-named since it has the appearance of a tiny 1 to 2 mm crab. The lice reside on the terminal hairs in the pubic region and may be seen as small bluish spots on the skin. The life cycle of the crab louse is about 30 days. The eggs, or nits, are 0.5 mm translucent egg-like structures clustered at the base of the hairs. The symptoms consist of *intense pubic, genital, and perianal itching,* some *erythema,* and excoriation of the skin due to the patient's persistent scratching.

The treatment usually consists of only one application of a 1% gamma benzene hexachloride (lindane 1%) (Kwell) shampoo to dry pubic hair, allow to remain for four minutes, add water, lather, and rinse thoroughly. Comb hair with a nit comb. Contacts should be treated and the patient's clothing should be sterilized. **Kwell should not be used on children under 10 years of age or on pregnant or lactating women.** A 1% rinse of permethrin (Nix) has been used in treating lice, ticks, mites, and fleas. It also appears to be quite effective in treating Pediculus humanus capitis. It is listed as a Category B type of drug in regard to its use in pregnancy.

*Reprinted with permission from Robert Bennett Bean, *Sir William Osler: Aphorisms from His Bedside Teachings and Writings,* William Bennett Bean, ed. Springfield, Ill.: Charles C Thomas, Publisher, 1968, p. 63.

137

2) Sarcoptes scabiei (itch mite)

Sarcoptes scabiei, the scabies itch mite, burrows into the stratum corneum of the skin, where it deposits its eggs within a burrow. These burrows, or tunnels, become elevated and have a small vesicle at the open end. When the larvae hatch, they migrate out onto the skin and congregate around the hair follicles, where they mature over the next six days. The mites then mate and the cycle begins all over again. The skin eruption develops in the webbing of the fingers, along the flexor surfaces of the wrists, and on the various areas of the body where the clothing may bind, such as the waist, the groin, or the axillae. The infected patient will tend to scratch these areas due to intense itching, especially when in bed, which may cause the skin to become excoriated and a secondary infection to occur. The mite or the eggs may be detected by using a hand magnifying lens and locating the burrows with the terminal papule over the open end. *If you scrape these burrows and place the material in saline or in mineral oil on a glass slide, you will be able to detect the larvae upon microscopic examination.*

The treatment of scabies consists of the application of a 25% suspension of benzyl benzoate, or a 1% gamma benzene hexachloride (Kwell) cream or lotion to all of the infected areas after a hot soapy bath in which the burrows have been thoroughly scrubbed. The medication should be applied after the skin has been thoroughly dried and then washed off in eight hours. **This agent is not recommended for use in pregnant women.** A 10% solution of crotamiton (Eurax) should be applied to the skin for two nights and then washed off 48 hours after the last application. **Crotamiton (10%) may be used in children under 10 years of age and in pregnant or lactating women.** Permethrin (Nix) has also been stated to be effective in the treatment of mites. All clothes and bed linens should be washed or dry cleaned. Due to the ease of transmission of scabies to other household members, the entire family should be treated; however, recurrences are common. Repeat treatment of all contacts may need to be carried out in one or two weeks, if the lesions recur. Antipruritic creams and lotions may be used, and if a secondary infection is present, systemic antibiotics may be necessary.

b. Foliculitis (furunculosis)

Occasionally, an infection of the hair follicles of the pubic and perianal hair may occur. *Staphylococcus* *aureus* is the usual organism involved in these furuncles. An acute lesion consists of a raised inflammatory nodule or a pustule about the hair root. The treatment consists of hot soaks to cause the pustule to "point" and then to drain. Systemic antibiotics such as cloxacillin or erythromycin, 250 mg q.i.d., p.o., should be administered.

c. Condyloma acuminatum

1) Incidence

The incidence of **human papilloma virus (HPV)** infections has increased 10-fold since the 1940s. **Condyloma acuminatum is a DNA viral skin lesion that is transmitted sexually to produce a warty excrescence in about three months (with a range of three weeks to eight months) after exposure.**

2) Types

The anogenital human papilloma viruses (HPV) consist of **types 6 and 11,** which are usually found in condyloma acuminatum, and **types 16 and 18, which have been implicated in the development of genital dysplasia and carcinoma, since up to 90% of these lesions have HPV-specific DNA present.** Type 16 is more common, whereas type 18 is apparently the more lethal virus. **Types 31, 33 and 35 have also been demonstrated in over 90% of significant cervical and vulvar dysplasias and cancers.** You should consider women with condylomata of the cervix to be at a high risk for the development of carcinoma of the cervix. This risk is increased even more if the male sexual partner has an HPV infection. It has been recommended that you should biopsy all of these lesions since there are frequently areas of neoplasia present. This may be particularly true in immunosuppressed patients. It has been estimated that as many as 5% of vulvar carcinomas may arise in persistent genital warts.

There are 35 serotypes of the human papilloma virus that have been identified. The other types of human papilloma viruses that have been found in various lesions are: (1) types 1 (a, b, c) and 4—**plantar warts,** (2) type 2 (a–e)—**hand warts,** (3) types 3 (a, b), 10 (a, b), and 41—**flat warts,** (4) type 7—**Butcher's warts,** (5) types 5 (a, b), 8, 12, 15, 17 (a, b), and 19–29—**warts in patients with epidermodysplasia verruciformis,** (6) types 13 and 32 (Heck lesions)—**oral focal hyperplasia,** (7) types 16, 33, and 34—**Bowenoid papulosis,** (8) types 6 (a–f), 11 (a, b), 16, 31, 33, and 35—**cervical intraepithelial neoplastic (CIN) lesions,** and (9) type 36—**actinic keratosis.**

3) Symptoms

The condylomatous lesion soon develops adjacent satellite lesions, which may then coalesce to form a continuous sheet of cauliflower-like warts over broad areas of the skin or the cervical and vaginal membranes. The moist, warm conditions present in the genital areas, coupled with poor hygiene, provide an ideal environment for this viral disease. These lesions occur almost exclusively in the anogenital region rather than in other areas of the body. Vulvar itching, dyspareunia, and rectal pain may be present in patients who have condylomatous lesions. The Papanicolaou smear may often be abnormal and may contain atypical cells. Histologic sections of the involved mucous membranes of the vagina or cervix will demonstrate vacuolated cells with large nuclei **(i.e., koilocytes)** in the upper layers of the epithelium.

A variant lesion that has been attributed to the human papilloma virus is the **vulvar papillomatosis lesion of the vaginal vestibule.** This lesion was described in patients with long-standing recalcitrant vulvar burning and pain, which usually occurs after intercourse or postmenstrually. Upon colposcopic examination of the vestibule, **pink soft lesions** will be noted that have three different characteristics: (1) Arizona cactus–like projections, (2) camel hump–like projections, and (3) stony colonial pavement–like projections. Histologic examination of these lesions reveals virally induced basal hyperplasia and atypia, papillary elongation, dyskeratosis, binucleation, and koilocytosis.

4) Treatment

The treatment of condyloma acuminatum in the nonpregnant state may be carried out by using frequent applications of 10–25% podophyllin in a tincture of benzoin, which will gradually eradicate the disease. In infants and in pregnancy, however, podophyllin is contraindicated. TCA (trichloracetic acid in a 50% solution in water) may cause burns on the skin, so caution should be exercised when using this modality. Carbon dioxide laser vaporization, cryosurgery, elec-

trocautery, or surgical excision has also been utilized with about an 80–90% success rate. The antimetabolite 5-fluorouracil (5-FU) acts by blocking nucleic acid synthesis. A 5% topical 5-FU cream can be used successfully on vaginal condylomata. Since it denudes the skin, it results in an extensive erosion of the vagina or vulva. This agent also has fetotoxic effects. A new approach to the treatment of condyloma acuminatum has been the introduction of interferon as either a topical, intralesional, or parenteral medication. The biological side effects of this drug are fever, chills, nausea and vomiting, fatigue, malaise, and headache. This treatment has apparently been successful in many cases. If the vaginal lesions are very extensive in pregnancy, cesarean delivery may be necessary.

The newborn children of mothers who have genital warts have been noted on occasion to develop papillomas on their vocal cords (i.e., **juvenile laryngeal papillomatosis**), which involves the human papilloma virus types 6 (a–f) and 11 (a, b), presumably acquired at the time of their passage through the birth canal. These lesions may progress to malignancy.

d. Chancroid

This disease in the past has been rarely seen in the United States, with only 878 cases having been reported from 1971 to 1980. In 1983, 90.1% of all reported cases (847) were seen in just four states: Florida, Georgia, California, and New York. The increasing incidence of this disease is reflected in the fact that more than 2,000 cases were reported in 1985. Furthermore, in 1986, 3,418 cases were reported—the largest number of cases since 1952. Chancroid occurs mainly in men who patronize prostitutes or who have imported the disease from countries outside of the United States. The causative organism is **Haemophilus ducreyi.**

1) Clinical findings

In chancroid, a "soft chancre" ulcer occurs on the perineal, vaginal, or cervical surfaces. These saucer-shaped inflammatory ulcers are usually very tender and produce a foul discharge. Obtaining a positive culture of the H. ducreyi organism is difficult and requires a special medium; less than 80% of the cases test positive. Recently, a dot-immunobinding serologic test, and a technique in which the H. ducreyi organism may be detected in the ulcer discharge material by immunofluorescence, have both proven to be helpful.

2) Treatment

The treatment of chancroid has primarily consisted of administering sulfonamides; however, recently the administration of erythromycin, 500 mg q.i.d. p.o. for 7–10 days, or trimethoprim-sulfamethoxazole tabs, 1 (160/800) b.i.d. for 7–10 days, have been used. Tetracycline, 500 mg q.i.d. p.o. for 14 days, or in combination with one of the above regimens, has also been recommended. Recently, two other antibiotic regimens have been advocated in resistant cases. The use of ceftriaxone, 250 mg I.M. in a single dose, has been suggested. The combination of amoxicillin, 500 mg, and clavulanic acid, 125 mg, t.i.d. for seven days, has also been effective if resistance to amoxicillin is present due to beta-lactamase production.

e. Granuloma inguinale

1) Etiology

Granuloma inguinale is a granulomatous disease of the genitalia caused by Calymmatobacterium granulomatis and transmitted by sexual intercourse. The lesion contains the characteristic *Donovan bodies,* which are intracytoplasmic coccobacillary organisms in the mononuclear cells. The disease is not usually found in the United States but is prevalent throughout India and the Orient.

2) Clinical findings

The organism seems to be rare in prostitutes and perhaps is more common in homosexual individuals who practice sodomy. It is thought that the organism may originate in the bowel. The usual incubation period for granuloma inguinale is about 8–12 weeks. The initial lesions are skin papulonodules that ulcerate and become infected with a malodorous discharge. Inguinal buboes may occasionally be present, and the healing of the lesions is slow. Due to autoinoculation, other perineal lesions may develop. Other sexually transmitted diseases, such as syphilis, may also be present.

3) Diagnosis

Calymmatobacterium organisms may be identified on crushed-tissue preparations stained with Wright or Giemsa stain. Biopsies may show granulation tissue with large macrophages that have rod-like inclusion

bodies (Mikulicz's cells) and plasma cells. **The microscopic identification of the cystic purplish-stained Donovan bodies in the large mononuclear cells on either Wright- or Giemsa-stained slides is characteristic of the disease.**

4) Treatment

The treatment of granuloma inguinale with tetracycline hydrochloride, 500 mg q.i.d. p.o. for 2–3 weeks, has been effective, as has treatment with streptomycin; however, these agents should be not be used in pregnancy, since they may endanger the fetus. Erythromycin, 500 mg q.i.d. p.o. for 2–3 weeks, may be used in pregnancy.

f. Oxyuriasis

1) Symptoms

While *oxyuriasis* is an intestinal infestation by Enterobius vermicularis (i.e., *pinworm*) and is not a disease that involves the vulva per se, it does cause considerable perianal itching as its major symptom. The pinworm is very common in young children, especially in those who reside in institutions. *Contact with the perianal region, or with the patient's bedding or clothing, may transfer the ova to the mouth, where they are swallowed.* The parasite then matures in the lower gastrointestinal tract over a period of several weeks. **The female pinworm then migrates to the perianal area and emerges from the anal canal at night to lay her eggs in the perianal skin folds.** When the larvae hatch, they may migrate back into the rectum and lower intestine to produce a retro-infection.

2) Diagnosis

The diagnosis of oxyuriasis may be made by trapping the ova on a piece of transparent adhesive tape that has been applied to the perianal area just after arising in the morning. The strip of tape is then placed upon a microscopic slide, the mucilage dissolved by a drop of toluene, and the ova identified.

3) Treatment

The treatment of oxyuriasis consists of meticulous hand washing and careful handling of the patient's clothing and bedding. *A single dose of pyrantel pamoate will generally eradicate the worms.* The whole family will usually be infested and should be treated. The use of *antipruritic creams or ointments* (e.g., ammoniated mercury ointment) may be necessary to control the pruritus.

A synthetic broad-spectrum antihelmintic, mebendazole (Vermox), comes in chewable tablets. The dosage is one chewable tablet for either an adult or a child. If a cure is not effected, a second course may be given in three weeks. This is a Pregnancy Category C drug.

g. Syphilis

1) Primary syphilis

a) Clinical findings

Syphilis is due to the spirochetal organism Treponema pallidum, which gains entrance into the human body through the mucous membranes by sexual contact. The organism rapidly invades the lymphatics and the blood vessels to spread to all organs of the body. The **primary syphilis** chancre develops when the treponemes reach a concentration of 10^7 per gram of tissue. **The luetic chancre is usually an indurated, painless, well-defined ulcer surrounded by an indurated rim.** There may be enlarged groin lymph nodes. The primary lesion may occur on the vulva, the vagina, the cervix, the breast, the nose, or any other skin or mucous membrane area of the body.

b) Antigens

Two antigens are elicited by the treponemes: the nontreponemal lipoidal antigens (i.e., cardiolipin) and the specific treponemal antigens. *The level of the cardiolipin antibodies, or Wasserman antibodies, is a reflection of the amount of inflammation that is produced by the treponemes.* Nontreponemal antibody tests used for screening consist of the VDRL slide test and the RPR test. In some situations **these tests may be falsely positive, including those in which mononucleosis, malaria, leprosy, and collagen diseases are present.**

The fluorescent treponemal antibody absorption (FTA-ABS) test is widely used to detect the presence of a false screening test, since it measures the specific antibodies to T. pallidum and thus identifies the presence of an actual infection. Once this test is positive, however, it will remain positive for life. *The effec-*

tiveness of the treatment of syphilis is monitored by repeated nontreponemal antibody tests (e.g., VDRL or RPR).

c) Incubation period

The incubation period of syphilis is generally about 21 days; however, depending upon the size of the inoculum, it may range from 10–90 days. **The development of an antibody titer requires about three to six weeks following the initial infection.** Thus, although there may not be a positive serologic titer present at the time that the chancre appears, there is almost always one by the time the chancre heals. The chancre will persist for about 1–5 weeks, after which it will heal spontaneously.

2) Secondary syphilis

The manifestations of secondary syphilis appear about 6 weeks after the initial infection (with a range of 2–24 weeks). The secondary lesions tend to be smaller and more generalized mucocutaneous, maculopapular, or pustular lesions that are not ulcerated or indurated. The development of alopecia of the scalp may accompany these lesions. The moist papules that appear in the mouth and other mucous membranes are called **condylomata lata.** The T. pallidum organism may be recovered from these lesions, and lymphadenopathy may be present. These lesions disappear over a period of 2–6 weeks; however, succeeding crops of them may recur during the first two years, secondary to repeated episodes of spirochetemia. The patient will be infectious during this time. *At this point, the disease is balanced by the host resistance, and two-thirds of the patients will have no further difficulties with the disease, while one-third will develop the late disease some three to thirty years later.*

Syphilis has been divided into two periods: the early phase with a duration of less than one year; and a late latent phase with a duration exceeding one year.

3) Tertiary syphilis

The manifestations of late disease (tertiary syphilis) are of two types: the first is a gumma, and the second is a granulomatous degeneration of the media of the large arteries, especially the vasa vasorum of the aorta, and a perivascular

granulomatous involvement of the meninges and the parenchyma of the central nervous system.

4) Pregnancy and syphilis

a) Fetal effects

Pregnancy in association with syphilis may result in a late abortion, a stillbirth, a congenitally infected infant, or an uninfected infant. The infant has the greatest chance of being infected during primary or secondary syphilis, when recurrent episodes of spirochetemia take place, whereas if the mother has had the disease for a longer period of time, with fewer or no episodes of spirochetemia, then there is less of a chance that the fetus may die in utero and a greater chance that it will be either congenitally infected or totally unaffected **(Kassowitz's law or Diday's law).** If the fetus is exposed to a large inoculum early in the pregnancy, it may be aborted. While the treponemes may cross the placenta at any time during pregnancy, the involvement of the fetus is said to be unusual before about 18 weeks' gestation. This has been attributed to a supposed immunologic incompetence on the part of the fetus; however, immunologic competence in the fetus has been described by at least one investigator as occurring as early as the 13th week.

b) Diagnosis

The diagnosis of syphilis during pregnancy is made in the same way as in the nonpregnant woman. **Suspicion should be directed toward any painless, indolent lesion that occurs in the genital area that does not heal within two weeks.** Scrapings from the base of the lesion should be examined for spirochetes under a darkfield microscope. Sometimes there may be multiple lesions that go unnoticed by the patient. In asymptomatic patients without lesions, serological tests for syphilis (STS) (e.g., VDRL, RPR) should be obtained initially and at about 36 weeks' gestation in every pregnant woman. *If the serological test is positive, then a fluorescent treponemal antibody absorption (FTA-ABS) test should be obtained.* If this test is positive, then the patient should be treated, unless she has had syphilis previously, in which case the FTA-ABS test is of no help, since once it has turned positive, it remains positive. **Repeated quantitative STS may show a rising titer of at least a two-tube dilution in women who have been reinfected; these patients should be retreated.** With the initial infection, quantitative STS values, and

perhaps a lumbar puncture, should be performed to stage the infection prior to treatment. Following treatment, the quantitative STS should be followed in order to determine the response to therapy.

c) Neonatal infection

The clinical recognition of syphilis in the neonate is usually not possible until 2–4 weeks or more after delivery. **Syphilis presents in the infant as hepatosplenomegaly, hemolysis, and hyperbilirubinemia, much like infants of mothers who have erythroblastosis fetalis, toxoplasmosis, or cytomegalovirus.** The lesions may occur either during the first two years, or they may not appear until the third year of life or later. The lesions may include interstitial keratitis or nerve deafness. The STS results may be confusing in the neonate. On one hand, the maternal immunoglobulin IgG antibody may cross the placenta and produce a positive STS result in an infant that may not be infected. On the other hand, if the fetus is indeed infected, then it will produce its own IgM antibodies but will also have maternal IgG antibodies. Thus, the fetus will show a positive STS in either instance, and will have to be retested after the maternal antibodies have disappeared in order to determine its true status.

d) Treatment

The treatment of syphilis in the nonpregnant and the pregnant woman should follow the guidelines issued by the Centers for Disease Control (CDC) (Table 11-1, Table 11-2, and Table 11-3).

TABLE 11-1. Early syphilis (primary, secondary, latent syphilis of less than 1 year's duration) should be treated with:

Benzathine penicillin G, 2.4 million units total I.M. at a single session.

OR

if the patient is allergic to penicillin, and this allergy is confirmed, then treat with:

Tetracycline HCL, 500 mg by mouth 4 times daily for 15 days.

OR

Erythromycin, 500 mg by mouth 4 times a day for 15 days.

Adapted from *Morbidity and Mortality Weekly Report Supplement,* vol. 34, no. 4S, October 18, 1985.

TABLE 11-2. Syphilis of more than one year's duration, except neurosyphilis (latent syphilis of indeterminate or more than one year's duration, cardiovascular, or late benign syphilis), should be treated with:

Recommended regimen:

Benzathine penicillin G, 2.4 million units I.M. once a week for three successive weeks (a total of 7.2 million units).

Penicillin-allergic patients: Perform pretherapy cerebral spinal fluid examination with these regimens.

Tetracycline HCL, 500 mg by mouth four times daily for 30 days. (Patient compliance with this regimen may be difficult, so care should be taken to encourage compliance.)

OR

If the patient cannot tolerate tetracycline and if this allergy is confirmed, then treat with erythromycin, 500 mg by mouth four times daily for 30 days.

Cerebrospinal fluid examination:

Cerebrospinal fluid examination should be performed in patients with clinical symptoms or signs consistent with neurosyphilis. In patients with syphilis of greater than one year's duration, a cerebrospinal fluid examination should be performed to exclude asymptomatic neurosyphilis.

Neurosyphilis:

Published studies show that a total dose of 6.0–9.0 million units of penicillin G over a three- to four-week period results in a satisfactory clinical response in approximately 90% of patients with neurosyphilis.

Potentially effective regimens, although none have been adequately studied, are:

Aqueous crystalline penicillin G, 12–24 million units I.V./day (2–4 million units every four hours) for 10 days, followed by benzathine penicillin G, 2.4 million units I.M. weekly for three doses.

OR

Aqueous procaine penicillin G, 2.4 million units I.M. daily plus probenecid, 500 mg by mouth four times daily, both for 10 days, followed by benzathine penicillin G, 2.4 million units I.M. weekly for three doses.

OR

Benzathine penicillin G, 2.4 million units I.M. weekly for three doses.

Adapted from *Morbidity and Mortality Weekly Report Supplement,* vol. 34, no. 4S, October 18, 1985.

h. Acquired immune deficiency syndrome (AIDS)

1) General considerations

Since 1980, the human T-cell lymphotropic virus type III (HTLV-III) has exploded on the medical scene as one of the most devastating infectious diseases of this century. It is caused by a **retrovirus** that uses its RNA to produce DNA, which in turn results in the production of RNA that is responsible for the viral proteins. The surface markers on the lymphocytes are T4 and T8, which can be recognized by monoclonal antibodies. The **T4 are the helper cells,** while the **T8 are the suppressor**

TABLE 11-3. Syphilis in pregnancy

All pregnant women should have an initial VDRL or RPR test performed at the time of the first prenatal visit. An additional test should be performed in high-risk patients in the third trimester. Cord blood should be tested for syphilis antibodies. Seroreactive patients should be evaluated promptly with a history and physical examination, a quantitative nontreponemal test, and a confirmatory treponemal test. If the treponemal test is nonreactive, and there is no clinical evidence of syphilis, then treatment is unnecessary. These tests should be repeated in four weeks. If the patient has been adequately treated in the past, then no treatment is indicated unless there is evidence of reinfection, such as darkfield-positive lesions, a four-fold titer rise of a quantitative non-treponemal test, or history of recent sexual exposure to a person with syphilis.

Recommended regimens:

Penicillin should be administered in the appropriate dosage according to the stage of syphilis as recommended for nonpregnant women. In patients who are allergic to penicillin, erythromycin should be utilized. Infants born to mothers treated during pregnancy with erythromycin for early syphilis should be treated with penicillin. **Tetracycline is not recommended in pregnant women because of potential adverse effects on the fetus.** Monthly quantitative non-treponemal tests should be obtained throughout the pregnancy, and if there is a four-fold rise in titer, they should be retreated. Furthermore, those women who do not show a four-fold decrease in titer in a 3-month period should be re-treated.

All infants of mothers who have had adequately treated syphilis during pregnancy should be followed at 1 month of age and then every 3 months for the first 15 months, and then every 6 months until the nontreponemal serologic tests are negative or stable at low titer. If the serologic test is positive at 3 months of age, the infant should be treated for congenital syphilis. A CSF examination should be performed on infants with congenital syphilis.

Recommended regimens for symptomatic or asymptomatic infants:

Aqueous crystalline penicillin G, 50,000 units/kg I.M. or I.V. daily in 2 divided doses for a minimum of 10 days,

OR

Aqueous penicillin G procaine, 50,000 units/kg I.M. daily for a minimum of 10 days.

Adapted from *Morbidity and Mortality Weekly Report Supplement,* vol. 34, no. 4S, October 18, 1985.

cells. An infection with HTLV-III results in a reversal of the usual T4:T8 ratio of 1.5 to a ratio of 0.6–0.8. This reversal is not specific to AIDS; it may also occur with acute cytomegalovirus, the Epstein-Barr virus, and hepatitis infections.

This retrovirus is the cause of the acquired immune deficiency syndrome (AIDS) and AIDS-related complex (ARC), which includes lymphadenopathy, malaise, fever, nausea and vomiting, and immune dysfunction and was initially seen in a few homosexual men before the onset of opportunistic infections.

Lymphadenopathy-associated virus (LAV) is probably the same as HTLV-III. These AIDS viruses are now referred to as the **human immunodeficiency viruses (HIV).** The human immunodeficiency virus has now been separated into HIV-1 and HIV-2, since 58% of the nucleotide sequence of HIV-2 is different from that of HIV-1. It was initially estimated that 29,000 people in the United States received blood products infected with HIV-1. With the widespread use of antibody tests, the risk of HIV-1 transmission from screened blood was thought to be extremely low;

however, with the recent identification of HIV-2, a closely related retrovirus that was first linked to AIDS in West Africa, this concern has again resurfaced, since the HIV-1 screening tests currently being used for blood donors may fail to detect HIV-2. Furthermore, a new related retrovirus that is serologically distinct from both HIV-1 and HIV-2 was recently isolated from a Nigerian patient with AIDs, and so the AIDS story is still unfolding. AIDS has become manifest in 54,233 victims in the United States (as of March 21, 1988) and has infected many more persons worldwide. It has been estimated that there are about 270 cases per 1 million population in the United States; however, this estimate is changing rapidly as more and more cases are identified. The average life span after the onset of the initial hospitalization for clinical AIDS has been estimated to be about 224 days.

The incubation period of AIDS may last up to 7–10 years, with about 10% of the infected individuals in any given year developing clinical symptoms. AIDS is transmitted sexually by both homosexual and heterosexual contact. It may also be spread by needle-stick injuries among health-care workers who are exposed to the blood of patients with AIDS (percutaneous transmission). It appears that AIDS may also be passed on to women who receive artificial insemination. The infection of the fetus has also occurred in cases where the mother was infected (perinatal exposure). The population at risk includes Haitians, health-care workers, intravenous (I.V.) drug abusers, recipients of blood products, homosexuals, bisexuals, and more recently, the heterosexual population. The presence of serological evidence of HIV antibodies in homosexual and bisexual men ranges from 10–70%, with most of the studies showing a 20–50% incidence. In intravenous drug abusers in New York City, the incidence was 50–65%. In patients with hemophilia A, the incidence was 70%, whereas in those with hemophilia B, it was 35%, and this prevalence holds true throughout the United States. In heterosexual partners of infected persons, the incidence ranges from 10 to 60%. In contrast, the prevalence of HIV in other groups within the general population was as follows: blood donors, 0.04%; candidates for military service, 0.15%; Job Corps applicants, 0.33%; and among patients of family planning clinics and women's clinics, less than 1%.

Most of the evidence indicates that the disease is not transmitted by casual public contact, toilet seats, aerosol spread, or by being exposed to sneezing or coughing. Recently, however, there has been some concern expressed about the risk of contracting AIDS from blood contact on the abraded skin or by splashes of infected blood or secretions in the eyes of health-care workers who are treating AIDS patients. Some experts have suggested that goggles, double gloves, and waterproof aprons should be worn at the time of a delivery or during a surgical procedure on such patients.

2) Clinical findings

AIDS causes the destruction of the individual's immune response, which in turn allows other opportunistic infections to develop. Infections such as disseminated histoplasmosis, bronchial or pulmonary candidiasis, and aspergillosis have been identified in AIDS patients. In addition, non-Hodgkin's lymphoma of a high-grade pathologic type, and **Kaposi's sarcoma of the skin** in patients over 60 years of age, have also been noted. **The presence of serum antibodies to the HTLV-III virus is indicative of AIDS infection.**

The most common clinical symptoms include febrile episodes and malaise, associated with a weight loss of as much as 20–30% of the body weight. Many patients may have **cytomegalovirus** in their blood, the presence of Epstein-Barr virus in their lymphocytes and pharynx, and **Mycobacterium avium and Mycobacterium intracellulare** in their blood and bone marrow. The insidious development of dyspnea and progressive hypoxemia may be secondary to **Pneumocystis carinii,** although **Cryptococcus neoformans** is also common. Watery diarrhea with nausea is frequently seen in AIDS patients. **A variety of enteric organisms,** such as Giardia lamblia, Entamoeba histolytica, Shigella, and Salmonella species may be involved. Neurological symptoms with a loss of mentation and a withdrawal of the patient from social situations occurs in about 10% of patients. Toxoplasma gondii is often seen, and, cryptococcal meningitis may also occur.

Early markers of a possible HIV infection in gynecologic patients are Candida infections, condyloma acuminatum, herpes simplex virus, and perhaps some of the other sexually transmitted diseases. Women constitute only about 7% of the AIDS patients in the United States. Candidiasis is a common organism present when there is T-cell dysfunction, especially if it is chronic, but it may occur either as a chronic vaginal infection or as a persistent oral thrush. The presence of chronic anogenital condylomata is also commonly seen in immunodeficient situations, such as with the use of immunosuppressive therapy for organ transplantation or in patients with lymphomas. While condylomata may not be clearly associated with AIDS, one should nonetheless be suspicious of severe anogenital warts in this context. Severe ulcerative genital herpetic lesions were one of the first recognized clinical signs of an AIDS infection, but only occur in about 2% of patients with AIDS.

3) Diagnosis

Several test kits have been used in the diagnosis of AIDS, one of which is based upon the *enzyme-linked immunosorbent assay (ELISA) technique,* which is quite effective (with a sensitivity of 93% and specificity of 99.8%). Positive tests should be repeated, and if still positive, or if uncertain, then an additional test, called the *Western blot test,* an assay of the antibody to the major viral antigens, should be utilized. A third test that may be used is a *radioimmunoprecipitation assay (RIPA),* which is an assay of the suspected major core protein.

Many laboratories are attempting to develop further tests to identify the multiple virus-specific protein bands, such as p17 (core protein), p24 (core protein), p31 (endonuclease component of polymerase translate), gp41 (transmembrane envelope glycoprotein), p51 (reverse transcriptase component of polymerase translate), p55 (precursor of core protein), p66 (reverse transcriptase component of polymerase translate), gp120 (outer envelope glycoprotein), and gp160 (precursor of envelope glycoprotein). **The licensed Western blot test measures p24, p31, and either gp41 or gp160.** If all bands are present, then the test is considered to be positive. If not all of these bands are present, then the results are indeterminant. If no bands are present, then it is negative. Other unlicensed tests use different bands to determine positivity.

The Centers for Disease Control (CDC) has published a case definition for AIDS for surveillance purposes (Fig. 11-1) as follows:[1]

---

[1] Reprinted from *Morbidity and Mortality Weekly Report,* vol. 36, no. 15, August 14, 1987.

I. Without laboratory evidence regarding HIV infection.

A. Causes of immunodeficiency that disqualify diseases as indicators of AIDS in the absence of laboratory evidence for HIV infection.

1. High-dose or long-term systemic corticosteroid therapy or other immunosuppressive/cytotoxic therapy for less than or equal to three months before the onset of the indicator disease.

2. Any of the following diseases diagnosed less than or equal to three months after the diagnosis of the indicator disease: Hodgkin's disease, non-Hodgkin's lymphoma (other than primary brain lymphoma), lymphocytic leukemia, multiple myeloma, any other cancer of lymphoreticular or histiocytic tissue, or angioimmunoblastic lymphadenopathy.

3. A genetic (congenital) immunodeficiency syndrome or an acquired immunodeficiency syndrome atypical of HIV infection, such as one involving hypogammaglobulinemia.

B. Indicator diseases diagnosed definitively.

1. Candidiasis of the esophagus, trachia, bronchi, or lungs.

2. Cryptococcosis, extrapulmonary.

3. Cryptosporidiosis with diarrhea persisting for more than one month.

4. Cytomegalovirus disease of an organ other than the liver, spleen, or lymph nodes in a patient more than one month of age.

5. Herpes simplex virus infection causing a mucocutaneous ulcer that persists longer than one month; or bronchitis, pneumonitis, or esophagitis for any duration affecting a patient more than one month of age.

6. Kaposi's sarcoma affecting a patient less than 60 years of age.

7. Lymphoma of the brain (primary) affecting a patient less than 60 years of age.

8. Lymphoid interstitial pneumonia and/or pulmonary lymphoid hyperplasia (LIP/

PLH complex) affecting a child less than 13 years of age.

9. Mycobacterium avium complex or Mycobacterium kansasii disease, disseminated (at a site other than or in addition to the lungs, skin, or cervical or hilar lymph nodes).
10. Pneumocystis carinii pneumonia.
11. Progressive multifocal leukoencephalopathy.
12. Toxoplasmosis of the brain affecting a patient more than one month of age.

II. With laboratory evidence of HIV infection.
A. Indicator diseases diagnosed definitively.

1. Bacterial infections, multiple or recurrent (any combination of at least two within a two-year period), of the following types affecting a child less than 13 years of age: septicemia, pneumonia, meningitis, bone or joint infection, or abscess of an internal organ or body cavity (excluding otitis media or superficial skin or mucosal abscesses) caused by Haemophilus, Streptococcus (including pneumococcus), or any other pyogenic bacteria.
2. Coccidioidomycosis, disseminated (at a site other than or in addition to the lungs, or cervical or hilar lymph nodes).
3. HIV encephalopathy (also called "HIV dementia," "AIDS dementia," or "subacute encephalitis due to HIV").
4. Histoplasmosis, disseminated (at a site other than or in addition to the lungs or cervical or hilar lymph nodes).
5. Isosporiasis with diarrhea persisting for more than one month.
6. Kaposi's sarcoma at any age.
7. Lymphoma of the brain (primary) at any age.
8. Other non-Hodgkin's lymphoma of B-cell or unknown immunologic phenotype and the following histologic types:
   a. Small noncleaved lymphoma (either Burkitt or non-Burkitt type).
   b. Immunoblastic sarcoma (equivalent to any of the following, although not necessarily all in combination: immunoblastic lymphoma, large-cell lymphoma, diffuse histiocytic lymphoma, diffuse undifferentiated lymphoma, or high-grade lymphoma). Note: Lymphomas are not included here if they are of T-cell immunologic phenotype or their histologic type is either not described or is described as lymphocytic, lymphoblastic, small-cleaved, or plasmacytoid lymphocytic.

9. Any mycobacterial disease caused by mycobacteria other than M. tuberculosis, disseminated (at a site other than or in addition to the lungs, skin, or cervical or hilar lymph nodes).
10. Disease caused by M. tuberculosis, extrapulmonary (involving at least one site outside of the lungs, regardless of whether there is concurrent pulmonary involvement).
11. Salmonella (nontyphoid) septicemia, recurrent.
12. HIV wasting syndrome (emaciation, "slim disease").

B. Indicator diseases diagnosed presumptively.

1. Candidiasis of the esophagus.
2. Cytomegalovirus retinitis with loss of vision.
3. Kaposi's sarcoma.
4. Lymphoid interstitial pneumonia and/or pulmonary lymphoid hyperplasia (LIP/PLH complex) affecting a child less than 13 years of age.
5. Mycobacterial disease (acid-fast bacilli with species not identified by culture), disseminated (involving at least one site other than or in addition to the lungs, skin, or cervical or hilar lymph nodes).
6. Pneumocystis carinii pneumonia.
7. Toxoplasmosis of the brain affecting a patient more than one month of age.

III. With laboratory evidence against HIV infection.
When the laboratory tests are negative for an HIV infection, a diagnosis of

Text continues on p. 150

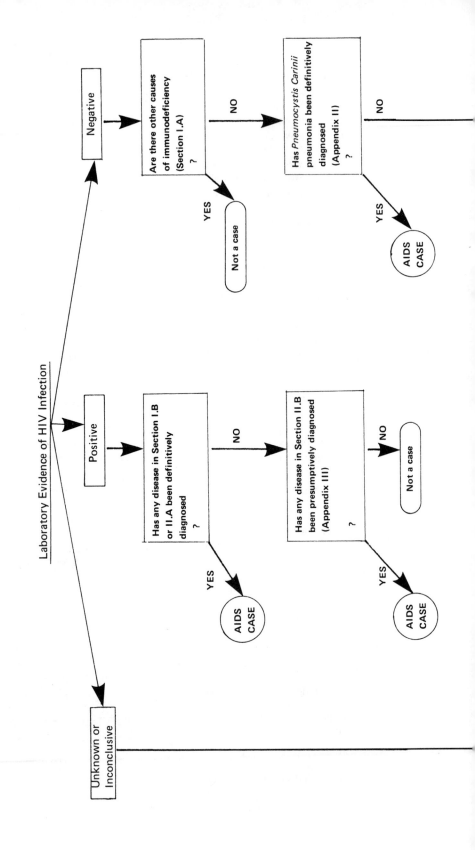

Laboratory Evidence of HIV Infection

Negative

Positive

Unknown or Inconclusive

Are there other causes of immunodeficiency (Section I.A) ?

Has *Pneumocystis Carinii* pneumonia been definitively diagnosed (Appendix II) ?

Has any disease in Section I.B or II.A been definitively diagnosed ?

Has any disease in Section II.B been presumptively diagnosed (Appendix III) ?

YES → Not a case

YES → AIDS CASE

YES → AIDS CASE

YES → AIDS CASE

NO → Not a case

NO

NO

NO

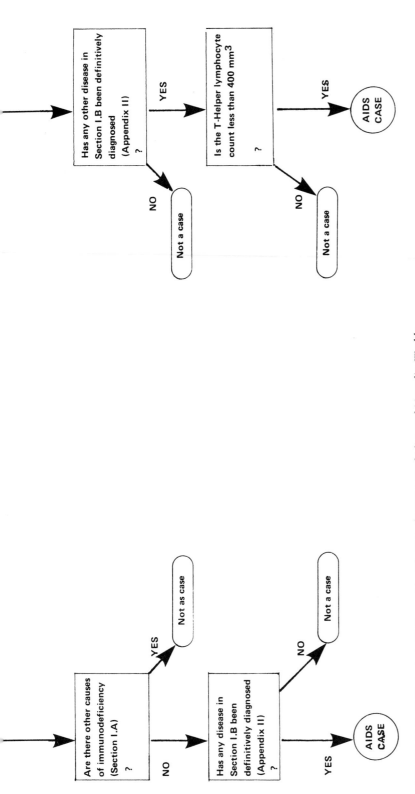

FIGURE 11-1. CDC chart of AIDS case identification. (*Source: Morbidity and Mortality Weekly Report*, vol. 36, nos. 15–95, August 14, 1987.)

AIDS for surveillance purposes is ruled out unless:

A. **All other causes of immunodeficiency listed in Section I.A. are excluded; and**

B. **The patient has had either:**
   1. Pneumocystis carinii pneumonia diagnosed by a definitive method; or
   2. Both of the following:
      a. Any of the other diseases indicative of AIDS listed in Section I.B. diagnosed by a definitive method; and
      b. A T-helper/inducer (CD4) lymphocyte count of less than 400/mm^3.

4) Recommendations

It has been recommended that patients who have persistent positive tests for HTLV-III, but who have no known risk factors and no symptoms of AIDS or ARC (i.e., at low risk), should be educated about the disease and observed closely by a physician for the onset of signs of infection. These individuals should not donate blood, plasma, or sperm. While sexual relations probably should not be restricted, condoms should be used. The sexual partner should also be tested at intervals, since the occurrence of HTLV-III positive in the consort would provide evidence of a probable true-positive test in the patient. According to some authors, postponement of pregnancy should perhaps not be recommended; however, since there is an increased risk of transmission to the fetus (perhaps as high as 65%) if the individual does have the disease, each case should be considered individually. These patients should inform their medical or dental health care personnel of the fact that they have tested positive for HIV. It should be kept in mind, however, that many of these asymptomatic patients may turn out to have a false-positive test. On the other hand, many individuals die over about a 10-year period from the onset of a positive test; thus, it may turn out that there is a long incubation period involved and that once the test is positive it may be only a question of time until clinical symptoms and death occur. Employment, education, or other social contacts in general should not be restricted; however, again, each case should be considered on an individual basis.

Patients who have repeatedly tested positive for HIV infection, and who are known to have been exposed to AIDS, are at high risk for developing the disease and transmitting it to others. Individuals who have had exposure to intravenous drugs of abuse, or to men and women who are known to have had a positive HIV test, and hemophiliacs, who are exposed to blood transfusions, are all at high risk. These patients should also obtain the services of physicians who specialize in the various manifestations of AIDS and should have a close follow-up examination to determine whether they have any evidence of the disease. They should be instructed to seek immediate medical attention if any clinical manifestations of AIDS or ARC occur, or to have routine semi-annual checkups if asymptomatic. Many of these people seem to remain asymptomatic, but the long-term prognosis is unknown. Personal items, such as toothbrushes and razors, should not be shared with other people because of the risk of transmitting the disease. Deep kissing and sexual relations without a condom should be avoided. Pregnancy is to be avoided, but if it occurs, the infant should be checked for the disease after birth. Other household contacts of these people do not necessarily have to be tested. If blood or body fluids are spilled, they should be washed off with a 1:10 dilution of household bleach, and all needles that are used on such patients should be sterilized or disposed of correctly. If the individual works in a situation in which his blood or body fluids might contaminate other people, precautions to prevent such transmittance should be carried out. Medical personnel with repeatedly positive HIV tests who are at high risk should protect their patients in the same manner as they would if they had a hepatitis B infection.

5) Classification of human immunodeficiency virus (HIV)

The CDC has suggested that adult patients with AIDS should be classified as follows:[2]

a. **Group I:** Acute infection.
b. **Group II:** Asymptomatic infection.
c. **Group III:** Persistent generalized lymphadenopathy.
d. **Group IV:** Other disease.
   1) **Subgroup A:** Constitutional disease.
   2) **Subgroup B:** Neurological disease.

---

[2] Reprinted from *Morbidity and Mortality Weekly Report,* vol. 35, no. 20, May 23, 1986.

3) **Subgroup C:** Secondary infectious disease.
   a. **Category C-1:** Specified secondary infectious diseases listed in the CDC surveillance definition of AIDS.
   b. **Category C-2:** Other specified secondary infectious diseases.
4) **Subgroup D:** Secondary cancers.
5) **Subgroup E:** Other conditions.

The **group I** patients have a mononucleosis-like syndrome, with or without an aseptic meningitis, associated with seroconversion for the HTLV-III/LAV antibody. In **group II,** the patient is asymptomatic and has never had any of the signs or symptoms of active disease that appear in groups III and IV. Patients classified as being in **group III** have unexplained palpable lymphadenopathy with nodal enlargements of greater than 1 cm at two or more extra-inguinal sites that persist for longer than three months. In **group IV,** the patient may be assigned to a subgroup with constitutional disease, such as in **subgroup A,** in which an unexplained persistent fever, weight loss greater than 10%, and diarrhea have been present for one month. Patients assigned to **subgroup B** have an unexplained dementia, myelopathy, or peripheral neuropathy. In **subgroup C,** opportunistic infections indicative of a defect in the cell-mediated immunity are present. These might include, in **category C-1,** Pneumocystis carinii, chronic toxoplasmosis, cryptococcosis, histoplasmosis, myobacterium, cytomegalovirus, herpesvirus, and other opportunistic infections. In the **category C-2** patients, one of six other diseases must be present: salmonella, nocardiosis, tuberculosis, oral candidiasis, multidermatomal herpes zoster, or hairy leukoplakia. In **subgroup D** patients, secondary cancers that are known to be associated with HTLV-III/LAV infection are present, such as Kaposi's sarcoma, non-Hodgkin's lymphoma, or a primary lymphoma of the brain. In **subgroup E** patients, other diseases that cannot be classified in the above groups of opportunistic infections are included. Chronic lymphoid interstitial pneumonitis would be included in this group, for example.

In children who are less than 13 years of age, the classification is as follows:[3]

---

[3] Reprinted from *Morbidity and Mortality Weekly Report,* vol. 36, no. 15, April 24, 1987.

Class P-0. Indeterminate infection.
Class P-1. Asymptomatic infection.
   Subclass A. Normal immune function.
   Subclass B. Abnormal immune function.
   Subclass C. Immune function not tested.
Class P-2. Symptomatic infection.
   Subclass A. Nonspecific findings.
   Subclass B. Progressive neurological disease.
   Subclass C. Lymphoid interstitial pneumonia.
   Subclass D. Secondary infectious diseases.
      Category D-1. Specified secondary infectious diseases listed in the CDC surveillance definition for AIDS.
      Category D-2. Recurrent serious bacterial infections.
      Category D-3. Other specified secondary infectious diseases.
   Subclass E. Secondary cancers.
      Category E-1. Specified secondary cancers listed in the CDC surveillance definition for AIDS.
      Category E-2. Other cancers possibly secondary to HIV infection.
   Subclass F. Other diseases possibly due to HIV infection.

6) Treatment

Currently, there is no known effective treatment for HIV infections. A number of antiviral agents are under investigation, such as ribavirin (Virazole) and alpha-2a recombinant interferon (Roferon-A). The latter is a leukocyte-derived protein with antiviral properties. **Recently, Retrovir (zidovudine), which is azidothymidine (AZT) has been released for the treatment of AIDS.** In the initial studies with this drug, it was found that it significantly reduced the probability of these patients acquiring an opportunistic infection. Hematologic toxicity, including granulocytopenia and severe anemia, have been noted as side effects with AZT. This drug is indicated in the patient who has symptoms of AIDS or advanced ARC with a history of a cytologically confirmed Pneumocystis carinii or an absolute CD4 (T4 helper/inducer) lymphocyte count of less than 200/mm^3 in the peripheral blood prior to the beginning of therapy. The usual dosage is 200 mg p.o. every four hours around the clock.

If the patient is pregnant and has AIDS, the opportunistic infections may prove difficult to manage, and vertical transmission of AIDS to the fetus may occur. It is unknown whether a cesarean section will reduce this risk of transmission, as some infants who have been delivered by cesarean section have developed the disease.

i. Herpesvirus infections

1) General considerations

A Herpesvirus hominus type II infection of the vulva has become a common STD that has assumed increasing importance over the past few years because it may recur and it is essentially incurable. There are two serotypes, type I and type II. The **type I virus** is commonly seen in "cold sores" of the lips, and the **type II virus** is more commonly found in the lower genital tract (85%). Antibodies to these DNA viruses share a cross-reactivity. The incubation period is 2–7 days and the virus is transmitted by sexual contact. The antibodies develop about 21 days after the patient acquires the primary infection.

2) Clinical findings

The initial herpetic lesions consist of vesicular eruptions that appear as 1- to 3-mm blisters on the skin or mucous membranes. The initial tingling and itching are replaced by irritation and pain as the vesicles rupture and ulcerate. In some cases, the ulcers may coalesce to form an extensively ulcerated area, which will subsequently scab over and then re-epithelialize. At times, the lesions may be so extensive about the vulva and the urethra as to cause urinary retention due to the edema of the introitus and the urethra. In some patients, the presence of an inflammatory involvement of the sacral portion of the spinal cord may result in an **increased cerebrospinal fluid cell count and an elevated protein content,** due to a polyradiculitis, which also may result in urinary retention **(Elsberg's syndrome).** In about 40–50% of those patients who have primary lesions, fever, malaise, photophobia, myalgia, and a tender lymphadenopathy may occur, lasting approximately 4–6 days. Viral meningitis may occur in 4–10% of patients, and lower motor neuron dysfunction with urinary retention (neurogenic bladder), impotence (in men), constipation, and perineal numbness may occur in 1–3%.

A *primary infection* of Herpes simplex virus (HSV)

will classically produce ulcerative lesions that may last for 16–21 days in men and 10–16 days in women. The shedding of the virus has been noted to last for about 9.1–11.6 days in men and 8.0–14.7 days in women. Patients may also shed the virus and be asymptomatic.

Between recurrent infections, the virus resides in the sensory sacral ganglia, where they remain for life. *Recurrent infections are common during the first six months,* although the lesions tend to be smaller and more localized than those that occur with the initial infection. Systemic symptoms usually do not recur with subsequent recurrences of the infection. Physical, psychological, and emotional events may trigger a recurrence of an HSV infection.

3) Diagnosis

The diagnosis of a herpesvirus infection should be verified by identifying *multinucleated giant cells on a Papanicolaou smear,* or more specifically by **viral cultures,** which have a sensitivity of 95%. Rising antibody titers may also be determined. ELISA techniques (i.e., enzyme-linked immunosorbent assay) have a sensitivity of about 70–80%.

4) Treatment

The use of **acyclovir (Zovirax)** in the nonpregnant patient, topically administered to the lesions q.i.d. for seven days, will often assist in the healing and will usually decrease the duration of symptoms in a primary infection. The use of acyclovir, 200 mg five times daily orally for ten days, when administered within six days of the onset of the lesions, seems to be effective in the initial and recurrent episodes of genital herpes. It also seems to reduce the viral shedding, itching, pain, and the healing times when taken within six days of the appearance of the primary disease. In severe cases, acyclovir, 5 mg/kg I.V. q8h for five days, has been advocated. In some patients, this agent will shorten recurrent disease episodes by one day when the patient is placed on an oral dosage regimen of 200 mg five times daily for five days, if it is started within two days of the onset of the lesions. Acyclovir topical ointment is not indicated in recurrent infections. The use of acyclovir in pregnancy has not yet been defined as being safe for the fetus. Acyclovir apparently acts by inhibiting viral replication. Intravenous acyclovir should be reserved for severely affected hospitalized patients, such as immunocompromised individuals or those with disseminated disease.

The transmission of herpes to a sexual consort is common; therefore, the use of a condom should be encouraged even when the patient is asymptomatic. Over 60% of the women who deliver infected infants are asymptomatic. The risk of the infant developing infection after a vaginal delivery in a patient with an **active recurrent herpesvirus infection** is about 5%. If the patient delivers with a **primary infection,** however, then there is about a **50% risk of transmission of the disease to the infant,** and if a disseminated herpesvirus infection does occur in the infant, then there is about a **50% neonatal mortality rate.** Neonatal infections may take one of three forms: (1) asymptomatic, (2) a localized infection of the skin, nervous system, or eyes, and (3) a generalized systemic involvement of the major organ systems. The onset of disseminated disease occurs on the average at about 16 days postdelivery. Localized disease occurs at 11 days postdelivery.

Herpesvirus cultures that are performed at weekly intervals from about 36 weeks of gestation until term have not been shown to be cost-effective in identifying the patient who may be shedding the virus and thus allow for a cesarean delivery. Patients who have no suspicious genital lesions at the time of labor should be allowed to deliver vaginally. If the patient has genital herpetic lesions, however, then it is recommended that a cesarean section be performed in an effort to protect the infant from acquiring the virus during its passage through the birth canal. The length of time that the membranes have been ruptured in relation to the choice of whether or not to use a vaginal or cesarean section delivery has not been determined. In one multicenter report, an ascending infection was noted to infect the fetus with intact membranes in 12% of the cases. Patients who have nongenital herpetic lesions and no evidence of genital involvement may be delivered vaginally, however, the infant should be protected from contact with such lesions in the neonatal period.

j. Molluscum contagiosum

These umbilicated lesions are due to a mildly contagious virus. The symptoms consist of a mild pruritus only. The multiple growths vary from a few millimeters to as large as 1 cm. The treatment of molluscum contagiosum consists of the destruction of the base of the lesion with trichloroacetic acid or a silver nitrate application. One recent report of the use of the CO_2 laser to destroy these lesions on the thighs noted a high incidence of keloid formation, so this treatment modality should probably not be used.

k. Intertrigo

The inflammation of the body folds due to moisture and chafing has been called intertrigo. In these cases, a secondary bacterial or fungal infection may occur. Treatment consists of keeping the area dry and combating local infectious invaders with antibiotic creams or antifungal ointments.

l. Behcet disease

This condition is uncommon and consists of the presence of *oral and genital lesions associated with ocular inflammation.* It has been suggested that this condition may be due to an autoimmune phenomena. The extent of the vulvar destruction and scarring may be severe. Treatment with high dosage oral contraceptives has been suggested.

m. Fox-Fordyce disease

This disease affects the **apocrine sweat glands,** which become plugged with keratin. Both the axillae and the vulva may be affected with these tiny papules. The pruritus is apparently related to the level of estrogen in the menstrual cycle, with remissions occurring during pregnancy. The treatment consists of topical estrogens and acne medications.

n. Hidradenitis suppurativa

This chronic disease consists of the inflammation and blockage of the apocrine sweat glands of the vulva. The symptoms consist of itching and burning associated with skin abscesses, which periodically recur, coalesce, and drain, with the development of scarring and sinus tracts. The treatment consists of administering an appropriate antibiotic, such as tetracycline, and the use of hot sitz baths. The incisional drainage of the abscesses should be carried out as necessary. The administration of oral contraceptives may decrease the apocrine glandular secretions.

2. Benign conditions

a. Imperforate hymen

The incidence of an **imperforate hymen** would be difficult to determine, since many cases are not reported. Frequently, the hymen has one or more small perforations in it; however, in some instances, the hymen may be completely intact. The patient may be brought to you at the age of menarche, but she will not have yet begun to have menstrual periods; however, she will report having abdominal cramps and pelvic pain for several days each month. These symptoms are due to the accumulation of blood behind the hymen *(i.e., hematocolpos)*. In time, the accumulation of blood may result in the retrograde passage of the menstrual blood into the fallopian tubes *(i.e., hematosalpinx)*, and out into the peritoneal cavity. On rare occasions, a massive dilatation of the tubes may result in an adnexal torsion and even the death of the patient. The treatment of an imperforate hymen consists of the excision of the hymenal membrane and the release of the hematocolpos. Care must be taken with the incision, however, in order to avoid undue scarring and the subsequent development of dyspareunia.

b. Epidermal inclusion cysts

The occlusion of the pilosebaceous ducts, or the turning under of an epithelial surface secondary to trauma or surgical suturing, may result in the development of small cystic structures that are filled with an oily material and desquamated epithelial cells. Upon incision, or needling, an inspissated whitish material may be expressed.

c. Bartholin's duct cyst

If the Bartholin's duct is obstructed, either by infection or by trauma, a cystic dilatation will result. If there is an infection, the patient will complain of tenderness and swelling, and an abscess will be present. While Neisseria gonorrhoeae organisms may be the cause of an abscess in many instances in the nonpregnant woman, other infections and trauma (e.g., postepisiotomy) perhaps are more common etiologies in the postpartum patient.

The primary treatment of an abscess of Bartholin's duct is incision and drainage, with the installation of a one-quarter inch iodoform gauze wick left in the cavity, or the placement of a Word catheter, which is then left in place for one to two weeks to keep the cavity

patent to the outside. Alternatively, a *marsupialization* of the Bartholin's gland may be performed. This operative procedure has the advantage over the *complete excision of the gland* in that there is a preservation of the glandular secretions. In women who are over forty years of age, a swelling of the Bartholin's gland should alert you to the possibility of a carcinoma.

d. Dystrophy

In the past, the terms leukoplakia and kraurosis were used to describe white lesions on the vulva, regardless of their etiology. In 1966, the term **dystrophy** was first used to describe these lesions. **There are two basic types of dystrophy: hypertrophic and atrophic. When they occur together, they are referred to as a "mixed dystrophy," with or without atypicality.**

Those vulvar lesions that have an increased amount of nuclear activity will take a 1% toluidine blue stain (wash area with stain for three minutes and then rinse it off with 1–2% acetic acid) and thus may be more easily identified; however, this test has both a high false-positive and a high false-negative rate. **The diagnosis of dystrophy must be obtained by the histologic evaluation of a vulvar biopsy specimen.**

1) Hypertrophic dystrophy

Hypertrophic dystrophy histologically shows a thickened epithelium, with an elongation of the rete pegs (acanthosis) and a chronic leukocytic infiltrate in the underlying tissues. Often this raised white lesion is the result of chronic infection or irritation. This chronic dermatitis may be treated by the application of a *cortisone cream* to control the pruritus. The premalignant potential of this lesion is unknown.

2) Atrophic dystrophy

Atrophic dystrophy occurs with aging and is due to a decrease in the estrogenic stimulation of the vulvar tissues. The vulvar skin becomes thinned out and is easily traumatized. Pruritus is common, as is dyspareunia. Estrogen creams are effective in restoring the thickness of the atrophic epithelium.

a) Lichen sclerosis et atrophicus

One example of an atrophic lesion of the vulva is the lesion called **lichen sclerosis et atrophicus,** which is characterized by hyperkeratosis, a thin epithelium, and an underlying acellular collagenization and leukocytic infiltration of the dermis. This thin whitish lesion is benign and of unknown etiology. It is easily treated with testosterone ointment, which restores the epithelial thickness and provides relief of the symptoms. Hydrocortisone may also be beneficial, if pruritus is present.

3) Atypical dystrophy

Atypical dystrophy is largely due to chronic irritation. In these cases, the epithelium will contain evidence of an atypical maturation, and abnormally keratinized cells may occur in the basal cell layer of the epithelium. In atypical lesions, wide excision, or a local vulvectomy, should be performed. **If both lichen sclerosis and hyperplastic lesions are found together, they are referred to as a "mixed dystrophy," with or without the presence of atypical hyperplasia.** Atypical lesions occur mostly in postmenopausal patients.

e. Fibroma/lipoma

Several kinds of tumors, such as fibromas (fibroblastic tumors), fibromyomas (fibromuscular tumors), and lipomas (fatty tumors) may occur on the vulva. These tumors should be completely excised. Fortunately, most of these tumors are benign; however, occasionally a sarcoma may arise from such lesions.

f. Hidradenoma

A hidradenoma of the vulva is a rare, raised, ulcerated, sessile tumor that is generally only about 1 cm in diameter. This solid apocrine tumor is benign and is found on the labia majora or on the perineum. Since it is asymptomatic, it is often an incidental finding during the performance of a routine pelvic examination. The treatment consists of the local excision of the lesion.

g. Granular cell myoblastoma (schwannoma)

The granular cell myoblastoma is a benign, painless, nodular lesion of the vulva that measures about 1 to 4 cm. It may frequently recur after excision. Since the myoblasts actually arise from the nerve sheaths, the designation of **schwannoma** is probably a more ac-

curate term. In rare instances, this type of lesion may become malignant. Treatment consists of a wide excision of the tumor.

h. Nevi

A vulvar nevus may appear as a pigmented flat or elevated papillomatous mass. These lesions are suggestive of a malignant melanoma and should be completely excised and examined closely to be certain that they are not malignant.

i. Labial fusion

Recently, it has been suggested that the presence of labial fusion in prepubescent girls may be an indication that sexual abuse has occurred and that it may be caused by the irritation that occurs with penile-labial intercourse or masturbation. It should also be remembered that the administration of androgenic substances during pregnancy between the 9th and 13th week may produce both clitoromegaly and labial fusion in the fetus, whereas after the 13th week, such agents will cause clitoromegaly only.

3. Premalignant conditions

a. Carcinoma-in-situ of the vulva

J. D. Bowen in 1912 was the first to call attention to what he described as a precancerous dermatosis in two of his cases. This lesion of the vulva has since been called **Bowen's disease;** however, more recently, others have suggested that the term **carcinoma-in-situ** is probably a more appropriate term. The human papilloma virus (HPV) and the herpesvirus have been suggested as possible etiological factors in this lesion.

1) Clinical findings

Most patients with this condition are either in their thirties or in their sixties, so apparently two different age groups are affected. Those in **the early age group tend to have a multifocal disease, whereas the older patients more commonly have a unifocal disease.** *Pruritus* appears to be the most prominent symptom, and it is also associated with the presence of a lump, pain, or bleeding of the vulva. Occasionally it may be asymptomatic and may be found on the external genitalia during a routine examination. The use of 1% toluidine blue staining has been successful in detecting this lesion. A biopsy specimen will reveal, on histologic examination, the presence of individual cell keratinization, *corps ronds*, nuclear graining, and clumping *(i.e., so-called bowenoid changes)*. In some instances, the immature cells may extend from the basal cell layer to the surface, while in others there may be keratinization of the rete tips. The presence of carcinoma-in-situ (CIS) of the vulva, or vulvar intraepithelial neoplasia (VIN), should alert you to the association of this lesion with similar neoplastic lesions of the perianal, cervical, and vaginal tissues. The use of washings of 3% acetic acid may accentuate the surface epithelial findings. Interestingly, about 20–40% of patients with CIS of the vulva will have either a prior, concurrent, or subsequent development of a neoplasia of the anogenital tract.

2) Treatment

The treatment of carcinoma-in-situ of the vulva consists of a *local wide excision,* unless the lesion is very extensive, in which case it is recommended that a simple skinning vulvectomy, with a 1.5–2.0 cm margin around the tumor, should be performed. Skin grafts may be necessary to repair the defect. The use of a skinning vulvectomy for smaller lesions, however, produces an increased amount of unnecessary scarring and may result in a possible constriction of the vaginal outlet, without adding any benefits in terms of cure, since the recurrence rate is the same as that associated with a simple local excision. Although *carbon dioxide laser therapy* can eradicate the lesion, the recurrence rate will still be of the order of 33%. With the exception of hyperkeratotic lesions, about 50–60% may be cured by the use of 5% *5-fluorouracil* cream. This agent causes a denudation of the skin similar to that produced by applying *dinitrochlorobenzene* locally to the lesion.

A simple vulvectomy is generally reserved for patients 60–75 years of age who have premalignant lesions, such as those who have: (1) granulomatous diseases, (2) recurrent carcinoma-in-situ lesions, and (3) atypical hyperplastic dystrophic lesions.

b. Paget's disease

This lesion was first described by **Sir James Paget** in 1874. Initially, the lesion was noted to affect the skin overlying a ductile breast cancer. **Extramammary Paget's disease (i.e., the vulvar location) has also been found to be of apocrine origin, with nests of epithelioid-like, apocrine, clear cells invading the basal layer of the skin. The hair follicles may be involved in 75–90% of these cases.** The characteristic **Paget's cell** has a large pale nucleus, a nucleolus, and a clear cytoplasm that reacts positively with mucicarmine stain (which stains the intracellular mucopolysaccharide).

1) Clinical findings

The clinical findings consist of a velvety, ill-defined red lesion found on the labia in white women during the early postmenopausal years. **The patient will generally complain of itching. About 70% of these cases may be classified histologically as a carcinoma-in-situ and may be treated by local excision. The remaining 30% of Paget's disease cases will constitute an invasive cancer of the vulva.**

2) Treatment

Recurrences of Paget's disease are common following a local excision and may require further multiple local excisions. In addition, breast neoplasia may develop at a later time, and therefore the breasts should be monitored during follow-up treatment of the patient with Paget's disease. In patients with invasive disease, the prognosis is poor. A radical vulvectomy, a groin dissection, and the use of irradiation seems to be the best form of treatment.

4. Malignant vulvar conditions

a. Basal cell carcinoma

A basal cell carcinoma of the vulva is a slow-growing neoplasm that rarely metastasizes. The lesion is slightly elevated and has a rolled edge that surrounds a superficial ulceration of the skin. Histologically, there are basal cells that extend into the stroma from the epithelium. Although these lesions are multicentric in origin and may recur quite frequently, the simple excision of each lesion provides essentially a 100% cure.

b. Squamous cell carcinoma

Squamous cell carcinoma is the most common type of vulvar cancer. Vulvar carcinoma occurs more commonly in women who have had prolonged vulvar irritation and poor perineal hygiene than in others. About two-thirds of these cases occur in women between 61 and 80 years of age; when it occurs in the younger patient, it is usually in association with a tropical granulomatous disease.

1) Clinical findings

A complaint of *vulvar itching* of some considerable duration is usually elicited from the patient with a vulvar carcinoma. A whitened area of the vulva with a raised nodule or ulceration may be noted on examination. About 70% of these lesions will occur on the labia, with most of them being on the labia majora.

2) Staging

The staging of carcinoma of the vulva is based upon a classification system suggested by the Cancer Committee of the International Federation of Gynecology and Obstetrics (FIGO) (Table 11-4). Unfortunately, the error rate in the clinical staging of carcinoma of the vulva may be as much as 25–40%, since the nodes cannot be well assessed by palpation. The use of a postoperative staging system has been shown to be a more accurate method of evaluating nodes, but it cannot be applied to the nonsurgical candidate.

3) Treatment

The lymphatic drainage of the vulva is through the inguinal and femoral nodes to the iliac and other pelvic lymph nodes. Based upon this observation, it would seem obvious that an en bloc radical vulvectomy with a groin dissection of the lymph nodes would be the preferred method of therapy for invasive carcinoma of the vulva; however, recent evidence indicates that this approach should be modified. In midline or clitoral lesions, it was originally thought that a pelvic lymphadenectomy should be carried out; however, this procedure is no longer recommended. Some surgeons will do the superficial and deep inguinal lymphadenectomy and a radical vulvectomy initially, and then reserve the pelvic lymphadenectomy for those patients who have positive inguinal

TABLE 11-4. FIGO classification of vulvar carcinoma

Stage 0	Carcinoma-in-situ. (e.g., Bowen's disease, noninvasive Paget's disease).
Stage I	Tumor confined to vulva, 2 cm or less in diameter. Nodes not palpable or are palpable in either groin, not enlarged, mobile (not clinically suspicious of neoplasm).
Stage II	Tumor confined to the vulva, more than 2 cm in largest diameter. Nodes are not palpable or are palpable in either groin, not enlarged, mobile (not clinically suspicious of neoplasm).
Stage III	Tumor of any size with (1) adjacent spread to the urethra, all of the vagina, perineum, or anus, or (2) nodes palpable in either or both groins (enlarged, firm, and mobile, not fixed but clinically suspicious of neoplasm).
Stage IV	Tumor of any size (1) infiltrating the bladder mucosa, the rectal mucosa, or both, including the upper part of the urethral mucosa, or (2) fixed or ulcerated nodes in either or both groins, or distant metastases.

Source: Reprinted with permission from FIGO, *Annual Report on the Results of Treatment in Gynecologic Cancer,* vol. 19, 1985.

nodal involvement. If the deep inguinal nodes (e.g., Cloquet's node) are not involved, then generally there will not be involvement of the pelvic nodes, since the tumor sequentially involves the superficial and then the deep inguinal nodes before it spreads to the external iliac, hypogastric, presacral, and obturator nodes. *Unfortunately, if the pelvic lymph nodes are involved, the prognosis for survival is poor.* As a consequence, the pelvic lymphadenectomy may be deleted in some patients. In young women who have a minimal lesion of the posterior vulva, the anterior vulva and clitoris may be preserved and sampling of the inguinal nodes may be carried out.

In patients who are found to have less than a *5-mm penetration* into the stroma, or a "microinvasive" lesion, wide local excision (with a 3-cm margin) and superficial groin node dissection have been utilized. However, metastases to the regional lymph nodes have been shown to occur in 10% of these cases. In another study, as many as 29% of patients with less than 5 mm of invasion had metastases; however, on microscopic examination it was found that they had *vascular space and lymphatic involvement,* which were not present in those microinvasive cases that had a more favorable outcome. Furthermore, in those lesions that were deeper than 5 mm, as many as 61% of the patients had nodal involvement. Recently, it has been suggested that if the lesion does not extend more than 1 mm below the level of the adjacent normal dermal papillae, and if it is not anaplastic or associated with lymphatic invasion, then the patient will be at minimal risk. It has been suggested that the concept of "microinvasion" should be applied to the vulvar lesions very cautiously.

The histologic type and the tumor differentiation also influence both the lymph node involvement and the five-year survival rates. If the tumor is well differentiated, lymph node involvement has been noted to occur in about one-third of cases, whereas if it was poorly differentiated, then more than two-thirds of the cases have had metastatic lymph node involvement. The tumor volume forms the basis for the classification system, with a *2-cm diameter* being the dividing line between stage I and stage II lesions. The incidence of node metastases also increases in association with lesions larger than 2 cm. In some series, 3 cm has also been found to be an effective dividing line, in that the incidence of lymph node metastases was about 19% in tumors smaller than 3 cm and 72% in those larger than 3 cm.

The overall surgical mortality rate in patients treated for vulvar carcinoma is about 2.2%. While a low dosage of prophylactic heparin therapy has decreased the incidence of postoperative pulmonary embolism, it has perhaps also increased the incidence of groin lymphocysts. *According to one report, the overall five-year survival rate, after correction for intracurrent disease, was of the order of 90% (stage I), 81% (stage II), 68% (stage III), and 20% (stage IV). The incidence of positive groin node metastases in two other reports was 5–10.5% (stage I), 18.5–29.8% (stage II), 60–66% (stage III), and 84–100% (stage IV).* In patients who did not have regional and pelvic node metastases, the overall survival rate was about 91%, whereas in those who did have inguinal-femoral nodal metastases, the five-year survival rate dropped to 30%. **Deep lymph node metastases do not oc-** **cur unless the groin nodes are first involved.** In the treatment of patients with recurrent vulvar carcinoma, the patient's management must be individualized according to the location and extent of the tumor. Irradiation, radical vulvectomy, lymphadenectomy, or exenteration may be necessary in some cases.

c. Malignant melanoma

A malignant melanoma is a rare neoplasm of the vulva. Melanomas occur on the vulva in 8% of melanoma cases. It may occur any time after puberty, with a peak incidence at the age of 55. These tumors are rarely found in black women. It is thought that most malignant melanomas do not arise in an already existing melanocytic nevus (i.e., a mole), but rather arise de novo and have a similar histologic appearance to that of a nevus during certain phases of their development. **The lesion is most commonly found on the labia minora, the clitoris, the fourchette, and the areas about the introitus.** This is in contrast to squamous carcinoma, which is more commonly found on the labia majora. It is thought that there are two melanoma cell types: *the keratinocyte and the melanocyte.* The pigment production is in the melanocyte, while the pigment storage is in the keratinocyte.

The lentigo maligna melanoma (10%) and the superficial spreading melanoma (80%) have an in-situ stage that may continue for as long as five years. A nodular melanoma (10%) does not have an in-situ phase and appears to penetrate the basement membrane and the underlying stroma rapidly.

The treatment of a malignant melanoma is dependent upon the staging and the depth of invasion. Local excision with wide margins should be performed in most cases, as radical surgery does not seem to offer any benefit over local wide excision in levels 1 and 2. The *inguinal-femoral lymph nodes should be sampled to determine the extent of the disease.* The use of the chemotherapeutic agent dimethyl-triazene-imidazole-carboxamide (DTIC), has produced regression of the tumor in up to 20–25% of patients who had disseminated disease. If the subcutaneous fat has been invaded, only about 40% of the patients will survive for five years.

CHAPTER 12

Vaginal disease

. . . .

The processes of disease are so complex that it is excessively difficult to search out the laws which control them, and, although we have seen a complete revolution in our ideas, what has been accomplished is only an earnest of what the future has in store.

—*Sir William Osler**

. . . .

1. Vaginal disorders

Vaginitis is a very common complaint in the outpatient setting. Because the vagina has minimal nerve endings present, the symptoms of perineal itching and burning that occur with vaginitis usually result when the irritating vaginal secretions excoriate the vulva. Normally the vagina cleanses itself by the discharge of secretions. **The normal vaginal flora maintains the pH of the vagina at about 3.5 to 4.5.** The glycogen present in the surface epithelium is utilized by the lactobacilli to produce the lactic acid that helps to maintain this level of acidity, which generally is antagonistic to harmful bacterial organisms.

Many factors may change the vaginal pH or the glycogen levels and lead to a vaginal infection. Both pregnancy and oral birth control pills will increase the glycogen content of the vaginal epi-

thelium and allow the overgrowth of yeast organisms, such as Candida. Oral-genital sexual contact may also be a source of infection, as the Candida organism is common in the mouth, the throat, and the large intestine. Diabetes is often associated with infections by this organism, as is the use of antibiotics. The alkaline pH of semen may also change the pH sufficiently to allow a vaginal infection to develop.

Educating the patient as to the principles of vaginal hygiene is important with regard to the prevention of vaginitis. Even the normal vaginal pH and glycogen levels may be overwhelmed by a large inoculum of virulent bacteria. **It is easy and convenient for the female to wipe the anal area in a frontward manner following a bowel movement.** In doing so, however, it is difficult if not impossible to prevent the contamination of both the vaginal orifice and the urethra. Many woman develop frequent vaginal and bladder infections as a consequence of this habit.

Douching is another technique that has often been utilized inappropriately. Most women begin douching after they become sexually active (perhaps because they subconsciously believe that sex is "dirty"), and douching then becomes a habit. But this practice repeatedly upsets the natural flora of the vagina and allows infections to occur. While there is little clinical evidence to prohibit douching for health reasons, there is an equal lack of evidence that it is beneficial. There is also much concern that if douching is incorrectly performed, it may be dangerous or even fatal (e.g., death from air embolism). In addition, recent evidence indicates a higher incidence of ectopic pregnancy in women who douche. Certainly, douching should not be performed at all during pregnancy.

---

*Reprinted with permission from Robert Bennett Bean, *Sir William Osler: Aphorisms from His Bedside Teachings and Writings,* William Bennett Bean, ed. Springfield, Ill.: Charles C Thomas, Publisher, 1968, p. 62.

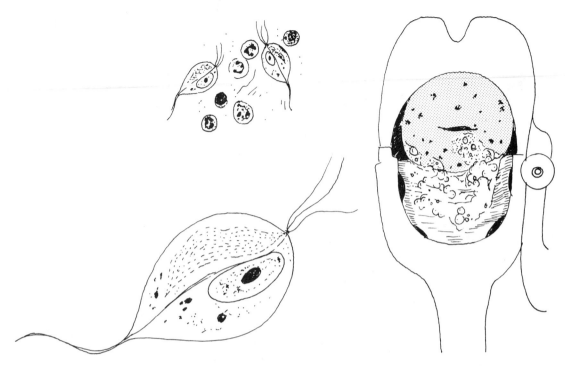

FIGURE 12-1. Trichomonas vaginalis. *Lower left:* Normal trophozoite. *Upper left:* Trophozoites compared to white blood cells. *Right:* The so-called "strawberry spots" on the cervix.

2. Infections

a. Trichomonas vaginitis

1) Clinical findings

Approximately 25% of all cases of vaginitis are due to the sexually transmitted, unicellular, flagellate organism Trichomonas vaginalis. The vaginal discharge in this infection will usually be *frothy* and greenish. *There may be peculiar erythematous spots present on the vaginal epithelium, which have been referred to as "strawberry spots."* The vaginal pH is alkaline (i.e., 5.0–5.5), and many polymorphonuclear leukocytes are commonly present. The infection may often become worse during pregnancy or just after menstruation. You should always check the *pH of the vaginal secretions* with litmus paper (i.e., with a pH range of 3.5 to over 6.5) in patients who complain of a trichomoniasis. In a saline wet smear, the typical motile *tear drop–like protozoan*, with its constantly moving flagellae, may be easily identified (Fig. 12-1).

A Gram-stained preparation of the vaginal secretions provides an excellent means of diagnosing the organisms involved. The **Gram stain procedure** may be performed as follows: (1) briefly heat-fix the slide that contains the smear of vaginal secretions, (2) flood the slide with gentian violet stain solution for 10 seconds, (3) wash it in water, (4) flood it with Gram's iodine solution for 10 seconds, (5) wash it again in water, (6) decolorize it with acetone/alcohol solution for 10 seconds, (7) flood it with safranin stain for 10 seconds, (8) wash it in water a third time, and (9) cover it with a glass coverslip and view it under a microscope. The addition of a drop of saline on top of the coverslip will allow you to use the oil emersion lens of the microscope without adding oil.

2) Treatment

The treatment of choice for trichomoniasis is *oral metronidazole* (Flagyl), which may be given in a variety of ways. **Commonly, 2 gm p.o. in a single dose may be used; however, alternately, metronida-**

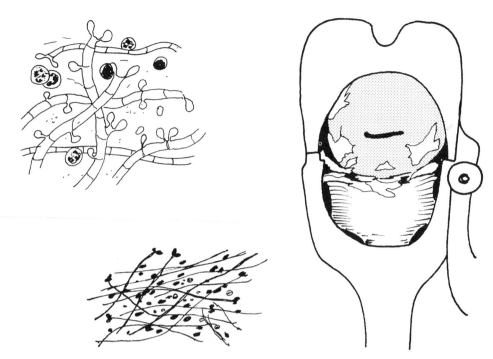

FIGURE 12-2. Candida albicans. *Lower left:* Filamentous pseudohyphae forms of Candida albicans. *Upper left:* Magnified pseudohyphae and blastospores. *Right:* White plaques of Candida albicans on the cervix and vagina.

zole 250 mg t.i.d. p.o. may be given for seven days. Since this drug has an antabuse-like effect, *patients who drink alcoholic beverages should abstain from drinking while on this medication. Further, metronidazole is contraindicated during the first trimester of pregnancy.* If the patient is nursing, the usual single 2.0-gram dose of metronidazole p.o. may be administered; however, the nursing should be interrupted for 24 hours after treatment. The male partner should also be treated with a single 2.0-gram dose of metronidazole p.o., and should have a follow-up examination for other coexistent sexually transmitted diseases.

Clotrimazole (Gyne-Lotrimin), 100 mg tablets intravaginally, may also be of benefit in treating trichomoniasis, and the use of clotrimazole vaginal cream has been effective.

Although douching with specific agents may be helpful in the treatment of a patient with a vaginitis, this practice should generally be avoided, since the normal ecology of the vagina may be upset by indiscriminate douching. Repeated episodes of trichomon-

iasis infections may be due to the survival of the organism in tap water, swimming pools, saunas, and bubble baths.

b. Monilial vaginitis

1) Clinical findings

Patients who have a thick, white, cheesy discharge that burns and itches, associated with a beefy red erythema of the vulva, will almost always have an infection involving Candida albicans, Candida tropicalis, or, in 10% of the cases, Candida (previously Torulopsis) glabrata. These yeast organisms produce *mycelia, pseudohyphae, and yeast buds* that are easily identifiable on saline wet smears, or, if there is a large amount of cellular debris, in a 10–20% potassium hydroxide wet smear (Fig. 12-2). **The pH of the vaginal secretions in Candida infections is 4.0 to 4.5.** While cultures can be obtained using Sabouraud's dextrose agar, it is usually unnecessary in an initial infection to go to this length to make the diagnosis. An exact culture identification becomes important, however, in difficult or recurrent cases.

The **lactobacilli-overgrowth syndrome** may mimic a Candida infection in the production of a thick, pasty discharge. There is usually no odor or vaginal irritation present in this condition; however, the patient may complain of a burning sensation following coitus. The pH of the vaginal secretions will be 4.0–4.5. On a wet smear, there will be many rod-shaped organisms, stripped nuclei, epithelial cells, and cytoplasmic debris. It has been recommended that baking soda douches (1 or 2 tablespoons to a quart of warm water) may be beneficial.

2) Treatment

A 2% miconazole nitrate vaginal cream (Monistat 7), one applicatorful (100 mg) daily for 7 days, or **butoconazole nitrate (Femstat),** one vaginal applicatorful at bedtime for 3 days, or **clotrimazole cream (Gyne-Lotrimin** or **Mycelex-G),** one applicatorful at bedtime for 7–14 days, or **terconazole vaginal cream (Terazol 7),** one applicatorful at bedtime for 7 days, are all effective in the treatment of most patients with monilial vaginitis. Tablets or suppositories are also available for Monostat, Gyne-Lotrimin, and Terazol. These drugs should not be used during the first trimester of pregnancy (Pregnancy Category C). The use of **boric acid gelatin capsules (600 mg of powder),** one capsule nightly for 14 days, is also effective. In resistant or severe cases, the use of a topical application of a **1% gentian violet dye** is very effective. The patient's entire vagina and vulva should be painted with this dye under direct vision through a speculum. On occasion, it may be necessary to paint the vagina and the vulva twice each week for one or two weeks in order to completely eradicate the infection. The consort should be cautioned to use a condom during the treatment period to avoid reinfecting the patient.

c. Gardnerella vaginitis
1) Clinical findings

Next to Candida organisms, Gardnerella vaginalis (previously Haemophilus vaginalis or Corynebacterium vaginale) is a common cause of vaginitis in the United States. **The patient who has a Gardnerella vaginalis infection will complain of a thin, greyish-white, watery discharge that has a fishy or stale odor, which is due to the amines and fatty acids that are present.** Recently, it has been suggested that trimethylamine may be the primary cause of the fishy odor associated with bacterial vaginitis. This odor may be released by the addition of a 10% potassium hydroxide solution to a drop of the vaginal secretions on a glass microscope slide ("whiff test"). **The vaginal pH in a Gardnerella vaginalis vaginitis, which is greater than 5.0, may be determined by applying a nitrazine paper to the vaginal mucous membranes and noting the color change.** The speculum examination does not usually reveal any specific vaginal changes, such as erythema or irritation. A saline smear, however, will reveal the presence of mature vaginal squamous cells with small, pleomorphic, gram-negative Gardnerella coccobacilli adhering to their surfaces. These cells have been called **clue cells** (Fig. 12-3).

2) Treatment

The treatment of choice for Gardnerella vaginalis vaginitis is metronidazole (Flagyl), 500 mg b.i.d. for 7 days; shorter courses are usually ineffective. Alternative regimes include ampicillin, 500 mg q.i.d. for 7 days; amoxicillin, 500 mg t.i.d. for 7 days; or cephradine, 500 mg q.i.d. for 7 days. The use of a condom by the patient's consort should be encouraged until the vaginitis has been eradicated in an effort to prevent reinfection, and treatment of the male partner is also advised.

d. Chlamydia trachomatis infections
1) Incidence

Infections due to Chlamydia trachomatis are now thought to be the most prevalent of the sexually transmitted diseases in the United States. About 3 million cases of Chlamydia trachomatis infections have been documented annually. In addition, it is associated with gonorrhea in at least 25–45% of cases. There are actually two species of Chlamydia: Chlamydia psittaci and Chlamydia trachomatis. The different serotypes of C. trachomatis may be demonstrated by immunofluorescent techniques. These organisms may cause trachoma (particularly in Third World countries), lymphogranuloma venereum, and other infections. **Of the 15 recognized serotypes, L1, L2, and L3 are associated with lymphogranuloma venereum; A, B, C, and**

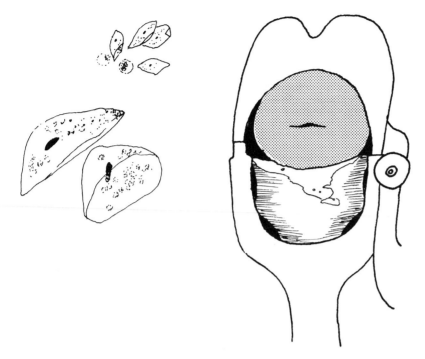

FIGURE 12-3. Gardnerella vaginalis. *Lower left:* "Clue cells" are epithelial cells with attached gram-negative bacteria. *Upper left:* "Clue cells" compared to other superficial epithelial cells. *Right:* Greyish-white discharge with no other vaginal changes.

Ba are seen in trachoma; and D, E, F, G, H, I, J, and K are involved in inclusion conjunctivitis and pneumonia in the newborn, urethritis and epididymitis, cervicitis and salpingitis, and the acute urethral syndrome. These obligate intracellular organisms (elementary bodies) usually penetrate the host epithelial cell and grow within a cytoplasmic vacuole (lysosome) over a period of about 48–72 hours. The infective particles are then released when the host cell dies. The organisms are transmitted by skin-to-skin contact. Only 50% of women who are infected with Chlamydia will manifest symptoms; about 33% will carry the organism in their urethras, and another 20% will suffer from a purulent cervicitis.

2) Clinical syndromes

a) Lymphogranuloma venereum

Lymphogranuloma venereum (LGV) is common in tropical climates and is found in the United States among sexually promiscuous individuals. The acute infection with this organism, an L serotype of Chlamydia trachomatis, is accompanied by regional lymphadenopathy, fever, arthralgia, headache, meningismus, erythema nodosum, and erythema multiforme.

b) The inguinal syndrome

The inguinal syndrome may begin with a small erosion or papule that heals and is followed by inguinal adneopathy and the appearance of a genital ulceration. In about 75% of these cases, the nodes ultimately drain pus from multiple fistulous tracts.

c) The genitoanorectal syndrome

The genitoanorectal syndrome occurs in 25% of Chlamydia cases and has fewer constitutional symptoms. The anorectal mucosa becomes friable and edematous and begins to bleed. Ulcerative lesions of the vulva and vagina also may occur, with destruction of the tissues and, at times, of the urethra, accompanied by enlarged inguinal nodes. In time, the extensive destruction and scarring of the lymphatics of the vulva will result in the development of elephantiasis. Inflammation and scarring of the rectal tissues may result in perirectal abscesses, rectovaginal fistulas, and perirectal strictures. As long as there are ulcerations present on the anogenital tissues, the disease may be transmitted to other persons. The organism apparently does not cross the placenta.

d) The female cervicitis/PID

Usually, you should suspect a C. trachomatis infection of the cervix in the patient who: (1) is less than 24 years of age, (2) is single, (3) has had multiple sexual partners (with a new one within the preceding two months), (4) has not used a barrier contraceptive, and/or (5) has a mucopurulent cervical erosion, which bleeds upon examination. If two or more of these criteria are present, then a screening test for Chlamydia trachomatis should be performed. You should be able to detect over 90% of the cases of Chlamydial infection if you use these criteria.

Chlamydia trachomatis may produce a genital infection that involves the cervix and endocervix in the female. It has been suggested that as many as two-thirds of these cervical infections may be asymptomatic. In addition, in 25–32% of the cases, this organism has been implicated in salpingitis, and indeed, it may produce pelvic pain, fever, and tenderness that is identical to the **pelvic inflammatory disease (PID)** produced by N. gonorrhea. Even the **Fitz-Hugh-Curtis syndrome** may be caused by this organism.

e) Nongonococcal urethritis syndrome (NGU)

Acute dysuria is a common gynecological complaint. If the urine culture shows more than 100,000 colonies/ml (i.e., 10^5 colony-forming units), then the diagnosis of cystitis may be made, whereas with a lesser number of colonies present, the patient should be diagnosed as having the **urethral syndrome.** In most cases, the urethral syndrome is produced by vaginal and urethral infections.

In many instances, the urethral syndrome precedes a urinary tract infection. In the initial cultures, the colony counts may be less than 10^5; however, in some reported studies, over 50% of these patients later developed a significant bacteriuria. The treatment of the urethral syndrome with antibiotics improves most patients' symptoms. Escherichia coli has been commonly cultured in 46% of patients with the urethral syndrome. **Vaginal and periurethral colonization with E. coli apparently precedes the infection and the development of the urethral syndrome.** If the female patient has the habit of wiping frontwards after a bowel movement, it is possible that this deposits a significant inoculum of bacteria in the urethra and the vagina. Patients with cystitis may have either an infection of the bladder or one primarily in the kidneys, even though they may have no symptoms of pyelonephritis.

Sexually transmitted diseases such as Neisseria gonorrhoeae and Chlamydia trachomatis may be found in patients with the urethral syndrome. In some studies, it has been suggested that as many as one-third of indigent patients who are seen in the emergency room have an acute urethral syndrome associated with either Neisseria gonorrhoeae or Chlamydia trachomatis organisms. Herpes infections initially may be associated with dysuria in 80% of patients. Vaginitis with Candida albicans, Trichomonas vaginalis, and Gardnerella vaginalis have all been associated with dysuria and cystitis in some women. The presence of a typical vaginal discharge and symptoms of itching associated with dysuria should alert you to this possibility. The association of Ureaplasma urealyticum or Mycoplasma hominis infections with dysuria, however, is controversial. These organisms seem to be present in equal numbers in both symptomatic women and in control subjects.

Anaerobic bacteria and microaerophilic bacilli have been suggested as possible causes of the urethral syndrome; however, the evidence is not very convincing. Allergies, emotional stress, trauma, and obstruction have all been suggested as other possible causes. Frequent or traumatic intercourse may cause enough urethral mucosal irritation to produce dysuria.

Nongonococcal urethritis in men has also been associated with Chlamydia trachomatis. The main symptom in males is **dysuria,** and there is usually no urethral discharge or bacteriuria.

f) Neonatal conjunctivitis/pneumonia

Chlamydia trachomatis has been implicated in as many as 73% of the infants who have neonatal purulent conjunctivitis. In general, 20–50% of these infants will develop chlamydial conjunctivitis and 10–20% will develop pneumonia. Other pathogens that may be involved singly or collectively in neonatal conjunctivitis are Staphylococcus aureus, Haemophilus, Streptococcus pneumoniae, enterococcus, and Branhamella catarrhalis.

3) Diagnosis

Chlamydia trachomatis may be cultured using cycloheximide-treated McCoy cells in much the same manner as in culturing viruses. This technique is a sensitive, albeit a slow method of making the diagnosis. Recently, two new tests have become available. The Chlamydiazyme test is an enzyme-linked immunosorbent assay (ELISA) that is read with a spectrophotometer. The other test is a direct slide test utilizing *fluorescein-conjugation* that stains the elemental bodies of the C. trachomatis monoclonal antibodies [i.e., direct immunofluorescent monoclonal antibody stain (DFA)]. This test requires a fluorescent microscope, which is quite expensive. Both of these tests have a sensitivity of over 90% and a specificity of about 95%. It has been suggested that if the prevalence of Chlamydia trachomatis is less than 10%, then a tissue culture technique should be utilized.

4) Treatment

Specific treatment regimens have been recommended by the Centers for Disease Control (CDC) in pregnant women who have a culture-proven C. trachomatis infection, or in the woman's sexual partners, if they have a nongonococcal urethritis syndrome (NGU). The treatment consists of erythromycin base, 500 mg, q.i.d. p.o., on an empty stomach for at least 7 days, or erythromycin ethylsuccinate, 800 mg q.i.d. p.o. for 7 days. If this dosage is not tolerated, then a dose of 250 mg of erythromycin base, or 400 mg erythromycin ethylsuccinate q.i.d. p.o. for at least 14 days, should be given. *The nonpregnant patient or the sexual partner may also be treated with tetracycline hydrochloride, 500 mg p.o. q.i.d. for at least 7 days, or doxycycline, 100 mg p.o. b.i.d. for 7 days.* If the lymphogranuloma venereum serotype is involved, the treatment should be extended to at least 14 days. Sulfamethoxazole, 1.0 gram b.i.d. p.o. for at least 2 weeks, is an alternative treatment regimen.

e. Toxic shock syndrome

1) Historical aspects

Vaginal or perineal menstrual blood collectors have been in use for over 3,000 years. Rolls of papyrus,

cotton cloth, flannel, soft wool, grass, and even elongated labia minora in women of a South African tribe, have all been utilized. In the 1700s, medicated tampons that had been dipped in copper sulfate or vinegar were used. In 1896, Lister towels made of gauze and cotton were the first disposable perineal pads to be manufactured. In 1933, a Denver physician patented the first vaginal tampon, which was bought by the Tampax Corporation in 1936 and sold commercially.

The toxic shock syndrome (TSS) has occurred in both men and women; however, the majority of cases (95%) have occurred in white women and have been associated with menstruation and the use of vaginal tampons. The incidence of TSS in the United States is 6.2 per 100,000 menstruating women per year. Although it was initially shown that a large number of TSS cases were associated with the Rely brand of tampons, the major problem appeared to be due to the use of a superabsorbant material in the tampon, which provided an environment favorable for the growth of **Staphylococcus aureus.** Since TSS may also occur in nonmenstruating females and in men, it is obvious that factors other than the use of absorbant tampons are involved. Apparently, a negative association also exists between TSS and the use of oral contraceptives.

Once a woman has been colonized with S. aureus, the bacteria and its toxins (i.e., TSS-toxin 1) may enter the bloodstream in two different ways: (1) through a reflux of menstrual blood from the uterus and out through the tubes, with the absorption of the toxin through the peritoneum (due to the obstruction of the menstrual flow by the tampon), or (2) through surface abrasions of the vaginal wall.

2) Clinical findings

TSS usually has an abrupt onset with a high fever (102° F, or 38.9° C), chills, diarrhea, sore throat, headache, vomiting, hypotension (less than 90 mm Hg), a palmar erythema, and a diffuse macular rash that has been described as being similar to a *sunburn. The rash begins to desquamate after several days (for up to two weeks) and involves the palms of the hands and the soles of the feet.* Hyperemia of the mucous membranes is also present. Almost all of these patients complain of myalgia, and in addition, dizziness is common. An involvement of the other organs, such as the CNS, the renal, and the pulmonary systems, may also occur. *In the presence of the adult respiratory distress syndrome (ARDS), the prognosis is poor.*

3) Treatment

The treatment of TSS consists of *supportive fluid therapy* to restore the circulating blood volume and to provide for an adequate perfusion of the vital organs. The placement of a Swan-Ganz catheter allows for a rational monitoring of the patient's condition. The administration of intravenous dopamine and the use of Military Anti-Shock Trousers (MAST) may help to maintain the blood pressure. Hypocalcemia is usually present and may be partly responsible for the hypotension. The administration of intravenous calcium chloride will correct this deficiency. While the use of corticosteroids is controversial, the use of *antistaphylococcal antibiotics,* such as nafcillin, is recommended. Oxygen and adequate ventilation (PEEP) may prevent irreversible hypoxic pulmonary damage and the development of ARDS.

3. Other types of vaginitis

a. Allergic vaginitis

Contact dermatitis, or allergic vaginitis, may involve either the vulva or the vagina and is often caused by clothing dyes, synthetic fabric undergarments, tight jeans, perfumed sprays or soaps, tampons, or commercial douche medications. The removal of the offending agent, plus the use of topical corticosteroids, is usually an effective treatment. An accurate history of the patient's use of new clothing or feminine hygiene products is important in detecting this type of vulvitis or vaginitis.

b. Psychosomatic vaginitis

An excessive vaginal discharge, or a **leukorrhea** (i.e., an excessive clear or lightly clouded discharge without itching or irritation), may be due to a cervical ectropion, to excessive anxiety and nervousness, or to a psychosomatic disorder that is secondary to a deeper psychological problem. Repeated office visits for "vaginitis," with minimal or no positive findings, should alert you to the possibility that the patient may have a **psychosomatic vaginitis.** For example, a woman might develop a vaginitis after she finds out that her husband is seeing another woman. Often the patient will complain of feeling "dirty" and will report

excessive douching. In any case, it is essential that the physician examine a wet smear on each occasion, or obtain a specific culture to test for vaginal organisms, in order to rule out an actual infectious agent. The treatment of psychosomatic vaginitis consists of exploring the patient's reactions and feelings with regard to the precipitating event. In severe cases, it may be necessary to refer the patient for psychiatric counseling.

c. Foreign body vaginitis (nonspecific vaginitis)

On occasion, a patient may complain of having a vaginal odor and irritation but will be found on examination to have a *forgotten tampon* in the vagina. In patients with psychiatric problems, other foreign objects may also be found in the vagina; however, this situation is not as common. **More commonly, vaginal foreign bodies are found in young children.** Often, the mother will note either a pus-like discharge or blood on the child's panties and will bring the girl in for examination. Frequently, it is difficult to carry out a vaginal examination on a very young child, even with a small nasal speculum, and an examination under anesthesia will be necessary. A rectal examination may allow the palpation of an intravaginal object, and the use of a small metal probe may locate a plastic or metallic object in the vagina by "clicking" against it. Other objects, however, may not be identified quite as easily. A flat plate (x-ray) of the pelvis may detect a radiopaque object. **Removal of the object almost always requires that the child be under general anesthesia in the operating room.** An antibiotic such as a sulfa drug, penicillin, or ampicillin will usually be necessary to treat the associated infection.

4. Pelvic relaxation

a. Cystocele/urethrocele

1) Etiology

The pelvic floor is chiefly made up of the levator ani muscular sling, which is composed of three muscles: the iliococcygeus, the pubococcygeus, and the puborectalis. In addition, the bulbocavernosus muscles and the superficial transverse perineal muscles insert into the midline of the perineum (i.e., the perineal body), posterior to the vaginal introitus and anterior to the rectum. The

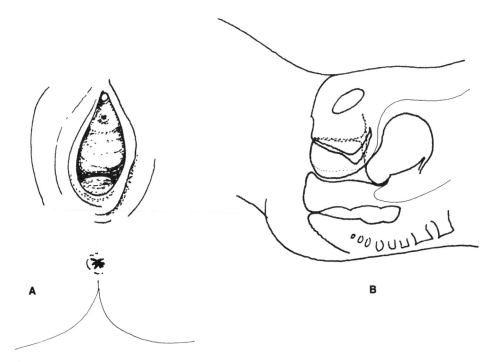

FIGURE 12-4. Cystocele. (A) The bulging of the anterior vaginal wall, due to the loss of supporting fascia, is obvious on examination. (B) The lateral view shows the bulging of the anterior vaginal wall and the detachment of the urethra from its normal position.

anal opening is surrounded by the interdigitating muscles of the external sphincter. The lower rectum and vagina are thus supported by the bulbocavernosus, the transverse perineal muscles, and the puborectalis muscle of the levator ani sling. In addition, the urethra, vagina, and rectum are invested with endopelvic fascia, which supports these organs in the middle of the pelvis. The cardinal ligaments and the uterosacral ligaments assist in suspending the uterus and adjacent organs so that they do not prolapse whenever there is an increase in intra-abdominal pressure.

With each successive vaginal delivery, stress is transmitted to the musculofascial supporting structures of the bladder and the pelvic floor. **Excessive stretching and trauma may result in tears in this supporting tissue (i.e., endopelvic fascia), which allows the base of the bladder to drop posteriorly (i.e., forming a cystocele) and the urethra to fall away from its normal position behind the symphysis pubis (i.e., forming an urethrocele, or detached urethra)** (Fig. 12-4) (see Chapter 2).

The fascial support in the pelvis of caucasian women seems to be more susceptible to being damaged than that of oriental or black women. The loss of the normal anatomical relationships of the urethra and the bladder may or may not affect the function of the bladder. As a consequence, in the presence of a cystourethrocele, the patient may be completely asymptomatic or may experience an uncontrollable loss of urine under stressful conditions such as coughing, sneezing, or running (i.e., stress incontinence).

2) Historical aspects

The interest in gynecologic urology by physicians in this country began with the appointment of **Dr. Howard A. Kelly** (1858–1943), who was recruited to Johns Hopkins University in 1889 at the age of 31 by **Dr. William Welch. The four most illustrious physicians of this era were Dr. Welch (pathology), Dr. William S. Osler (medicine), Dr. Kelly (gynecology), and Dr. William S. Halsted (surgery).** Dr. Kelly subsequently appointed **Dr. J. Whitridge Williams** to the Obstetrics Department. Dr. Williams's textbook on obstetrics, and its 18 up-

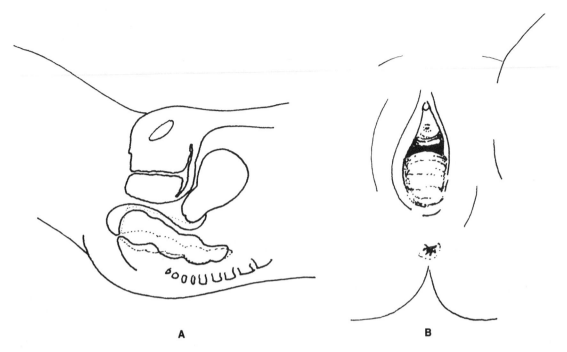

A   **B**

FIGURE 12-5. Rectocele. (A) Lateral view showing the rectum bulging up into the vagina. (B) The bulging of the posterior vaginal mucosa is obvious on examination, due to the herniation of the anterior rectal wall through the pararectal and paravaginal fascia of the rectovaginal septum.

dated editions, has endeared him to generations of medical students since then.

Dr. Kelly's main interest was the female urinary system. He introduced the air cystoscope and published a textbook on *Operative Gynecology* illustrated by Max Brödel. This book, which detailed the Richardson technique of total abdominal hysterectomy, was very instrumental in establishing the total procedure rather than the subtotal hysterectomy in clinical practice. Dr. Kelly was the first surgeon to plicate the tissues under the urethrovesical junction for the correction of stress incontinence. Dr. Kelly's establishment of a long-term training period later formed the basis for the formal residency training programs in the specialty of obstetrics and gynecology.

3) Classification

The classification of the degree of cystocele that may be present is as follows: (1) a mild cystocele is one in which the anterior vaginal wall prolapses to the introitus upon straining; (2) a **moderate cystocele is one in which the vaginal wall extends beyond the introitus with straining; and (3) a severe cystocele is one in which the vaginal wall extends beyond the introitus in the resting state.**

b. Rectocele/enterocele (cul-de-sac hernia)

When the musculofascial support between the vagina and rectum is unduly stretched or lacerated in childbirth, there is a herniation of the rectum into the posterior wall of the vagina to form a bulging mass. Most commonly, the muscular defect that allows the development of a *rectocele* occurs in the lower portion of the vagina (Fig. 12-5).

If the cul-de-sac of Douglas deepens owing to the effects of intra-abdominal pressure on the weakened or lacerated rectovaginal endopelvic fascial tissues, then a loop of small bowel may herniate between the uterosacral ligaments and extend down the rectovaginal septum to the introitus (i.e., forming an enterocele). This entity is initially most noticeable in the upper half of the posterior vagina.

The usual symptoms associated with a rectocele are a feeling of rectal pressure, or a feeling of pelvic pressure, and some difficulty in completely evacuating the lower bowel. At times, the patient will relate that she must insert her finger into her vagina in order to splint or brace the posterior vaginal wall when straining at stool in order to assist in completely evacuating her bowel. An enterocele is generally asymptomatic, except for some pressure and heaviness in the pelvis toward the end of the day after prolonged standing.

c. Uterine prolapse

1) Etiology

Various stresses, including childbirth, heavy physical work, and aging, may stretch the cardinal ligaments and weaken the endopelvic fascial planes in such a manner as to cause the uterus to descend. In rare cases, there is a congenital weakness of these tissues. The cardinal ligament, the vesicouterine ligaments, and the uterosacral ligaments are the main supporting ligaments; however, the connections of the vaginal muscles to the cardinal ligaments also play a role in stabilizing the uterus in its midpelvic position. **As these supports give way, the uterine corpus moves backward into a retroverted, or retroflexed, position.** In doing so, the round ligaments gradually stretch and fail to hold the uterine corpus in the normal anterior anteverted or anteflexed position. **At this point, the uterus moves backward and aligns itself with the axis of the vagina. Any increase in intra-abdominal pressure may then cause the entire weight of the uterus to descend down the vaginal canal, similar to the action of a piston in a cylinder.** In time, the entire uterus may descend down the vaginal barrel and may extend outside of the vaginal introitus (i.e., uterine prolapse, or procidentia) (Fig. 12-6) (see Chapter 2).

2) Clinical findings

The symptoms of a uterine prolapse consist of *pelvic pressure, low backache,* and the inconvenience of hav-

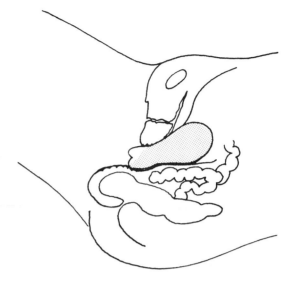

FIGURE 12-6. Prolapsed uterus. When the cardinal ligaments and uterosacral ligaments are weakened or disrupted, the uterus may descend to the introitus and beyond to produce a uterine prolapse, or procidentia, of a first, second, or third degree. There is an enterocele present also with a loop of bowel prolapsed into the rectovaginal septum from the cul-de-sac of Douglas.

ing the uterus protrude between the labia. Often, in a third-degree prolapse, the cervix may become eroded and may bleed due to the drying effect on the mucous membranes, and the effect of trauma to these tissues. Also, due to the uterine procidentia, the ureters may prolapse and obstruct causing hydronephrosis to occur. While these changes are usually asymptomatic, repeated bouts of urinary tract infections may occur. These patients will also complain of dyspareunia, which is due to the trauma to the cervix during coitus.

5. Physiology of micturition

a. Neurologic control

The bladder muscle (*i.e., the detrusor*) and the urethral muscle are controlled by various neural elements, from the cerebral cortex to the local motor and sensory nerves of the pelvis, including the autonomic nervous system. It is important for every practicing physician to have an understanding of the neurologic control of micturition. The voiding process is initiated by the sensation of bladder fullness that is transmitted to the central nervous system by the proprioceptor nerves, which results in the relaxation of the pelvic floor via the pudendal nerve. Following this relaxation, there is a contraction of the detrusor muscle and the smooth muscle of the trigone. Almost simultaneously with the contraction of the detrusor muscle of the bladder, there is a reciprocal relaxation of the smooth muscle of the urethra, which then allows the voiding process to begin.

An understanding of the neurologic arcs involved in this process is most helpful in the diagnosis and management of problems of the lower urinary tract of the female patient. This circuitry involves **four basic loop mechanisms** (Fig. 12-7), the **first** of which originates in the frontal lobes of the cerebral cortex and terminates in the pontine-mesencephalic reticular formation of the brain stem. *This loop coordinates the voluntary control of the micturition reflex.* A number of disease states may alter this circuit, such as Parkinson's disease, brain tumors, cerebral vascular disease, and multiple sclerosis. Interruption of this circuit results in an autonomous bladder function. The test of integrity of this neural loop is the cystometrogram.

The **second loop** originates in the pontine-mesencephalic reticular formation of the brain stem and terminates in the sacral micturition area. As part of this loop, sensory afferent fibers originate in the bladder musculature and travel directly to the brain stem without synapse. A total interruption of this circuit would result in an absence of detrusor contractions; this condition is seen in patients who have had spinal cord trauma, for example, or in those who have multiple sclerosis. Again, the cystometrogram is the primary test used to define abnormalities in this loop, since the patient so afflicted will be unable to initiate a detrusor contraction when instructed to do so.

The **third loop** originates in the sensory afferents of the detrusor muscle and travels to the sacral micturition center. The interneurones of this loop are located close to the pudendal motor nucleus and therefore *allow for the relaxation of the pelvic floor to initiate the voiding reflex.* If this loop malfunctions, the urethral muscles are unable to relax during the micturition process, which results in hesitancy and prolongation of the voiding time. This particular loop

is difficult to evaluate clinically, and diagnosis requires sophisticated neurophysiologic techniques.

The **fourth loop** originates in the frontal lobe of the cerebral cortex and terminates in the pudendal nucleus of the sacral micturition area. *It is this last loop that is essential for the voluntary control of the striated external urethral sphincter muscle.* As with the other loops, malfunction may occur with spinal cord trauma, tumors, cerebral vascular disease, and on occasion, with lower urinary tract disease. When this loop is abolished, difficulty in the initiation of the voiding process results. In order to test this circuit, it is necessary to utilize electromyographic techniques.

Both the sympathetic and the parasympathetic nervous systems have a strong influence over the control of micturition and the entire lower urinary tract (Fig. 12-8). *The parasympathetic fibers originate from S2, S3, and S4 (i.e., the pelvic nerve) and function by stimulating the detrusor muscle to contract and to inhibit the contraction of the urethral muscles.*

The sympathetic nervous components originate from thoracic spinal cord segments T10–T12 through the second lumbar segment (L2). Stimulation of the sympathetic nerve trunk causes a contraction of the trigone and a reciprocal inhibition of the detrusor contraction. *Since sympathetic nervous stimulation may inhibit parasympathetic transmission, it acts as a modulator of the autonomic system.*

Stimulation of the alpha receptors, which are located primarily in the urethra, causes contraction of the urethra; when they are blocked, relaxation of the urethra occurs. Conversely, the stimulation of beta receptors, located primarily in the dome of the bladder, causes the bladder to relax.

b. Urinary incontinence

1) Historical aspects

During the nineteenth century, a vesicovaginal fistula was considered a repugnant affliction because of its intolerable ammoniacal urine odor. In 1845, **Dr. James Marion Sims** (1813–1883), a young physician in Montgomery, Alabama, surgically experimented on three slaves (Anarcha, Betsy, and Lucy) who suffered from vesicovaginal fistulas in an effort to find a proper method of repairing these lesions. In 1855 he founded a hospital for women in New York City, where, in cooperation with T. Gaillard Thomas, Thomas A. Em-

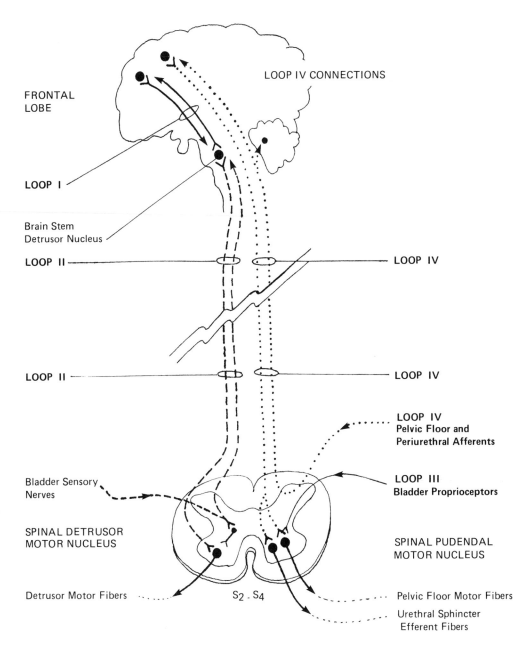

FRONTAL LOBE

LOOP IV CONNECTIONS

LOOP I

Brain Stem
Detrusor Nucleus

LOOP II

LOOP II

LOOP IV

LOOP IV

LOOP IV
Pelvic Floor and
Periurethral Afferents

Bladder Sensory
Nerves

LOOP III
Bladder Proprioceptors

SPINAL DETRUSOR
MOTOR NUCLEUS

SPINAL PUDENDAL
MOTOR NUCLEUS

Detrusor Motor Fibers

$S_2 - S_4$

Pelvic Floor Motor Fibers

Urethral Sphincter
Efferent Fibers

FIGURE 12-7. The central nervous system control of the bladder and the periurethral musculature. The I, II, III, and IV control loops are shown. (Reproduced, with permission, from M. E. Williams and C. P. Fitzhugh, "Urinary Incontinence in the Elderly," *Ann Intern Med.,* 97 (1982), pp. 895–907.)

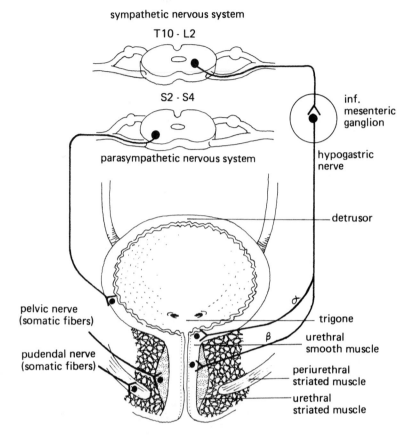

FIGURE 12-8. The peripheral innervation of the bladder and the urethral musculature. (Adapted from D. N. Danforth and J. R. Scott, eds., *Obstetrics and Gynecology,* 5th ed. Philadelphia: J. B. Lippincott Company, 1986, p. 950.)

met, and E. R. Peaslee, he perfected his fistula repair procedure, which involved using the knee-chest position and silver wire sutures. For his work in vaginal surgery, **Dr. Sims came to be known as the Father of American Gynecology.** In 1894, a statue of him was erected in Bryant Park; it was moved to Central Park across from the New York Academy of Medicine in 1936.

2) Fistula

During early infancy, voiding is frequent and uninhibited. Between the ages of two and three years, there is a gradual development of bladder continence, so that by the end of this time, most individuals will have developed voluntary control of the bladder.

A constant leakage of urine night and day, without any associated sensation of voiding, is usually due to a *vesicovaginal fistula.* These fistulas may be congenital, but they usually develop following pelvic surgery, irradiation, or childbirth. If the fistula is not visible, it may be diagnosed by first emptying the bladder and then filling it with a dilute solution of methylene blue (i.e., 250 ml). A tampon then placed in the vagina will be stained at the site of the fistula. Another technique that may be utilized is the administration of phenazopyridium HCl (Pyridium), two tablets, with observation of the vaginal tampon over 1–2 hours for the appearance of orange staining. In instances in which the fistula is very tiny and cannot be located by means of the tampon test, another approach may be utilized. The patient can be placed in the knee-chest position, a

CO_2 cystoscope placed in the bladder, the vagina filled with saline, a vaginal speculum inserted, and the bubbles of CO_2 observed over the site of the fistula (i.e., the "flat tire test").

3) Urgency incontinence (urgency syndrome)

Some patients note a frequent urge to urinate that may be exaggerated during the evening hours and especially during the sleeping hours. This condition may be due to a learned response upon the part of the patient and may be corrected by retraining the bladder to retain urine for longer periods of time—**the bladder drill.** On the other hand, if the patient voids with the slightest amount of bladder tension, then a chronic urinary tract infection must be considered. If pyuria is noted on urine analysis, but without a positive urine culture, then an infection with Chlamydia trachomatis should be suspected. Cystoscopic examination in these patients will reveal erythema of the bladder mucosa, which will have a trabeculated appearance. The trigone area may have a whitish covering (i.e., "cake frosting"). Urine cultures should be obtained to identify the organism and the patient treated with the appropriate antibiotics. The patient's symptoms should improve with the antibiotic treatment, and using the bladder drill method, she should be able to void every two hours on schedule.

4) Anatomic incontinence

Urinary incontinence is the involuntary loss of urine, which may be socially embarrassing to the patient. **The leakage may occur with coughing, sneezing, a sudden change of position, or with a variety of exercise maneuvers (i.e., stress incontinence).** This incontinence of urine is due to the loss of the proximal urethral support with the resultant downward displacement of the urethra. As a result of these changes, the urethra is unable to function in its normal capacity. With an increase in intra-abdominal pressure, the pressure in the bladder exceeds that of the urethra and the urine is lost.

5) Unstable bladder (detrusor dysynergia, detrusor over activity syndrome)

An unstable bladder results in involuntary contractions of the bladder with a sudden loss of urine without warning and may be associated with stress phenomena such as coughing, sneezing, or a change of position. The etiology of this condition is unknown, but it is associated with urinary tract infections in many instances and may be associated with anatomic changes. The treatment of this disorder consists of the administration of parasympatholytic agents, such as oxybutynin chloride (Ditropan), dicyclomine hydrochloride (Bentyl), or propantheline bromide (Pro-Banthine). Neuropsychiatric tricyclic drugs are also effective in the treatment of this problem, as they have a parasympatholytic action and also have alpha adrenergic stimulating effects to increase urethral tone. Imipramine hydrochloride (Tofranil) is the most commonly used agent in this category.

6) Neurogenic bladder

This type of incontinence is usually due to neurological disease. It is also associated with atherosclerosis. The usual presentation is that of an older patient, who may or may not be a diabetic, who experiences a loss of urine on an intermittent basis, unrelated to stress or other activities. The patient will be noted to have either a very small bladder capacity (e.g., volume of less than 150 ml) with an elevated bladder pressure, or she may have a very large bladder capacity (i.e., over 500 ml) with an absence of bladder contractions. These latter patients frequently have a residual urine volume of over 200 ml. On neurological examination, there may be an absence of the **bulbocavernosus and anal sphincter reflexes;** however, it should be remembered that in about 15% of normal patients this reflex may be absent. The treatment consists of instructing the patient to void every two hours, followed by an attempt to void after about 20 minutes. If this approach is unsuccessful, then the patient may be taught how to catheterize herself. This procedure should be performed at least twice each day, preferably after voiding in the morning upon arising and again at bedtime before going to sleep.

c. History, physical examination, and urodynamic testing

The urologic history is very helpful in determining the severity of a patient's urinary incontinence problem. The loss of urine with exercise, coughing, and sneezing, and without nocturia, frequency, or dysuria, should suggest to you that the patient has an anatomical incontinence. Frequent urination during the daytime, and nocturia at night, should alert you to the possibility of either an unstable bladder and/or a urinary tract infection. The patient's age, parity, the type of delivery of her previous children, and any previous pelvic surgical procedures are also important factors in evaluating the patient.

The physical examination should include a detailed description of the degree of relaxation of the apex of the vagina, with or without the uterus being present. The amount of relaxation of the anterior and posterior walls of the vagina also should be carefully noted. The description of the amount of cystocele, rectocele, enterocele, and uterine prolapse will provide you with a clear picture of the status of the endopelvic fascial supporting tissues (see Chapter 2). The **Q-tip test** will determine the degree of the detachment of the proximal urethra: This test is accomplished by placing a Q-tip into the mid-urethral area and then having the patient perform a Valsalva's maneuver (i.e., holding her breath and bearing down); the change in the angle of inclination of the Q-tip (normally 10–15 degrees) from the horizontal position is then recorded. In patients who have a significant urethral detachment, this angle will exceed 30–35 degrees. If the clitoris is stroked or gently squeezed, you should elicit the **bulbocavernosus reflex,** which involves the contraction of the bulbocavernosa and ischiocavernosus muscles. The **anal reflex,** or anal sphincter contraction, occurs when the skin lateral to the anus is stroked. These two tests indicate that the neuronal supply to the sacral dermatomes S2, S3, and S4 are intact (Fig. 12-9C). The use of the Marchetti test to reposition the upper urethra in its normal position with the fingers, or with clamps, and then testing the patient's ability to remain continent by having her cough, is of little value. Both of these procedures cause compression of the urethra and provide a false sense of security that surgical therapy will be successful in correcting the problem.

Without a doubt, the most important evaluation of the patient's bladder function is obtained by performing a **cystometrogram.** In this procedure, the patient's bladder should be filled with either carbon dioxide or saline at a steady rate through a urethroscope or a catheter. **The two main parameters to be evaluated are the "first urge" and the "bladder capacity" (i.e., first pain). The normal patient will have a sense of fullness with an urge to void at about 150–200 ml, and a bladder capacity (first pain) at approximately 300–500 ml.** An unstable bladder will usually have a capacity of less than 200 ml and will exhibit detrusor contractions (i.e., bell-shaped) provoked by heel-bouncing or coughing with the patient in a standing position. A simultaneous recording of the intra-abdominal pressure, via a rectal or vaginal probe, will rule out changes in pressures that are not related to bladder activity. When carbon dioxide is used in place of saline, as many as 30% of patients may have false bladder contractions. In addition, the cystometric volumes will be in the lower range (i.e., 150 ml for fullness and 300 ml for bladder capacity), due to the irritating effect of the carbon dioxide on the bladder.

Prior to performing the cystometrogram, you may have your patient void in your presence, while you time the flow (i.e., uroflow test). This method allows you to determine the degree of dysfunction of the voiding mechanism. **A normal patient should be able to have 15–25 ml per second of urine flow.** A flow rate of less than 15 ml per second suggests that the patient may have an inadequate voiding mechanism (e.g., inflammatory, or dysfunctional). A flow rate of 25 ml or more per second should suggest both anatomic and unstable bladder problems. **The residual amount of urine left in the bladder after voiding should be less than 50–100 ml.** A urinalysis and culture should be obtained on this specimen in all patients. After the above studies have been obtained, the urethra and bladder may be visualized with a cystourethroscope using either saline or CO_2. After the urethral orifices and the bladder wall have been visualized, the cystourethroscope is then retracted to approximately 0.5–1.0 cm below the ure-

FIGURE 12-9. Urologic pelvic examination. (A) Visual examination with a vaginal speculum of the anterior vaginal wall for the presence of a cystourethrocele. (B) The pelvic muscle tone may be assessed by having the patient "squeeze" while you palpate the levator ani muscle. (C) Stroking the clitoris will elicit the bulbocavernosa muscle reflex. (D) Stroking the skin lateral to the anus will cause an anal sphincter contraction. (E) The "Q-tip" test may be used to determine the degree of detachment of the proximal urethra.

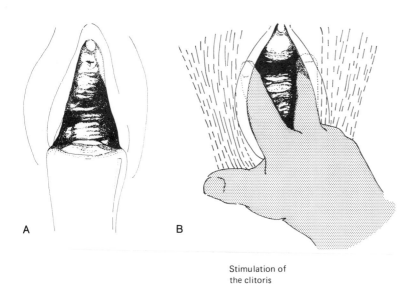

A

B

Stimulation of
the clitoris

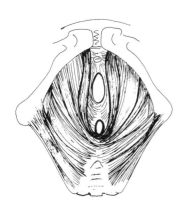

C

Relaxed vaginal
oulet

Bulbocavernosa
Muscle Reflex

Perianal stimulation

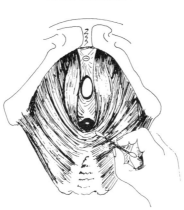

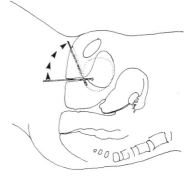

D

Relaxed anus

Anal sphincter
contraction

E

throvesical neck and the orifice. The urethral sphincter should close tightly. On one hand, if the patient is anatomically continent, episodes of coughing or bearing down will not cause the lower portion of the bladder to funnel or allow the urethrovesical sphincter to open. On the other hand, in patients with an unstable bladder, or those with an anatomical incontinence, the urethrovesical sphincter will open widely with a Valsalva's maneuver or with coughing. If anatomical incontinence is present, the sphincter will open and then rapidly close after the provocation, whereas in the patient with an unstable bladder, the sphincter will remain open for several seconds.

d. Treatment of urinary incontinence

All urinary tract infections should be treated with antibiotics, and then the patient should be reevaluated after a full course of therapy to determine if there are any residual symptoms of bladder dysfunction. If an unstable bladder is found, then the patient should be taught the bladder drill and treated with anticholinergic agents. On occasion, the patient may need to try different drugs in order to find the one that is just right for her. The use of **Kegel's perineal exercises** to strengthen the perineal muscles may be of value in some patients. A **transvaginal electronic pelvic floor stimulator** (Vagitone) may be of benefit in exercising the perineal muscles in patients with mild urinary stress incontinence.

A large neurogenic bladder should be managed by having the patient void at frequent, timed intervals. Self-catheterization may become necessary in these cases. Patients who have a small bladder capacity are best managed with parasympatholytic drugs; however, this condition responds poorly to treatment. A common cause of bladder symptoms that is frequently overlooked in the menopausal patient is that of estrogen depletion. Intermittent short-term estrogenic vaginal cream therapy is often of benefit, since the bladder has estrogen receptors like the genital structures. The lack of estrogen is easily detected on vaginal examination, since the vaginal rugae will be absent when there is no estrogen stimulation.

Surgical therapy is reserved primarily for patients with anatomical incontinence. Surgery is recommended only when the loss of the urethrovesical angle is present, with or without a clinically significant cystocele. The patient with a neurogenic bladder is not a candidate for surgical therapy, but the patient with a minor unstable bladder problem, who also has a major anatomical defect, may be a candidate for surgical correction.

The goal of all surgical therapy is to restore the proximal urethra to its normal position. In addition, almost all of the surgical procedures compress the urethra to some extent as well. When the urethra is replaced in its normal position, the urethral pressure returns to a level of more than 20 cm of water above that of the bladder during increased intra-abdominal pressures.

Surgery may be performed via the abdominal route (i.e., Marshall-Marchetti-Krantz procedure, Burch procedure, or the Richardson paravaginal procedure), or by the vaginal approach (i.e., Stamey procedure, Pereyra procedure, or the Kelly plication procedure). Since a hysterectomy is usually performed at the time of the corrective surgery on the bladder, the surgical correction of the bladder neck is usually delayed until the patient has completed her childbearing. Subsequent deliveries are thereby prevented so as to not disrupt the repair procedure.

6. Carcinoma of the vagina

a. Incidence

Primary carcinoma of the vagina is quite rare, whereas secondary carcinomas (i.e., metastases) are not uncommon. When cancer of the vagina does occur, it is usually a squamous carcinoma occurring in the upper half of the vagina. It generally occurs between the ages of 35 and 70.

The extension of carcinoma of the vagina, and its clinical staging, is usually in the same pattern as with carcinoma of the cervix when it occurs in the upper portion of the vagina, and like the extension of vulvar carcinoma when it arises in the lower part of the vagina (Table 12-1).

During the past 30 years, a clear-cell adenocarcinoma of the vagina has been found in women whose mothers were given diethylstilbestrol during pregnancy (see Chapter 13). More than 500 of these cancers have been reported since 1940, with an age range of 7–34 years. The highest clinical use of DES in pregnancy was in the early 1950s, and it was discontinued in 1971. The treatment of these clear-cell carcinomas by radical hysterectomy and lymphadenectomy has resulted in a five-year cure

TABLE 12-1. FIGO classification
of vaginal carcinoma

Classification	Description
	Preinvasive carcinoma
Stage 0	Carcinoma-in-situ, intraepithelial carcinoma
	Invasive carcinoma
Stage I	Carcinoma limited to vaginal wall
Stage II	Carcinoma involving the subvaginal tissue, but not extending onto the pelvic wall
Stage III	Carcinoma extending onto the pelvic wall
Stage IV	Carcinoma extending beyond the true pelvis or involving the mucosa of the bladder or rectum. Bullous edema as such does not permit a case to be allotted to Stage IV
Stage IVa	Spread of growth to adjacent organs
Stage IVb	Spread to distant organs

Reproduced with permission from FIGO, *Annual Report on the Results of Treatment in Gynecologic Cancer,* vol. 19, 1985.

rate of about 88%. Although these tumors are similar to squamous carcinomas of the cervix, they metastasize to the lungs more often than squamous carcinomas. The overall survival rate for all stages of patients with a clear-cell carcinoma is about 78%, instead of the lower salvage (55%) seen in cervical squamous cancer.

b. Symptoms

The symptoms of vaginal cancer consist of a vaginal discharge and bleeding. If the lesion is anteriorly located, there may be urinary tract symptoms secondary to compression. Occasionally, in postmenopausal patients, the lesion may be asymptomatic and only detected on the routine annual pelvic examination.

c. Management

In small tumors (stages I and II) located in the upper vagina, a hysterectomy, partial vaginectomy, and pelvic lympadenectomy may be performed. The majority of carcinomas of the vagina, however, can be treated by radiotherapy. If the upper vaginal carcinoma is large and bulky, external irradiation will shrink the tumor sufficiently to employ local radiation therapy.

On occasion, interstitial needle implants may be required. Bulky stage III and IV lesions may be treated with 5,000 rads of external irradiation over 5–6 weeks. Additional irradiation through reduced fields may also be used in some cases. In one study, the five-year survival of patients who were treated with radiotherapy was 83% (stage I), 63% (stage II), 40% (stage III), and 0% (stage IV).

7. Sarcoma botryoides

Sarcoma botryoides consists of a rare lesion that occurs in young children. These tumors arise from the anterior wall of the vagina in a multicentric fashion. They present with reddish, grape-like lesions that protrude from the vagina, or on occasion, they may erode through the base of the bladder and present as a reddish polypoid lesion at the urethral orifice.

Sarcoma botryoides is highly malignant. In the past, exenterative surgery has been performed; however, recent studies have shown that comparable results can be obtained with less radical surgical procedures by utilizing chemotherapy and/or radiotherapy.

CHAPTER 13

Cervical disease

Look wise, say nothing, and grunt. Speech was given to conceal thought.

—*Sir William Osler**

1. Infection

a. Acute cervicitis

Acute cervicitis is an acute inflammation of the cervix that is usually due to a cervical/vaginal infection. Candida, Trichomonas, and Gardnerella vaginalis are all common pathogens that involve the cervix. Recently, **Chlamydia trachomatis has been noted to primarily involve the cervix, and indeed the cervix may actually be the reservoir for this organism.** Neisseria gonorrhoeae may also infect the cervix and is frequently found in association with Chlamydia. Herpes simplex type II, as well as condyloma acuminatum, are very common invaders, and there seems to be a high incidence of cervical dysplasia associated with these two viruses. Rarely, syphilis, tuberculosis, or granuloma inguinale may infect the cervix.

Acute cervicitis often appears as a reddened **erosion;** however, in many instances, this so-called erosion is actually an **ectropion,** or an outfolding of the normal columnar epithelium from the endocervical canal. In patients who are pregnant, or in those who

have been taking birth control pills, a proliferation of the endocervical glands (microglandular hyperplasia) may be found to be present on histologic examination. This finding is usually associated with an increased amount of a clear mucoid secretion (leukorrhea). **In a true cervical erosion, the surface epithelium of the cervix is actually denuded.** With an ectropion, the patient will usually complain of only a (leukorrhea) (i.e., a clear vaginal discharge), whereas in an acute cervicitis, a purulent discharge with an odor as well as itching and irritation may be present, depending upon the causative organism.

In an acute cervicitis, you should culture the cervix to test for Chlamydia trachomatis and Neisseria gonorrhoeae organisms (see Chapter 12). If one or both of these organisms are present, then you should also obtain a serologic test for syphilis. A Gram-stained smear may provide you with a tentative diagnosis of gonorrhea. A wet smear of the vaginal secretions will usually detect Candida, Trichomonas, or Gardnerella infections. If cancer is suspected, then you should obtain a Papanicolaou smear. If the patient complains of dysuria, a urinalysis and culture should also be obtained to rule out an associated urinary tract infection.

b. Chronic cervicitis

Evidence of **chronic cervicitis** may be found on histologic examination of almost every cervix. All of the organisms that may be involved in acute cervicitis may also be involved in chronic cervicitis. Clinically, there may be an erosion and hypertrophy of the cervix with the presence of multiple nabothian cysts. A purulent vaginal discharge may often be the only symptom, and the cervix may show areas of attempted healing by

---

*Reprinted with permission from Robert Bennett Bean, *Sir William Osler: Aphorisms from His Bedside Teachings and Writings,* William Bennett Bean, ed. Springfield, Ill.: Charles C Thomas, Publisher, 1968, p. 130.

squamous metaplasia. The Papanicolaou smear may be mildly abnormal and show evidence of inflammation. The treatment of a very severe chronic cervicitis consists of systemic antibiotic therapy; however, in most cases local vaginal treatment is effective. In rare cases, cryosurgery may be necessary to cure a badly infected cervix.

2. Benign conditions

a. Dysplasia/carcinoma-in-situ

It has been thought in the past that there was about a 10–15 year difference in the mean ages of women who have cervical dysplasia and those who have invasive squamous cell carcinoma of the cervix. This long preinvasive phase in the natural history of cervical cancer provided a window in which cervical neoplastic disease could be detected and eradicated prior to the development of the more lethal invasive disease. Recent evidence concerning the human papilloma virus (HPV), however, indicates that this window may be as short as three years. Patients who have cervical lesions with HPV serotypes 16 and 18 seem to be the ones that progress to cancer, whereas those with serotypes 6 and 11 almost never develop cervical cancer.

1) Papanicolaou smear

Since the introduction of the annual Pap smear technique, American women have been taught to obtain a Pap test and an examination at periodic intervals. While most patients will generally comply and have an examination at intervals of about twenty-two months, this procedure also allows the physician the opportunity to examine patients at regular intervals and perhaps diagnose ovarian lesions, breast masses, and other illnesses at an earlier stage. Thus, while cervical cancer has been the main focus of these annual checkups, they have served the patient in many other ways as well.

There is no doubt that Pap smears have detected a significant number of cervical intraepithelial neoplastic (CIN) lesions. **The current recommendation is that the Pap screening should commence when the female becomes sexually active, or when she reaches the age of 18, and** **that it be repeated at one-year intervals thereafter. After three or more consecutive normal annual Pap smears, the Pap smear may then be performed at less frequent intervals at the physician's discretion.**

A report by the Canadian Task Force on Cervical Screening Programs in 1976 (i.e., the Walton Report) recommended that if the initial smear in women over the age of 18 and the subsequent one-year Pap smear was negative, then repeat Pap smears could be obtained at intervals of one to three years up to the age of 35, and if still negative at that time, then at five-year intervals until the age of 60, after which they could be discontinued entirely. The American College of Obstetricians and Gynecologists, in its Periodic Cancer Screening for Women policy statement released in 1980, disagreed with this approach and specified that patients should have annual Pap smears because the transit time from CIS to invasive cancer could occur within three years or less in 5% of cases. A second Walton Report published in 1982 recommended annual Pap smears between the ages of 18 and 35, and then at five-year intervals until the age of 60. Subsequently, the American Cancer Society recommended that if the initial two annual smears were negative, then, in the low-risk patient, the Pap smear could be performed every three years thereafter. **Currently, the gynecologists in this country follow the recommendations of the American College of Obstetricians and Gynecologists and usually obtain a Pap smear on their patients at annual intervals.** *Patients who are at high risk include those who have had early sexual contacts (less than age 20), multiple partners, HPV group 16 and 18 cervical lesions, or herpetic lesions; these patients should definitely be screened with a Pap smear at yearly intervals.*

It is important to recognize the existence of the **false-negative Pap smear.** Some authors have noted that the incidence of a negative Pap smear within one year of the development of a stage I carcinoma may be as high as 40%. **In most studies, however, the false negativity rate for cytology smears has been reported to be between 8 and 20%.** In the past, the inadequate training of pathologists in the cytologic interpretation of Pap smears may have contributed to this problem. Although this should not be the case today, it should be kept in mind that the pathologist cannot read on a slide something that is

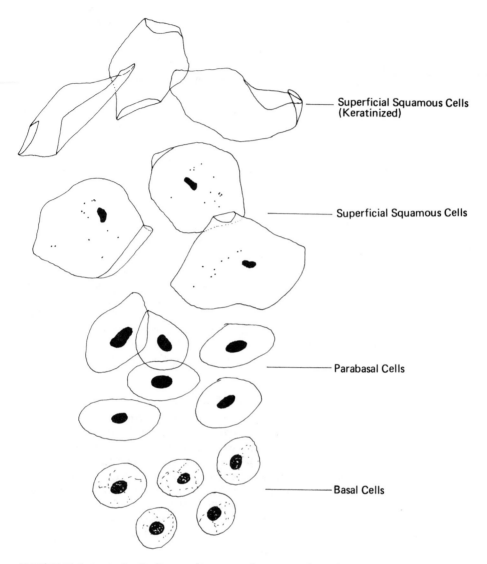

Superficial Squamous Cells
(Keratinized)

Superficial Squamous Cells

Parabasal Cells

Basal Cells

FIGURE 13-1. Normal cells that may be seen in the Papanicolaou smear.

not there, and therefore *when you take the smear on your patient, you must be careful that you obtain an adequate sampling of the cervical and endocervical areas* (Fig. 13-1).

In view of the increasing availability of the colposcope in the offices of private practitioners, and the reputed false negativity rate for the cytologic smears, one might consider the possibility of doing **routine colposcopy** screening as part of the annual checkup along with the Pap smear; however, this approach has

not been generally advocated by experts in the field as yet. Due to the close association of the human papilloma virus (HPV) with cervical neoplasia, a DNA screening test for HPV may also be included in the annual checkup of the patient in the future.

Recently, the use of **cervicography,** where a photograph or a **cervigram** is taken of the cervix after two applications of 5% acetic acid, has been advocated. Any white lesion thus detected on the cervix would be designated as a suspicious lesion. While

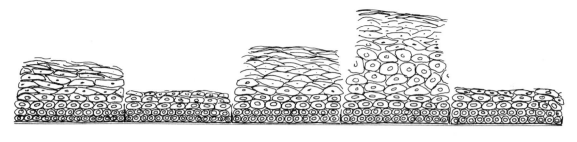

NEWBORN   CHILDHOOD   ADULT   PREGNANCY   POSTMENOPAUSE

FIGURE 13-2. Schema showing the changes in the vaginal and cervical epithelium due to the hormonal milieu. *From left to right:* The newborn shows an estrogen effect from the mother. The prepubertal child has no estrogenic stimulation. The adult has normal estrogen stimulation. The pregnant woman demonstrates an increased estrogen level. The postmenopausal woman shows an atrophic vaginal mucosa secondary to the loss of estrogenic stimulation.

there seems to be a high false-positive rate associated with the cervigram, it remains a sensitive screening method for cervical dysplastic lesions.

2) Dysplasia

The term *dysplasia* is derived from *dys,* meaning *bad,* and *plassein* meaning *to form;* thus, an *abnormal formation of tissue.* **The normal stratified squamous epithelium of the cervix is composed of four layers:** (1) a one- to two-cell layer of basal cells, (2) a three- to four-cell layer of parabasal cells, (3) a wider zone of intermediate cells, and (4) a superficial layer of cells having minimal or no nuclei present and that show evidence of some degree of keratinization (Fig. 13-2). Dysplasia results when there is a delay in the maturation of the basal cells as they attempt to move toward the surface; as a result, the cells with abnormally large nuclei and minimal cytoplasm will appear to be closer to the surface of the epithelium on histologic examination.

a) Classification of dysplasia

If a biopsy reveals that the larger nucleated cells are present in the **lower third** of the stratified squamous epithelium, the lesion has been called **mild dysplasia (cervical intraepithelial neoplasia, or CIN I).** If these cells appear to be in the **lower half** of the epithelium, then **moderate dysplasia (or CIN II) is** present. If these immature cells extend **almost full thickness** through the epithelium, leaving only a few

mature cells on the surface, **then severe dysplasia (or CIN III) is present.** If the abnormal cells extend from the basal cell layer all the way to the surface, with no maturation of the cells at all, then the lesion is called **carcinoma-in-situ, but it is still part of the CIN III classification.** It is thought that a developmental continuum takes place from mild dysplasia to invasive carcinoma.

In many dysplastic cervical lesions, there is evidence of a human papilloma virus infection. Indeed, the incidence of other sexually transmitted diseases, such as herpesvirus type II, syphilis, gonorrhea, and trichomoniasis, have all been noted to be higher in patients with cervical neoplastic lesions. **A history of having had intercourse at an early age, having had multiple partners, being black, and being poor are all high-risk factors for the development of cervical cancer.**

Because these viruses are intracellular parasites and may therefore interfere with the replication of DNA in the cell, they have the potential for being oncogenic. Indeed, a number of tumors in lower animals are thought to be due to herpesvirus type II. **The serotypes 6 and 11 of the human papilloma virus have been associated with condylomatous cervical lesions, whereas serotypes 16 and 18 (also serotypes 31, 33, and 35) have been found in in-situ and invasive carcinomatous lesions of the genitalia** (see Chapter 11). Cellular changes commonly noted with viral infections and CIN lesions include cells with large dark nuclei and a clear perinuclear cytoplasm (i.e., vacuolization) found in the outer layers of the squamous epithelium; these are called **koilocytotic cells.**

b) Colposcopic diagnosis

Colposcopy complements and extends the value of the Pap smear in detecting cervical dysplasia. A Pap smear relies on cytology, which consists of the microscopic evaluation of individual cells that have been exfoliated from the cervix. Their nuclear and cytoplasmic morphology are indicative of their maturation. Nuclei that are bizarre in size, staining qualities, or abnormal configurations may be seen more commonly in CIN III lesions or invasive carcinoma.

Colposcopy utilizes a **stereoscopic microscope** that is capable of visualizing the cervix (i.e., 6× to 40× magnification) under proper artificial lighting conditions. This procedure is accomplished by inserting a self-retaining vaginal speculum and positioning the colposcope so as to examine the cervix. The cervix should be cleaned with a dry sponge, and then again with a swab that has been moistened with saline. A solution of 4% acetic acid on a swab will coagulate the remaining cervical mucus and allow for its removal. In addition, it will slightly dehydrate any dysplastic cells so that they may become whiter and more visible. The use of a *green filter* on the colposcope will allow the viewer to see the underlying vascular network.

The metaplastic junctional area between the columnar epithelium of the endocervix and the original stratified squamous epithelium of the ectocervix has been termed the **transformation zone.** When cervical dysplasia/carcinoma occurs, it will almost always be within this zone.

Abnormal colposcopic findings consist of a **mosaic pattern, punctuation,** and an **aceto-white epithelium.** In addition, there may be **abnormal vascular patterns with changes in the intercapillary distances,** and an elevated or **uneven surface contour** of the lesion. **The presence of sharp borders between the normal tissue and the abnormal tissue may be seen in advanced dysplasias.** If the squamocolumnar junction cannot be seen (which occurs in perhaps 15% of patients), the colposcopic procedure should be considered to be an *unsatisfactory colposcopic examination.* In these cases, a cold conization of the cervix must be considered in severe dysplasias to rule out any advanced endocervical lesions, such as carcinoma-in-situ or invasive carcinoma (see Chapter 18).

b. Endocervical polyps

Most cervical polyps arise from the endocervix, and only rarely from the ectocervix. This tumor may be either a pedunculated or a sessile growth composed of a vascular, fibrous stromal core that is covered by epithelium, either columnar or squamous. The histologic criterion in diagnosing a polyp is the finding of a finger-like piece of tissue **with an epithelial surface on at least three sides.** The polyp is usually a fragile, red, finger-like tumor extending from the cervical os. It may be as small as a few millimeters or as large as 2–3 cm in diameter and 5–7 cm long. Most polyps, however, are about 0.25–0.5 cm broad and perhaps 2–3 cm long. *The incidence of malignancy in an endocervical polyp is less than 1%, with squamous carcinoma being the most common type.* On rare occasions, multiple polypoid tumors of **sarcoma botryoides** may be seen in the vagina of a young girl. These tumors are highly malignant (see Chapter 12).

Since inflammation and necrosis are often present at the tip of an endocervical polyp, intermenstrual spotting and postcoital bleeding are common complaints. The treatment of an endocervical polyp consists of simple excisional removal. If the base of the polyp is thin, it can be grasped by a hemostat and twisted off with minimal bleeding. The use of a *silver nitrate cautery stick* will generally control any ooze from the base. The use of *Monsel's solution* on a cotton swab will also stop the bleeding. In those cases in which the polyp is sessile with a broad base, the removal should be carried out in the hospital by an electrosurgical or sharp-knife excision, with suture control of the bleeding if necessary. The polyp should always be evaluated histologically to be certain that there has been no malignant change.

c. Cervical leiomyoma

Cervical leiomyomas are relatively uncommon because there is very little smooth muscle present in the cervix. These small muscular tumors are generally asymptomatic. **Larger tumors become symptomatic because of their pressure upon the surrounding organs.** For example, an anterior leiomyoma may cause urinary retention, frequency, or urgency because of the pressure on the bladder or the urethra. In some instances, there may be compression of the ureters sufficient to result in a hydroureter with hydronephrosis. A large posterior leiomyoma may result in constipation because of its compression of the bowel. Dystocia in labor may occur in the presence of a large cervical leiomyoma.

The treatment of small leiomyomas is merely observation in order to detect any increase in size. In larger tumors, myomectomy or hysterectomy may become necessary, depending upon the degree of clinical difficulties encountered and the desire of the patient for continued fertility.

d. Congenital/DES changes

1) Congenital changes

The congenital absence of the cervix is rare. In some instances, the cervix may be shortened or only partially absent. If the cervical canal is absent and there is a functioning endometrium and ovaries, then retrograde menstruation may occur at menarche, which may eventually result in pelvic endometriosis. The patient may complain of cyclic lower abdominal pain and amenorrhea. Occasionally, the cervical os may be involved in a congenital stricture or conglutination.

2) DES changes

In the daughters of women who received **diethylstilbestrol (DES)** during their pregnancy, there is an increased risk of genital abnormalities. In addition, these individuals carry a risk of a 0.14:1,000 to 1.4:1,000 for developing a clear-cell carcinoma of the vagina. A definite history of DES exposure has been found in about 60–65% of these cases, with another 10% giving a history of exposure to some kind of unknown medication (see Chapter 12).

A number of cervical changes have been associated with DES syndrome. In perhaps one-third of these patients (range 20–60%), anatomical changes of the cervix occur. These changes include: (1) a circular sulcus about the endocervical os, (2) columnar epithelium on the portio vaginalis of the cervix, and (3) hypertrophy and pseudopolyp formation of the endocervical tissue and of the anterior lip of the cervix. **These findings have been called cervical hoods, collars, vaginal ridges, and cockscomb formations.** Interestingly, they seem to regress spontaneously with time. Furthermore, there is an extension of the endocervical epithelial tissue onto the vaginal fornices (i.e., **adenosis**) in some 50–75% of these patients, where it is eventually covered over by squamous metaplasia. These patients were all exposed to DES prior to the 19th week of gestation. This extensive **transformation zone** can become the site of later epithelial dysplasia (in 4–12% of cases) and neoplastic changes.

Some of these patients will experience pregnancy losses in the second trimester due to an incompetence of the internal cervical os. If cervical conization or cryosurgery is used to treat dysplastic lesions of the cervix in these patients, cervical stenosis will often occur (70%), since the cervix does not heal normally.

In 40–70% of these patients, there is a distortion of the uterus, with a T-shaped or constricted cavity, uterine hypoplasia, or cornual bulbs; however, these findings do not necessarily indicate that the woman will have a complicated pregnancy. Preterm delivery and ectopic pregnancy (6–10%), however, have apparently been more common in these patients.

3. Malignant conditions

a. Squamous carcinoma

Squamous cell carcinoma of the cervix accounts for about 85% of the cases of malignant cervical disease, with the remainder being due to adenocarcinomas and mixed tumors. Next to carcinoma of the breast and the endometrium, carcinoma of the cervix is the most common type of cancer in the female. As many as 2–3% of women over the age of 40 will develop cancer of the cervix. In general, the peak incidence of in-situ lesions is between 30 and 40 years of age, whereas invasive lesions occur between 40 and 50 years of age; however, cases of invasive carcinoma may be seen in women as early as 18 years of age.

1) Etiology

While the etiology of cervical cancer is unknown, women with early sexual exposure, who have multiple partners, and who are of high parity seem to be at high risk. Although the human papilloma virus (HPV) and the herpesvirus type II have been implicated in the genesis of this type of lesion, a causal relationship has not yet been proven. It has also been suggested that male semen might contain a specific oncogenic protein that might be capable of producing such a neoplasm.

TABLE 13-1. FIGO classification of carcinoma of the cervix (with 1987 revisions)

Classification	Description
Stage 0	*Preinvasive carcinoma* Carcinoma-in-situ or intraepithelial carcinoma, not to be included in any statistics for invasive carcinoma.
Stages I–IV	*Invasive carcinoma*
I	Carcinoma strictly confined to the cervix (extension to the corpus should be disregarded).
Ia	Preclinical carcinomas of the cervix; that is, those diagnosed only by microscopy.
Ia1	Minimal microscopically evident stromal invasion.
Ia2	Lesions detected microscopically that can be measured. The upper limits of the measurement should not show a depth of invasion of more than 5 mm taken from the base of the epithelium, either surface or glandular, from which it originates; and a second dimension, the horizontal spread, must not exceed 7 mm. Larger lesions should be staged as Ib.
Ib	Lesions of greater dimensions than stage Ia2, whether seen clinically or not. Preformed space involvement should not alter the staging but should be recorded specifically so as to determine whether it should affect treatment decisions in the future.
II	The carcinoma extends beyond the cervix, but has not extended onto the pelvic wall.
IIa	The carcinoma involves the vagina, but not the lower one-third. No obvious parametrial involvement.
IIb	Obvious parametrial involvement.
III	Carcinoma extends onto the pelvic wall or lower one-third of vagina. All cases with hydronephrosis or nonfunctioning kidney should be included, unless known to be due to other causes.
IIIa	The tumor involves the lower one-third of the vagina, with no extension onto the pelvic wall.
IIIb	Extension onto the pelvic wall. Rectal examination demonstrates no cancer-free space between the tumor and the pelvic wall.
IV	Carcinoma has extended beyond the true pelvis or has involved the mucosa of the bladder or rectum. Bullous edema alone does not permit a lesion to be categorized as Stage IV.
IVa	Spread of growth to adjacent organs.
IVb	Spread to distant organs.

Reprinted with permission from FIGO, *Annual Report on the Results of Treatment in Gynecological Cancer,* vol. 19, 1985. The recent changes in the FIGO staging are reprinted with permission from the American College of Obstetricians and Gynecologists, W. T. Creasman, "Changes in FIGO Staging," *Obstetrics and Gynecology* 70 (1987), p. 138.

2) Pathophysiology

Squamous cell carcinoma begins in the epithelium of the **transformation zone** of the cervix, either on the portio of the cervix, or in the endocervical canal. Carcinoma is thought to develop over the course of many years from a preinvasive lesion, such as dysplasia. In time, the **dysplasia (i.e., mild, moderate, or severe)** may progress to **carcinoma-in-situ** and then eventually to an early stromal invasion of less than 3 mm below the basement membrane **(microinvasion).** As the tumor spreads to the deeper structures, it also spreads to the lymphatic channels and then ultimately to the vessels, from which it is then spread to distant sites (i.e., **invasive disease with metastases to other organ systems**). When the carcinoma is confined to the cervix (stage 1), the incidence of regional nodal metastases is about 15–20%. In stage IIB cases, this nodal involvement may increase to as much as 40%, with 10% of patients having involvement of the para-aortic nodes. In stage III lesions, the para-aortic nodes may be involved in as many as 45% of cases (Table 13-1).

3) Histology

Squamous carcinoma has been classified both by cell type and by the degree of differentiation. **The cell types include: (1) the large-cell nonkeratinizing carcinomas, (2) the large-cell keratinizing carcinomas, and (3) the small-cell carcinomas. The nonkeratinizing large-cell type seems to have the best prognosis, whereas the small-cell tumor has the worst. When classified according to the degree of differentiation, the cells are graded according to the presence of well-defined intracellular bridges, keratinization, epithelial pearls, and the number of mitoses per high power field. In grade I well-differentiated tumors,** there are less than two mitoses per high power field and the cells look mature and have intracellular bridges and cytoplasmic keratohyalin. There may be epithelial pearls present. In **grade II moderately differentiated tumors,** there may be fewer intracellular bridges and epithelial pearls present. In addition, there are 2–4 mitoses per high power field. The cells usually vary somewhat in size and shape. In **grade III tumors, which are poorly differentiated,** cells are present in nests and cords. The nucleocytoplasmic ratio is increased, and there is more disparity in the size and shape of the nuclei. Giant cells may be numerous, and keratinization is essentially absent. There will be more than four mitoses per high power field.

The less differentiated the tumor is, the worse the prognosis. The involvement of the vascular spaces and the lymphatic spaces increases the chance of lymph node involvement and distant metastases. A marked lymphocytic response in the cervical stroma, however, is evidence of a good host response and perhaps of a better prognosis.

b. Adenocarcinoma

Adenocarcinoma of the cervix is usually derived from the columnar epithelium of the endocervix. In the clear-cell variety, a history of prior exposure in utero to DES may be found, although this lesion may also arise de novo. A rare form of adenocarcinoma derives from the wolffian (mesonephric) duct remnants. The cells of this tumor are generally cuboidal and may have a minimal glandular pattern. The staging and management of adenocarcinoma of the cervix is essentially the same as with squamous carcinoma.

c. Treatment of cervical carcinoma

The diagnosis of carcinoma of the cervix has been greatly aided by the introduction of the Pap smear. Abnormal Pap smears are now evaluated by colposcopy and by directed cervical and endocervical biopsies. If the biopsies are inadequate, or if carcinoma-in-situ is suspected, then a conization of the cervix may be necessary for a thorough evaluation.

1) Carcinoma-in-situ

If carcinoma-in-situ is found, the treatment is based upon the patient's desires with regard to further childbearing. *If she wishes further children, after being apprised of the risk of developing a possible invasive carcinoma, then the pregnancy should be initiated as soon as possible.* Close follow-up of these patients is absolutely necessary after the initial treatment to oblate the cervical lesion (i.e., conization, laser therapy, cryosurgery, or electrocautery). About 1–2% of these patients will eventually develop invasive carcinoma. *If the patient has completed her childbearing, then a vaginal hysterectomy should be considered.*

2) Microinvasive carcinoma

If microinvasive carcinoma of the cervix is present (i.e., stromal penetration of the tumor to less than 3 mm below the basement membrane, and without lymph space involvement or confluence of the tumor), then a simple hysterectomy should be done.

3) Invasive carcinoma

In invasive carcinoma, either radical surgery or irradiation may be used for treatment. *Surgery is usually confined to stage IIA lesions and below, with radiation therapy being utilized for advanced lesions.* The results of either type of treatment modality are essentially the same.

In early invasive lesions (stage I, IIA) of the cervix, a radical hysterectomy and a lymph node dissection may be carried out. **In this operation, the external and internal iliac lymph nodes are removed en bloc with extensive dissection of the bladder and ureters. The lateral uterine supporting en-**

dopelvic fascial structures are removed from the lateral pelvic walls at the same time that the uterus is removed. The ovaries may be retained in the young patient. Due to the extensiveness of the surgery, ureterovaginal, vesicovaginal, or rectovaginal fistulas may occur in about 1–2% of patients.

In patients who have a *central recurrence* of their disease, a total or partial *exenteration* may be performed. In this formidable procedure (i.e., total exenteration), the rectum, vagina, bladder, and vulva may be removed en bloc, with the construction of an ileal conduit for urinary diversion and a rectosigmoid colostomy for fecal diversion. The surgical mortality of this procedure is about 2.5%.

4) Follow-up care

In any patient in whom the diagnosis of cancer has been made, continued follow-up must be carried out at specific intervals for the rest of the patient's life. This follow-up care requires periodic tests and studies that are essential for the safety of the patient. While the private gynecologic practitioner often feels that he or she is qualified to perform the radical cancer surgery, few practitioners have the expertise to undertake the follow-up care. Such follow-up should not be undertaken lightly, since these patients are at high risk for a recurrence of their tumor, which must be detected early if the patient is to have any chance of survival. These patients are better managed by gynecologic oncologists, who are specifically trained in radical operative procedures, radiation therapy, and chemotherapy and are willing to maintain a "tumor registry" of such patients as they follow them throughout the remainder of their lives.

CHAPTER 14

Disease of the uterus and fallopian tubes

The physician must be able to tell the antecedents, know the present, and foretell the future—must meditate these things, and have two special objects in view with regard to diseases, namely, to do good or to do no harm.

—Hippocrates (460–370 B.C.)*

1. Infection

a. Acute/chronic salpingo-oophoritis

In the past, the diagnosis of acute salpingo-oophoritis was universally attributed to the organism **Neisseria gonorrhoeae.** While it was generally accepted that in chronic salpingo-oophoritis, opportunistic secondary invader organisms were involved, the basic disease process was still considered to be a continuation of the gonorrheal infection or a reinfection by this organism.

It has become increasingly recognized that an acute pelvic inflammatory disease (PID) may frequently be due to a coexisting infection with both N. gonorrhoeae and Chlamydia trachomatis. Chlamydia trachomatis, an obligate intracellular bacterial parasite, is associated with Neisseria gonorrhoeae in pelvic inflammatory disease in at least 25–45% of the cases and perhaps even in as many as 80%.

*Reprinted with permission from Encyclopaedia Britannica, Inc. *Great Books of the Western World,* vol. 10, "Hippocrates and Galen," Robert Maynard Hutchins, ed. Chicago: William Benton, Publisher, 1952, p. 46.

b. Initial infection

1) Symptoms

Gonorrhea is one of the most common sexually transmitted diseases and is caused by the organism **Neisseria gonorrhoeae.** There are perhaps as many as 3–5 million new cases of gonorrhea in the United States each year. *Gonorrhea is transmitted by skin-to-skin contact during sexual relations.* **The patient will usually present with complaints of dysuria and an increased frequency of urination in association with a purulent vaginal discharge.** *The initial infection usually becomes manifest about 3–5 days after contact.* The spread of an infection with Neisseria gonorrhoeae occurs as the result of an ascending infection from the surface of the cervix/endocervix to the surface of the uterine endometrium and out onto the mucosa of the fallopian tubes, where it spreads to the ovaries. The onset of symptoms often occurs *during or just after a menstrual period;* however, if the patient has an intrauterine contraceptive device (IUD) in place, the infection may ocur at any time during the menstrual cycle. In some cases, however, the patient is totally asymptomatic. The organisms may also attach themselves to the spermatozoa and may be transported to the upper genital tract by this means. The patient usually develops a **fever of greater than 38° C (100.4° F), a leukocytosis (WBC > 10,000/mm³), and lower abdominal cramps and pain,** which may become severe if not treated promptly. *Chronic pelvic inflammatory disease (PID)* may present with symptoms identical to those of the acute infection.

2) Clinical findings

Upon examination, you will note the presence of erythema of the vaginal mucous membranes and a purulent cervicitis. The abdomen will have tenderness in the lower quadrants and occasionally rebound tenderness. **The cervix will elicit tenderness on motion, and the adnexal regions will also be tender.** Occasionally, a unilateral Bartholin's gland will be involved and a tender, swollen abscess may be present. If anal intercourse has been performed, acute proctitis may be noted. Patients who frequently practice anal intercourse will have a loose anal sphincter that relaxes quickly and easily during the rectal examination. Pharyngeal gonorrheal inflammation may occur after fellatio, and petechiae of the soft palate may be present. *The N. gonorrhoeae organism produces an infection of the fallopian tubes and ovaries in perhaps 15% of patients if the initial infection is left untreated.*

One of the most common hematogenous complications of gonorrhea is the involvement of the skin and joints—the **arthritis-dermatitis syndrome.** The individual develops fever, chills, and myalgia, which are followed in 2–4 days by a polyarticular tenosynovitis of the extensor tendons of the fingers, and an erythematous papular rash of the extremities and joints. Joint cultures may be positive for N. gonorrhoeae in about 50% of these cases.

Other complications of gonorrhea include **endocarditis, meningitis, and pericarditis. Perhaps the most common complication of pelvic inflammatory disease is tubal occlusion and infertility.** Adhesions within the lumin of the fallopian tube, as well as those occurring between the tube and the adjacent pelvic organs, may obstruct the tubal lumin and either prevent the zygote from being transported to the uterine cavity (i.e., ectopic pregnancy) or prevent the sperm from traversing the fallopian tube to fertilize the egg (i.e., infertility).

Perhaps as many as 2–5% of these patients, and especially those who are pregnant, exhibit no symptoms of gonorrhea at all. Prematurity and intrauterine growth retardation, however, in addition to the risk of chorioamnionitis in cases of prolonged rupture of membranes, have been linked to gonorrheal infections in pregnancy. Gonorrheal infection of the eyes (*neonatal gonococcal ophthalmia*), of the ear canal, of the oropharynx, and of the anal canal may provide sites for the hematogenous spread of the organism to cause meningitis and arthritis in the neonate.

3) Diagnosis

A tentative diagnosis of gonorrhea requires obtaining a Gram-stained smear of the cervix or endocervix and demonstrating the presence of **intracellular gram-negative diplococci in the leukocytes.** Mimeae and Herrellea organisms may mimic N. gonorrhoeae, so cultures should also be obtained from the endocervix (positive in 80–90% of gonorrhea cases), the urethra (positive in 50–60%), the pharynx (positive in 10%), and the anus. Since the organism is somewhat fastidious in its ability to grow, it should be immediately swabbed onto a Thayer-Martin medium. **The presence of one sexually trasmitted disease (STD) in a patient should alert you to the possibility that she may have another STD as well.** A serologic test for syphilis should be obtained, and a test for a possible Chlamydia trachomatis infection should also be carried out.

4) Treatment

It has been estimated that 15% of patients with gonorrhea are treatment failures, 20–25% have a recurrence, 20% become infertile, and that there is a six- to tenfold increase in the occurrence of ectopic pregnancy among these patients.

The treatment of PID has presented a difficult problem due to the fact that the vagina contains numerous organisms, some of which are pathogenic and some of which are not, which are so intertwined in acute and chronic PID with the Neisseria gonorrhea and Chlamydia trachomatis pathogens that the contributions of each organism to the disease are impossible to define. It has also been suggested that a bacterial synergism may be operating—a factor that would play a critical role in the development of a pelvic infection.

One concept of how these organisms might interact in a *postoperative gynecologic pelvic infection* involves an *anaerobic progression,* in which it has been postulated that the aerobic organisms use up most of the available oxygen in the infected tissue, and as they die off, they make room for those facultative bacteria that can exist on minimal oxygen. *In turn, these organisms use up the remaining oxygen, producing anaerobic conditions that are perfect for the growth of anaerobic organisms like those of the Bacteroides species.* Theoretically, the oxidation-reduction potential (i.e., the redox potential) of the diseased tissue decreases during the course of this progression from a value of about (+)150 mv (the value for healthy tissues) to about (−)150 mv. If this concept is true, then perhaps the success of the antibiotic regimen in pelvic infections is dependent upon: (1) the types of bacterial organisms present at any given time, (2) the oxygen conditions in the tissue, and (3) the effective spectrum of the antibiotics being used.

Some authors have advocated cefoxitin (Mefoxin) and doxycycline (Vibramycin). If the Gram stain of the cervix was negative, then perhaps the organism involved was other than N. gonorrhoeae, in which case the combination of clindamycin (Cleocin) and gentamicin (Garamycin) could be administered. Other authors have advocated using a cefoxitin and clindamycin combination. Since the infection is **polymicrobic,** the treatment should take into consideration the fact that the gonococcus may be present in 30–40% of PID cases, the chlamydial organisms in 20–60%, and other bacteria in almost all cases, including the gram-negative aerobes, the gram-positive and gram-negative anaerobes, and Mycoplasma hominis. It is important to reexamine the patient frequently during the early course of therapy to watch for the development of a tubo-ovarian abscess. Furthermore, all patients should be recultured about one month after treatment begins in order to make sure that the infectious agent(s) have been truly eradicated.

In 1985, the Centers for Disease Control (CDC) published suggested regimens for the ambulatory and inpatient treatment of PID (Table 14-1). While other regimens have been tried or are being considered, at the present time many physicians are following the CDC recommendations.[1]

c. Tubo-ovarian abscess

A severe acute or chronic salpingo-oophoritis (PID) may be associated in perhaps 15% of cases with the subsequent development of a tubo-ovarian abscess. This is more frequently the case when the institution of the appropriate antibiotic therapy has been delayed or when there have been repeated episodes of the disease over a period of time (i.e., chronic salpingo-oophoritis). A pelvic abscess may also occur in association with gastrointestinal infections, such as with a ruptured appendicitis or a diverticulitis.

1) Diagnosis

The presenting symptoms of a pelvic abscess are usually the same as those of acute pelvic inflammatory disease (PID). **In contrast to the usual PID, however, the diagnosis is based not only on the**

---

[1] See *Morbidity and Mortality Weekly Report Supplement,* vol. 34, no. 4S, October 18, 1985.

TABLE 14-1. Acute pelvic inflammatory disease

Acute inflammatory disease of the pelvis involves many different organisms, and thus the treatment regimens must cover a broad spectrum of bacteria. Hospitalization is almost always necessary. The treatment of choice has not been established.

Suggested treatment regimens:

If the patient is hospitalized:

1. Doxycycline, 100 mg I.V. b.i.d. daily, PLUS cefoxitin, 2.0 grams q.i.d. I.V. per day. Maintain therapy for at least 4 days and until the patient is afebrile for 48 hours. Continue doxycycline, 100 mg p.o. b.i.d., to complete 10–14 days of treatment. (Doxycycline is contraindicated in pregnancy), OR,
2. Clindamycin, 600 mg I.V. q.i.d. daily, PLUS gentamycin, 2.0 mg/kg I.V., followed by 1.5 mg/kg I.V. t.i.d. if the renal function is normal. Continue the antibiotics for 4 days and at least 48 hours after the patient becomes afebrile. Continue clindamycin, 450 mg p.o. q.i.d., to complete 10–14 days of therapy.

If the patient is not hospitalized:

1. Cefoxitin, 2.0 grams I.M., or amoxicillin, 3.0 grams p.o., OR ampicillin, 3.5 grams p.o., OR aqueous procaine penicillin G 4.8 million units I.M. at 2 sites, OR ceftriaxone, 250 mg I.M. Probenecid, 1.0 gram p.o., is administered with all of the above regimens except ceftriaxone.

The above regimen is followed by:

Doxycycline, 100 mg p.o. b.i.d., for 10–14 days.
While tetracycline HCl, 500 mg q.i.d., may be substituted for doxycycline, it is not as effective.

Adapted from *Morbidity and Mortality Weekly Report Supplement,* vol. 34, no. 4S, October 18, 1985.

symptoms of fever and pelvic pain but also on the clinical finding of a palpable tubo-ovarian abscess. Supporting evidence includes an elevated leukocyte count with a left shift and an elevated erythrocyte sedimentation rate (ESR). While the use of ultrasonography and CT scans may be helpful in some cases in which the pelvic contents have been poorly defined on examination, in most instances these tests are not necessary.

2) The Fitz-Hugh-Curtis syndrome

In 15–30% of patients with PID and/or a tubo-ovarian abscess, **infectious perihepatitis,** or the Fitz-

Hugh-Curtis syndrome (FHCS), may occur. The patient with this syndrome will usually complain of a pleuritic right upper quadrant (RUQ) pain that limits chest expansion, which is associated with symptoms and findings of PID. An inflammation of Glisson's capsule of the liver and of the undersurface of the diaphragm with the development of adhesive bands account for these symptoms. The condition is thought to be due to N. gonorrhea and/or C. trachomatis in almost all cases. It is unknown whether the infection is transmitted by the pelvic **lymphatics** to the subdiaphragmatic lymphatics, by a **hematologic spread** to the liver or diaphragm, or by **direct extension** via the paracolic gutters to the liver and the diaphragm. In the reported cases of FHCS in men, either the hematogenous mechanism or the lymphatic extension may be operative.

d. Medical management of PID

The patient with acute PID should be hospitalized immediately and treated with broad-spectrum intravenous antibiotics. Hot sitz baths and a modified Fowler's position (i.e., the head of the bed is raised slightly more than the usual 20 inches above the horizontal—**semi-Fowler**) will assist in containing the infection in the pelvis and will provide comfort to the patient. The increased vascularity and congestion that occurs secondary to the local heat of the hot sitz bath may also be of value in allowing the antibiotics to reach the infected areas in a higher concentration. You should monitor your patient's electrolytes and fluid requirements closely. If a severe *anemia* (i.e., hemoglobin less than 6 gm/dl) is present and the patient is not responding well to therapy, then she should receive a blood transfusion to reach a hemoglobin level of more than 10 gm/dl in order to enhance her ability to combat the infection.

A triple antibiotic regimen using ampicillin (or penicillin), gentamicin, and clindamycin has been found to be an effective combination in treating a tubo-ovarian abscess. Other regimens that have been suggested include doxycycline and cefoxitin, and clindamycin and tobramycin (or gentamicin) (see CDC recommendations). **Clindamycin has been of particular value because of its unique ability of being able to penetrate an abscess cavity in therapeutic concentrations.**

In some patients with fever and symptoms beyond 5–6 days who do not have an abscess, and who are unresponsive to antibiotic therapy, **pelvic thrombophlebitis** may be present. If so, a *test course of intravenous heparin* may be added to the regimen for 48 or 72 hours. If the patient's fever responds to this treatment, then the full heparin dosage should be continued for a total of seven days.

e. Colpotomy drainage

Often during the course of therapy, the pelvic or tubo-ovarian abscess will point into the cul-de-sac. Although it is rare for the abscess to rupture spontaneously into the rectum, it more commonly becomes fluctuant and cystic and bulges or points into the posterior fornix of the vagina. *When this occurs, a posterior colpotomy may be performed to allow for drainage of the abscess cavity.* Loculi within the cavity should be broken up digitally and a Malecot catheter placed to allow continued drainage over the next few days. Usually, the patient's temperature decreases dramatically after the abscess has been drained and the other symptoms improve rapidly. Surprisingly, a small percentage of these patients will later become pregnant and have successful deliveries, so neither you nor the patient should have a completely bleak outlook with regard to her future fertility.

If the patient with a suspected tubo-ovarian abscess does not respond to appropriate broad-spectrum antibiotic therapy within 48–72 hours, a change in the antibiotic regimen or surgery should be considered.

f. Definitive surgical management

In a small number of patients, medical management fails and surgery becomes necessary. Usually, a **total abdominal hysterectomy and a bilateral salpingo-oophorectomy** will be necessary; however, if the patient desires continued fertility, and if one side appears normal, a unilateral salpingo-oophorectomy may be performed. *If surgery is undertaken during the acute phase of the tubo-ovarian abscess, there will be an increase in the morbidity and in the risk of bowel and bladder injury.* **In most cases, however, medical management will be effective and the surgery can be delayed until 4–6 weeks or more after the acute episode.** The erythrocyte sedimentation rate will gradually return to normal over perhaps 4–6 weeks as the inflammatory process heals, and as such, it provides a useful gauge in following these patients. Antibiotics should be administered orally during the first two weeks after discharge from the hospital (e.g., tetracycline to cover for Chlamydia) or at any time that a bimanual pelvic examination elicits a febrile response.

g. Rupture of a tubo-ovarian abscess

The most serious complication associated with a tubo-ovarian abscess is the **rupture of the abscess** into the peritoneal cavity, which results in the development of a generalized peritonitis and may lead to shock and death. This complication occurs in about 10% of patients. The patient will usually complain of a sudden increase in pelvic pain, associated with fever, chills, tachycardia, hypotension, and evidence of peritoneal irritation. **As soon as this diagnosis is strongly considered, it is essential that surgery not be delayed.** Shock should be rapidly corrected with intravenous lactated Ringer's solution, normal saline, or with packed red blood cells if the patient is anemic. A midline vertical incision should be utilized, in case it becomes necessary to explore the upper abdomen. Aerobic and anaerobic cultures and Gram-stained smears should be obtained upon entry into the abdomen. The patient should not be placed in a Trendelenburg's position until after the purulent material has been cleansed out of the pelvis. Peritoneal lavage, utilizing saline or a gentamicin solution, has been advocated by some authorities. Following the hysterectomy, a retroperitoneal vaginal drain should be placed, in addition to the drains that are placed above and below the abdominal wall fascia. Stay sutures should be placed, or the abdominal wall above the fascia should be left open for later closure, to allow the wound to heal by third intention. Broad-spectrum antibiotics should be continued until the patient is afebrile for at least 24–48 hours.

2. Benign conditions

a. Acute/chronic pelvic pain

Pelvic pain is a common gynecologic complaint and is present in perhaps a third of all gynecologic patients. It may be part of an acute process, such as an ectopic pregnancy or a ruptured corpus luteum cyst, or it may be a chronic process, in which case it may be related to other pelvic pathology.

1) History

It is very important to take an **adequate history** in the patient who has pelvic pain, including a detailed analysis of the pain: (1) the time sequence of the onset of the pain, (2) the location, (3) the intensity and duration, (4) whether it remains localized or radiates, (5) what relieves it or exacerbates it, and (6) its relationship to activities such as eating, sleeping, or having intercourse. Furthermore, it is important to determine the patient's cultural, social, sexual, and marital situation, since pelvic pain may provide the patient with certain emotional or psychological benefits—such as being "too sick to go to work," or "having too much pain to have intercourse," or other secondary gains that may not be immediately apparent. A general evaluation of the patient's level of maturity and psychological make-up should be carried out in an effort to determine how much "psychological overlay" she may place upon the pain. **Hypochondriasis, depression, and other unconscious needs may be uncovered in your psychological evaluation. A psychiatric consultation may be helpful in defining these problems.**

2) Periodic pain

Pelvic pain may be classified as being periodic or continuous. **Periodic pain** is often related to a specific event or to a certain time of the month. Pain (or cramping) that occurs only with menstrual periods may be ascribed to anything from normal ovulation to primary dysmenorrhea; on the other hand, it may be caused by secondary dysmenorrhea due to such conditions as endometriosis, adenomyosis, or pelvic inflammatory disease. When periodic pain occurs only at midcycle and is accompanied by a 2–3 day history of pelvic pressure and a clear, mucoid vaginal discharge, it is almost certainly due to ovulation *(i.e., mittelschmerz)*. When periodic pain occurs with intercourse (dyspareunia), it should be further determined whether it occurs on deep penetration or upon initial vaginal entry. **Vaginismus** usually occurs upon the initial entry of the penis into the vagina and has a strong psychological component, most likely representing a conditioned response to pain experienced at some earlier time, and as such, may be a defensive reaction. Women who habitually "tense up," making it difficult to perform a pelvic examination, should be questioned, with sensitivity, as to whether they have ever been raped or molested in the past. In addition, in patients who experience pain during intercourse because of minor gynecologic conditions such as cervicitis or vaginitis, a psychological response may develop sufficient to set up an involuntary vaginal introital or levator ani muscle contraction with subsequent episodes of coitus. While **deep dyspareunia is often due to organic pathology,** at times it may only be due to the deep thrusting of the penis against the cervix during intercourse, which may be painful for some women. You should advise the woman that closing her legs slightly during coitus may prevent this undue depth of penetration. Moreover, since the uterus rises in the pelvis and the vagina lengthens with sexual excitement, premature vaginal entry before the woman is sufficiently stimulated may cause a painful penile-cervical contact.

3) Continuous pain

Continuous pelvic pain (i.e., pain that has been present for more than three months) is often not truly continuous but occurs often enough and in a random enough fashion that it cannot be mistaken for periodic pain. **Continuous pain seems to be related to changes in the anatomic relationships of the pelvic tissues and to the amount of vascular congestion present.** *Adhesions* may occur between the ovaries and the bowel, which may lead to pelvic pain as bowel peristalsis occurs. Furthermore, adhesions may frequently trap gas in pockets of the large bowel at the flexure areas, due to a minor degree of obstruction, and allow distension of the gut, which may then result in pain. A history of a gradually developing pain toward the end of the day in a nervous woman who also smokes may indicate this diagnosis. An enlargement of the ovary with cystic changes, in which the ovary becomes distorted because it is encased in adhesions too tight to accommodate any increase in size, may produce pain. Adhesions secondary to *endometriosis* may also cause pain.

The **pelvic congestion syndrome (i.e., Taylor's syndrome)** may occur in a number of situations. **The Allen-Master's syndrome,** a form of the pelvic congestion syndrome, occurs in women who have had a traumatic or precipitate delivery of a large infant. Usually, the patient dates the onset of her symptoms from her delivery. The uterus is usually found to be retroverted, tender, and boggy, and at laparotomy, is found to be congested (i.e., bluish). There will

be **tears in the posterior leaf of the broad ligaments. In these patients, large varicosities are present in the rents of the posterior leaf of the broad ligament, and the infundibulopelvic ligaments will also be found to contain large varicosities.** With the repair of the tears, the uterus becomes anteverted, shrinks to a normal size, and turns pink, and the varicosities throughout the pelvis disappear. In patients in whom this diagnosis has been verified, a repair of the broad ligament tears usually produces complete relief of the pain. In those patients who do not desire continued fertility, a hysterectomy may be performed.

Continuous pelvic pain may occur in women who do not have a regular orgasmic release. **It is postulated that the pelvic congestion that occurs with sexual excitement requires an orgasm to relieve the congestion.** If a woman has frequent sexual excitement without having a climax, and is too fastidious to masturbate, pelvic pain may result.

The presence of continuous pelvic pain in patients who have a high degree of anxiety has also been thought to be due to pelvic vascular congestion. Psychological problems may produce a "pelvic migraine" picture clinically. **Some authors have identified myofascial "trigger points" in the pelvic tissues, that when injected with local anesthetic solution seems to result in the relief of pain.**

Whether most patients with the pelvic pain syndrome have their symptoms because they have psychologic problems, or whether they have the pain from other causes and then have the psychologic problems, is difficult to determine. **Certainly, these patients deserve to have a thorough psychologic evaluation.** This approach should not be presented to the patient in the sense that you think that she is "crazy," but rather it should be presented as part of the basic evaluation to determine if there are any other factors in her life that may be aggravating her pain.

Prolonged pelvic pain, either localized or generalized, should alert you to the fact that the patient might have a psychosomatic disorder. The psychodynamics of the patient's problem may be quite variable; however, they are often related to a **long-standing emotional problem.** The degree of severity of the symptoms that the patient experiences is often related to the amount of turmoil in her life at any given point in time. It is often helpful to explore the possibility that the patient's parents or her spouse may be *very critical of her.* **The patient is usually psychologically and emotionally immature, with a history of a chaotic home life as a child and as an adult. Depression is common in these patients.** The patient should be closely evaluated for any evidence of inappropriate behavior or abnormal thought content, since some of these patients may actually be psychotic.

Although there is a large psychologic component in many patients who have pelvic pain, as many as 83% may have pelvic pathology, most commonly pelvic adhesions, as the possible cause of their pelvic pain. Certainly, a laparoscopic evaluation should be performed in all patients with this complaint.

4) Diagnosis

The diagnosis of the chronic pelvic pain syndrome depends upon the history, the physical examination, the psychological assessment of the patient, and finally, the results of a laparoscopic evaluation of the pelvis for organic disease. Medical or psychological measures should be utilized initially, unless there is demonstrable organic pathology found in the physical examination. Obviously, if organic pathology has been found to be present, such as an ovarian mass, then the appropriate therapy should be carried out. Recently, **pelvic venography** has been utilized in patients with pelvic pain in an effort to identify varicosities of the ovarian veins. Tenderness over the course of the ovarian veins (i.e., lateral and inferior to the umbilicus) may be noted in these patients during an abdominal examination. In patients who have no obvious pathology, and in whom all other approaches, including medical therapy for pain relief, have been tried without effect, it is essential that you perform a laparoscopy to be certain that there are no surgically correctable organic lesions present.

b. Endometriosis/adenomyosis

Endometriosis may be defined as the presence of endometrial tissue in an ectopic location. When the endometrial tissue locally invades the myometrium from the endometrial surface, the condition is called internal endometriosis, or **adenomyosis.** When the endometrial tissue is found in other pelvic locations or is disseminated to other parts of the body, it is called external **endometriosis.**

1) Internal endometriosis (adenomyosis)

Endometrial tissue may either invade the myometrium from the endometrial surface in a diffuse manner **(adenomyosis)** or, more rarely, may produce a mass of endometrial tissue within the myometrium **(adenomyoma).**

In adenomyosis, the endometrium invades the myometrium by a direct downgrowth of the basalis layer of the endometrium, which may extend all the way to the serosal surface of the uterus. Like the basalis, the endometrium in the depths of the myometrium may be somewhat unresponsive to hormonal influences, although the effects of both estrogen (i.e., cystic hyperplasia) and progesterone (i.e., decidual changes of the stroma) may be seen. The responsiveness of any individual implant is probably related to the number of hormone receptors present. The diagnosis may be made on histologic examination by the identification of both glands and stroma at least 8 mm, or two low power fields, below the basalis layer, according to one strict criterion. Others have utilized a somewhat less strict criteria, which consists of finding glands and stroma at only one low power field below the junction of the myometrium and the endometrium (i.e., 2–3 mm).

The patient with adenomyosis is usually in her 40s or 50s and usually complains of **menorrhagia** and **dysmenorrhea** that has gradually developed over the past several years. On examination, the uterus will be symmetrically enlarged to the same size as in the 8th week of gestation and will be globular and softened. **If the patient is examined during a menstrual period, the uterus will usually be tender to palpation.** The diagnosis is based upon the clinical assessment of the patient and the pathologic examination of the uterus. In patients with severe, persistent dysmenorrhea and menorrhagia, a vaginal hysterectomy may be performed as definitive therapy.

2) External endometriosis

Perhaps as many as 5–15% of all premenopausal women have endometriosis. It has been noted that 8–10% of female first-degree relatives of these patients will also have endometriosis, which is probably handed down on the basis of a polygenic-multifactorial form of inheritance. Endometriosis seems to be increasing in frequency. It has been found to be present in a significant number of black and oriental

other factors
- pt never pregnant

women, contrary to previous opinion, which held that it was more common in caucasian women. Also, endometriosis has been found in teenagers, in spite of the fact that the peak incidence of the disease is in the fourth decade. It has been well recognized that pregnancy seems to decrease the incidence of the disease.

a) Theories of histogenesis

The classic theory of John A. Sampson, first promulgated in 1921, is still attractive and has stood the test of time. **This theory holds that endometriosis is caused by retrograde menstruation and subsequent bleeding from the fallopian tubes into the abdomen.** The desquamated endometrium is then implanted on the pelvic peritoneum and on other pelvic viscera to produce endometriosis. In support of this theory, blood has been observed to be flowing from the fallopian tubes during surgical procedures that were carried out at the time of menstruation. Moreover, desquamated cells from the endometrium have been shown to be capable of growth and development on the peritoneal surfaces. Endometriosis in other parts of the body (e.g., the umbilicus, or lung), however, cannot be readily explained by this hypothesis.

A second theory on the etiology of endometriosis was that of R. Meyer, who proposed that endometriosis develops as the result of a metaplastic change in the coelomic epithelium of the peritoneal cavity.

Finally, J. Halban suggested that endometriosis might be disseminated by means of the lymphatic and vascular system. This theory could explain the presence of endometriosis in the umbilicus and the presence of endometriosis in the forearm or thigh.

b) Clinical findings

Nearly 60% of patients with endometriosis have pelvic pain that is not related to just the menstrual period (i.e., dysmenorrhea). It may be unilateral or bilateral, and it is often accentuated by menstruation. *Dysmenorrhea* occurs in 28–63% of the patients with endometriosis. *Dyspareunia* is also common in these patients (12–27%), especially if the uterosacral ligaments and the cul-de-sac are involved. Low backache around the time of the menses is quite common (25–31%). In patients who have cyclic pelvic pain, endometriosis must be considered as a possible diagnosis. Catamenial hemoptysis may result from a metastatic pulmonary endometriotic implant. Periodic hematuria or rectal bleeding may also be due to endometriosis.

Infertility occurs in about 30% of patients with endometriosis. Often the fallopian tubes may be obstructed by adhesions, or the ovaries may be so involved with endometriotic scarring that ovulation, or ovum pickup by the ovarian fimbria, may be impeded. Theoretically at least, the retrograde peristalsis that occurs in the fallopian tubes might not only explain the development of endometriosis, but could also explain the associated infertility, since ovum transport might be adversely affected.

c) Diagnosis

The finding of nodules on the uterosacral ligaments, in association with a retroverted and somewhat fixed uterus, is highly suggestive of endometriosis. At the time of menstruation, the nodules may become quite tender. Occasionally, a small bluish cyst may be found on the cervix or in the vaginal fornix, which reveals endometriosis on biopsy. While the diagnosis of endometriosis may be strongly suspected if nodularity of the uterosacral ligaments or cul-de-sac thickening is found, final confirmation by means of laparoscopy is usually still required. At the time of surgery, endometriosis most commonly involves one or both ovaries (55%), the broad ligament (35%), the posterior cul-de-sac (34%), and the uterosacral ligaments (28%).

d) Staging

The variety and extent of the physical findings present in endometriosis has complicated any meaningful comparisons between one series of patients and another in terms of fertility, treatment regimens, or the alleviation of symptoms. In an effort to standardize these variables, the American Fertility Society has proposed a *staging scheme for endometriosis* (Table 14-2). The disease may be separated into mild, moderate, or severe stages, and scores may be assigned according to these stages.

e) Treatment

The mere presence of endometriosis is not necessarily an indication that treatment should be started. Indeed, severe symptoms may occur

with minimal disease, and minimal to no symptoms may occur with severe disease. In general, the severity of the patient's symptoms, her age, and her desire for further childbearing are all important considerations in the management of the individual patient. Any of three therapeutic approaches may be used in these patients: (1) observation, (2) the use of hormones, and (3) surgery.

(1) Observation. **Observation** is called for in patients who have minimal to no symptoms and who do not desire to improve their fertility. This approach is only recommended when there are no pelvic masses present on examination that could turn out to be ovarian neoplasms.

(2) Hormones. The purpose of **hormone treatment** is to suppress ovulation and menstruation. This could be accomplished either by a natural pregnancy or by the creation of a **pseudopregnancy** through the use of exogenously administered hormones. *Diethylstilbestrol,* 0.5 mg/day, may be administered for a few days and then increased slowly to as much as 100 mg/day, which will suppress menstruation for 3–6 months. This technique has not been very successful, however. Another technique utilizes *methyltestosterone,* 5–10 mg/day, to suppress menstruation. While this approach is successful in eliminating the symptoms in many patients, it carries a risk of inducing virilization at the higher dosage levels.

One of the most common hormonal approaches consists of administering *progestational agents,* such as medroxyprogesterone acetate (Depo-Provera, Provera, Curretab, Provera Dosepak), or norethynodrel with mestranol (Enovid). Birth control pills may also be used to suppress menstruation. The usual dose is doubled after one month and then increased as necessary thereafter to prevent breakthrough bleeding. The result of such treatment is a pseudopregnancy effect in which the endometrial implants undergo decidual changes. About 50% of patients experience an improvement of their symptoms or become pregnant following the cessation of the treatment; however, a recurrence of symptoms is common.

The treatment of choice for endometriosis currently involves the use of the drug danazol (Danoerine). Danazol, 200–800 mg b.i.d. or less, when administered for six months, is effective in relieving pain in 72–100% of patients, with an improvement in other symptoms occur-

ring in 85–95% of cases. A barrier form of contraception should be utilized during therapy, since if pregnancy should occur, the drug would have a masculinizing effect on the female fetus. **This agent has resulted in a 46% incidence of pregnancy (28–60%), after stopping the drug, although the recurrence rate may be of the order of 33%. This medication is expensive and has been reported to have side effects in up to 85% of patients.**

(3) Surgery. In patients who are over 40 years of age, in those who have a **severe** form of the disease, or in those who have adnexal masses, surgery should be carried out and a total abdominal hysterectomy and bilateral salpingo-oophorectomy performed. The use of replacement estrogen and progesterone should not be withheld, since the incidence of reactivation of the endometriosis in these patients is less than 5%.

Younger patients who have a **mild** form of the disease and are infertile may be candidates for **conservative surgery.** In these patients, laparotomy, with fulguration of minimal superficial implants in the cul-de-sac and on the other pelvic organs, resection of endometriomas, lysis of adhesions, and a uterine suspension should be carried out. A presacral neurectomy may be advisable if pelvic pain or dysmenorrhea are prominent symptoms. Following surgery, conception will occur in about 75% of the patients with mild disease, in 60% with moderate disease, and in 40% with severe disease. About 80% of the conceptions will occur within the first 18 months after surgery.

c. Uterine synechiae (Asherman's syndrome)

Destruction of the endometrium may result in scarring and the development of bands of scar tissue, or synechiae, within the uterine cavity. *This destruction may occur as a result of an overzealous curettage of the uterus following an abortion, or more commonly, after a curettage of a more advanced pregnancy, or in the postpartum period.* In rare cases, tuberculosis may cause uterine synechiae, and in some instances, the causes are unknown. Amenorrhea or oligomenorrhea, in association with infertility following a D&C, are the usual presenting complaints.

The treatment of Asherman's syndrome consists of

Text continues on p. 198

TABLE 14-2. The American Fertility Society revised classification of endometriosis

Patient's Name _____ Date _____

Stage I (Minimal) 1–5
Stage II (Mild) 6–15
Stage III (Moderate)16–40
Stage IV (Severe) >40
Total _____

Laparoscopy _____ Laparotomy _____ Photography _____
Recommended Treatment _____
_____
Prognosis _____

	ENDOMETRIOSIS	<1 cm	1–3 cm	>3 cm
PERITONEUM	Superficial	1	2	4
	Deep	2	4	6
OVARY	R Superficial	1	2	4
	Deep	4	16	20
	L Superficial	1	2	4
	Deep	4	16	20

	POSTERIOR CUL-DE-SAC OBLITERATION	Partial	Complete
		4	40

	ADHESIONS	<1/3 Enclosure	1/3–2/3 Enclosure	>2/3 Enclosure
OVARY	R Filmy	1	2	4
	Dense	4	8	16
	L Filmy	1	2	4
	Dense	4	8	16
TUBE	R Filmy	1	2	4
	Dense	4*	8*	16
	L Filmy	1	2	4
	Dense	4*	8*	16

*If the fimbriated end of the fallopian tube is completely closed, change the point assignment to 16.

Additional endometriosis: _____
_____
_____
_____

Associated pathology: _____
_____
_____
_____

To be used with normal
tubes and ovaries

L   R

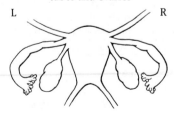

To be used with abnormal
tubes and/or ovaries

L   R

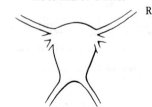

196

EXAMPLES & GUIDELINES

STAGE I (MINIMAL)

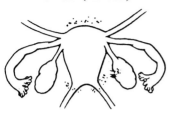

PERITONEUM
Superficial Endo	—	1-3 cm	2
R. OVARY			
Superficial Endo	—	<1 cm	1
Filmy Adhesions	—	<1/3	1
		TOTAL POINTS	4

STAGE II (MILD)

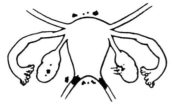

PERITONEUM
Deep Endo	—	>3 cm	6
R. OVARY			
Superficial Endo	—	<1 cm	1
Filmy Adhesions	—	<1/3	1
L. OVARY			
Superficial Endo	—	<1 cm	1
		TOTAL POINTS	9

STAGE III (MODERATE)

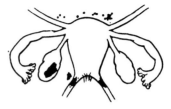

PERITONEUM
Deep Endo	—	>3 cm	6
CUL-DE-SAC			
Partial Obliteration			4
L. OVARY			
Deep Endo	—	1-3 cm	16
		TOTAL POINTS	26

STAGE III (MODERATE)

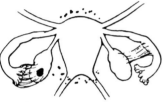

PERITONEUM
Superficial Endo	—	>3 cm	3
R. TUBE			
Filmy Adhesions	—	<1/3	1
R. OVARY			
Filmy Adhesions	—	<1/3	1
L. TUBE			
Dense Adhesions	—	<1/3	16*
L. OVARY			
Deep Endo	—	<1 cm	4
Deep Adhesion	—	<1/3	4
		TOTAL POINTS	29

STAGE IV (SEVERE)

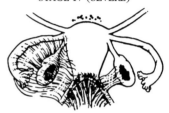

PERITONEUM
Superficial Endo	—	>3 cm	3
L. OVARY			
Deep Endo	—	1-3 cm	32**
Dense Adhesions	—	<1/3	8**
L. TUBE			
Dense Adhesions	—	<1/3	8**
		TOTAL POINTS	51

STAGE IV (SEVERE)

PERITONEUM
Deep Endo	—	>3 cm	6
CUL-DE-SAC			
Complete Obliteration			40
R. OVARY			
Deep Endo	—	1-3 cm	16
Dense Adhesions	—	<1/3	4
L. TUBE			
Dense Adhesions	—	>2/3	16
L. OVARY			
Deep Endo	—	1-3 cm	16
Dense Adhesions	—	>2/3	16
		TOTAL POINTS	114

*Point assignment charged to 16.
**Point assignment doubled.

Determination of the stage or degree of endometrial involvement is based on a weighted point system. Distribution of points has been arbitrarily determined and may require further revision or refinement as knowledge of the disease increases.

To ensure complete evaluation, inspection of the pelvis in a clockwise or counterclockwise fashion is encouraged. Number, size, and location of endometrial implants, plaques, endometriomas and/or adhesions are noted. For example, five separate 0.5 cm superficial implants on the peritoneum (2.5 cm total) would be assigned 2 points. (The surface of the uterus should be considered peritoneum.) The severity of the endometriosis or adhesions should be assigned the highest score only for peritoneum, ovary, tube, or cul-de-sac. For example, a 4 cm superficial and a 2 cm deep implant of the peritoneum should be given a score of 6 (not 7). A 4 cm deep endometrioma of the ovary associated with more than 3 cm of superficial disease should be scored 20 (not 24).

In those patients with only one adenexa, points applied to disease of the remaining tube and ovary should be multiplied by two. **Points assigned may be circled and totaled. Aggregation of points indicates stage of disease (minimal, mild, moderate, or severe).

The presence of endometriosis of the bowel, urinary tract, fallopian tube, vagina, cervix, skin etc., should be documented under "additional endometriosis." Other pathology such as tubal occlusion, leiomyomata, uterine anomaly, etc., should be documented under "associated pathology." All pathology should be depicted as specifically as possible on the sketch of pelvic organs, and means of observation (laparoscopy or laparotomy) should be noted.

Source: Fertility and Sterility 43 (1985), p. 351. Reprinted with permission from the publisher, The American Fertility Society, 2131 Magnolia Avenue, Suite 201, Birmingham, Alabama 35256.

dividing the synechiae, either by hysterography or by a D&C. Following surgery, the uterine cavity should be kept open by the placement of a pediatric Foley catheter for the first week. The patient should be treated with broad-spectrum antibiotics and placed on high doses of estrogens [e.g., conjugated estrogens, (Premarin), 10 mg p.o. daily for 21 days per month, with medroxyprogesterone acetate (Provera), 10 mg per day from day 15 to day 25 of the cycle]. Cyclic therapy with estrogens should be continued for six months to assist in reforming the endometrial lining of the uterus.

d. Endometrial hyperplasia

Endometrial hyperplasia may be classified as: (1) cystic hyperplasia, and (2) adenomatous hyperplasia. Cystic hyperplasia is often seen in patients who have anovulation and is therefore thought to be secondary to unopposed estrogen stimulation. While cystic hyperplasia frequently precedes adenomatous hyperplasia, it has a low malignant potential and is not thought to be a premalignant lesion. It has been estimated that less than 1% of patients with cystic hyperplasia will develop endometrial carcinoma. On histologic examination, *large, dilated endometrial glands,* which have been likened to Swiss cheese in appearance, are found to be present in a hyperplastic stroma. The stroma may appear as an endometrial polyp.

Adenomatous hyperplasia has been considered to be a premalignant lesion that may progress to atypical adenomatous hyperplasia, then to carcinoma-in-situ, and finally, to an invasive carcinoma. Adenomatous hyperplasia consists of many closely packed glands with a *minimal amount of intervening stroma.* This *"back-to-back" gland pattern* is characteristic of this lesion. The cells of the glands become more active and tend to pile up to form "tufting" within the glands. Atypical adenomatous hyperplasia includes all of the above findings, and in addition will have cells with a more anaplastic appearance and enlarged, vesicular, variable staining nuclei with prominent nucleoli. Adenocarcinoma of the endometrium may be only slightly more "atypical," with the loss of the polarity of the nuclei, the development of gland-in-gland formation, and lymphatic and vascular invasion.

Distinguishing between these lesions is difficult, and there is often major disagreement, even among very experienced pathologists, as to which lesion is hyperplasia and which is cancer. **It is thought that 20–25% of patients with adenomatous hyperplasia will ultimately develop endometrial carcinoma.** This incidence is doubled if the atypical hyperplasia is left untreated.

The treatment of a young woman with these lesions requires a D&C, followed by progesterone therapy to counteract the stimulating effects of the estrogens. Close follow-up, with repeated endometrial biopsies, should then be carried out to be certain that the lesion has regressed with the progesterone therapy. In the older patient with adenomatous hyperplasia, a hysterectomy and a bilateral salpingo-oophorectomy is the treatment of choice.

e. Endometrial polyps

Endometrial polyps have a highly vascular stromal core that is covered by endometrial tissue. They are usually finger-like tumors that project above the endometrial surface, are often multiple, and may grow to become rather large, fleshy, smooth, reddish-brown tumors. Examination may reveal ulceration of the distal tip of the polyp, with cystic hyperplasia of the glandular elements and squamous metaplasia of the overlying epithelium. If there are considerable amounts of smooth-muscle bundles present in the polyp, the diagnosis is that of a *pedunculated adenomyoma* instead of an endometrial polyp. The base may be small with a thin stalk, or it may be more sessile with a broad base. They may occur throughout the reproductive years, but are more common near menopause. The etiology of these tumors is unknown. *The malignant transformation of a polyp is rare.* While an endometrial polyp may prolapse through the cervix and be visible on pelvic examination, most of them do not. Usually, pre- or postmenstrual spotting occurs, or there may be a history of menorrhagia, which should alert you to the possibility of this diagnosis. Endometrial polyps may be diagnosed through the use of a hysterosalpingogram (HSG), and may be visualized and removed by means of a hysteroscopic instrument. Polyps are frequently missed with the curette knife; thus, in order to detect and remove them at the time of a D&C, it is necessary to thoroughly explore the uterine cavity with polyp forceps.

f. Leiomyomas

1) Incidence

Leiomyomas (fibroid, myoma, fibromyoma) are benign tumors primarily made up of _smooth muscle_ with some connective tissue. They may arise in any part of the body where there is smooth muscle. While these tumors are well circumscribed in the uterus, they do not have a true capsule; rather, they only condense and compress the surrounding tissues to produce a **pseudocapsule.** These tumors are the most common type involving the uterus and are probably present to some degree in nearly 40% of all women over the age of 40. They are two to five times more common in black and oriental women than in white women.

2) Pathogenesis

Leiomyomas are thought to be dependent upon estrogen secretion and thus tend to regress in the postmenopausal period. Further, during pregnancy, they are frequently stimulated to grow to a larger size and demonstrate degenerative changes, such as _red or carneous degeneration._ It has been demonstrated that many estrogen receptors are present in leiomyomas; a direct cause-and-effect relationship between estrogen and the development of leiomyomas, however, has not been demonstrated.

3) Location

These tumors are usually multiple and affect the uterine fundus (95%) more often than the cervix (5%). They may lie immediately beneath the endometrium _(submucosal),_ within the uterine wall _(intramural or interstitial),_ or beneath the serosa _(subserosal)_ (Fig. 14-1). If a leiomyoma extends between the leaves of the broad ligament, it is called an _intraligamentary leiomyoma._ Other subserosal leiomyomas may be _pedunculated_ on a long narrow stalk, or they may actually develop a blood supply from an adjacent organ and become completely detached, forming a _parasitic leiomyoma._ Submucosal pedunculated fibroids may occasionally prolapse through the cervix and deliver, and if the base is broad, then an _inversion of the uterus_ may occur. Due to the fact that a submucosal leiomyoma contains more muscular tissue than a subserosal leiomyoma, sarcomatous change is more common in the former.

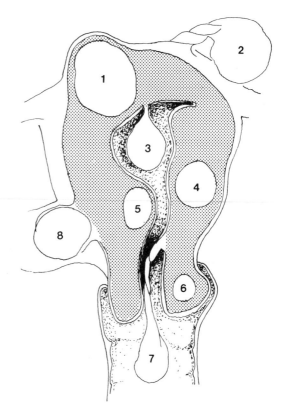

FIGURE 14-1. The possible sites of leiomyomas of the uterus. (1) A subserous leiomyoma. (2) Torsion of a pedunculated abdominal leiomyoma. (3) A pedunculated endometrial leiomyoma. (4) An intramural leiomyoma. (5) A submucosal leiomyoma. (6) A cervical leiomyoma. (7) Torsion of an endometrial leiomyoma that has prolapsed into the vagina. (8) An intraligamentous leiomyoma. Note the distortion of the endometrial cavity and the increased endometrial surface area.

4) Degenerative changes

On cross-section, the leiomyoma is firm and has a pinkish-white whorled appearance. _Hyaline degeneration is the most common degenerative process in leiomyomas (63%), followed by myxomatous degeneration (13%), and calcific degeneration (8%). Fatty degeneration and cystic or red (carneous) degeneration are less common. In about 0.01–0.5% of cases, sarcomatous degeneration may occur._ The number of mitotic figures present in a cellular leiomyoma is used to determine malignancy. _If there are less than 5_ *mitotic figures per 10 high power fields, the tumor will be benign. If the tumor has more than 10 mitotic figures per 10 high power fields, then it will be malignant.* Other histologic characteristics of note are nuclear hyperchromatism, nuclear pleomorphism, and other bizarre cellular shapes, including giant cells, in addition to the invasion of blood vessels.

5) Rare types of leiomyomas

a) Intravenous leiomyomas

The *intravenous leiomyoma* develops projections into the venous system of the uterus and the parametrial tissues, such as the broad ligaments. On occasion, this type of leiomyoma may progress up the inferior vena cava to the heart. It is unknown whether these lesions develop from a leiomyoma that invades the veins or whether they develop de novo from the walls of the parametrial and uterine veins.

b) Benign metastasizing leiomyomas

Nearly 24 cases have now been reported in which a *benign leiomyoma has metastasized* to other tissues, such as the periaortic lymph nodes, omentum, ovaries, or lungs.

c) Leiomyomatosis peritonealis disseminata

Leiomyomatosis peritonealis disseminata is a benign local dissemination of the leiomyoma to adjacent pelvic organs. It is usually either found in patients who were recently pregnant or were taking birth control pills. It is thought that these tumors may be derived from the smooth muscles of the blood vessels.

6) Signs and symptoms of leiomyomas

Many leiomyomas manifest no symptoms at all. Observation of those tumors that do not exceed 12 weeks' gestational size is all that is needed clinically, since the risk of sarcomatous degeneration is of the order of 0.1–0.5%. When the uterus is **larger than 12 weeks' gestational size,** the evaluation of the adnexal regions may become quite difficult, if not impossible. In such patients, the uterus should be removed, since its presence could obscure an ovarian neoplasm, which, if malignant, could jeopardize the life of the patient.

Probably less than 50% of patients with leiomyomas will have symptoms. In patients who have red or carneous degeneration, an infected leiomyoma, or a torsion of a pedunculated leiomyoma, then *fever and pain* may be prominent presenting symptoms. **Patients who become pregnant with a leiomyoma may have a higher incidence of red degeneration with pain, tenderness, and fever.** Usually, the patient's symptoms will gradually subside over a few days with supportive medical therapy.

In about 33% of patients, *abnormal uterine bleeding* (i.e., menorrhagia, or menometrorrhagia) will be present; this symptom is most common with the submucosal type of leiomyoma. A number of reasons have been advanced to explain the excess bleeding that occurs in association with leiomyomas. It has been demonstrated, for example, that the area of the normal uterine cavity (15 cm^2) may be increased to as much as 200 cm^2 by a leiomyoma that encroaches into the uterine cavity. **If the bleeding of menstruation is related to the amount of surface area of the uterine cavity, then this increase in size might account for the excess bleeding.** Another theory is that the presence of an intramural leiomyoma might **restrict uterine contractions** and thus interfere with the contraction of the spiral arteries in the basalar endometrium, which would allow for excessive bleeding. Finally, endometrial changes in the vicinity of the submucosal leiomyoma, such as atrophy, necrosis, or hyperplasia, might affect the amount of blood loss and thus allow for excessive bleeding.

Occasionally, pelvic *pressure symptoms* may occur in association with leiomyomas. If the bladder is compressed, such symptoms may consist of urinary frequency or chronic urinary tract obstruction. About 5% of leiomyomas are associated with ureteral compression or obstruction, with hydronephrosis.

Patients with uterine leiomyomas should be followed closely to determine any change in the size of the leiomyomas. The *rapid growth of a leiomyoma* in a premenopausal patient usually indicates that the patient is pregnant; however, in the postmenopausal patient, it generally signifies the presence of a malignancy.

Uterine leiomyomas have been thought to be responsible for an *increase in abortion.* Because of the space it occupies, the lesion may distort the uterine cavity; it may also cause alterations in the blood supply, or result in endometrial changes that interfere with the implantation of the fertilized ovum and with subsequent placental development. Torsion of a pedunculated leiomyoma is also more common in pregnancy than in nonpregnant women. Finally, large leiomyomas may not only cause a fetal malposition during pregnancy, but may also obstruct the inlet and interfere with the descent of the fetal presenting part (i.e., soft tissue dystocia).

7) Treatment

Myomectomy may be indicated in the patient who has repeated spontaneous abortions in the presence of one or more significant leiomyomas. While a myomectomy should generally not be performed because of infertility, some studies show that as many as 54% of these patients conceive following a myomectomy. Therefore, it would seem that in carefully selected cases, in which all other causes of infertility have been ruled out, such therapy may be of benefit. In the past, if the endometrial cavity was entered during the removal of the leiomyoma, then the uterus was considered to be scarred and therefore all subsequent pregnancies were delivered by cesarean section. In light of the newer concept of allowing vaginal deliveries following previous cesarean sections, this management approach may need to be revised.

The indications for hysterectomy in patients with leiomyomas are generally as follows: (1) the presence of significant leiomyomas associated with bleeding to the point of anemia, (2) the presence of leiomyomas of 12 weeks' gestational size or greater in which the pelvic structures cannot be adequately defined on pelvic examination, and (3) the rapid growth of a leiomyoma of any size. The ovaries should not necessarily be removed at the time of hysterectomy, unless there are other reasons for their removal.

If the patient has significant leiomyomas and/or bleeding problems and wishes to be **sterilized** (but does not meet the above criteria), a hysterectomy should be considered. Without these other considerations, hysterectomy should probably not be done for sterilization alone, since this operation carries significant morbidity and mortality rates. Some authors have suggested that when there are no clear-cut indications for performing a particular surgical procedure, but there are other associated diagnoses, none of which by themselves would be an indication for the surgery (i.e., the so-called **X factors**), then the combination of diagnoses may be sufficient to justify performance of the surgery. Caution should be exercised, however, whenever these X factors are added to the decision-making process.

Prior to performing a hysterectomy, it is essential to be certain that there is no other pathology present in the uterus. A *Papanicolaou smear* of the cervix, and perhaps a *multiple-sampling endometrial biopsy,* should be obtained to be sure that there is no evidence of carcinoma present. In patients over 40 years of age with a history of abnormal bleeding, a *fractional D&C* should be performed. On occasion, endometrial polyps will be found to be the cause of bleeding and not a leiomyoma. In other patients with an enlarged uterus (and a negative pregnancy test), an adenocarcinoma of the endometrium will be found at D&C.

g. Abnormalities of the uterus

1) Types of abnormalities

The incidence of uterine anomalies is about 0.13–0.4% of women who are in their childbearing years. The most common anomalies are due to an incomplete fusion of the müllerian ducts, accompanied by a failure of the intervening septum to be resorbed (Fig. 14-2). In cases involving complete nonfusion of the müllerian ducts, **uterus didelphys and a septate vagina** result. In this situation, there are two uterine horns, two uterine cervices, and two vaginas.

On occasion, one horn of the uterus (i.e., one müllerian duct) may fail to develop completely. When this situation occurs, a **rudimentary horn** results. This horn may or may not communicate with the other uterine horn (i.e., the uterine cavity). If there is a complete absence of one müllerian tube, a **uterus unicornis** results. When there is only a partial resorption of the intervening walls of the two müllerian ducts, a **uterus bicornis** results, with either one or two cervices, depending upon the amount of resorption of the uterine septa. The uterine **septus** and **subseptus** varieties occur when there is a variable resorption of the uterine septa. When there has been almost maximal resorption of the intervening septa, a heart-shaped, or **arcuate,** uterus is formed. Another type of abnormality is the **T-shaped** uterine cavity, which has been described in association with diethylstilbestrol exposure of the fetus prior to birth.

2) Diagnosis

The diagnosis of a uterus didelphys is usually made at the time of a speculum examination. If a vaginal septum is present, however, this type of defect may be

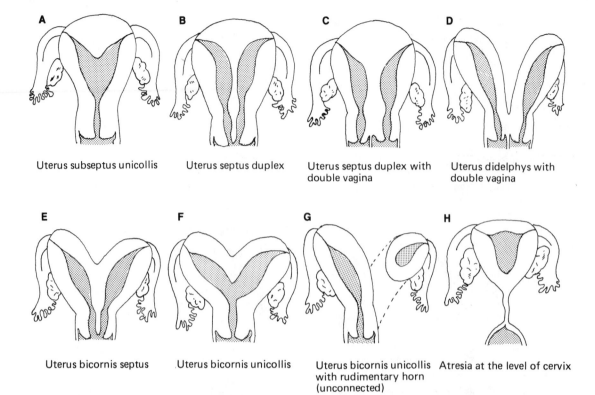

FIGURE 14-2. Schematic diagrams showing the various types of congenital abnormal uteri.

difficult to identify because the speculum may be alternatively placed in one or the other vagina without the septum being recognized. When there is no vaginal septum, it is obvious that two cervices are present. Lesser abnormalities may be diagnosed at the time of a D&C, or they may be detected with a hysterosalpingogram. During pregnancy, a heart-shaped uterus may be detected during the performance of Leopold's maneuvers. Direct observation of the uterine cavity with a hysteroscope, or of the uterus at the time of laparoscopy, may also lead to a diagnosis. Finally, the uterine septum may be demonstrated during manual uterine exploration at the time of delivery.

3) Clinical problems

Uterine anomalies may cause problems in the nonpregnant patient, such as amenorrhea, dysmenorrhea, and infertility. During pregnancy, however, patients with uterine anomalies have experienced first- and second-trimester fetal losses, preterm labor, fetal malpresentation, and retained products of conception. Generally, midtrimester fetal losses are more common in patients who have uterine abnormalities. In the postpartum period, retained placenta, hemorrhage, and subinvolution may occur. The septate or subseptate uterus seems to be associated with a poorer obstetric performance than the other abnormalities.

In 20% of patients who have unilateral renal agenesis, there is also a major genital anomaly present. In 10% of patients who have uterine abnormalities, renal abnormalities are present. Therefore, patients with uterine anomalies should also be investigated for **urinary tract anomalies.**

4) Treatment

The treatment of an abnormal uterus is dependent upon the fertility history of the patient. A rudimentary horn, along with its tube, should be excised. If the patient has difficulty with fertility, a **Tompkin's me-**

troplasty, using a sagittal incision, may be performed. The **Jones's metroplasty** involves the removal of a wedge of the septum. The **Strassmann's procedure** may also be used to unite the two halves of a uterus bicornis. About an 85% success rate for future pregnancies has been reported with each of these procedures.

3. Malignant conditions

a. Adenocarcinoma of the endometrium

1) Incidence

Endometrial adenocarcinoma occurs in about 1:1,000 postmenopausal women per year and is the fourth most common malignancy in the female, being exceeded only by carcinoma of the breast, the bowel, and the lung.

It has been found that the postmenopausal woman converts about 1% of the available androstenedione to estrone in the adipose tissue. This percentage of conversion increases in direct proportion to the individual's weight. The obese patient is at risk for hypertension and diabetes and may also be at an increased risk for the development of adenocarcinoma of the endometrium, presumably due to the increased levels of estrone.

In women who are receiving unopposed exogenous estrogen therapy in the postmenopausal period, the risk of developing endometrial carcinoma may be increased by as much as eight-fold over those who do not receive estrogens. The relationship of estrogens, especially when they are not opposed by progesterone, and the development of endometrial cancer would seem to be a strong one, although a true cause-and-effect relationship has not been proved. Patients with granulosa-cell tumors of the ovary, which secretes estrogens, have been shown to have a 3.5–27% risk of developing endometrial carcinoma. In contrast, endometrial carcinoma has never been found in patients with gonadal dysgenesis, a condition in which there is no estrogen secretion.

It is recommended that if estrogens are utilized in the postmenopausal patient (i.e., estrogen replacement therapy, or ERT), then they should be administered in a low dose, such as 0.625 mg/day of conjugated estrogen (Premarin), in an interrupted pattern (i.e., 25 out of each 30 days), and that a progestin (i.e.,
Provera, 10 mg/day) should be given from day 13 to day 25 of each month. This regimen should be used even in the absence of the uterus, since recent evidence has suggested that progestin therapy may also protect against the development of breast carcinoma.

2) Staging

The clinical staging of malignant disease is important from both a therapeutic and a prognostic viewpoint (Table 14-3). If it is diagnosed early and its histologic pattern is well differentiated, endometrial cancer has a relatively good prognosis. In general, about 20–25% of patients with endometrial cancer are diagnosed prior to the menopause, and it has been thought that these patients may have a more favorable prognosis than those who develop cancer in the postmenopausal period. Also, women who have a late-onset menopause seem to be at greater risk for developing endometrial carcinoma.

3) Histology

Carcinoma of the endometrium may have several histologic subtypes, such as: (1) an adenocarcinoma, (2) an adenoacanthoma, (3) an adenosquamous carcinoma, (4) a clear-cell carcinoma, or (5) a papillary carcinoma. The first three types together comprise about 92% of all endometrial epithelial malignancies, with the adenosquamous carcinoma occurring in less than 25% of the cases. In general, pure adenocarcinoma, adenoacanthoma (i.e., malignant glandular and benign squamous elements), and adenosquamous carcinoma (i.e., with both glandular and squamous elements being malignant) have essentially the same prognosis. The papillary carcinoma is usually much more aggressive and anaplastic than the other types, with a five-year survival rate of only 51%. **The five-year survival rates in patients who have the first three types of tumors are directly related to the degree of histologic differentiation of the tumor. The survival rates are 81% (grade 1), 74% (grade 2), and 50% (grade 3).**

The original Broder classification (1941) has since been changed and includes three grades: highly differentiated (grade 1), moderately well differentiated (grade 2), and poorly differentiated (grade 3). **The involvement of the lymph nodes is also related**

TABLE 14-3. Definitions of the clinical stages in carcinoma of the corpus uteri (Correlation of the FIGO, UICC and AJCC nomenclatures)

Classification	Description
Stage 0	Atypical endometrial hyperplasia. Carcinoma-in-situ. Histologic findings are suspicious of malignancy. Cases of Stage 0 should not be included in any therapeutic statistics.
Stage I	The carcinoma is confined to the corpus.
Ia	The length of the uterine cavity is 8 cm or less.
Ib	The length of the uterine cavity is more than 8 cm.
Stage II	The carcinoma has involved the corpus and the cervix, but has not extended outside the uterus.
Stage III	The carcinoma has extended outside the uterus, but not outside the true pelvis.
Stage IV	The carcinoma has extended outside the true pelvis, or has obviously involved the mucosa of the bladder or rectum. A bullous edema as such does not permit a case to be allotted to Stage IV.
IVa	Spread of the growth to adjacent organs as urinary bladder, rectum, sigmoid, or small bowel.
IVb	Spread to distant organs.

Histopathology—Degree of Differentiation

Cases of carcinoma of the corpus should be grouped with regard to the degree of differentiation of the adenocarcinoma as follows:

G1—Highly differentiated adenomatous carcinoma.
G2—Moderately differentiated adenomatous carcinoma with partly solid areas.
G3—Predominantly solid or entirely undifferentiated carcinoma.
GX—Grade not assessed.

Reproduced with permission from FIGO, *Annual Report on the Results of Treatment in Gynecological Cancer*, vol. 19, 1985.

to the grade of the tumor, and in one study was found to be 2.2% in grade 1, 11.4% in grade 2, and 26% in grade 3. **The depth of the tumor's invasion into the myometrium** is also an important prognostic factor. When the cervix is involved, the rich complex of lymphatics in the cardinal ligaments increases the involvement of the pelvic lymph nodes. The **usual lymphatic drainage** routes are: (1) by means of the paracervical and parametrial lymph channels to the internal iliac nodes, (2) via the ovarian nodes in the infundibulopelvic ligament superiorly to the para-aortic nodes, and (3) through the lymph nodes of the round ligament to the external iliac and femoral lymph nodes. The tumor may also be spread to distant organs by hematogenous means.

4) Diagnosis

The diagnosis of endometrial cancer is usually suggested by a history of abnormal bleeding in the peri- or postmenopausal woman. The Pap smear will only detect about 20–30% of endometrial carcinomas, so it should not be relied upon in the diagnosis of this disease. An endometrial multiple-sample biopsy is a better diagnostic modality; however, even this method is not as effective as a **fractional D&C.** By fractionating the procedure, endocervical tissue can be obtained separately from the endometrial tissue in order to detect whether there is any spread of the disease to the cervix. The depth of the endometrial cavity should also be noted. The endometrial tissue should be evaluated for progesterone receptors, since recurrent disease may respond to progesterone if high levels of progesterone tissue receptors are present. The use of the hysteroscope to define the extent of the disease and the cervical involvement has also been advocated by some authors.

5) Treatment

Depending upon (1) the depth of the uterine cavity, (2) the histologic grade of the tumor, (3) the extent of myometrial involvement, (4) the stage of the disease, and (5) whether the nodes are positive, the treatment profile may be modified to utilize surgery, intracavitary radiation, and/or external pelvic irradiation.

The basic treatment of carcinoma of the endometrium is total hysterectomy and bilateral salpingo-oophorectomy. About 48–72 hours prior to surgery, intracavitary or external irradiation may be instituted, since this procedure has been shown to decrease the incidence of central cuff recurrences from about 10% to less than 5%. The use of this combination of both surgery and irradiation is probably most significant in controlling the disease and improving the five-year survival rates when grade 3 lesions are present. **The overall five-year survival rate of patients with carcinoma of the endometrium in one FIGO study of 69 institutions was: stage I, 73.1%, stage II, 54.8%; stage III, 27.5%; and stage IV, 8.7%.**

Recurrent carcinoma may be treated with additional radiation; however, if radiation was used in the initial treatment, then the dosage must be restricted to a lesser amount. In patients with a high tumor level of progesterone receptors, progesterone may be used. Other chemotherapeutic agents, such as doxorubicin, melphalan, 5-fluorouracil, cyclophosphamide, and cisplatin, have been used with limited success in patients with poorly differentiated tumors.

b. Uterine sarcoma

One classification of uterine sarcomas defines the tumor by the cell type and the site of origin. Sarcoma of the uterus includes: (1) tumors of *myometrial origin* (i.e., sarcomatous degeneration of a leiomyoma, primary leiomyosarcoma, and intravenous leiomyomatosis), (2) tumors of *stromal origin* (i.e., stromatosis, stromal sarcoma), and (3) tumors of *mixed mesodermal origin* (i.e., hemangiopericytoma, leiomyomatosis peritonealis disseminata). The classification of uterine sarcomas by the Gynecologic Oncology Group lists: (1) leiomyosarcomas, (2) endometrial stromal sarcomas, (3) mixed homologous Müllerian sarcomas (e.g., carcinosarcoma), (4) mixed heterologous Müllerian sarcomas (e.g., mixed mesodermal sarcoma), and (5) other uterine sarcomas.

1) Myometrial sarcomas

It was previously believed that sarcoma of the myometrium most commonly arose in preexisting leiomyomas, since sarcomatous degeneration occurred in about 0.1–0.5% of all leiomyomas; however, recent studies indicate that mixed mesodermal sarcomas may be the origin of 40% of all sarcomas, in contrast to leiomyosarcomas, which account for only 16%.

Patients who have leiomyosarcomas have symptoms of bleeding in about 60% of the cases, abdominal pain in 50%, and genitourinary or gastrointestinal problems in about 30% of the cases. This type of tumor tends to occur at about the age of 50, but when it occurs at a younger age, the prognosis seems to be better. On occasion, *the tumor may prolapse through the cervix.* **It would appear then that those tumors with less than 5 mitoses per 10 high power fields are truly benign (group 1), whereas if the tumor is highly cellular with at least 10 mitoses per 10 high power fields (group 3), then it is usually highly malignant with a five-year survival rate of less than 20%. Tumors with between 5 and 10 mitoses per 10 high power fields (group 2), are prognostically indeterminant, unless atypicality is present, in which case they are considered to be malignant. A primary sarcoma** of the myometrium tends to metastasize early and carries a poor prognosis.

The treatment of myometrial sarcoma of the uterus consists of performing a total abdominal hysterectomy and a bilateral salpingo-oophorectomy. The overall five-year survival rate in patients with leiomyosarcomas is about 39%.

Intravenous leiomyomatosis is usually a benign proliferation of the tissue into the vascular channels. Although this condition would seem to increase the risk of thromboembolism, this apparently has not been a problem. These tumors tend to recur locally.

2) Stromal sarcomas

Endolymphatic stromal myosis is considered to be an adenomyosis-like lesion that consists of the stromal component without the glandular element. There are fewer than 10 mitoses per 10 high power fields present in this type of lesion. These rare tumors invade locally and may eventually metastasize to distant organs. While they have the histologic characteristics of malignant tumors, they are only considered to be low-grade malignancies. Treatment consists of total abdominal hysterectomy and bilateral salpingo-oophorectomy. If more than 50% of the myometrium is involved with the tumor, progestational steroids (megestrol 80 mg/day) should be administered. The 10-year survival rate is nearly 100%.

A true endometrial stromal sarcoma, although similar to endolymphatic stromal myosis, is usually a highly aggressive tumor with a poor prognosis. On histologic examination, these tumors contain more than 10 mitoses per 10 high power fields. A total abdominal hysterectomy and bilateral salpingo-oophorectomy is followed in most cases with chemotherapy. Radiation therapy has not improved survival.

3) Mixed mesodermal tumors

Mixed mesodermal tumors (mixed müllerian tumors) may develop after pelvic irradiation in 12–20% of patients. Patients with these tumors are usually postmenopausal and present with bleeding and abdominal discomfort. The tumors are highly anaplastic with bizarre nuclei. If they are homologous with stromal and epithelial elements, they are called carcinosarcomas, whereas if they are heterologous, then cartilage, bone, or skeletal muscle may be present. The prognosis is the same for homologous and heterologous sarcomas. **Fibrosarcomas, hemangiopericytomas,** and other bizarre uterine sarcomas are quite rare. They are usually moderately aggressive, and the treatment should be individualized.

In general, the treatment of uterine sarcoma involves the initial control of the acute vaginal bleeding and then definitive therapy of the disease. Since the hemorrhage from these tumors may be quite severe, consideration should be given to the use of irradiation (400–500 rads each day) over a 2–3 day period, embolization of the pelvic vessels, or hypogastric and uterine artery ligation. In high-grade malignant sarcomas, a simple hysterectomy and a bilateral salpingo-oophorectomy is advocated, owing to the early dissemination of the tumor locally as well as distally to other organs. In selective cases, pelvic and para-aortic lymphadenectomy may be performed. Chemotherapy with such agents as progesterone, or doxorubicin combined with vincristine or decarbazine (DTIC), have been used, but with variable and generally poor results. Radiation therapy has generally not been successful except for tumors localized to the pelvic region.

CHAPTER 15

Ovarian disease

. . . .

On Christmas morning, 1809, in Danville, Kentucky, Dr. Ephraim McDowell (1771–1830), assisted by his nephew and colleague, James McDowell, operated on Mrs. Jane Todd Crawford without anesthesia and removed an ovarian tumor that consisted of fifteen pounds of gelatinous material and seven pounds of ovarian sac. The patient survived and was sent home in 25 days. Dr. McDowell has been called the Father of Abdominal Surgery.

—D. R. Dunnihoo

. . . .

1. Benign ovarian lesions: general considerations

When the ovary is found to be enlarged on pelvic examination, it is important for you to define its size in centimeters, its consistency, and its location. You should keep in mind that the upper limits of the normal size of the ovary may be as large as 5 cm in diameter. *In a premenarcheal or postmenopausal woman, the ovaries should not be palpable at all on a bimanual pelvic examination. Thus, any ovarian enlargement in these patients should be considered abnormal.*

In a woman in the reproductive age group, the diagnosis of an ovarian enlargement is frequently a benign physiologic corpus luteum cyst. This type of functional cyst will usually disappear in about a month. Since women on birth control pills have their ovarian function already suppressed by the hormones, functional cysts should not occur. Consequently, it was previously thought that any ovarian masses that were found in such patients were presumably neoplastic and deserved further evaluation. While these statements were correct when high-dose oral contraceptives

were being used, they may not be true with the low-dose birth control pills, since functional cysts have been described in the ovaries of patients on triphasic pills.

Large ovarian cysts (i.e., more than 7 or 8 cm) also indicate the possibility that a true neoplastic cyst may be present. If the ovarian mass has a *palpable solid component,* the possibility of a malignancy must be strongly considered. If an ovarian mass is very large, if it *increases in size* during the observation period, or if it does not disappear after observation through one complete menstrual cycle, then a laparotomy is indicated.

2. Malignant ovarian lesions: general considerations

A woman has a 1.4% chance of developing carcinoma of the ovary during her lifetime. The American Cancer Society has estimated that in 1987 there will be 19,000 new cases of ovarian cancer and that as many as 11,700 women will die of this disease. Protective factors include: (1) multiparity, with more than five children and (2) the use of oral contraceptives for prolonged periods (i.e., more than five years). These factors remove the stimulation of FSH and LH on the ovary and perhaps prevent the formation of inclusion cysts and their subsequent transformation into a malignancy.

One author has suggested that there are three hereditary syndromes: (1) women who are at risk for the development of ovarian cancer only, (2) women who are at risk for the development of breast cancer as well as ovarian cancer, and (3) women with the cancer family syndrome who are at risk for the development of cancer of the colon, the ovary, and the uterine endometrium. Risk factors include: (1) a high-fat diet, which may double the risk, (2) environmental pollutants and chemicals, such as smoking, alcohol, and perhaps talc exposure, (3) a history of two first-degree relatives that have had cancer of the breast or ovary, and (4) a history of the patient having had cancer of the colon, breast, or endometrium.

Ovarian carcinoma is difficult to diagnose because of its intra-abdominal location. By the time it is palpable, it is often far advanced. The overall five-year survival rate is still only about 37%. The staging of an ovarian carcinoma is helpful in determining the patient's prognosis (Table 15-1).

The initial therapy for ovarian carcinoma involves determining the extent of the ovarian lesion. This step is accomplished by surgically exploring the abdomen and collecting peritoneal fluid or washings in order to detect the presence of tumor cells through cytologic examination of a **cell block.** At the time of the initial surgery, an attempt should be made to surgically remove as much of the tumor as possible. This is called **cytoreductive surgery, or a "debulking procedure."**

Following chemotherapy for ovarian cancer, a **second-look operation** is often performed after the treatment regimen has been completed in order to assess the results of the therapy, especially when toxic chemotherapeutic agents have been used, such as melphalan (Alkeran) and cis-platin. This second-look operation allows for a **restaging** procedure to be undertaken, which consists of the collection of peritoneal washings from each paracolic gutter for cytologic examination and a meticulous examination of the peritoneal surfaces of the abdominal and pelvic cavities.

Recently, **flow cytometry** and **the imaging cytometer** have been applied in second-look procedures. In the technique of *flow cytometry,* applied to peritoneal washings, the cells are labeled with a fluorescent stain and then passed through a light source that excites the labeled nuclei. These cells are then passed through a photomultiplier tube for the quantification of the emitted fluorescence. This method had a sensitivity of 84.5% and a specificity of 97% in one study. The *imaging cytometer* scans the specimen under the microscope and measures the DNA content. Both of these techniques analyze the amount of DNA present. The readout establishes whether the cells are euploid (normal) or aneuploid (dysplastic).

The abdominal organs should be palpated in a second-look operation and evaluated for the presence of tumors, and **multiple random biopsies** of the peritoneum should be obtained if there are no visible lesions. In general, representative biopsy specimens should be obtained from: (1) the cul-de-sac, (2) the lateral side walls, (3) the bladder surface, (4) the right and left inferior hemidiaphragm, (5) the residual omental tissue (i.e., the omentum is usually removed during the initial surgical procedure), (6) the left and right infundibulopelvic ligaments, (7) the left and right round ligaments, (8) the sigmoid peritoneum, (9) the vaginal cuff, (10) the large and small bowel serosa, (11) the large and small bowel mesentery, and (12) any suspicious pelvic or para-aortic lymph nodes. Silastic catheters may be left in place in the paracolic gutters if radioactive phosphate (^{32}P) is to be instilled postoperatively.

3. Benign adnexal problems

a. Functional cyst

1) Follicle cyst

Follicle cysts often occur when there has been a failure to ovulate. The cysts form when the atretic follicles fill with a clear, straw-colored fluid. These cysts are not uncommon in infancy and childhood, and they are usually less than 3 cm in size. No treatment is necessary since they disappear in a short time.

2) Corpus luteum cyst

Depending upon the amount of fluid or blood that accumulates in the follicle after ovulation, the ovary may increase in size up to 7–8 cm or more. The distension of the ovary by this accumulation of blood may cause lower abdominal discomfort in the patient. If the corpus luteum is defective and begins to fail in its production of progesterone, premature vaginal bleeding may occur. If the corpus luteum persists beyond its normal 14-day life span, then a triad of symptoms may occur, consisting of a period of amenorrhea, followed by vaginal bleeding and lower quadrant abdominal pain (i.e., **Halban's disease**), which may lead you to initially suspect that the patient may have an ectopic tubal pregnancy. **A culdocentesis may return a clear yellow or serosanguineous fluid, which is pathognomonic of a leaking corpus**

TABLE 15-1. FIGO clinical classification of carcinoma of the ovary (with 1987 revisions)

Stage I	Growth limited to the ovaries.
Ia	Growth limited to one ovary; no ascites. No tumor on the external surface; capsule intact.
Ib	Growth limited to both ovaries; no ascites. No tumor on the external surfaces; capsule intact.
Ic	Tumor either Stage Ia or Ib, but with tumor on the surface of one or both ovaries; or with capsule ruptured; or with ascites present containing malignant cells; or with positive peritoneal washings.
Stage II	Growth involving one or both ovaries with pelvic extension.
IIa	Extension and/or metastases to the uterus and/or tubes.
IIb	Extension to other pelvic tissues.
IIc	Tumor either Stage IIa or IIb, but with tumor on the surface of one or both ovaries; or with capsule(s) ruptured; or with ascites present containing malignant cells; or with positive peritoneal washings.
Stage III	Tumor involving one or both ovaries, with peritoneal implants outside the pelvis and/or positive retroperitoneal or inguinal nodes. Superficial liver metastasis equals Stage III. Tumor limited to the true pelvis but with histologically proven malignant extension to small bowel or omentum.
IIIa	Tumor grossly limited to the true pelvis, with negative nodes but with histologically confirmed microscopic seeding of abdominal peritoneal surfaces.
IIIb	Tumor of one or both ovaries with histologically confirmed implants of abdominal peritoneal surfaces, none exceeding 2 cm in diameter. Nodes are negative.
IIIc	Abdominal implants greater than 2 cm in diameter and/or positive retroperitoneal or inguinal nodes.
Stage IV	Growth involving one or both ovaries with distant metastases. If pleural effusion is present, there must be positive cytology to allot the case to Stage IV. Parenchymal liver metastases equals Stage IV.
Special category	Unexplored cases that are thought to be ovarian carcinoma.

Reprinted with permission from FIGO, *Annual Report on the Results of Treatment in Gynecological Cancer,* vol. 19, 1985. The recent changes in the FIGO staging are reprinted with permission from the American College of Obstetricians and Gynecologists, W. T. Creasman, "Changes in FIGO Staging," *Obstetrics and Gynecology* 70 (1987), p. 138.

luteum cyst. Such a finding, however, does not rule out the presence of a concomitant tubal pregnancy.

In the presence of a small ovarian cyst, if the beta-hCG is negative, then birth control pills may be utilized to suppress the FSH and LH support for the functional ovarian cyst, which will cause it to resolve over the course of one menstrual cycle. Indeed, mere observation throughout one cycle will often be sufficient, as this type of cyst often disappears in that time. If the cyst increases in size or does not disappear within one menstrual cycle, then the diagnosis of a neoplastic cyst of the ovary must be considered. In young girls, functional cysts and benign neoplastic tumors are common. An x-ray flat plate of the abdomen may detect a dermoid cyst (i.e., benign teratoma) by demonstrating the presence of a tooth. In older women, greater consideration should be given to the possibility that the mass may be malignant than in younger women.

b. Adnexal torsion

The first case of adnexal torsion, reported in 1890 by **J. Bland Sutton,** involved the torsion of a hydrosalpinx. Since then, well over 300 cases have been reported in the world literature, and there have probably been many others that have not been reported. There have been more than 15 cases of bilateral adnexal torsion reported.

There are many reasons for the development of adnexal torsion. Some of the factors that have been implicated as the cause of torsion in either pregnant or nonpregnant women are: (1) a spasm of the fallopian tube, (2) developmental abnormalities of the adnexa, such as an absent mesosalpinx or an excessively long tube, (3) excessive tortuosity of the veins of the fallopian tube, (4) enlargement of the fallopian tube, (5) enlargement of the ovary, (6) trauma, and (7) a tubal ligation.

When normal tubes and ovaries are involved in torsion, it has been postulated that tubal spasm may have been the inciting factor. Pelvic congestion, such as may be found during pregnancy, may cause an excessive tortuosity of the veins. The twisting or coiling effect of these vessels might be sufficient to cause a torsion of the tube. The loss of a stabilizing mesosalpinx, the presence of a very long tube, or the interruption of the tube by tubal ligation may allow the tube to rotate freely in any direction and lead to torsion. When there is an enlargement of either the tube or the ovary, a **pendulum-like** action may occur, which may lead to torsion. This pendulum-like effect is probably the most common etiology for this entity. Trauma or sudden changes in body motion may also cause torsion.

Interestingly, the direction of the rotation of the torsion often follows **Küstner's law,** which may be stated as follows: If the observer views the pelvis from the front, with the uterine end of the adnexal pedicle base pointing downward and away from the observer, then the patient's right adnexa will rotate in a clockwise direction and the left adnexa will rotate in a counterclockwise direction. The surgeon will generally view the pelvic contents from this perspective during surgery.

Adnexal torsion often presents with an abrupt onset of lower abdominal pain associated with nausea and vomiting and a low-grade fever. A tender mass may be palpable during the pelvic or abdominal examination. Significantly, the diagnosis of appendicitis or acute pelvic inflammatory disease (PID) is usually made. The diagnosis of adnexal torsion has been considered in only about one-third of the cases. *These patients quite frequently have had previous episodes of lower abdominal pain, which, in contrast to PID or appendicitis, may completely disappear overnight, only to recur again at a later time.*

The treatment of adnexal torsion consists of a laparotomy and the excision of the twisted adnexa, which is generally infarcted and necrotic. If an unduly mobile adnexa is present, a future occurrence of the same lesion on the other side may occur unless the adnexa is stabilized by a few well-placed sutures. Rarely, autoamputation of one or both adnexa may occur; in such cases, the stumps of the fallopian tubes will be found at the time of surgery as mute evidence of the event.

c. Polycystic ovary syndrome

1) Pathophysiology

The polycystic ovary syndrome (PCO), or the variant, Stein-Leventhal syndrome (SLS), was first described in 1935 as a syndrome of secondary oligomenorrhea, infertility, and obesity associated with bilaterally enlarged ovaries and anovulation. Hirsutism was later noted in up to 50% of the patients. **The cause of this syndrome is chronic anovulation in which the normal hormonal fluctuations that occur during the menstrual cycle have become static and enter a steady state (i.e., elevated LH and normal or low FSH).** In addition, the serum levels of testosterone, dehydroisoandrosterone (DHA), dehydroisoandrosterone sulfate (DHAS), androstenedione, and estrone are elevated. DHAS is produced by the adrenal gland, whereas DHA, testosterone, and androstenedione are secreted by the ovary. The conversion of androstenedione in the peripheral adipose tissue stroma to estrone accounts for the increased levels of estrone. The sex hormone–binding globulin (SHBG) is decreased by about 50% in these patients. The FSH level is decreased because of the increased amount of estrone secretion and the increased free estradiol that is present secondary to the decreased SHBG. As a consequence, these patients carry an increased risk of developing hyperplasia or adenocarcinoma of the endometrium owing to the unopposed estrogen stimulation of the endometrium.

The partial FSH suppression results in continued stimulation of the ovarian follicles, and these cystic follicles then increase in size and may have a life span that persists for several months, resulting in the **polycystic ovary syndrome.** Repeated episodes of follicular atresia and follicular cyst production maintain the ovary at its increased size.

In response to elevated LH secretion, the ovarian stroma is stimulated to produce androstenedione and testosterone. The theca cells in some cases are stimulated to produce a layer of **hyperthecosis around the follicles.** The increased circulating levels of androgen cause hirsutism and perpetuate the blockage of normal follicular development that is causing the anovulation.

In a recent study, hyperprolactinemia was noted in 45% of patients with polycystic ovary syndrome, and a relative deficiency in dopamine was postulated as the cause. The treatment of these patients with bromocriptine was effective in reestablishing menstruation and ovulation. It would appear that anovulation may have a number of different causes, any of which may result in polycystic ovary syndrome.

2) Therapy

If the patient wishes to become pregnant, then the therapy of the PCO syndrome should be directed at the induction of ovulation. **Clomiphene citrate (Clomid),** 50–100 mg each day for 5 days each cycle (from day 5 to day 9), may be administered to these patients in an effort to stimulate ovulation. GnRH, gonadotropins, and dexamethasone have been utilized successfully to induce ovulation. If pregnancy occurs after ovulation is induced, then there should be no further concern about the PCO syndrome. If pregnancy is not the goal, then the uninterrupted estrogenic stimulation of the breast and endometrium should be counteracted by the administration of a progestin. **Medroxyprogesterone acetate (Provera),**

10 mg/day, may be administered from day 13 to day 25 of each month to mature the endometrium and to counteract the unopposed estrogen stimulation. If menstruation occurs at the expected time each month (i.e., 3–5 days posttherapy), then there should be no real concern about the development of endometrial cancer; however, an initial endometrial biopsy and then later periodic endometrial sampling has been recommended in order to monitor the response of the endometrium. If hirsutism is of concern, then the administration of low-dose birth control pills will suppress the gonadotropins and decrease the production of androgens.

d. Theca lutein cysts

Theca lutein cysts may occur as the normal corpus luteum that is formed after ovulation, may be associated with a hydatidiform mole, or may occur after the administration of clomiphene citrate or chorionic gonadotropin for ovulation induction.

Following ovulation, the ovarian follicle fills with blood **(forming a corpus hemorrhagicum)** and the lining granulosa cells begin to produce progesterone. Under the continued tonic secretion of luteinizing hormone (LH), the corpus luteum lasts for about 9–11 days, after which its function begins to decline just prior to the next menstrual period, unless a pregnancy should intervene.

The **theca lutein cysts** that occur in association with a mole or ovulation induction medication are usually large bilateral cysts containing a clear straw-colored fluid. These tumors occur as the result of **hyperstimulation of the ovaries** due to high levels of hormones. If the ovaries are greatly enlarged, ascites and torsion of the adnexa may occur. Following the removal of the trophoblastic disease, these tumors disappear spontaneously. Cysts associated with ovulation induction will disappear after the medication has been discontinued.

e. Endometrioma

In the presence of endometriosis, the ovary may be involved with endometrial tissue in about 50% of cases, often bilaterally. This condition produces enlargement of the ovaries with a cystic structure that is filled with old, dark, hemolyzed blood. **These cysts have been called "chocolate cysts."** Due to the fact that these ovarian masses may become quite large, they are often confused with other ovarian neoplasms. Occasionally, these chocolate cysts will rupture, releasing the old blood into the peritoneal cavity, which will cause the development of a chemical peritonitis.

f. Parovarian cysts

The remnants of the wolffian duct lie within the broad ligament and are referred to as the epoophoron, or organ of Rosenmüller, and Gartner's duct. Small tubules (tubules of Kobelt) extend from the duct toward the hilum of the ovary and the fallopian tube. Cysts that arise in any of these ducts or tubules are called **parovarian cysts.** Although they may remain small, some of them may be as large as 8–12 cm in size. These benign, thin-walled cysts are filled with a clear liquid and have a lining consisting of a single layer of cuboidal epithelium. On pelvic examination, the presence of a fixed cystic mass that is contiguous with the uterus may alert you to the possible presence of a parovarian cyst. Surgical removal should be carried out.

4. Ovarian neoplasms derived from the coelomic epithelium

Ovarian tumors may be classified according to their tissue of origin (Table 15-2).

a. Ovarian inclusion cysts

These microscopic cystic lesions occur in older women and are due to the invagination of the coelomic epithelium of the ovarian surface, which then becomes sealed off to allow small cysts to form in the depths of the ovarian stroma. This remodeling of the convoluted surface of the ovary may also involve portions of the fallopian tube. These cysts are benign and generally are of no consequence clinically, unless metaplasia occurs, in which case they may become a serous, a mucinous, an endometrioid tumor, or a Brenner tumor.

b. Serous cystadenoma

Serous cystadenomas occur between the ages of 20 and 50 years. **These tumors are one of the most common types of benign epithelial tumors of**

TABLE 15-2. Classification of ovarian tumors

1. Ovarian tumor-like conditions
   a. Functional cyst
   b. Ovarian torsion
   c. Polycystic ovarian syndrome
   d. Theca-lutein cysts
   e. Endometrioma
   f. Paraovarian cysts
2. Ovarian neoplasms derived from the coelomic epithelium
   a. Germinal inclusion cysts
   b. Serous cystadenoma
   c. Serous carcinoma
   d. Cystadenofibroma
   e. Mucinous cystadenoma
   f. Mucinous carcinoma
   g. Endometrioid carcinoma
   h. Clear-cell carcinoma (mesonephroma)
   i. Brenner tumor
3. Neoplasms derived from germ cells
   a. Dysgerminoma
   b. Endodermal sinus tumor
   c. Benign cystic teratoma (dermoid cyst)
   d. Immature teratoma
   e. Embryonal carcinoma
   f. Choriocarcinoma
   g. Gonadoblastoma
4. Neoplasms derived from gonadal stroma
   a. Granulosa cell tumor
   b. Thecoma
   c. Fibroma
   d. Sertoli-Leydig cell tumors (androblastoma, arrhenoblastoma)
   e. Gynandroblastoma
   f. Lipid cell tumor
5. Neoplasms that are metastatic to the ovary
   a. Breast
   b. Intestine (Krukenberg tumors)

the ovary and are usually relatively large (i.e., 5 to 15 cm). Commonly, they are unilocular and filled with a straw-colored fluid, and 10–20% are bilateral. They are usually smooth and lobulated, but in 10–30% of cases, they have a few small papillary excrescences on their external surfaces. The presence of numerous papillary excrescences is suggestive of a malignant transformation, and the presence of hemorrhage within the cyst is also a sign of possible malignancy.

The lining cells of the cyst are usually cuboidal or columnar in type, and are usually only one cell in thickness. These cells may resemble those found in the fallopian tube. Both ciliated and nonciliated cells may be present. Calcareous deposits in the tissue, called *psammoma bodies (psammos*—G. "sand"), are the end result of the degeneration and calcification of the papillary implants. These deposits may be visible in an X-ray examination of the pelvis, appearing as many small calcified dots.

The treatment of a benign serous cystadenoma consists of a unilateral salpingo-oophorectomy, unless the patient is beyond the childbearing age, in which case a total abdominal hysterectomy and a bilateral salpingo-oophorectomy should be carried out.

c. Serous carcinoma

Serous carcinomas are much more common than mucinous carcinomas and also grow to a large size. **This type of tumor is a smooth, multiloculated, cystic mass, with some solid components, having papillary excrescences upon its surface.** Hemorrhage and necrosis may be present. Microscopically, the lining epithelium of the cyst may be stratified, with tufting and papillary overgrowth into the cystic spaces. This overgrowth sometimes fills these spaces completely, producing a solid-appearing mass of tissue. Invasion of the stroma may also be present. **Other characteristics include nuclear pleomorphism, atypicality, a piling up of the epithelial cells, and an increased number of mitotic figures. In about 60% of these cases, the tumor occurs bilaterally.**

The tumor is derived from the coelomic epithelium of the ovary and thus shares a common origin with the lining mesothelium of the peritoneal cavity, the endometrium of the uterus, the endocervix, and the fallopian tube. **The differentiation of the tumor (i.e., the histologic grade) is more important than the cell type in terms of prognosis. This guideline applies to all epithelial tumors.**

The treatment of a malignant serous carcinoma of the ovary consists of complete extirpation of the lesion by performing a total hysterectomy and bilateral salpingo-oophorectomy. In addition, an omentectomy is usually performed.

d. Cystadenofibroma

A variant of the serous cystadenoma is the cystadenofibroma, which is much less common than the former.

This type of tumor may be cystic and/or solid. It is greyish in color and contains many cystic and solid lobulated areas. A clear, straw-colored fluid is present in its many cysts. Histologically, the cut tissue shows whorls of fibrous connective tissue with cystic cavities that have the appearance of a serous cystadenoma. Treatment requires surgical removal of the tumor.

e. Mucinous cystadenoma

The mucinous cystadenoma is a benign ovarian tumor that is almost as common as the serous cystadenoma. **It may reach truly gigantic proportions; tumors measuring up to 50 cm and weighing as much as 200 pounds have been reported.** They are smooth, bluish, unilateral, multilocular cysts filled with a clear viscid fluid similar to the mucinous material that is produced by the intestinal mucosa. These tumors are rarely bilateral (5–7%), and they occur most commonly between the ages of 30 and 50. These tumors may arise from a teratoma (as a single remaining tissue) or may develop from the surface epithelium of the ovary.

Microscopically, the locules, or cysts, have a tall, columnar epithelium with a basally located nucleus ("picket-fence"), goblet cells, and a mucinous secretion. The cells resemble those of the endocervix or those of the intestinal lining mucosa. The stroma is usually scant.

In about 2–3% of patients with this condition, the tumor will either be found to be ruptured or it will rupture during the course of the resection. When this happens, the spilled material may stimulate the development of mucin-secreting cells in the peritoneal mesothelium to produce mucin. This complication is known as **pseudomyxoma peritonei.** If such spillage occurs during surgery, it has been suggested that the peritoneal cavity be flushed with 5% glucose in water or a 2–10% solution of dextran sulfate. The glucose solution should have a mucolytic effect and will allow the removal of the spilled or implanted material after an hour or so. Often, however, the mucinous material will eventually reaccumulate in the abdominal cavity. Although this condition is benign, it acts in a malignant manner and leads to emaciation and malnutrition in the patient. Chemotherapy may be required to control this problem.

The treatment of a mucinous cystadenoma of the ovary is unilateral oophorectomy, unless the other ovary is also involved or the patient is beyond 40 years of age, in which case a total abdominal hysterectomy and a bilateral salpingo-oophorectomy should be performed.

f. Mucinous carcinoma

Mucinous carcinomas of the ovary are epithelial tumors that are often quite large and are usually multilocular. The lining epithelium resembles the mucosa of the intestine. The treatment of these tumors consists of a hysterectomy, a bilateral salpingo-oophorectomy, and an omentectomy. The lymph node chains, the paracolic gutters, and the diaphragm should be thoroughly inspected for any evidence of advanced disease at the time of surgery. In tumors that have 2–5 mitoses per high power field, the five-year survival rate is about 50%. Chemotherapy or radiation may offer an additional treatment modality. **The tumor may secrete carcinoembryonic antigen (CEA); thus, testing for these secretions can be used as a marker in the follow-up care of the patient.**

g. Endometrioid carcinoma

It is thought that this type of malignant epithelial tumor of the ovary may be derived from metaplasia of the coelomic epithelium. This histogenetic concept would be compatible with the coelomic metaplasia theory for the development of endometriosis. **The fact that endometriosis is present in 28% of patients with endometrioid carcinoma** lends further support to this concept. **This tumor has also been associated with adenocarcinoma of the endometrium in 15–26% of cases, which poses a problem in determining the origin of the primary tumor.** There are three different possibilities: (1) an ovarian endometrioid carcinoma with metastases to the endometrium, (2) an adenocarcinoma of the endometrium with metastases to the ovary, or (3) two separate primaries, one in the ovary, and the other in the endometrium. The microscopic findings of an endometrioid carcinoma are similar to those of an adenocarcinoma of the endometrium, and the tumor is usually well differentiated. The treatment of an endometrioid carcinoma of the ovary consists of a hysterectomy and a bilateral salpingo-oophorectomy and omentectomy, with the removal of the tumor tissue. Chemotherapy with progesterone has been of benefit in those tumors that are well differentiated. Chemotherapy and radiation therapy have been used in the undifferentiated lesions. The five-year survival rate for patients with this tumor has been reported to be about 50–60%.

h. Clear-cell carcinoma (mesonephroma)

The clear-cell carcinoma of the ovary (previously known as a mesonephroma) is an epithelial tumor that is similar (if not the same) to the endometrioid carcinoma; however, in contrast, it is usually quite **undifferentiated** histologically. *It is seen in association with endometriosis and may arise from this lesion in 25% of the cases.* This highly malignant tumor has two basic patterns: **a solid clear-cell pattern,** and a **hobnail pattern.** *Hypercalcemia occurs in 30% of these patients.* The relatively good prognosis of these tumors is due to the fact that most patients present with stage I tumors.

i. Brenner tumor

While almost all Brenner tumors of the ovary are benign, solid epithelial tumors, malignant transformation has been reported in a few cases. These tumors have been noted in all age groups, but about 50% of them occur in the postmenopausal patient. *They are bilateral in about 6–13% of cases.* The size may vary from a microscopic tumor, which may be found incidentally in a histologic examination of the ovary, to ones as large as 30 cm. They are smooth, greyish-white, lobulated tumors, which on cut surface show a white, whorled appearance.

Microscopically, there is an abundance of fibrous connective tissue stroma with well-defined islands of epithelial cells. Histogenetically, these tumors have been variously thought to be derived from the granulosa cells (by **Fritz Brenner, who first described this tumor**), and then later from the Walthard's cell rests, and are now thought to be *derived from the surface epithelium of the ovary (since the Walthard's rests themselves are thought to be derived from the germinal epithelium).* Interestingly, **Meig's syndrome,** consisting of a hydrothorax and ascites, has been reported with Brenner tumors. The coexistence of mucinous cystadenomas with Brenner tumors would lend credence to their origin from the germinal epithelium of the ovary. Treatment consists of oophorectomy.

5. Neoplasms derived from germ cells

a. Dysgerminoma

This small (3–5 cm), solid, bosselated tumor *occurs bilaterally in 11–15%* of cases and is one of the most common types of germ-cell tumors. It may grow rapidly to a large size, which often results in hemorrhagic and central necrotic areas being present within the tumor. Histologically, it tends to reproduce the primitive gonad. There are nests of germ cells in bands of fibrous trabeculae, associated with lymphocytic infiltration and the formation of an occasional giant cell. Most of the patients with these tumors are young; some are asymptomatic while others have pain (50%) secondary to the rapid growth of the tumor with its accompanying hemorrhage and necrosis. On occasion, the tumor ruptures and causes intraperitoneal bleeding. In 3–5% of cases, the tumor is associated with a teratoma.

While unilateral salpingo-oophorectomy may be performed if there are no nodal metastases to either the pelvic or to the para-aortic nodes, and the tumor mass is less than 10 cm, *there is a propensity for this type of tumor to metastasize to the lymph nodes early.* Some studies have shown an overall five-year survival rate of 75–90%. These tumors are sensitive to aggressive chemotherapy, and an excellent five-year survival may be obtained with conservative surgery, appropriate staging with lymph node sampling, and chemotherapy. Radiation therapy can be used if chemotherapy fails.

b. Endodermal sinus tumor

The endodermal sinus tumor is a common germ-cell tumor of the ovary that is highly malignant. It occurs in young girls ages 17–24 and grows to a size of 15–30 cm. It is encapsulated, lobulated, and smooth, and on cut surface it appears tan-colored and variegated with cystic and other areas of extensive necrosis and hemorrhage. The other ovary is rarely involved.

This type of tumor is currently thought to derive from the cells that arose from the extraembryonic tissues, such as the yolk sac and the vitellus, which then migrated toward the caudal region in the embryonic stages to lie in the gonadal anlage. *The tumor produces alpha-fetoprotein (AFP).* Histologically, five different subtypes have been described: (1) reticular (most common), (2) festoon, (3) alveolar-glandular, (4) solid, and (5) polyvesicular vitelline.

The surgical removal of the tumor should be accomplished; however, there are frequently metastases to the lymph nodes and the liver, and thus, multiagent chemotherapy using such combinations as vincristine, actinomycin-D, and cyclophosphamide (VAC) and velban, bleomycin, and cis-platin (VBP) has achieved a much better survival rate. Alpha-fetoprotein levels can be monitored during the treatment period and in the follow-up care of the patient.

c. Benign cystic teratoma (dermoid cyst)

The mature teratoma or dermoid of the ovary is a very common type of germ-cell tumor. It is a benign, cystic tumor that occurs during the reproductive years. **The contents of the cyst resemble components of the skin and consist of balls of hair, clumps of squamous epithelium, an oily sebaceous material, and occasionally a piece of bone or a tooth.** *The incidence of malignancy is of the order of 1–2%.* These tumors should be removed to avoid torsion with infarction, as well as to avoid the risk of rupture with a resultant chemical peritonitis.

Often these tumors are found to be about 6–10 cm in size, and on a pelvic examination they tend to be located anteriorly in the pelvis. A flat plate x-ray of the abdomen may reveal a calcified mass that resembles a *tooth within the cyst.* In addition, there may be a *halo effect* within the cyst due to the sebaceous material within the tumor cavity. *About 5–10% of these tumors are bilateral.* The histologic findings consist of completely **mature elements** of mesodermal, endodermal, and especially, ectodermal tissues. On rare occasions, thyroid tissue may predominate, which suggests a **struma ovarii,** if it is metabolically active (i.e., about 10%).

The treatment involves the "shelling out" of the tumor (i.e., cystectomy) from the normal ovarian tissue. Although the thin shell of ovarian tissue that remains may appear to be insufficient, the careful placement of sutures to eliminate the dead space and to attain hemostasis will usually salvage the ovary. The opposite ovary should be palpated to detect the presence of another teratoma; however, it is not necessary to bivalve a normal-appearing opposite ovary to examine it, since this procedure may result in the development of adhesions and possible infertility.

d. Immature teratoma

Immature or malignant teratomas of the ovary, like most germ-cell tumors, are rarely bilateral. They contain one or more immature elements of mesoderm, endoderm, or ectoderm. **The immaturity and the quantity of the neuroepithelial component that is present is of prognostic significance.** Occasionally this tissue will mature in extragenital sites, and chemotherapy may prolong the survival time long enough for this maturation to occur.

These tumors are most commonly seen in young children. They show rapid growth, which often results in hemorrhage and central necrosis of the tumor. They are smooth and lobulated, and on cut surface show a grey to dark brown fleshy tissue with areas of necrosis and hemorrhage. Hair, cartilage, and bone may be present.

The treatment of a patient with an immature teratoma consists of a unilateral salpingo-oophorectomy followed by postoperative chemotherapy, since these tumors have generally been considered to be radioresistant. If the tumor is grade I, stage IA, then no adjuvant chemotherapy is necessary. Chemotherapy regimens using multiple agents, such as vinblastine, bleomycin, and cis-platin (VBP), or vincristine, actinomycin-D, and cyclophosphamide (VAC), have been administered for 12–24 months, usually followed by a second-look operation to determine the extent and histologic type of any residual disease. The patient's chance of survival is related to the histologic grade of the disease: 81% (grade 1), 60% (grade 2), and 30% (grade 3).

e. Embryonal carcinoma

This rare germ-cell tumor has been considered to be a stem-cell tumor from which other tumors, such as teratomas, endodermal sinus tumors, and choriocarcinomas, may develop. **This type of tumor produces both alpha-fetoprotein (AFP) and human chorionic gonadotropin (hCG).** It may develop into one of three histologic types: (1) embryonal, with teratomatous elements, (2) extraembryonal, with yolk sac or vitelline (endodermal sinus) elements, or (3) a choriocarcinoma. The tumor may grow to a large size (i.e., 5–25 cm), and it often contains areas of central necrosis and hemorrhage. In one-third of the cases, the tumor may even penetrate the capsule.

The treatment of an embryonal carcinoma consists of the surgical resection of the tumor followed by multiagent chemotherapy. If no residual tumor was left behind, then vincristine, actinomycin-D, and cyclophosphamide (VAC) may be utilized. In cases in which the tumor was incompletely resected, the combination of vinblastine, bleomycin, and cisplatin (VBP) has been used with success. *Para-aortic lymph node sampling is mandatory in all malignant germ-cell tumors because of their tendency to metastasize to the lymph nodes early in the course of the disease.* The levels of AFP and hCG should be monitored during the post-treatment period.

f. Choriocarcinoma

This rare type of tumor may occur as the result of trophoblastic disease or may be of germ cell derivation. On microscopic examination, sheets of cytotrophoblastic and syncytiotrophoblastic tissue can be seen. The serum levels of chorionic gonadotropin are elevated in these cases. When this tumor is primary and not of gestational origin, the prognosis is poor because it will fail to respond to chemotherapy and/or radiation therapy.

g. Gonadoblastoma

Most of these tumors are found in patients who have abnormal, or dysgenetic gonads. The most common karyotypes are 46,XY and 45,X/46,XY. While the patients may be phenotypically female in 80 percent of the cases, they will usually show evidence of masculinization. This tumor is composed of germ cells, sex cord elements, and stromal cells similar to lutein and Leydig cells. Usually the germ cells and Sertoli-Leydig or granulosa cells grow in well-demarcated groups or nests, which contain hyaline bodies much like the Call-Exner bodies. These nests of cells are surrounded by stromal cells of the Leydig or lutein type. These hyaline bodies may calcify. Treatment of these tumors requires removal of the dysgenetic gonad.

6. Neoplasms derived from gonadal stroma

a. Granulosa cell tumor

Granulosa cell tumors are derived from the stromal elements of the ovary. They are often

hormonally active and produce estrogens. If the tumor occurs prior to puberty, then the patient may present with precocious puberty. If the tumor occurs during the reproductive years, the patient will generally present with amenorrhea, since the persistent estrogenic stimulation leads to anovulation in 50% of the cases. Since about 66% of these tumors occur in the postmenopausal years, they are often associated with endometrial hyperplasia, or, in 5% of the cases, with adenocarcinoma of the endometrium. The usual presenting symptom in these patients is vaginal bleeding. These tumors utilize the delta (Δ)-5 pathway to produce estrogen instead of the normal delta (Δ)-4 pathway.

The granulosa cell tumor varies in size between 5 and 15 cm and may appear to be both cystic and solid, depending upon the amount of fibrous and cellular tissue present. *These tumors are unilateral in 92–97% of the cases.* **If rupture occurs, then in 10% of these patients intraperitoneal hemorrhage will occur. This is a complication to be avoided by examining the patient gently to prevent rupture.**

The microscopic examination of the granulosa cell tumor may show any of several patterns. The **microfollicular pattern** is the most distinctive, with its small cystic spaces that are filled with proteinaceous material and surrounded by granulosa cells with pale, grooved nuclei. These rosette-like structures have been called **Call-Exner bodies,** and they may be found in 50% of the tumors. The **macrofollicular pattern** consists of large cysts lined with granulosa cells and surrounded by theca cells. The other two patterns are the **trabecular** and the **insular** patterns, which are composed of ribbons or islands of granulosa cells in a fibromatous or thecomatous matrix.

The granulosa cell tumor is a low-grade malignancy that is marked by its long course, with recurrences developing as long as 15–20 years after the initial resection. The survival rate after 5 years has been reported to be 68–97%, after 10 years, 56–93%, and after 20 years, 50–60%. Older patients, those with large tumors, and those who show evidence of both local and remote disease appear to have the worst prognosis.

The treatment of choice for a patient with a granulosa cell tumor is a hysterectomy and a bilateral salpingo-oophorectomy, unless the patient has a unilateral, unruptured tumor and desires to bear children, in which case a unilateral salpingo-oophorectomy

may be performed. If rupture of the tumor has occurred, however, postoperative irradiation should be carried out. While the use of chemotherapy in the treatment of stromal tumors has been less effective than in the epithelial tumors of the ovary, the administration of more than one chemotherapeutic agent may be more effective.

b. Thecoma

Theca cell tumors of the ovary are benign, solid, stromal tumors that produce *estrogens.* They are most commonly seen in postmenopausal women who present with irregular bleeding that is secondary to adenomatous hyperplasia or adenocarcinoma of the endometrium. Microscopically, two histologic forms have been described: the **first type** is the most typical and consists of spindle-shaped cells with a vacuolated cytoplasm containing lipid material in a fibrous stroma; the **second** is the luteinized type, which is similar histologically to a fibroma except that luteinized cells are present. **The luteinized thecoma tends to occur at an earlier age and may secrete androgens in 25–50% of the cases.** Thecomas are usually unilateral. In the younger patient, since the incidence of malignancy is rare, a unilateral salpingo-oophorectomy is adequate; however, in the postmenopausal woman, a total hysterectomy and a bilateral salpingo-oophorectomy are preferred.

c. Fibroma

Fibromas are most commonly found in women over the age of 40. These tumors are solid and almost always unilateral. **There are two syndromes that have been identified with fibromas: (1) the Meig's syndrome, and (2) the basal-cell nevus syndrome.** Meig's syndrome consists of an ovarian fibroma in association with a pleural effusion and ascites. While the full syndrome occurs in only 1% of fibroma cases, ascites may be present in up to 15% of the cases. *The basal-cell nevus syndrome* is a hereditary condition that is transmitted as an autosomal dominant characteristic. It is characterized by the association of bilateral (rather than unilateral) ovarian fibromas with basal cell carcinomas and keratocysts of the jaw.

Fibromas of the ovary have a glistening, white appearance on cross-section, in contrast to thecomas, which usually have a golden yellow color due to the lipid content of the cells. In tumors that are quite cellular, the histologic finding of more than 4 mitotic figures per 10 high power fields indicates a fibrosarcoma rather than a fibroma. About 10% of fibromas have characteristics that are intermediate between a fibroma and a thecoma. The sclerosing form of fibroma, a benign, unilateral tumor that rarely has any endocrine activity, occurs in patients between 20 and 30 years old.

d. Sertoli-Leydig cell tumors

These rare stromal tumors of the ovary differentiate along male lines and contain Sertoli cells and/or Leydig cells. If germ cells are present, the diagnosis may actually be that of an intra-abdominal testis or a gonadoblastoma. "Arrhenoblastomas" or "androblastomas" are other terms that have been used for some of these poorly differentiated tumors. **They are more commonly found between ages 20 and 30, and about 50–80% of these tumors are associated with virilization due to the secretion of androstenedione and testosterone.** In the pure Sertoli tumor, estrogen may be secreted. The "folliculoma lipidique," a variant Sertoli cell tumor that contains a great amount of cellular lipid and variable amounts of Leydig cells, is also associated with estrogen secretion.

If the tumor is composed entirely of Leydig cells, then it is called a **hilar cell tumor,** and is considered a variant of the Sertoli-Leydig cell tumor. Well over 50 hilar cell tumors have been reported in the literature; however, fewer than this number have been noted to contain **Reinke crystalloids** in the cytoplasm of the cells, which are similar to the mature Leydig cell of the testes. **These tumors are about 3–5 cm in size, unilateral, reddish-brown in color, and are usually found in the hilus region of the ovary.** (Note: **Hilar cell hyperplasia** is said to be present when the hilar cell mass is not grossly visible.) Hilar cell tumors are associated with masculinization in most instances, but mild estrogenic effects have been noted in a few cases. The hilar cell tumor is of low malignant potential, with only one malignant tumor having been reported.

A variety of the Sertoli-Leydig cell tumors have been found with bizarre, poorly differentiated cells that may be *sarcomatoid* or even have a retiform pattern in which there is an attempt to simulate the rete testis. *Heterologous elements,* such as gastrointestinal epithelium, may also be present, which have led some authorities to believe that these tumors are teratomas.

While most Sertoli-Leydig tumors are benign (90%), it is not possible to predict their behavior from the tumor pattern or from the degree of differentiation. Those tumors that are intermediate or poorly differentiated have a malignancy rate of about 11%, with a mortality rate of about 3–34%. If heterologous elements are present, the prognosis in one series is very poor with a 70% mortality rate.

The treatment of a patient with a Sertoli-Leydig cell tumor consists of a hysterectomy and a bilateral salpingo-oophorectomy; however, due to the low incidence of bilaterality, a unilateral salpingo-oophorectomy may be done to preserve fertility in young patients. If there has been a rupture of the tumor, or if it has been incompletely resected, then postoperative irradiation should be considered.

e. Gynandroblastoma

When there are elements of granulosa cell tumors, as well as elements of an arrhenoblastoma, such as Leydig cells and tubules present, then the tumor has been called a gynandroblastoma. They may be clinically associated with either estrogenic or androgenic effects, and they have a low-grade malignancy rate. These tumors are exceedingly rare.

f. Lipid cell tumors

Lipid cell tumors include a type that resembles hilar cell tumors as well as stromal luteomas, masculinovoblastomas, and adrenal rest cell tumors. All of these tumors are unilateral, and histologically they have polygonal cells containing lipid. Those tumors that cannot be proven to be either a Leydig cell tumor, an adrenal rest cell tumor, or a stromal luteoma should be included in the lipid or lipoid cell tumor category. Leydig cell tumors may be diagnosed by the presence of cytoplasmic Reinke crystalloids.

Adrenal rest cell nests are found in the region of the broad ligament (mesovarium) in 25% of hysterectomy and bilateral salpingo-oophorectomy cases. The tumor cells usually have a clear cytoplasm and a vesiculated nucleus. These tumors produce androgens. The stromal luteoma arises within the ovarian stroma and consists of nests of lutein cells in the stroma. The lipid cell tumors are usually androgenic but occasionally may show estrogenic manifestations.

They are unilateral, and if they attain the size of 8 cm or more, then about 25% will be malignant.

7. Neoplasms that are metastatic to the ovary

a. Breast

In about 6–10% of the cases in which an ovarian carcinoma is found, the cancer will be noted to be metastatic from some other organ. One of the most common tumors to metastasize to the ovaries is carcinoma of the breast. Since these metastases are generally small, they are usually found incidentally during pathologic examination after the removal of the ovaries for other reasons.

b. Intestines

Metastatic tumors to the ovary from the stomach or intestines usually produce bilateral ovarian masses called **Krukenberg tumors.** These large, solid tumors are usually found to contain **signet ring cells** that are similar to those seen in the stomach, or they may have large ascini present, which are characteristic of intestinal carcinomas. Carcinoma of the endometrium may also metastasize to the ovary quite frequently, but it is often difficult to determine which tumor is the primary one (the ovary vs. the endometrium) (see "Endometrioid Tumor"). While the method of spread of a breast cancer or an intestinal cancer to the ovary is unknown, it is suspected that it occurs by means of the lymphatic channels.

CHAPTER 16

Breast disease

The art consists of three things—the disease, the patient, and the physician. The physician is the servant of the art, and the patient must combat the disease along with the physician.

—*Hippocrates (460–370 B.C.)**

1. Inflammatory breast disease

a. Puerperal mastitis

Puerperal mastitis occurs in about 2–3% of nursing mothers. During lactation, the breast may become infected by the entry of bacteria through cracks in the nipple. The systemic symptoms in these patients usually consist of chills, fever (102°–104° F), and a flu-like syndrome. **The infection causes local swelling, erythema, and increased heat over the infected portion of the breast, which, if untreated, may progress to the development of a frank abscess.** The most common organism involved is **Staphylococcus aureus;** however, β-hemolytic streptococci, Haemophilus influenzae, Haemophilus parainfluenzae, Klebsiella pneumoniae, and Escherichia coli have also been found in these infections. Simple breast engorgement will have no systemic or local findings other than swelling and tenderness. If the leukocyte count of the milk is less than 10^6/ml and the bacterial count is less than 10^3/ml, then the diagnosis is milk stasis. Hot compresses and manual or mechan-

ical pumping of the milk may give relief. If the bacterial count remains low and the leukocyte count of the milk increases to more than 10^6/ml, then there is about a 50% chance that clinical infectious mastitis may later develop.

Therapy for this infection consists of administering penicillin, 250 mg q.i.d. for seven days. If the patient is allergic to penicillin, then erythromycin, 250 mg q.i.d., should be used. The treatment of the penicillin-resistant staphylococci consists of the administration of dicloxacillin, 125–250 mg q.i.d. depending on the seriousness of the infection. If an abscess develops, then incision and drainage must be performed.

b. Periareolar mastitis

Inflammation may occur beneath the areola in nonlactating women. This condition is usually recurrent in nature and is caused by the periodic obstruction of the nipple ducts with squamous metaplasia and the accumulation of keratin, followed by the fistulous release of the material through the areolar margin. After the acute inflammation subsides, the involved duct should be excised.

2. Benign breast lesions

a. Fibrocystic disease

Nearly 50% of all women in the reproductive age group have been found to have fibrocystic disease of the breasts. Women with these lesions have multiple, painful masses in their breasts that become more symptomatic just prior to and during the menses. These lesions occur usually between 30 and 50 years of age and are rare in the postmenopausal

---

*Reprinted with permission from Encyclopaedia Britannica, Inc., *Great Books of the Western World,* vol. 10, "Hippocrates and Galen," Robert Maynard Hutchins, ed. Chicago: William Benton, Publisher, 1952, p. 46.

patient. **Estrogen is thought to be the etiologic factor in the development of this condition.** Fibrocystic dysplasia may consist of simple cysts, sclerosis, sclerosing adenosis, duct ectasia, or apocrine metaplasia, all of which have been considered to be proliferative lesions of the breast that are at a low risk for the development of carcinoma, whereas *hyperplastic lesions* of the ducts or of the lobular units, with or without atypia, are thought to carry a higher risk for the development of breast carcinoma.

The theory that **methylxanthines stimulate the release of catecholamines,** which then stimulate the cyclic adenosine monophosphate (cAMP) in the breast, may perhaps be correct, since 82.5% of the patients in one study had a complete remission of their symptoms when coffee, tea, and chocolate were eliminated from their diets.

b. Fibroadenoma

A fibroadenoma of the breast is a slow-growing, well-defined, rubbery, mobile, benign tumor that is commonly found in patients who are about 20–30 years of age. The tumor may remain the same size for many years, or it may be stimulated by the hormonal changes during the menstrual cycle, or it may be stimulated by pregnancy to grow to a considerable size. In about 10–15% of women, there may be multiple tumors in both breasts. The removal of the tumor through a circumareolar incision is the treatment of choice.

c. Intraductal papilloma

The intraductal papilloma is a benign tumor that occurs in women who are in their late forties and usually presents with a bloody brownish or greenish nipple discharge. The tumor is slow growing and is generally only 3–4 mm in size, so it is usually not palpable. Cytologic examination of the nipple discharge should be performed to rule out cancer. Local excision of the tumor is the treatment of choice.

d. Lipoma

The most common type of breast lesion is the benign lipoma, a fatty tumor that grows slowly, is encapsulated, and has a soft consistency. The treatment consists of excision.

e. Duct ectasia

An obstruction of the terminal collecting ducts of the breast will cause dilatation of the duct, which then fills with material. The local inflammation that occurs will result in fibrosis and scarring.

f. Fat necrosis

Trauma to the breast may cause fat necrosis. In these cases, the release of fatty acids into the surrounding breast tissue causes an inflammatory response, which then results in fibrosis and calcification.

g. Mondor's disease

Mondor's disease is a benign disease that may be confused with an infiltrating carcinoma of the breast. It is secondary to thrombosis of the thoracoepigastric vein, which may traverse across the breast or laterally into the axilla. A tender fibrotic cord may be felt that attaches itself to the skin to produce a puckering. It is a self-limited condition.

3. Malignant breast lesions

a. High risk factors

1) Incidence

The incidence of breast carcinoma in the United States is about 1:11 women. About 130,000 new cases of breast cancer are reported each year, along with about 40,000 deaths. Furthermore, it has been suggested that there is probably a significant breast lesion in about 1:100 pregnant women. A high index of suspicion is necessary in order to make an early diagnosis and institute adequate treatment of this disease. There are certain historical findings that indicate whether a woman may have an increased risk of developing breast cancer.

2) Risk factors

There is an increased incidence of breast cancer in association with **meat consumption,** and in those countries in which meat is seldom eaten, the incidence of breast cancer has been found to be low. **The total fat intake, especially of polyunsaturated fat,** may also be a factor. There is a **strong associa-**

tion between the patient's weight and the development of breast cancer after the age of 50. If a patient's weight exceeds 60–70 kg, then the risk of developing breast cancer increases by 80%. Recently, alcohol ingestion has also been linked to an increased incidence of breast carcinoma; however, the evidence is tenuous at this time. Women who go through menopause after the age of 55 have twice the risk of developing breast carcinoma than those women who enter menopause before the age of 45. Thus, risk of developing breast cancer seems to be related to the total number of years of menstrual activity and perhaps the duration of estrogen exposure. Probably one of the most significant factors is a history of having had a previous cancer in one breast. In this situation, there is a 8–15% chance that a cancer will develop in the remaining breast. This risk increases by about 1% per year thereafter, so if a woman has a breast cancer in one breast at an early age, her risk could become substantial for the development of cancer in the other breast as she gets older.

Breast cancer in a family member may double or triple a woman's risk of dying from breast cancer. This risk may increase to more than eightfold if the disease was bilateral and occurred prior to the age of 50. No recognizable pattern of inheritance has been found in these families; however, since these patients tend to live in the same areas, there may be an environmental or infectious etiology involved. The B-type RNA virus particle has been found in the milk of some of these patients.

There is a high risk of developing breast cancer in women who begin menarche at an earlier than average age. Since the breast tissue develops with menarche, secondary to estrogen stimulation, the additional length of estrogen exposure might explain this increased risk of developing breast cancer. The incidence of breast carcinoma increases up to the age of 40, after which it levels off with only a gradual increase thereafter into old age. While it was once thought that there was a decreased risk of breast cancer associated with increasing parity, and that nulliparous women had an increased risk, this has not been proven to be true. The woman who has had her first child under the age of 20 has about a 50% lower risk of eventually developing breast carcinoma than the nulliparous woman.

There has been some interest in the association of anovulation with breast cancer. *Recent evidence indicates that the use of exogenous progesterone in post-menopausal women may be protective against the development of breast carcinoma.* Elevated prolactin levels have been found in the daughters of patients with breast carcinoma; however, these data are conflicting. Certainly, elevated levels of estrogen do seem to increase the risk of developing breast cancer; however, it is possible that estrogen may merely play a permissive or preparatory role in this disease.

The risk of breast carcinoma in patients with fibrocystic disease and fibroadenomas of the breast was thought to be significant in the past; however, it is currently believed that these conditions probably do not predispose the woman to breast carcinoma unless there are hyperplastic or atypical changes present histologically.

b. Types of carcinoma

About 90% of breast carcinomas are first detected by the patient, who has usually found a lump in the upper, outer quadrant of her breast. Nearly 80% of these lesions will have no evidence of metastatic disease. An infiltrating ductal carcinoma is the most common type of breast carcinoma, since it is present in 80% of the cases. These breast tumors include: (1) the papillary carcinoma, (2) the colloid carcinoma, (3) the medullary carcinoma, and (4) the intraductal carcinoma. The remaining 20% of cases of breast carcinoma include: (1) the lobular carcinoma, (2) the sweat gland carcinoma, (3) the tubular carcinoma, (4) the sarcoma, and (5) the lymphoma. The stage of a breast tumor should be determined since the staging has considerable significance in terms of the patient's long-term prognosis (Fig. 16-1). The percentage of patients with disseminated disease who survive even five years is less than 10%, as opposed to about an 85% survival in those who have localized disease.

c. Diagnostic techniques

1) Diagnosis

The optimum time to examine the breasts is during the days immediately following menstruation, since during the latter half of the menstrual cycle an increasing amount of engorgement develops that precludes

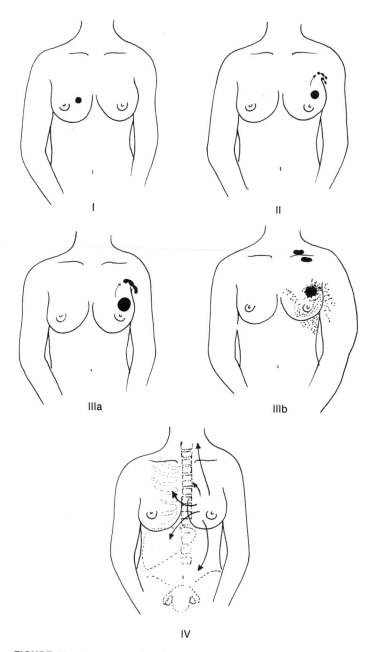

FIGURE 16-1. Schematic classification of the stages of breast carcinoma. Breast carcinoma has been divided into four clinical stages by The International Union Against Cancer and The American Joint Committee on Cancer. Stage I—Tumors less than 2.0 cm in diameter that are confined to breast. Stage II—Tumors of less than 5 cm, or smaller tumors with small, mobile axillary lymph nodes. Stage IIIa—Tumors greater than 5 cm, or tumors with enlarged, axillary lymph nodes fixed to one another or adjacent tissues. Stage IIIb—More advanced lesions with satellite nodules, fixation to the skin or chest wall, ulceration, edema, or with clinically apparent supraclavicular or infraclavicular nodal involvement. Stage IV—All tumors with distant metastases. (Adapted from D. N. Danforth and J. R. Scott, eds., *Obstetrics and Gynecology,* 5th ed. Philadelphia: J. B. Lippincott Company, 1986, p. 1172.)

an adequate examination. Once a breast mass has been found, its size, shape, consistency, location, and mobility should be carefully defined. Cystic lesions and fibroadenomas tend to be well defined and mobile, whereas cancer is usually fixed with ill-defined borders. The axillary and supraclavicular nodal areas should also be examined for suspicious lymph nodes. **Monthly breast self-examinations should be carried out by the patient from the age of 20 onward** (Fig. 16-2). **Between 20 and 40 years of age, a breast examination should be performed by a physician every three years, while after 40 years of age, the physician's examination should be done every year.** Many physicians make a point to include the breast examination on every annual routine Pap smear evaluation of their patients.

2) Needle aspiration

Simple cysts of the breasts may be diagnosed and treated by needle aspiration. If the cyst contents are greenish, with or without a brownish tinge, and the cyst collapses completely, then the cyst is probably benign. Confirmation can be obtained by submitting the cyst's contents to the laboratory for cytologic examination. The patient should return in two weeks, at which time the cystic mass should not be palpable and the pathology report should show no evidence of cancer. If the mass does not initially collapse, if it is solid, or if it recurs, then an excisional biopsy should be carried out. An intracystic neoplasm may be detected by performing a pneumocystogram after removal of the cystic fluid.

3) Breast biopsy

If a breast mass is to be excised, a *circumareolar incision* should be utilized whenever possible so as to provide for a good cosmetic result. In order to locate very small lesions, hookwires are usually inserted into the lesion under ultrasonic control prior to surgery to provide a guide for the surgeon. An open biopsy of a breast lesion of about 4 cm or less, under general anesthesia, should attempt to encompass the margins of the tumor. If a frozen section reveals cancer, then an axillary resection may be performed. Such tumors should be tested for the *presence of estrogen and progesterone receptors.*

4) Mammography

Mammography is a valuable tool in detecting early breast cancer. Indeed, it may uncover a malignant neoplasm that is asymptomatic and nonpalpable. As a consequence, mammography has assumed an important place in the management of patients with breast lesions and in the evaluation of patients who are at high risk for developing breast carcinoma. **The American Cancer Society has recommended that any asymptomatic woman over 35 years of age should have at least one mammogram initially, then have mammograms every one or two years between the ages of 40 and 49 and have annual mammograms thereafter beyond the age of 50.**

A malignant breast tumor will usually cause a distortion of the normal trabecular pattern of the breast on a mammogram and will generally have an irregular and ill-defined border that is characteristic of an infiltrative mass. The classic mammographic finding of a three-dimensional density with radiating spicules is almost diagnostic for breast cancer, with a 99% accuracy rate. *Fine groups of calcifications due to the calcification of necrotic intraductal material are present in about 30% of cases* (Fig. 16-3). These clustered microcalcifications may occur at a very early stage of breast cancer, even before a mass can be demonstrated, and they usually presage an early lesion and a good prognosis with no nodal metastases.

The mammogram has an estimated accuracy rate of 65–95%, varying according to the architecture of the breast and the experience of the operator. Certainly, the clinical detection of a palpable mass takes precedence over a negative mammogram; however, this type of conflicting data occurs only rarely (9%). Usually, the mammogram provides a more precise diagnosis of the exact pathology than clinical detection. Improvements in mammography techniques have included the use of xeromammography, which has good imaging with the new film techniques. The film/screen technique is commonly used today and results in approximately 160 millirads average absorbed dose to the patient.

Early detection is essential if the ravages of this disease are to be avoided. The average doubling time of breast carcinoma cells has been estimated at between 100 and 180 days. Thus, it would take about 20 doubling times to produce a tumor about 1 mm in size

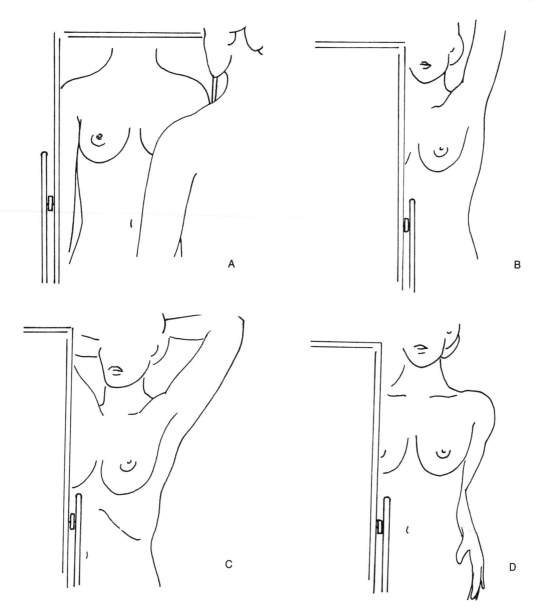

FIGURE 16-2. Breast self-examination. (A) Inspection in front of mirror. Look for dimples or retraction of the skin overlying the breasts. (B) Inspect with arms above head. (C) Pressure at the back of the head to tense the pectoralis major and underlying tissues. (D) Thumbs forward, hands on the hips, tense pectoralis major muscles by throwing back shoulders and elbows. (E) Examine breasts with the flats of the fingers in the shower using soapy water, and again while lying supine, in a methodical four-quadrant approach to the palpation of the breasts and beneath the nipples. Be sure to squeeze the nipples and attempt to express any secretion that may be present.

(continued)

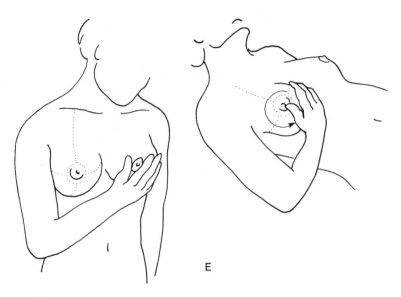

E

FIGURE 16-2. *(continued)*

(containing 1 million cells). A tumor would have to grow for more than five years before it would reach a size that could be detected on a mammogram. In order to reach the threshold of clinical detection, the tumor would have to have been present for about 8–9 years. The concept of "early" detection of breast cancer is therefore not very "early" in the true sense of the word. **If there is no nodal involvement, the five-year survival rate is about 85%; however, this rate decreases to about 65% when the nodes are involved.**

5) Clinical findings and the mammogram

The breast is made up of glandular, fibrous, and fatty elements that are in a state of dynamic flux according to the hormonal milieu. Nulliparous patients tend to have dense breast tissue that is primarily made up of glandular and fibrous tissue elements, whereas in the postmenopausal patient, the breast tissue mainly consists of a fatty component; however, these findings are highly variable from one patient to another. **The correlation of the clinical findings with the appearance of the breast on a mammogram has proven to be the most accurate approach to the diagnosis of breast lesions.** A palpable, firm mass (e.g.,

a fibroadenoma) without signs of skin retraction, skin thickening, nipple retraction, or increased vascularity may show dense calcification on the mammogram, which is indicative of a benign lesion. On the other hand, a mammogram may not initially detect a duct ectasia or a papilloma in a patient with a nipple discharge. In these cases, with the instillation of a radiopaque dye into the involved duct (i.e., ductogram), filling defects may be readily apparent on *contrast mammography*.

6) Thermography

Thermography (i.e., heat detection) in the past was advocated as a screening device for carcinoma of the breast because cancer usually is associated with an increased amount of heat in the tissues, an effect probably due to the increased metabolism of the tumor tissue. It has been found that some cancers that are "cold" on the thermogram have a better prognosis than the "hot" ones. The accuracy of thermography, however, is poor compared to mammography, and the thermogram is normal in as many as 25% of patients who have a proven breast cancer. Currently, the use of thermography is being condemned as a screening technique for breast cancer.

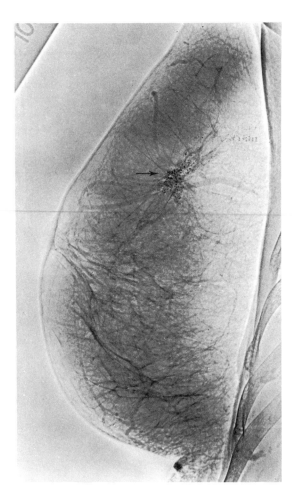

FIGURE 16-3. Xeromammogram shows malignant calcification in carcinoma of the breast. Calcified carcinoma (arrow) can be seen in upper part of breast. Malignant calcification is typically very fine and may be much more difficult to see than in this example. (Reprinted with permission from D. N. Danforth and J. R. Scott, eds., *Obstetrics and Gynecology,* 5th ed., Philadelphia: J. B. Lippincott Company, 1986, p. 1193.)

7) Adjunctive tests

If cancer is diagnosed, then a chest film and routine blood studies should be obtained. In patients with advanced disease (stage II), a metastatic bone survey with selective tomograms may be necessary, since about 20% of these patients will have lung involvement and 25% will have skeletal metastases.

4. Recent changes in surgical therapy

In recent years, the surgical treatment of breast cancer has undergone considerable changes. There still remains much controversy over whether a radical mastectomy, a modified radical mastectomy, or a local excision of the tumor (i.e., "lumpectomy") should be utilized. **Dr. William Halsted** first described the **radical mastectomy** for the treatment of breast cancer in 1894. This procedure included the removal of the breast, the underlying pectoralis major and minor muscles, and the nodal contents of the axillae. Recent evidence indicates that **conservative surgery** in the treatment of breast cancer is equally effective and is much less disfiguring than radical surgery. This procedure consists of the removal of the breast and axillary nodal tissue with the preservation of the pectoralis muscles. In some cases, a small, well-localized tumor that is located in the periphery of the breast may be removed with a 2-cm margin of surrounding normal tissue.

a. Hormonal receptors

A number of adjuvant treatment methods have been developed for breast cancer, and one of these involves determining the presence or absence of hormone receptors in the tumor tissue. **Estrogen receptors are present** in the breast tumor tissue in about 33% of the cases, and about 25% of these patients will respond to hormonal manipulation. In another 33% of patients, **both estrogen and progesterone receptors are present,** and of these patients, nearly 80% will respond to hormone treatment. The remaining one-third of the patients have **neither estrogen nor progesterone receptors present,** and in these patients, only about 5% will respond to changes in the hormonal milieu. In those patients who do have estrogen receptors, the administration of *tamoxifen citrate,* an antiestrogenic compound, has appeared to be an effective treatment.

Chemotherapy has been used in patients who do not have estrogen receptors. Agents such as prednisone, melphalan, vincristine, vinblastine, doxorubicin, and the nitrosoureas have been commonly utilized. **Combination chemotherapy,** using such agents as cyclophosphamide (Cytoxan), methotrexate, and fluorouracil have been proven to be effective in some patients. The use of **immunostimulating agents,** such as BCG (bacillus of Calmette-Guérin), have also been effective when combined with other chemotherapeutic regimens.

Radiation therapy has been used for the local control of tumors and for the treatment of metastases, especially to the brain, the lungs, and the bones. In general, the more extensive the surgical procedure, the less the radiation that is required. Conversely, conservative surgery (i.e., lumpectomy) is usually followed with postoperative radiation for local tumor control. A dose of 180–200 cGy per day is usually administered to the entire breast for a total dose of 4,500–5,000 cGy. Radiation dosage above this level may result in unacceptable fibrosis and retraction of the tissues; however, some authorities will boost this dose to a total of about 6,000 cGy in certain patients. A centiGray (cGy) is the recent terminology for the equivalent of 1 rad.

CHAPTER 17

Human sexuality

In 1954, Dr. William H. Masters and his research associate, Virginia E. Johnson, began their initial studies into the human sexual response cycle at the Washington University School of Medicine in St. Louis, Missouri. These studies were later carried out even more extensively at the Reproductive Biology Research Foundation in St. Louis, where they eventually culminated in a considerable body of knowledge concerning this most important aspect of human behavior.

—*D. R. Dunnihoo*

1. General considerations

a. Sexual development

At birth, there are two aspects of the infant's sexuality that may be identified: the **anatomical sex** and the **chromosomal sex.** By the age of two years, the child will have added another parameter, which is the sex of rearing, or the **psychological sex.** Of the three, the psychological sex is the strongest and the most important. If there are ambiguous genitalia anatomically, or if the child has been raised as a member of the opposite sex, then there may be considerable damage to the child's sexual self-image. After the age of **two years,** the psychological sex will be fixed and cannot be changed without paying a high emotional and psychological price, since the child will have adapted by this time to the male or female gender role. Furthermore, the parents will have dressed the child in a manner appropriate to the selected gender role and will have treated the child in a particular way according to that role, which will have defined the gender role even more strongly.

Most children are raised in the gender role of their anatomical and chromosomal sex, and they are taught their respective societal sexual roles by their parents and the other family members. The ensuing stages of psychosexual development are different for each individual and are dependent upon the sexual mores and attitudes of the society, the sexual beliefs and experiences of the family members, and the responses of the parents to the child's early genital exploration, masturbation, and sexual curiosity.

b. Pubertal sexual changes

Prior to puberty, there is little sexual attraction between the two sexes. With the onset of the pubertal changes in both the male and the female, the basic sexual drives begin to appear. To many young girls who are still dependent, insecure, and emotionally immature, the physical changes that occur with puberty can be very confusing. Initially, **seduction** develops as the first stage of sexual activity. As the child matures, the creation of **visual, olfactory, tactile, or auditory sensations that lead to sexual excitement** forms the next stage of the sexual response cycle. This stage then leads to the third stage of **sexual involvement,** which consists of the individual having physical contact with the opposite sex during **heavy petting,** and then eventually **coital activity.** Finally, the last stage of sexual activity development involves the individual's **interpretation of the sexual encounter.**

The young pubertal boy usually begins masturbatory activity relatively early and develops his "male" image according to what he has been taught constitutes "a real man." It has often been taught, if not overtly then covertly, that the female was someone who would satisfy the male's sexual needs. In some subcultures, it was expected that the man would learn all about sex prior to marriage, so that he could teach his "virgin wife" how to satisfy him. With the onset of dating, the male learns that the primary object is "to make out" with his date. Innocent "necking" often rapidly progresses to "heavy petting," which then leads to unprepared intercourse and occasionally to an unwanted pregnancy.

In contrast to the male's approach to the female/male relationship, the female's motives are usually directed toward the acquisition of "love and tenderness" and a feeling of being "wanted" by the other person. The desire for sexual release for the female apparently is not as strong as the need for "closeness" and "love." In time, the trust and faith that the female initially places in the male not to exploit and leave her is replaced by a realization that she is a grown woman with a sexual identity of her own. At this point, the male may also change and may begin to develop a more caring and loving approach toward the female. Eventually, the female learns to enjoy sex, perhaps as much as the male, and then may add some desires of her own to the shared experience. At this stage of sexual development, the various birth control methods are often explored in order to ensure that their future will not be complicated by an unwanted pregnancy.

c. Adult sexuality

The sexual act means different things to different people at different times. It may be an expression of love, a release of tension, or a mechanism by which one person controls the other. The *motives* of people with regard to sexual function may vary considerably, and as such they constitute the inner dynamics of the sexual relationship. The female may note changes in her sexual desires according to the day of her menstrual cycle, since, for example, an increased level of progesterone tends to decrease sexual interest, whereas the elevated levels of androgens at the time of ovulation may tend to increase sexual interest. If the woman fears becoming pregnant, then such concerns might interfere with her desire for sex. During pregnancy, if the woman has concerns about the safety of the fetus, then she may have a decreased desire for sex. Since sexual excitement may cause uterine contractions, if there are indications of a threatened abortion or of premature labor, then sexual activity should be avoided.

The presence of small children or of a crying baby in the next room may immediately remove any desire

for sex that the woman in the midst of the sexual act may have had. Worries about finances, family illness, or other crises may have a great influence on either of the individuals' desire for sex. The presence of fatigue in either party may also result in a loss of sexual interest. Certain sexual practices (e.g., fellatio, anal intercourse) may cause the woman to lose interest in sex if she does not wish to participate in these activities. If the husband is unfaithful, some women may lose all interest in sex, while others may "try even harder to please him" in an effort to keep him from straying from home and seeking out another woman.

Both the male's and female's interest in having sex may also vary considerably and may be dependent upon many factors. The presence of high tension in his job may drive the man to want increased sex as a way of reducing his nervous tension. In the case of the female, tensions about her career may interfere with her desire or enjoyment of sex. The presence of a pregnancy in his wife, however, may awaken concerns for the "mother image" of his wife. He may relate his wife to his image of his own mother, and since there is a strong aversion to incest in our society, he may lose all interest in sex during her pregnancy. If the woman is too aggressive in her approach to sex, the man may lose interest in sex, especially if he has any fears about being able "to keep up" with his wife's demands.

d. Sex and the senior citizen

As the couple approach their forties and fifties, the pattern of their sexual activities will gradually show a decrease in the frequency of sex, in the variety of sexual acts that are utilized, and in sex in general. The man may often go through a pseudomenopausal period much like that of the menopausal period in the female. During this period, the man may question his abilities, both in the business world and in the bedroom. He may feel disappointment in the goals that were or were not attained. He may show evidence of "burnout" in his job and may have episodes of depression, or he may have difficulty in reorienting himself as to the meaning of his life.

Similarly, the woman who is going through the perimenopausal period may begin to have hot flushes and may notice changes in her moods and in the way she handles stress. Her image of herself as a desirable woman may change, and she may feel that her life is over with the children "out of the nest." After having demands placed upon her by each of the children and by her husband for so many years, she may feel that she is now at a loss as to what to do, since she has too much time on her hands and her family no longer seems to need her attentions. The loss of her ability to bear children may also affect her psychologically, in spite of the fact the she would view another pregnancy at her age with horror. Women who have worked for a number of years may also share the burden of missed goals and career disappointments. Women who have not worked, however, may find that working or going back to college may assist them in their transition through these difficult years.

By the time the couple reaches their sixties and seventies, a further adaptation will have occurred and they will have settled into another existence in which the values and needs of the earlier years are no longer of concern. The constant striving for advancement and the acquisition of material things may no longer be of any interest. Indeed, the physical and financial upkeep on many material assets will tend to be more work than they are worth. Truly, when the beach cottages, boats, and other material goods require too much money and time to maintain, then they "own you" rather than the other way around. Sex at this time of life usually settles into a once or twice a month occurrence and loses almost all of the previous variations that may have been present in earlier years, except for rare occasions. It will still be enjoyed, but it tends to take on an aura of a "comfortable old shoe" in that it is comfortable and reassuring to both parties.

e. Communication

Couples who are having sexual problems are really having trouble with the rest of their relationship, and the sexual aspects merely reflect the greater problem. Behind most marriage or sexual problems is a lack of good communication. *This lack of communication may either be overt or nonverbal.* Each individual should learn her mate's moods and feelings and should learn to reflect appropriately her own moods and feelings in return. **Complete trust in one another is essential, and each partner must place the welfare of the other above his own. When there is good communication between the man and the woman, there is an ability on the part of each individual to "sense" the mood of the other mate.** This "sixth sense" provides them with the ability to know what to do, or not to do, in the marriage relationship.

The individuals in a marriage relationship must first "like themselves" as well as "liking" each other. **They**

must feel free to "expose" their feelings to each other without any fear of rebuke or censor. They should be able to let down their psychological barriers and be themselves. The discussion of sexual matters should always be open and free between the man and the woman. While some things are better left unsaid, the nonverbal communication approach can often convey far more than mere words. "Listening" to your partner and placing your partner's enjoyment and happiness above your own constitutes real communication.

2. The physiology of sex

The classic studies of William H. Masters and Virginia E. Johnson have clearly delineated the four stages of the sexual response cycle: (1) the excitement phase, (2) the plateau phase, (3) the orgasmic phase, and (4) the resolution phase (Fig. 17-1, Fig. 17-2).

a. Excitement phase

The early changes that occur with sexual excitement are similar in both the male and the female. The breasts in the female show some increase in size, and both the male and the female have an **erection of their nipples.** While the male has almost no sex flush or rash initially, the female will rapidly develop a **maculopapular rash** over the breasts. Both individuals will develop some **increase in generalized muscle tone** (i.e., myotonia), and both will experience increased blood pressures and pulse rates.

The penis and the clitoris become erect almost as soon as the sexual excitement begins. Vaginal lubrication develops soon after this initial response, and a reddish or purplish color change occurs on the vulva. **The testes will be drawn up into the scrotum** as the scrotal skin becomes more tense. **The sexual excitement results in an elevation of the uterus in the pelvis, where it becomes more irritable,** and the labia become congested and swollen.

b. Plateau phase

During the plateau phase of sexual excitement there is an increase in the breast changes, and **now the male develops a maculopapular rash** that spreads across the chest and face. **Increased muscle ten-**

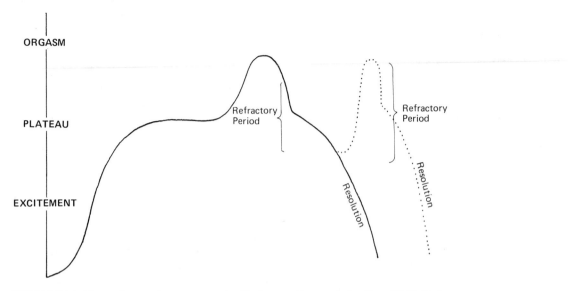

FIGURE 17-1. The male sexual response cycle. (Redrawn with permission from W. H. Masters and V. E. Johnson, *Human Sexual Response*. Boston: Little, Brown, 1966, p. 5.)

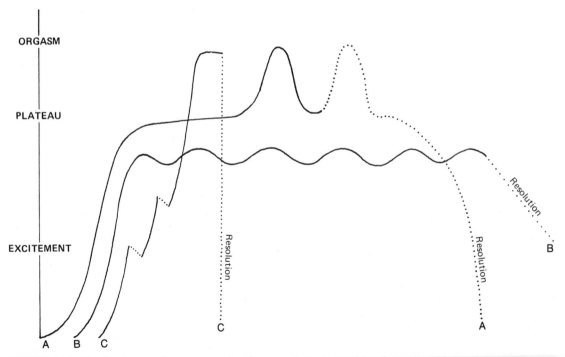

FIGURE 17-2. The female sexual response cycle. There are three types of female-type responses: (A) Multiple orgasms. (B) Prolonged plateau phase without orgasm. (C) Rapid excitement to orgasm with immediate resolution. (Redrawn with permission from W. H. Masters and V. E. Johnson, *Human Sexual Response*. Boston: Little, Brown, 1966, p. 5.)

sion is present in both the male and the female, and voluntary contractions of the rectal sphincter may be noted. **The blood pressure may increase** by as much as 80/40 mm Hg in the male and 60/20 mm Hg in the female, and both of them may experience **an elevation of the pulse rate** to as high as 175 beats per minute (bpm). The respiratory rate will also increase slightly.

The penile corona increases in its circumference and becomes more reddish-purple in color. The clitoris retracts under the clitoral hood, and is no longer easily palpable externally. The outer one-third of the posterior vagina then develops into an **orgasmic platform** in preparation for orgasm. There is an even greater **increase in the depth and width of the vagina** as the uterus elevates further out of the pelvis. By this time, in the male, the testes will have increased in size by 50% and will be fully elevated in the scrotum. **The labia will now be a deep purple color and will be even more congested and swollen.**

c. Orgasmic phase

During the orgasmic phase of the sexual response cycle, both the male and the female begin to have spontaneous spasms and involuntary contractions of some of the muscle groups. The rectal sphincter has involuntary contractions at 0.8-second intervals, similar to the contractions of the female vaginal **orgasmic platform** in the posterior vaginal floor **(i.e., the ischiocavernosus and pubococcygeal muscles).** In addition, there are contractions of the uterine corpus. The blood pressure may increase by as much as 100/50 mm Hg in the male and 80/40 mm Hg in the female, while the heart rate may increase to 180 bpm. The respiratory rate may briefly increase to as high as 40/min. **With the male ejaculation, the initial muscle contraction intervals are also at 0.8-second intervals and involve the ischiocavernosus and bulbocavernosus muscles.**

d. Resolution phase

During the resolution phase the female is only potentially refractory. If sexual stimulation is continued, she may have multiple orgasms with no discernible intervening refractory period. On the other hand, after ejaculation, the male im-

mediately enters the resolution phase and is almost always *refractory* to further stimulation for about thirty minutes. In both the male and the female, the breast changes, the rash, the muscular tension, and all of the other physiologic changes that have occurred in the previous phases rapidly regress. **While the male tends to sweat on his palms and soles, the female usually notes generalized sweating all over her body.**

The penis and the clitoris show gradual detumescence following the climax. The vaginal orgasmic platform disappears. The uterus then descends back into the pelvis, and the cervical os will be observed to be gaping. The testes return to their normal size with the subsidence of sexual excitement and descend back into the scrotum.

3. Sexual dysfunction

The human sexual response is a complex process that is made up of learned responses based on cultural, religious, and socioeconomic factors. It may be affected by organic disease, pharmacologic agents, or by the situational and psychological aspects of the individual's life. Furthermore, these factors may change considerably when placed in juxtaposition with the personality of their mate, who brings to the relationship an equally complicated set of sexual responses.

The modern trend for the female to carry on a career of her own has placed a significant stress upon the institution of marriage and upon the sexual expression of the couple. Not only may separate male and female careers interfere with the opportunity for sexual encounters, but the societal separation of the male and female roles also places an additional burden on the couple. In addition, the availability and effectiveness of oral birth control pills has allowed the female the freedom of pursuing her own sexual appetite in a manner that previously only the male had been allowed to do.

The woman may feel anger and frustration at the fact that the husband does not do his share of the home duties. She may feel that the household chores and the parenting have become her duties because she is a woman; although she is working at her profession as many hours as her husband is in his profession, the division of labor may not be equal. This frustration may result in an indifference to sex or may even cause an active attempt on the part of the woman to thwart her partner's sexual fulfillment.

An additional stress may be placed on the woman because of her guilt feelings concerning her career. She may have unrealistic expectations as to her ability to juggle her career, the children, and a husband and still fulfill all of her own professional needs and goals. The career woman's lack of authority in her job, her often low earnings, and the excessive work load that she must bear (both at home and at work) place a great burden on her. Truly, the professional woman must perform considerably better than her male co-workers to earn only half of what they are paid. Hypertension, ulcers, colitis, gastritis, and other psychosomatic illnesses are the price that the career mother must pay in our society today. Furthermore, the stresses of the marketplace and of a career may lead the woman to smoke, drink, or use drugs of abuse in order to alleviate her tensions.

a. Sexual phase dysfunction

It has been estimated that sexual dysfunction occurs in as many as 50% of U.S. couples. Certainly, it is a subject that many physicians fail to evaluate in their care of patients. You should make every effort to obtain an adequate sexual history from your patient, and in the process, you should allow her to ask questions and freely discuss her concerns about sexual practices. **It is very important in such an interchange that you remain nonjudgmental and that you do not attempt to force your morality or your religious beliefs upon those of the patient.**

There are three phases of sexual function that may lead to problems. These involve: (1) a lack of desire to have sex, (2) an inability to develop purposeful sexual activity, and (3) an inability to consummate the sex act.

1) Desire phase dysfunction

Sexual dysfunction that involves the initial phase of **the sexual drive (i.e., the desire for sex)** is frequently due to **psychological factors.** At times, however, the problem may be one of poor technique or ignorance of the sexual functions. If you take a good history concerning the couple's sexual activities, you may find that the **duration of foreplay** may be too short for the female to develop adequate vaginal lubrication and arousal, which may then lead to vagi-

nal dryness, irritation, and dyspareunia. The repetition of such an experience, with the associated pain and discomfort, may decrease the patient's desire to have sex at later times.

Some of these individuals, male or female, who have difficulty in the desire phase, are just not interested in sex, or tend to avoid intimate situations in order to avoid sexual contact. The male may have difficulties with his job, he may be under considerable strain for other reasons, or he may be just too fatigued and not physically up to having sex. Illness and other physical problems may also be involved in the loss of sexual desire. A loss of the male's ability to sexually fantasize about his mate may be noted in some instances in which there is very little sexual enticement and seduction remaining in the relationship. Anger that is directed at the mate may at times inhibit the individual's sexual desire. Inhibitory stimuli may also derive from a fear, on the part of the woman, of becoming pregnant.

2) Sexual excitement phase dysfunction

When the sexual problem occurs at the time of **purposeful sexual activity, or during the sexual excitement phase,** there may be either **psychological or physical** causes involved. Conditions such as *male impotence* or *female frigidity* are examples of types of dysfunction that can occur during the excitement phase. Failure to develop an erection or to maintain it, or the failure of the woman to maintain sufficient lubrication until the end of coitus, also constitutes excitement phase dysfunction. The onset of this type of sexual dysfunction is gradual in those who have an organic etiology and may be associated with an **increasing insensitivity** of the penis. In addition, in those individuals who have psychological problems there may be a similar problem, in that at first there may be a loss of the erection during intercourse, which progresses to a similar problem during foreplay, and then finally to an inability of the individual to perform at all.

3) Orgasmic phase dysfunction

Delayed or absent orgasm in the female is an example of orgasmic phase dysfunction. Psychological problems are often involved; however, drugs, alcohol, tranquilizers, or antihypertensive medications may also cause this kind of dysfunction. Occasionally, it may be necessary for you to give the patient "permission" to enjoy certain forms of sexual activity. Many women in the past were taught since childhood that sex was something that a "nice girl" did not do, and often the subsequent acquisition of a piece of paper (i.e., a wedding license) saying that they were now married, and that now sex was all right, did not change this conditioning overnight. In more recent times, with the more permissive sexual attitudes in our society, this kind of problem is no longer commonly encountered.

Moreover, resentment or anger against some aspect of the individual's life may carry over into the sexual relationship and inhibit orgasm. **If orgasm occurs with masturbation, then in almost all cases the cause of the anorgasmia with coitus is psychological.** In addition, illness and fatigue may produce a delayed or absent climax in both the male and the female.

Premature ejaculation is another form of orgasmic phase dysfunction. This problem usually occurs in men who are anxious and who do not make any effort to control the progression of their sexual response or to "pace themselves" with the woman. The hypersensitivity of the penis, coupled with an unwillingness on the part of the man to delay the ejaculation, results in a premature ejaculation and a failure to satisfy the woman. The use of the **squeeze technique,** in which the woman's thumb and forefinger are placed just beneath the corona of the penis and briefly squeezed, may decrease the male's sensation sufficiently to allow him to control his ejaculation for a longer period of time.

Vaginismus is almost always a psychological problem. The patient will have involuntary spasmodic vaginal contractions of the outer third of the vagina upon insertion of the penis, a finger, or a speculum. The pain that occurs in this condition may inhibit the orgasmic phase. Recent attempts to provide sex education to the public, as well as the increased premarital sexual activity that has occurred in our society, have served to decrease the incidence of this condition. If vaginismus should develop, the treatment consists of instituting a program of gradual vaginal dilatation. In addition, an attempt to psychologically desensitize the patient by the use of sexually explicit films has been of benefit in some patients.

The term **dyspareunia** is defined as "pain with intercourse," which may occur on either initial or deep penetration of the vagina. This condition may be due to local vaginal, cervical, or pelvic lesions or to psychological causes. You should try to rule out any organic cause for the pain before you attribute it to psychological problems. If the penile thrusting occurs before the vagina has elongated with sexual arousal, then the cervix may not withdraw out of the pelvis sufficiently and the pain may occur whenever the penis strikes the cervix. Prostatitis or epididymitis in the male may produce pain in the penis and testicles that may interfere with the male orgasm.

4) Interpretation of the sexual act

The interpretation stage of the sexual reponse cycle also involves the desire phase, since desire is based upon the person's previous sexual experiences. If the coital event was pleasurable, then the future desire for sex is accentuated. If the coitus was inadequate, or the person feels that she "failed to perform," then the desire may be tinged with the fear of "again failing to perform up to expectations" the next time. If the woman has a sense of shame or "dirtiness" following the sex act, due to the inappropriate association of "sin and sex," then this attitude also may affect the degree of her desire for the next sexual encounter. Homosexual tendencies might also play a role in the desire phase of the sexual response.

b. General treatment considerations

The treatment of sexual dysfunction problems requires mature judgment on the part of the physician. You should never automatically assume that the patient's complaint is psychological in origin. Instead, you should do a **thorough historic evaluation** of the patient, which should include all aspects of her psychological, socioeconomic, and medical health. A complete evaluation should be carried out in the male as well as in the female if at all possible. **A complete physical examination** may reveal evidence of physical disease, such as diabetes, hypertension, or other debilitating conditions that might be the cause of the patient's problem. The presence of other handicaps, such as a colostomy, a urinary catheter, or the presence of other physical problems that may interfere with the sexual act (e.g., amputees) should also be evaluated. You should encourage these patients to continue their sexual lives. An empathetic physician can provide valuable instruction to these individuals as to the various methods of sexual interaction that they might engage in to overcome these handicaps.

You should consider the **five "C's"** in approaching a sexual problem: **confidence, comfort, compassion, communication, and consultation.** You should feel confident that you have enough knowledge to be able to help the patient. You should feel comfortable in discussing sexual matters with her. You should be compassionate and realize that the problem may be a serious one for the marital unit. You should be able to take the time to communicate with the patient in a relaxed and unhurried manner without the press of a busy office. Finally, you should be able to recognize your limitations and know when to refer the patient to a consultant that specializes in sexual therapy. Those sexual counselors who belong to the American Society for Sex Education, Counseling, and Therapy (ASSECT) should be able to provide expert assistance in the management of your patient's sexual dysfunction.

The **PLISSIT model** has also been helpful in treating some patients. This acronym stands for **P (permission giving), L & I (limited information), SS (specific suggestions),** and **I & T (intensive therapy).** Initially, the physician gives the patient permission to discuss her sex life and lets her know that this is alright. Almost all patients are ignorant of the anatomical and physiological aspects of sexual problems and should be given limited basic information concerning such matters. **A determination of the degree and the amount of the patient's sexual knowledge is important, since frequently the patient's sexual concerns may arise strictly on the basis of ignorance.** You should make every effort to properly educate the patient about the medical aspects of sexual behavior and to reassure her concerning her fears and doubts. Keep in mind that the **communication problems** in sexual dysfunction involve both the man and the woman. The dual therapy approach that has been emphasized by Masters and Johnson seeks to determine not only the sexual concerns but also the dysfunction of the overall marriage relationship. It has been stated that when a marriage is good, sex only accounts for about 10% of it, whereas in a bad marriage, sex may account for 90% of it.

While you may not wish to extensively treat the couple who has a sexual dysfunction problem, you owe it to your patient to at least make a tentative diagnosis of the type of sexual problem and then refer the couple to a certified sex therapist for definitive treatment.

CHAPTER 18

Gynecologic procedures

In science the credit goes to the man who convinces the world, not to the man to whom the idea first occurs.
—*Sir William Osler**

1. Office procedures

a. Papanicolaou smear

The Papanicolaou smear was first introduced in 1943 to detect cervical cancer. The use of this test has provided not only an excellent screening test for cervical neoplasia but has also inculcated the need for periodic gynecologic examinations into generations of women in the United States.

1) Technique

The technique of obtaining a Papanicolaou (Pap) smear is simple. The patient should have refrained from douching within 24 hours of the examination. After the cervix is exposed with a bivalve speculum, the **endocervix and ectocervix** should be scraped with either a wooden or a plastic spatula, or with a saline-moistened cotton-tipped applicator, and an additional specimen should be obtained from the posterior fornix of the vagina. The specimen obtained from the squamocolumnar junction of the cervix should be smeared on one glass slide and the second posterior fornix specimen placed on a second glass slide. The

*Reprinted with permission from Robert Bennett Bean, *Sir William Osler: Aphorisms from His Bedside Teachings and Writings,* William Bennett Bean, ed. Springfield, Ill.: Charles C Thomas, Publisher, 1968, p. 112.

slides may then be sprayed with a preservative or immersed in a jar of ether/alcohol solution for transport to the laboratory, where the staining process may be carried out.

2) Interpretation

While many cytopathologists attempt to read the Pap smear in relationship to the suspected cervical lesion (e.g., whether there are cells present that are compatible with moderate dysplasia, etc.), others still read the Pap smear according to the old numerical classification, which is generally reported as follows:

Class I: Normal cells
Class II: Slightly abnormal cells with either mild dysplasia and/or inflammation
Class III: Suspicious of a greater degree of cellular abnormality, such as moderate dysplasia
Class IV: Suggestive of severe dysplasia or carcinoma-in-situ
Class V: Diagnostic for malignant cells, possibly invasive carcinoma

b. Schiller's test

Schiller's test relies upon the fact that Schiller's iodine solution (i.e., a weak iodine solution), or Lugol's iodine solution (i.e., a strong iodine solution) stains the glycogen present in the normal estrogen-stimulated vaginal mucosa to produce a mahogany-brown color. **If the vaginal mucosa is immature, scarred, or dysplastic, then it will not stain brown with the iodine solution.** This simple test serves to distinguish abnormal squamous epithelium from normal epithelium so that it may be further evaluated.

c. Colposcopy

While the Papanicolaou smear evaluates the exfoliated cells from the cervix, the technique of colposcopy examines the vascular network of the cervix and the cellular structure of the epithelial surface. Patients who have abnormal Papanicolaou smears should be further evaluated by colposcopy.

1) Technique

The colposcope is a stereoscopic microscope of 6× to 40× power of magnification that allows you to evaluate the surface of the cervix (Fig. 18-1). The cervix is initially visualized through a bivalve speculum and is cleaned of excess mucus with a cotton swab. The cervical blood vessels are then observed under a green filter after the surface is swabbed with a saline soaked swab. If the cervix is swabbed with a *3–4% acetic acid solution,* it will remove any remaining mucus and will also dehydrate the surface epithelium. In those areas of severe dysplasia that have a high nuclear-to-cytoplasmic ratio,

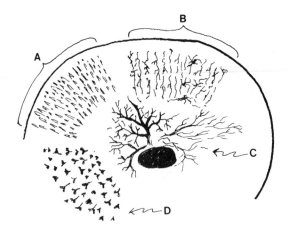

FIGURE 18-2. Schematic drawing of the different types of terminal vessels as observed in normal cervical epithelium. (A) Hairpin capillaries. (B) Network capillaries. (C) Branching vessels. (D) Double capillaries.

the cells will become white and will be well demarcated from the surrounding tissues. The region of most interest is usually the area of the cervix that was originally covered by columnar epithelium, but which has since been covered over by squamous metaplasia **(i.e., the transformation zone),** since the neoplasia will almost always develop within this zone.

Those abnormal colposcopic findings that are found in the transformation zone include mosaicism, punctation, white epithelium, and atypical blood vessels (Fig. 18-2). *If the entire squamocolumnar junction is visualized, then the colposcopy is considered to be "satisfactory."* In about 15% of patients under 45 years of age, however, the colposcopy examination will be found to be unsatisfactory and will usually require an additional evaluation, depending upon the degree and extent of the lesion. If severe dysplasia or carcinoma-in-situ is found to be present with an unsatisfactory colposcopic examination, then a diagnostic conization of the cervix should be performed.

Colposcopy provides a clinical appraisal of the type and extent of a cervical lesion and allows you the opportunity of obtaining a biopsy of the more severe areas of involvement. Such **directed biopsies** are superior to the random cervical biopsies that have been used in the past.

It should be recognized that dysplastic lesions can

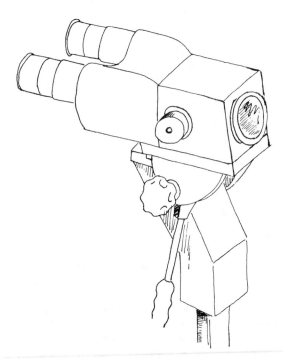

FIGURE 18-1. Zeiss colposcope.

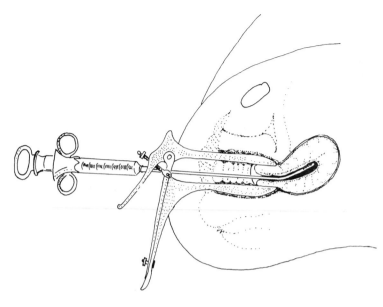

FIGURE 18-3. Technique of endometrial biopsy using a metal or plastic suction curette. The uterine cavity should be sampled throughout the full 360 degrees (multiple endometrial sampling technique).

occur in the vagina and on the vulva. The colposcope is a valuable diagnostic tool to evaluate these areas as well. The findings in the vagina are similar to those that are seen on the cervix. In patients who were exposed in utero to diethylstilbestrol (DES), there may be columnar epithelium in the vagina, which may be the first indication of the presence of adenosis. More than 500 cases of clear-cell carcinoma of the vagina or cervix have been reported since 1940 (see Chapter 13). Changes in the **vulva** due to dysplastic lesions are not as easily defined with the colposcope because of the increased thickness of the surface epithelium. The increased use of acetic acid washes, or alternatively, the application of oil, may make the underlying features of the epithelium more evident on colposcopic examination.

d. Cervical, endocervical, endometrial, and vulvar biopsies

1) Cervical biopsies

Currently, cervical biopsies are almost always obtained under **direct colposcopic control,** or lacking such a capability, they are obtained after identifying suspicious areas on the cervix by means of the Shiller's test. *Colposcopically "directed biopsies" are usually taken of those areas that appear to be the most abnormal* (e.g., whitened areas).

2) Endocervical biopsies

Endocervical scrapings (i.e., endocervical curettage, or ECC) are usually obtained at the same time as the cervical biopsies in order to detect any lesions that may be present high up inside the endocervical canal.

3) Endometrial biopsies

An endometrial biopsy should not be obtained if there is any possibility of a pregnancy being present. When an endometrial biopsy is performed, it should be obtained during the latter half of the menstrual cycle so that ovulation can be ascertained and the endometrium may be dated. If there is concern about a possible pregnancy, a beta–human chorionic gonadotropin (β-hCG) pregnancy test may be obtained, or the biopsy may be taken on the first day of menstruation. The uterus should be sounded, the depth in centimeters should be recorded, and the direction of the uterine cavity should be noted. A metal suction curette attached to a 10-cc syringe should be inserted slowly to the top of the uterine fundus and then somewhat forcefully scraped downward toward the endocervix, all the while with suction being maintained on the syringe. **This process should be repeated rapidly until the entire 360 degrees of the uterine cavity has been sampled (i.e., multiple-sampling technique, or MST)** (Fig. 18-3). The patient will usually tolerate this procedure quite well without anesthesia, but she should be warned that a few cramps may occur. The use of a thin plastic curette to obtain the biopsy may be less painful. The date of the patient's last menstrual period (LMP) and your clinical diagnosis should always be written on the laboratory request form so that the endometrium may be dated and evaluated appropriately.

4) Vulvar biopsies

If the vulva is stained with a 1% solution of toluidine blue dye and then washed with a 1% acetic acid solution, the nuclei of any abnormal dysplastic surface cells will retain the blue color, indicating the site for a possible biopsy. A biopsy of the vulva may be accomplished in the office under local anesthesia without difficulty. The lesion should be completely excised, and if necessary, a few 4-0 or 5-0 subcuticular chromic sutures may be placed. The use of the Keys cutaneous punch biopsy instrument may also be used to obtain a small biopsy. This instrument is similar to a cork borer. The skin specimen is bored out in a circular manner and the base of the specimen cut free.

e. Cryosurgery and cauterization

The diagnosis of cervical dysplasia by colposcopy and directed cervical biopsies will usually define the extent and type of the cervical lesion. **The term "cervical intraepithelial neoplasia" (CIN) has been applied to these colposcopic lesions, which may be divided into mild dysplasia (CIN I), moderate dysplasia (CIN II), and severe dysplasia/carcinoma-in-situ (CIN III). In the case of the vulvar lesions, the lesions are referred to as vulvar intraepithelial neoplasia (VIN) and are classified in a manner identical to that of the cervical lesions (i.e., VIN I, VIN II, and VIN III).**

The use of cryosurgery or hot electrocautery to obliterate these lesions has resulted in about a 90% cure rate. The cryosurgery refrigerants used are carbon dioxide ($-60°$ C), freon ($-60°$ C), nitrous oxide ($-80°$ C), and liquid nitrogen ($-90°$ C). While either a single or a double freeze technique may be used with the different refrigerants, it has been noted in the case of nitrous oxide that a single freeze is just as effective as a double freeze.

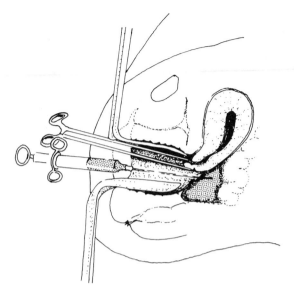

FIGURE 18-4. Technique of culdocentesis. The needle should be inserted in the midline of the posterior fornix. Sweeping motions with the needle in place should be avoided so as not to lacerate important structures.

f. Culdocentesis

The technique of culdocentesis, or a cul-de-sac puncture, consists of inserting a #20-gauge long spinal needle on a 10-ml syringe into the midline of the posterior fornix of the vagina and into the peritoneal cavity (Fig. 18-4). This technique is very valuable in detecting the presence of intra-abdominal problems. **The return of nonclotting blood is diagnostic of intra-abdominal bleeding and usually mandates either a laparoscopy or a laparotomy to determine the source and the amount of bleeding.** The most likely diagnosis when nonclotting blood is obtained is either a ruptured corpus luteum cyst or an ectopic pregnancy. It should be remembered, however, that in patients who have had abdominal trauma, a ruptured liver or spleen may be the source of such bleeding. Obtaining a **clear yellow serous fluid** is a normal finding, unless there is a large amount of it present, in which case it may represent a ruptured corpus luteum cyst without bleeding. Usually, **a serosanguineous fluid** (i.e., fluid with a hematocrit that is less than that of the patient) is obtained when there is a ruptured corpus luteum cyst with minimal bleeding. In such cases, close observation of the patient in the hospital overnight will usually be sufficient to be certain that there is no further intra-abdominal bleeding of consequence. The finding of serosanguineous fluid in a culdocentesis, however, does not rule out an ectopic pregnancy. If frank **pus** is returned on a cul-de-sac tap, then the diagnosis of an acute appendicitis or an acute salpingo-oophoritis must be strongly entertained.

Recently, this technique has been utilized in the follow-up of ovarian carcinoma patients. Cul-de-sac aspiration cytology may be of value in the evaluation of the patient who is on chemotherapy. One report has shown a 92% correlation between the cytology and the actual status of the patient as determined by a second-look operation.

g. Laser techniques

1) Terminology

There are **three different processes** that produce light waves: **spontaneous emission, absorption, and stimulated emission** of energy. When an electron falls to a lower energy orbit about its atom, **spontaneous emission** occurs; however, this emission has a low power density and must be focused. **Absorption** of light may occur whenever a photon strikes an atom and energy is absorbed. The light that is not absorbed is reflected in all directions, much as with spontaneous emission, but at a different frequency and wavelength. When an atom that is already in an excited state is hit with a photon of energy of a given frequency, a **stimulated emission** occurs, which is the release of two photons of energy with the same frequency and direction as the incident beam. As a consequence of this collision, there is an amplification of the original beam.

A laser (i.e., an acronym for "light amplification by stimulated emission of radiation") is a device that generates a monochromatic (equal wavelengths, same frequency and energy), **collimated** (parallel waves that do not cross one another), **coherent** (energy waves in phase along the beam) **electromagnetic radiation in the infrared, ultraviolet, or visible regions of the spectrum.**

The **power density** in watts/cm^2 is the amount of laser energy that is absorbed by the tissue. The **spot size** is the diameter of the focal point, which varies directly with the **focal length** (i.e., a short focal length corresponds to a small spot size and vice versa). With the power being constant, the smaller the spot size, the deeper the crater.

The beam may be delivered in a **continuous wave exposure** (laser energy is delivered for as long as the shutter is open) or by a **pulsed beam** (bursts of laser energy interspersed with refractory periods). **Gating** refers to the time period that the shutter is open regardless of how long the pedal is depressed. **Superpulsing** (a high energy pulse) is sometimes used to minimize heat effects on the tissue. The usual focal length for handpiece delivery is 50–100 mm; for micromanipulator delivery, it is 250, 300, and 400 mm. The spot size ranges between small (0.2–0.5 mm), medium (1.0–1.5 mm), and large (2–3 mm). Power settings usually range between a low of 10–15 W to a high of 20–30 W, with readings of more than 50 W being considered very high.

The laser beam is absorbed by the cell water, which instantly heats it to 100° C to form steam, which then causes the vaporization of the cell. There is no debris and no bleeding when this method is used. High power settings (superpulsing) and short operating times decrease the thermal damage to the surrounding tissue. If low power settings are used, there is a longer time involved and the tissue may attain temperatures as high as 1,000° C, which may cause thermal tissue injury to the adjacent tissues. A high flow vacuum pump may be used to remove the smoke from the field of operation.

2) Indications for laser technique

The laser technique may be used to perform major surgery. **It may be used as a scalpel** to incise the skin, the underlying fatty layers, and the fascia. A tightly focused beam acts as a knife, whereas a defocused beam functions as a blood vessel coagulator. The end of the fallopian tube may be reconstructed by using a laser, which is capable of creating flaps to form a pseudofimbriated end of the tube. A laser can also be used to carry out a **linear salpingostomy** on an ectopic tubal pregnancy. **Adhesions** about the ovaries or the fallopian tubes can be easily vaporized. In order to limit the depth of destruction, **a light-absorbing laser backstop rod** (e.g., of quartz, Pyrex, titanium, or another metal) may be used when performing certain operations (e.g., adhesiotomy). **Endometriotic implants** may be vaporized in such a manner that the depth of the ablation may be controlled by intermittent time gating. In situations in which a light-absorbing laser backstop rod cannot be used, such as with endometriotic implants on the bowel or bladder, an underlying 1 ml of 1:30 vasopressin solution may be injected beneath the serosa of the implant to **produce a liquid cushion** to protect the underlying tissues. Leiomyomas can be excised with a laser by incising the myometrium over the surface of the myoma and then shelling the tumor out of its pseudocapsule.

Many colposcopes now have a laser attachment that produces an **infrared energy beam.** This beam may be directed at a tissue surface (e.g., the vulva, the vagina, or the cervix) so as to provide for the uniform destruction of the tissue by evaporation and necrosis to a precise depth. Since the amount of overall tissue destruction is less than that which occurs with cryosurgery, the healing is more rapid. With an adequate depth of tissue destruction (e.g., about 5–7 mm), the cure rate is equivalent to that obtained by cryosurgery (i.e., 90%).

The three main types of lasers that have been used in gynecologic procedures are: the **carbon dioxide,** the **argon,** and the **neodymium-yttrium-aluminum-garnet (Nd-YAG) techniques.** The CO_2 laser accomplishes its destruction of the tissue by the vaporization of the cells. The other two techniques (Nd-YAG, argon) primarily coagulate the proteins in the tissues and thus tend to produce a deeper penetration of the tissue. The argon and Nd-YAG techniques can be used with flexible fiberoptic systems, whereas the CO_2 laser beam cannot be delivered in this manner. **The CO_2 laser is the only one that can be used to make incisions.** The Nd-YAG technique has been more commonly used with the hysteroscope, since the beam will pass through fluid and has an excellent ability to stop bleeding.

h. Hysteroscopy

1) Types of hysteroscopy

Hysteroscopy may be performed by using a hysteroscope (i.e., a fiberoptic instrument) to examine the uterine cavity. There are two types of hysteroscopic techniques that have been described: **contact** and **panoramic** hysteroscopy.

a) Contact hysteroscopy

In **contact hysteroscopy,** the 6-mm hysteroscope makes a physical light contact with the mucous membrane of the uterus so that the tissue can be viewed for color, contour vascular pattern, and the "feel" of the surface. Blood does not obscure the endometrial surface. The findings are similar to those that may be seen during colposcopy. Anesthesia is not necessary in many patients, especially in cases where the cervix is quite patulous.

b) Panoramic hysteroscopy

In order to see within the uterine cavity during a **panoramic hysteroscopy,** it is necessary to inflate the cavity with carbon dioxide or with a fluid, such as saline or a dextran-70 solution (Hyskon). **The 5- to 7-mm hysteroscope can then scan the cavity and detect the presence of an abnormal septum, intrauterine synechiae, polyps, a lost intrauterine contraceptive device, or other abnormalities.** Polyps may be removed, and submucosal leiomyomas may be morcellated by a shaving technique. If bleeding becomes excessive during the removal of a submucosal leiomyoma, the insertion of a Foley catheter filled with 30 ml of fluid will compress the endometrial surface and control the bleeding. A septum of an abnormal uterus can also be surgically removed with a hysteroscope; however, laparoscopy should be performed at the same time in order to be certain that the uterus is not perforated. Direct visualization **chorionic villus sampling (CVS)** can also be performed with a hysteroscope. Hysteroscopy has not been used very often in the detection of endometrial cancer because of the risk of disseminating the tumor cells out through the fallopian tubes. Some physicians have managed patients with menorrhagia by destroying the endometrium with a Nd-YAG laser technique.

c) Complications

Pregnancy, profuse bleeding, and cervical malignancy are contraindications to performing hysteroscopy. In addition, previous pelvic inflammatory disease contraindicates the use of the hysteroscopy technique because of the risk of having a flare-up of the PID. While uterine perforation may occur, it is uncommon when the direct vision technique of insertion is used. If perforation should occur, laparoscopy may be necessary to assess the damage. **The use of the Hyskon so-**

lution has been associated with pulmonary edema and with allergic reactions; however, pulmonary edema should not occur if the total distending fluid is limited to no more than 400 ml. With the Nd-YAG laser, there is a risk of backscatter from the beam causing **retinal damage to the surgeon.** Finally, if CO_2 is used hysteroscopically, there is always the risk of CO_2 embolism.

i. Ultrasonography

Ultrasonography involves the use of sound with frequencies greater than 20,000 cycles per second (i.e., hertz). Most diagnostic ultrasound utilizes a frequency range of between 1–10 megahertz (i.e., 1–10 million cycles per second). These sound waves are reflected from tissue interfaces back to a receiver, which records the echo and its intensity. *Such reflections from tissues of different densities provide a "picture" of the structures and their relationships to one another.*

Ultrasonography has been used extensively in obstetrics to determine the presence of an early pregnancy, to date the pregnancy, and to extensively evaluate the anatomical condition of the fetus (see Chapter 26). The placenta can be localized by ultrasound and the amount of amniotic fluid may be evaluated. The technique of amniocentesis has been greatly facilitated by the use of ultrasound to locate a clear pocket of amniotic fluid for the insertion of the needle. Using the Doppler effect, an ultrasound detector can determine the presence of the fetal heart rate as early as 9 weeks' gestation. In gynecology, ovarian neoplasms may be evaluated as to their cystic or solid components. Other pelvic conditions, such as an ectopic pregnancy, may also be detected. Recently, with the increase in the popularity of the in-vitro fertilization technique, the ultrasonic monitoring of ovarian follicles to detect the time of ovulation has been effectively accomplished. The new vaginal ultrasonic transducers have opened the door to even further applications of ultrasound in the pelvis.

2. Minor procedures

a. Fractional dilatation and curettage (D&C)

A dilatation and curettage (D&C) of the uterus may be performed in the treatment of incom-plete abortions or as a diagnostic technique in postmenopausal bleeding. In the latter instance, it is essential that the uterine cavity be adequately sampled, and, in the case of an abortion, that it be evacuated completely. Under suitable anesthesia (i.e., general, regional, or paracervical block anesthesia), the anterior lip of the cervix should be grasped with a tenaculum and the uterine cavity sounded with a metal probe to determine the *depth of the uterine cavity, which should be about 6–8 cm.* The cervical os may then be gradually dilated with Hegar's dilators to allow the introduction of a curette and the polyp forceps into the endocervix and the uterine cavity.

The fractionation of the specimens in a diagnostic D&C should be as follows: (1) the **endocervical canal** should be scraped with a small sharp curette from the internal os down to the external os throughout 360 degrees and the specimen placed in a container of formalin; (2) the **uterine cavity** should then be systematically scraped with a sharp curette throughout 360 degrees beginning at the 12 o'clock position, and then anteriorly and posteriorly across the uterine fundus from one cornual region to the other, and the tissue then placed in another formalin container; and finally, (3) **the uterine cavity should be explored with polyp forceps,** and any tissue obtained should be placed in a third formalin container. The uterine cavity should then be resounded to verify the depth of the cavity and to make certain that uterine perforation has not occurred.

b. Dilatation and evacuation (D&E)

The dilatation and evacuation (D&E) procedure is an extension of the D&C procedure that is usually performed in abortions from the 13th to the 24th week of pregnancy. It is beneficial to define the gestational age by ultrasound prior to performing the procedure. Since wider dilatation is usually needed to utilize the suction equipment and to remove the larger fetal parts with sponge forceps in the more advanced pregnancies, it is advisable to gradually dilate the cervix with a *laminaria tent* prior to surgery. The laminaria tent consists of seaweed that absorbs water and becomes swollen. In doing so, the seaweed slowly and gently dilates the cervical os over the course of about 12–24 hours just prior to surgery. A new moisture-absorbing polymer (Dilapan) has been marketed that may provide even more dilatation of the cervix in less time, so that a significant dilatation occurs in three hours.

A 14-mm suction cannula will usually evacuate fetuses up to about the 16th week of pregnancy. In more advanced pregnancies, after the drainage of the amniotic fluid, the remainder of the tissue may have to be removed by means of forceps. The uterine cavity should be gently explored with forceps, or with a suction apparatus, to be certain that the evacuation has been completed.

c. Conization

Cervical cold conization is utilized primarily today for the diagnosis and treatment of dysplasias of the cervix. Rarely will a conization be necessary to treat chronic cervicitis. The procedure should be carried out under adequate anesthesia (i.e., general or regional). The anterior lip of the cervix should be grasped with a single-toothed tenaculum and a black silk suture placed at about the 12 o'clock position on the portion of the cervix that is to be excised in order to assist the pathologist in orienting the tissue. A chromic suture is placed on each side at the 3 and 9 o'clock positions on the lateral portions of the cervix to ligate the descending branches of the uterine artery and to provide for good hemostasis. Alternatively, a 1:200,000 solution of epinephrine may be injected at the operative site to provide hemostasis (i.e., 1% lidocaine solution with a 1:100,000 solution of epinephrine, diluted in half with saline to form a 1:200,000 solution of epinephrine). The uterine cavity should then be sounded with a probe and the depth recorded. The uterine probe may be left loosely within the endocervical canal to provide for additional orientation during the circumoral excision of a "cone" of tissue. Since there is no need to obtain a large amount of stroma, an effort should be made to keep the cone biopsy somewhat shallow, even in the endocervical canal. After its removal, the specimen should be firmly pinned to a tongue depressor to allow for adequate fixation and orientation for the pathologic examination. Sutures may sometimes be necessary to control the bleeding after the removal of the specimen. The invagination of the outer margins into the cervical os should be avoided. The complications of conization include postoperative cervical bleeding, cervical stenosis, cervical incompetence, and infertility.

d. Colpotomy

In patients who have pelvic inflammatory disease with a cul-de-sac abscess, the abscess will often eventually **"point"** into the posterior fornix of the vagina. At that time, the abscess may be felt upon vaginal examination as a boggy, fluctuant mass that projects into the posterior portion of the vaginal apex. In order to drain the abscess and effect a cure, it may be necessary to perform a **colpotomy incision.** This operation consists of making an incision into the posterior fornix of the vagina and thus into the cul-de-sac of Douglas of the peritoneal cavity.

The patient should be administered a general or regional anesthetic in the operating room, and an 18-gauge long spinal needle on a 10 ml syringe should be inserted into the midline of the bulging posterior vaginal fornix until pus is encountered. At that point, the vaginal wall should be incised down the needle tract until the abscess cavity is entered. Once the incision is made in the abscess cavity, the opening should be enlarged slightly and any loculi that are present should be disrupted with your finger to be certain that the entire abscess cavity has been opened up. A malecot catheter may then be placed in the cavity and one loose chromic suture placed in the vaginal wall to retain it in position. This cul-de-sac drain may be removed in several days after the drainage has essentially stopped. Colpotomy drainage of a pelvic abscess usually effects a prompt response in the patient's condition. The fever should subside and the signs of infectious toxicity should disappear within 24 hours. Antibiotic therapy, however, should be continued until the patient has been afebrile for at least 48 hours.

The colpotomy operation may also be used for sterilization purposes. By opening the posterior fornix, it is possible to grasp the adnexal structures and excise them or remove a portion of each of the fallopian tubes without difficulty (e.g., Pomeroy tubal ligation).

e. Magnetic resonance imaging

If a patient is placed in a magnetic field and bombarded with radio waves (i.e., radiofrequency energy), then the atomic nuclei in the patient's body will absorb energy that may then be radiated to appropriate sensors after the radio signal has been turned off.

The technique of magnetic resonance imaging (MRI) relies upon the fact that molecular nuclei are aligned in the same direction in a magnetic field and will absorb and resonate energy. **When the nuclei are allowed to return to their original nonaligned random directional state, they reemit electrical signals and radio waves.** The time differential in the realignment process can then be measured and reconstructed into an image by computer processing. There is no radiation involved, so the patient is not subjected to a hazardous procedure. **Since MRI relies on hydrogen density, blood flow, and the exponential time constants of hydrogen (T1 and T2), these parameters may be manipulated to produce a difference in contrast in the images.** As a consequence, T1-weighted images result in a picture with sharp contrast, while T2-weighted images reveal the tissue layers within the organs more clearly. T1-weighted imaging has a short repetition time (TR) and a short echo time (TE), whereas in T2-weighted imaging these times are long. It is possible to utilize T2-weighted spin-echo sequences (long TR and TE) to identify the layers of the uterus.

The earth's magnetic field is of the order of 0.5 to 1.0 G. The magnetic field strength of MRI ranges from 1,000 to 20,000 G (i.e., 0.1 to 2.0 tesla). Magnetic fields are quantified in units that are called **tesla,** where one tesla equals 10,000 G.

The **pulse sequence** may be defined as follows: When a patient is placed in a magnetic field and the nuclear particles with magnetic moments of interest (e.g., protons) are excited to high energy states by radiofrequency pulses, the kind of image obtained is dependent upon the types of pulses (i.e., the angle through which they move the magnetic moments) and the times between them **(i.e., the interpulse interval).** Commonly, spin-echo and inversion-recovery pulse sequences are utilized. **An inversion-recovery image** may be constructed when the pulse sequence consists of two pulses, one at 180 degrees followed by one at 90 degrees. **A spin-echo image** may be obtained when the pulse sequence consists of two pulses, but in this case there is one 90-degree pulse followed by a 180-degree pulse, and the information that forms the image is collected after the 180-degree pulse has been completed. That amount of time, which is called the "time-to-echo," is twice the interpulse interval. **The relaxation time** is the rate of relaxation of the atomic nuclear magnetic moments from a high to a low energy state. During the relax-

ation, the transfer of the energy may be to the surrounding spin **(spin-spin relaxation, or T2)** or to the surrounding molecules **(spin-lattice relaxation, or T1).** In other words, the transverse or spin-spin relaxation time refers to the rate of the signal loss due to the interaction of the affected atomic nuclei with each other, whereas the longitudinal or spin-lattice relaxation time refers to the time that is required for the atomic nuclei to realign themselves with the magnetic field after stimulation by the radiofrequency pulse has ceased.

MRI can detect a number of conditions in the gynecologic patient because of its inherent ability to show contrast between the different tissue planes. For example, the endometrium may not only be distinguished from the myometrium but can also be appreciated to be thicker in the secretory phase of the menstrual cycle than in the proliferative phase. Furthermore, endometriosis may be detected, due to the brightness of the blood present in the tissues on T1- and T2-weighted images. Simple cysts of the ovary may be differentiated from hemorrhagic cysts and endometriomas. Leiomyomas may be identified and their location within the myometrium defined. If degeneration of a leiomyoma is present, the MRI can differentiate it from one in which there is no degeneration present. Cervical cancer may be identified as a high-intensity area that deforms the normally low-intensity cervical stroma. The fetus and the placenta may be visualized in detail with the MRI technique. Fetal motion during the procedure, however, may obscure the imaging. The sedation of the fetus with the maternal administration of 2 mg of diazepam (Valium) I.V. was shown to improve the images in one study.

3. Major procedures

a. Laparoscopy

1) Technique

Laparoscopy (peritoneoscopy) is an endoscopic procedure used for the evaluation of the contents of the peritoneal cavity (Fig. 18-5). In this procedure, a long thin endoscope is inserted through a small periumbilical incision and the entire abdomen explored visually for pathology. Limited amounts of surgery may then be performed using a special biopsy or operating instrument that is inserted either through a separate

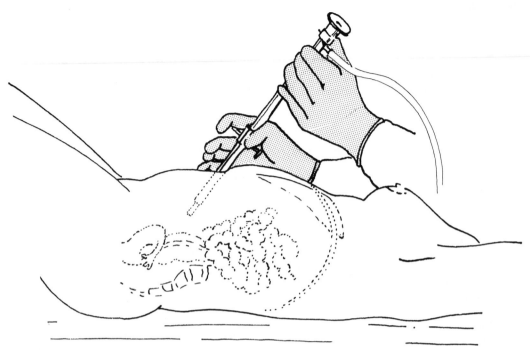

FIGURE 18-5. The technique of laparoscopy in Trendelenburg's position.

cannula or through the same cannula as the laparoscope.

After the induction of suitable anesthesia in the operating room, a laparoscope can be inserted into the abdomen through a 1–2 cm periumbilical incision, after the insufflation of about two liters of either CO_2 or N_2O to distend the abdominal wall and allow the intestinal contents to drop away from the point of the insertion of the trocar. Upon the entry of the laparoscope, a visual survey of the abdominal cavity above or below the umbilicus may be carried out. An olive-tipped cervical probe will allow the manipulation of the uterus in order to more fully evaluate the pelvic structures. The use of grasping forceps through the laparoscope, or through a second lower abdominal suprapubic incision, allows further evaluation of the pelvic structures, or the coagulation of the fallopian tubes for sterilization purposes.

The CO_2 laser has been used with laparoscopy as a cutting instrument, since it vaporizes the cells and penetrates to about 0.1 mm, whereas the argon laser penetrates to 0.8 mm and the Nd-YAG laser penetrates to 4.2 mm. The manipulation of the power settings, the duration of the exposure, and the use of appropriate backstops allow the operator to control the laser and accomplish a specific operative procedure. The accumulation of smoke and carbon debris during this procedure, however, may require that the abdominal cavity be flushed with as much as 30–80 liters of CO_2 during the course of an operation.

2) Indications

Laparoscopy with the electrocoagulation probe may be used for the fulguration of the fallopian tubes for sterilization, or for the fulguration of endometriotic implants. This procedure may also be used as a diagnostic aid in evaluating the pelvis in infertility cases, in detecting pelvic pathology in the patient with the pelvic pain syndrome, in identifying the presence of an ectopic pregnancy, and in many other situations where there is confusion as to the causes of pathology in the abdominal cavity. Laparoscopy should not be used in intestinal obstruction or generalized peritonitis.

3) Complications

The usual complications that may occur with laparoscopic procedures include: (1) hemorrhage from the laceration of the aorta, the inferior vena cava, or other vessels, (2) inadvertent puncture of the bowel, (3) the insufflation of gas into the retroperitoneal area, and (4) the occurrence of thermal burns of various pelvic viscera (more common with the unipolar equipment). Many patients complain of shoulder or chest pain secondary to the residual gas in the abdomen and the irritation of the diaphragm. Since most of the complications of laparoscopy occur as the result of the blind introduction of the Verres needle or the trocar, the **open technique of laparoscopy** was introduced in 1971. While the leakage of gas around the incision site and the difficulties in creating a pneumoperitoneum were noted with the open technique, both techniques have been found to be essentially the same with respect to the other technical difficulties and failure rates.

b. Laparotomy

An excision into the abdomen (i.e., laparotomy) carried a considerable risk in regard to infection in the days prior to antibiotics. The use of rubber gloves was a major step in preventing infection in surgical procedures. It is interesting that **Dr. William S. Halsted** of Johns Hopkins University is usually credited with the first use of rubber gloves in surgery, although they had been used by another surgeon some years before. **Dr. Horatio Robinson Storer** of Boston, who performed the first Porro cesarean section hysterectomy in 1869, actually wore the first rubber gloves in surgery. The story concerning Dr. Halsted probably came about because of Miss **Caroline Hampton** (who later married Dr. Halsted in 1890), who became the chief operating nurse upon the opening of Johns Hopkins Hospital in May of 1889. Miss Hampton apparently developed a severe case of dermatitis from some of the chemicals (e.g., carbolic acid) that were used in the operating room and had some rubber gloves made for her by the Goodyear Rubber Company to protect her hands. These gloves could be boiled and then used over and over for surgery. Later, Dr. Halsted began to use gloves in certain cases, but not in every case. The first surgeon to wear rubber gloves in every operation was **Dr. Joseph C. Bloodgood.**

An exploratory laparotomy (celiotomy) is the opening of the abdomen for exploratory purposes. The skin incision may be vertical or it may be horizontal (i.e., a slightly smiling incision). There are a number of incisional approaches that may be utilized in abdominal surgery (Fig. 18-6). In the lower abdomen, if the skin incision is horizontal, then the entry into the peritoneal cavity may be: (1) vertically through the midline between the rectus muscles *(i.e., Pfannenstiel's incision)*, (2) by means of a transverse incision across the rectus muscles *(i.e., Maylard incision)*, or (3) by means of a transverse incision through the tendinous insertion of the rectus muscles just above the pubis *(i.e., Cherney modification of Pfannenstiel's incision)*.

The layers of the abdomen that are traversed in a vertical incision below the umbilicus are: (1) the skin; (2) Camper's fascia, or the subcutaneous fat; (3) Scarpa's fascia, a thin fascial layer at the base of the fat layer; (4) the rectus fascia and muscle, or if the incision is vertical in the midline, the linea alba; (5) the transversalis fascia, or preperitoneal fat; and (6) the peritoneum. If the incision extends vertically down to the pubis, the small *pyramidalis muscle* may be seen on each side of the midline. If the skin incision is horizontal, then the inferior epigastric vessels may be seen coursing superiorly near the lateral margins of the incision between the fascial planes.

Upon entry into the abdomen, a systematic exploration of the peritoneal contents should always be carried out. In those cases in which there is an infection with obvious pus present, both aerobic and anaerobic cultures should be obtained upon entry into the abdomen. In those patients in whom carcinoma is suspected, saline washings of the abdomen and pelvis should be obtained initially for cytologic evaluation of the cell block. The upper abdomen should be explored manually on the **right side** to ascertain the condition of: (1) the diaphragm, (2) the liver, (3) the gall bladder, (4) the adrenal gland, (5) the kidney, (6) the para-aortic nodes, and (7) the appendix, the ascending colon, and the transverse colon. The **left side** is then manually explored to evaluate: (1) the diaphragm, (2) the spleen, (3) the adrenal gland, (4) the kidney, (5) the pancreas, (6) the stomach, (7) the para-aortic nodes, and (8) the transverse and the descending colon. The pelvis is then packed off with moist lap cloths and the pelvic structures individually identified on both sides.

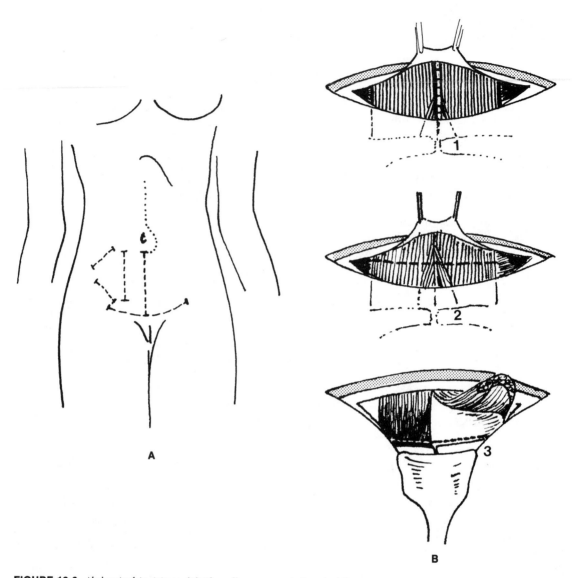

FIGURE 18-6. Abdominal incisions. (A) The off-center vertical and oblique incisions are often used for specific operations, such as an appendectomy or herniorrhaphy. The midline vertical incision should be utilized whenever exposure may be a consideration or the diagnosis is in doubt. The Kocher incision parallels the right costal margin. The McBurney incision overlies McBurney's point. The paramedian incision lies lateral to the midline vertical incision. The midline incision is a vertical incision between the pubis and the umbilicus. (B) Transverse incisions involve: (1) the midline vertical approach between the rectus muscles (Pfannenstiel), (2) a transverse incision of the rectus muscles (Maylard), or (3) a separation of the rectus muscles from their insertion on the pubic bone (Cherney).

c. Salpingostomy, salpingectomy, and salpingo-oophorectomy

The fallopian tube may be excised for a number of reasons, the most common one being an ectopic pregnancy. However, more recently, there has been a move in the direction of performing a salpingostomy rather than removing the entire tube. The technique of **salpingostomy** consists of making a linear incision over the top of the tube in order to remove the products of conception. The incision may either be left open or be repaired with very fine suture material to reconstruct the wall of the tube. It is essential that all of the products of conception be removed in a salpingostomy, since there have been cases in which the continued growth of the trophoblastic tissue has necessitated reoperation 4–6 weeks later for recurrent intra-abdominal bleeding (persistent ectopic syndrome).

If an ectopic pregnancy has ruptured and has destroyed the tube beyond repair, then a **salpingectomy** is indicated. In this procedure, the tube should be excised by clamping along the mesosalpinx between the tube and the ovary to the level of the uterine body. The cornual region may be superficially wedged out and carefully closed with figure-of-eight sutures **(i.e., cornual resection).**

In some instances, it may be necessary to remove both the fallopian tube and the ovary, often in conjunction with the removal of the uterus. **Salpingo-oophorectomy may be performed: (1) from the infundibulopelvic ligament toward the uterus, or (2) from the uterus toward the infundibulopelvic ligament.** The latter procedure is sometimes the easier of the two when there are large leiomyomas present that obstruct the exposure of the infundibulopelvic ligament area. By lifting up the uterine end of the broad ligament where it has been excised from the uterus (after the removal of the uterus), the retroperitoneal area in the region of the uterosacral ligaments may be visualized and the ureter easily identified. By incising the peritoneum above and lateral to the ureter up to the level of the ovarian vessels, the infundibulopelvic ligament with its ovarian vessels may be safely ligated and the adnexa removed.

In removing the adnexa from the infundibulopelvic ligament down toward the uterus, the peritoneum should be incised at the level of the round ligament and the incision carried up along the lateral pelvic wall peritoneum to the level of the infundibulopelvic ligament. When this lateral peritoneum is incised, the psoas muscle, the genitofemoral nerve, the external iliac vessels, and the external iliac lymph nodes become visible. A Kelly clamp should be placed on the medial peritoneal edge and another curved Kelly clamp slipped behind the peritoneum into the retroperitoneal space and lifted anteriorly against the posterior peritoneal surface. The ovarian vessels and the ureter will cling to the peritoneal surface, and when the peritoneum is lifted off the iliac vessels, the retroperitoneal Kelly clamp will easily expose the ureter by a gentle opening and partial closing of the clamp (i.e., dissecting motion). This clamp should then be inserted through the peritoneum above the ureter, and the infundibulopelvic ligament with its ovarian vessels clamped and doubly ligated. By carrying this peritoneal incision down to the level of the broad ligament and the uterus, the adnexa, along with its vessels, may be excised en bloc.

d. Hysterectomy

1) Morbidity and mortality of hysterectomy

Previously, about 700,000 hysterectomies were performed in the United States each year, but this number has declined somewhat in recent years. **The surgical mortality rate for hysterectomy in this country is less than 0.1%, while the overall morbidity is about 10%; however, it may be as high as 30–50% in indigent patients. The mortality rate for a hysterectomy associated with pregnancy is about 29.2:10,000. In those cases in which the hysterectomy is associated with cancer, the mortality rate is 37.8:10,000. If the hysterectomy is not associated with either of these conditions, then the mortality rate is 6.0:10,000.**

2) Infections

The majority of the morbidity associated with a hysterectomy consists of **febrile morbidity.** Vaginal hysterectomy was associated in one study with a 27% postoperative febrile morbidity, whereas 44% of the patients had febrile morbidity following an abdominal hysterectomy. Many of the postoperative infections are transient episodes of atelectasis. Infections are more common in indigent patients because of their

decreased resistance and poor nutrition. Other factors that predispose the patient to infection after a hysterectomy are: (1) the method of surgical skin preparation, (2) vaginal and rectal preparation, (3) the antiseptic scrubbing technique of the surgeon, (4) the placement of surgical drapes, (5) the length of surgery, (6) the inclusion of other procedures, (7) the use of packs or drains, (8) the use of a cautery, (9) the amount of dead space present, and (10) the surgical technique of the physician. Moreover, the presence of diabetes mellitus, obesity, recent cortisone administration, cancer, radiation treatment, and anemia have all been implicated as factors that are associated with a higher risk of postoperative infections. Major infections, such as a cuff and adnexal cellulitis, an infected cuff hematoma, or a pelvic abscess, are relatively common following this kind of surgery and are generally caused by organisms that are normally found in the vagina.

Numerous types of bacterial organisms are endogenous to the normal vagina and cervix. These include: (1) the common **aerobic gram-negative enteric bacilli,** such as the Klebsiella species, Escherichia coli, and Proteus mirabilis; (2) the **aerobic gram-positive cocci,** such as group B streptococci, Streptococcus viridans, and staphylococci; (3) the **enterococcus species;** and (4) **anaerobic organisms,** such as the Peptostreptococcus, the Peptococcus, the Bacteroides species, the Clostridium species, the Fusobacterium species, and the Actinomyces species. In addition to these endogenous species of bacteria, Neisseria gonorrhoeae, group A streptococci, Chlamydia trachomatis, and Mycobacterium tuberculosis may be involved in these infections. Other organisms may also become involved if a **nosocomial infection** (i.e., hospital-acquired infection) occurs.

With the incision into the vaginal cuff during a hysterectomy, there is an immediate introduction of bacteria into the lower pelvis. While cleansing vaginal douches and preoperative vaginal scrubbing may reduce the number of bacteria that are present, these procedures do not eliminate them completely.

In recent years, **antibiotics** have been **used prophylactically** in patients undergoing a hysterectomy to prevent postoperative pelvic infections. It has been demonstrated that if the antibiotic has attained an adequate concentration in the tissues by the time the contamination occurs, then the antibiotic is usually effective in preventing postoperative infection. The use of prophylactic antibiotics will decrease the

incidence of infection by about 50% of the usual incidence of infection in the population studied. In high-risk populations (i.e., patients in the lower socioeconomic strata), the concept of an **incipient infection,** or a "lowered host resistance," has been suggested. It would appear from the current studies that a single dose of an antimicrobial drug is as effective as multiple doses of the drug in preventing postoperative infections. Those drugs which have been used in a single-dose regimen are cefonicid sodium (Monocid), cefotaxime sodium (Claforan), and doxycycline hyclate (Vibramycin). Those antibiotics that have been used in *multiple-dose regimens* are cefamandole nafate (Mandol), cefoxitin sodium (Mefoxin), cefazolin sodium (Ancef or Kefzol), cephalothin sodium (Keflin), cephradine (Anspor or Velosef), and piperacillin sodium (Pipracil). Since these drugs have been shown to be highly successful in reducing the incidence of postoperative infectious morbidity, it has been suggested that prophylactic antibiotic therapy should also be used in patients undergoing radical gynecologic cancer surgery.

The **treatment of mild postoperative pelvic infections** generally involves the use of the extended spectrum cephalosporins or penicillins. If the patient does not respond appropriately within 48–72 hours, or if the infection is severe, then gentamicin and/or clindamycin should be added to the treatment regimen. Metronidazole may be utilized in place of clindamycin. If a Staphylococcus infection should be present, then nafcillin sodium (Unipen) or vancomycin hydrochloride (Vancocin) may be administered.

Although it was initially thought that antibiotic therapy for pelvic infections should be continued for 10–14 days, this procedure is not necessary in most instances. Rather, treatment should be administered until the patient has been afebrile for 24–48 hours and then discontinued.

In the presence of an acute pelvic inflammatory disease involving Neisseria gonorrhoeae, Chlamydia trachomatis, gram-negative enteric bacilli, the Bacteroides species, or the Actinomyces species, then the patient should be treated according to the guidelines recommended by the Centers for Disease Control (CDC).[1]

There is significant bacterial contamination of a cervical conization site within 48–72 hours postoperatively. As a consequence, if a hysterectomy is to be

---

[1] See *Morbidity and Mortality Weekly Report Supplement,* vol. 34, no. 4S, October 18, 1985.

performed following a cervical conization, it should be done within the first 48 hours of the conization surgery or it should be delayed for six weeks in order to avoid the risk of instigating a serious pelvic infection.

One of the most serious complications of abdominal surgery is the development of a **necrotizing fasciitis,** or synergistic bacterial gangrene of the skin. The organism that is most commonly involved in this type of infection is the **Group A beta-hemolytic Streptococcus;** however, secondary invaders, such as Staphylococcus aureus, Pseudomonas, and the Enterobacteriaceae species may be involved. In these cases, **the surgical wound edges have edema, a purplish skin discoloration, and an extensive loss of vascularity of the wound edges, which necessitates wide debridement of the skin, the subcutaneous fat, and the fascia to the point where the tissues show fresh bleeding.** High-dose wide-spectrum antibiotics should be given intravenously. Skin grafting will often become necessary because of the extensive debridement of the tissues that is required.

The surgical technique utilized by the surgeon is an important factor in the prevention of a postoperative infection. Whenever there is poor hemostasis and unnecessary crushing of the tissues, then conditions may be such that they provide an adequate culture medium for the growth of bacterial organisms. If the vaginal cuff is completely closed with sutures, then serum and blood may accumulate above the cuff and a cuff cellulitis or an abscess may form. In contrast, if the vaginal cuff is left open following a hysterectomy, the blood and serum will usually drain to the outside and infection will not occur. The placement of a special catheter drain with suction in the vaginal cuff postoperatively may also be of value in preventing the accumulation of blood or serous fluid and the subsequent development of a cuff abscess. One minor complication that may occur when the vaginal cuff is left open is that an increased amount of granulation tissue may form in the vaginal vault during normal healing, which will be noted four weeks later at the postoperative examination. This problem may easily be treated with a silver nitrate cauterization stick.

3) Hemorrhage

Postoperative hemorrhage after a hysterectomy has been reported in about 0.3–2.0% of cases. Often the bleeding site occurs at the vaginal cuff; how-ever, it may rarely involve the intra-abdominal vascular pedicles. This condition may require a reexploration of the abdomen in order to obtain hemostasis. It is important that all vascular pedicles be doubly ligated at the time of surgery in order to prevent this complication. *An elective hysterectomy should not be performed within three months of a pregnancy because of the increased pelvic vascularity and the greater risk of undue hemorrhage intraoperatively and postoperatively.*

4) The technique of abdominal hysterectomy

A simple abdominal hysterectomy is generally used for the management of benign disease. The tubes and ovaries may be left in situ, or if necessary, they may be removed along with the uterus. After opening the abdomen and identifying the pelvic contents, the uterine fundus should be grasped with a large multitoothed tenaculum in order to control the uterus and keep the *tissues on tension* during the operation.

If the adnexa are to be removed, then the operation begins with the round ligaments, which should be clamped, cut, and ligated bilaterally with no. 0 chromic or Vicryl suture. The peritoneum should then be incised toward the infundibulopelvic ligament, as in the technique of salpingo-oophorectomy, and the adnexa removed down to the uterine body, after which the uterine body is then excised as described below.

If the adnexa are to be retained, then following the ligation of the round ligament, the *anterior peritoneum should be incised bilaterally to just above the bladder reflection and the bladder flap reflected inferiorly* below the level of the vaginal fornix. A clear *vascular-free window* in the broad ligament may be developed beneath the fallopian tube and the ovarian ligament where they join the uterus. This area may then be bluntly penetrated with a finger or a clamp, with the tube and the ovarian ligament then doubly clamped, incised, and the pedicle doubly ligated. The broad ligament may then be opened up by blunt dissection alongside the uterine body, and the uterine vasculature may be "skeletonized" by removing the fibrinous areolar tissue about the vessels. The peritoneum along the posterior surface of the uterus and above the uterosacral ligaments should be incised and reflected inferiorly. The uterine vessels can then be clamped with a Heaney clamp in several small bites down to the level of the vaginal fornix on each side of the uterus. **At all times during the placement of these clamps, the uterus should be kept on tension by back pressure with the uterine tenaculum. In addition, it is very important that each bite of the clamp along the side of the uterus should always slide off the uterine body and should not be allowed to stray laterally away from the uterus.** If these two principles are adhered to, then the risk of clamping or cutting a ureter should be minimal.

When the uterus has been excised to the level of the vaginal fornix, then the vagina should be opened with heavy scissors and the uterus, tubes, and ovaries removed. The vaginal cuff edge should be sutured with a continuous lock-stitch to effect hemostasis and then left open for drainage. The posterior peritoneum should then be closed to cover the open vagina. Recently, some studies have shown that when the peritoneal surfaces are closed with sutures peritoneal adhesions may develop. Such adhesions are thought to lead to postoperative intestinal obstruction in some cases. As a consequence, many surgeons do not close the peritoneum upon leaving the abdomen. In the presence of an open cuff, my preference is to close the posterior peritoneum. Gentle handling of the tissues also aids in the prevention of adhesions, as does the use of wet lap cloths instead of dry lap cloths when trying to obtain exposure of the structures in the abdomen. Moist lap cloths do not scarify or abrade the tissues as much as the dry ones do.

5) The technique of vaginal hysterectomy

After the induction of adequate anesthesia in the operating room, the patient should be placed in a lithotomy position, the perineum prepped, and a weighted posterior speculum placed in the vagina. A narrow-bladed retractor should be placed anteriorly in the vagina and the cervix exposed. The cervix should then be grasped with a tenaculum and the loose reflection of the bladder identified by alternately pulling and pushing on the cervix. **In order to decrease the amount of bleeding and to facilitate the dissection, up to 100 ml of saline, or saline with a 1:200,000 Neo-Synephrine solution, may be injected into the anterior, posterior, and lateral tissues of the cervix where the circumoral incision is to be placed.** Some studies have shown that the use of epinephrine in the injection solution may impair the host tissue's defense mechanisms against infection and that it does not decrease the blood loss significantly. Other authors would perhaps disagree with this assessment. The cervical incision should be made with a sharp scalpel below the bladder reflection and continued circumferentially around to the posterior aspect of the cervix. The posterior vaginal mucosa may then be sharply dissected off the cervix and the peritoneum of the cul-de-sac of Douglas exposed. This peritoneal fold should be incised and the peritoneal cavity behind the cervix entered. A long-bladed weighted speculum should then be placed in the cul-de-sac to further facilitate the exposure.

The anterior vaginal mucosa should be sharply dissected to the level of the bladder reflection and then bluntly dissected between the bladder pillars to the level of the *vesicoperitoneal fold,* which should be incised to enter the abdominal cavity anterior to the uterus. If any difficulty is encountered in identifying this anterior peritoneal reflection, then this step may be delayed until later in the procedure, as long as due care is taken not to include this bladder fold in the subsequent vascular clamps.

With the uterus being pulled downward on tension with a cervical tenaculum, the uterosacral ligaments on each side should be grasped with a Heaney clamp (with the clamp sliding off the cervical body), cut on the uterine side, and suture-ligated with no. 0 Vicryl suture. The base of the broad ligament on each side should be grasped in a similar manner with a Heaney clamp, cut, and ligated. Each of these pedicles should be tagged with small clamps on long suture ends for later identification. The uterine vessels are then clamped, cut, and ligated bilaterally. At this point, if the anterior peritoneum was not previously identified and entered, it can now be easily incised and the peritoneal cavity entered. A long narrow-bladed anterior retractor (e.g., a narrow Deaver retractor) should be inserted into the peritoneal cavity in front of the uterus to assist in the further exposure of the uterus. The remainder of the broad ligament will be easily visualized and should be clamped, cut, and ligated in a stepwise fashion up to the junction of the round ligament, the ovarian suspensory ligament, and the fallopian tube, which should also be clamped, cut, and ligated in a similar manner bilaterally, and then the uterus should be removed.

The closure of the vaginal cuff has undergone many modifications since the original Heaney approach was promulgated. Classically, it has been thought that the broad ligament pedicles (containing the round ligament, the ovarian suspensory ligament, and the fallopian tube), the cardinal ligament, and the uterosacral ligaments, bilaterally, constituted the main ligamentous support of the uterus. It was thought that, after the removal of the uterus, these ligaments should support the vaginal cuff as well. These pedicles are usually plicated into several bundles on each side of the vagina and tied into the cuff with additional sutures. By doing so, not only is the cuff supported, but if postoperative bleeding should occur, the pedicles may be easily located. *The presence of the fallopian tube in the broad ligament pedicle could pose problems, however, in regard to a possible ectopic pregnancy at a later time, so the tube should not be included in this closure.* Since many physicians do not suture these pedicles to the vaginal cuff in an abdominal hysterectomy, one might question the value of doing so in a vaginal hysterectomy. Certainly, the inherent elasticity of the round ligament augurs against its ability to support the vaginal cuff. The other ligaments are really not disturbed in their relationship to the cuff, unless a large vaginal cuff was excised with the specimen. The main attachments of the cardinal ligaments are probably primarily to the cervical and uterine body; however, in view of the diffuse nature of these fascial and muscular tissues, it seems logical that the fornices of the vagina are also enmeshed in these supports. Thus, the resuturing of the vaginal cuff to these ligaments would seem to be a redundant procedure in some cases; however, it may provide additional support and is therefore usually performed.

The plication of the uterosacral ligaments is probably of value in preventing the future development of an enterocele. In addition, the placement of several pursestring sutures or plicating sutures **(i.e., Moschcowitz operation or the McCall procedure, respectively)** in the cul-de-sac to obliterate any tissue redundancy probably also reduces the probability of the future development of an enterocele.

The vaginal cuff peritoneum should be closed with a pursestring suture, and the vaginal cuff edge should be sutured with a continuous lock-stitch to obtain hemostasis and then left open for drainage.

4. Chemotherapy for malignancy

a. General considerations

Chemotherapy and radiation kill cells that are in the actively dividing phase (i.e., those in the growth fraction). **Since not all tumor cells are replicating at the same time, these treatment modalities can only kill a portion of the tumor at any one time.** Repeated applications of a chemotherapeutic agent or of radiation results in killing those replicating cells that were not killed in previous applications. The surgical excision of the bulk of a tumor results in an increase in the growth of the remaining tumor cells (an increased growth fraction). Excision, then, places a greater number of cells into the actively dividing phase, which thus makes them more susceptible to the effects of radiation and chemotherapy. The early growth of a tumor is exponential; however, as the cells begin to crowd each other (increasing bulk) and the vascularity in the depths of the tumor decreases, the doubling time of the tumor cells becomes longer and the growth fraction decreases.

Both chemotherapy and radiation therapy kill cells by affecting the deoxyribonucleic acid (DNA) so as to inhibit cellular replication. Both of these modalities have an effect on normal cells as well as on tumor cells, especially those that are rapidly reproducing, such as in the bone marrow, in the gastrointestinal system, and in the hair follicles. Not all tumors are susceptible to chemotherapeutic agents, and not all patients can tolerate the side effects of these agents.

The **mitosis (M) phase** is the process by which each cell divides into two daughter cells. The interval between mitotic divisions has been termed the "interphase." The **interphase period** may be divided into several other phases (Fig. 18-7). The first of these is the **G1 phase,** which is of variable duration (4–24 hours). During this phase there is a diploid content of DNA present as well as synthesis of ribonucleic acid (RNA) and of enzymatic proteins. The second phase is the **S phase** (about 10–20 hours) in which there is a duplication of the DNA content (i.e., DNA synthesis). The **G2 phase** (less than 2–10 hours) is a premitotic phase that continues the RNA and protein synthesis and where a tetraploid DNA content is present. The mitotic spindle apparatus is manufactured in this phase in preparation for the resumption of mitosis. The next stage of the mitotic division, the **M phase** (30–60 minutes), occurs with the division of the cell into two daughter cells. Following mitosis, some of the cells enter a **resting state (G_0),** a return to G1 in which there is no replication for a period of time. The cell in the G_0 resting phase is less susceptible to the damaging effects of radiation or chemotherapy. Usually, the majority of cells in a tissue are in the resting

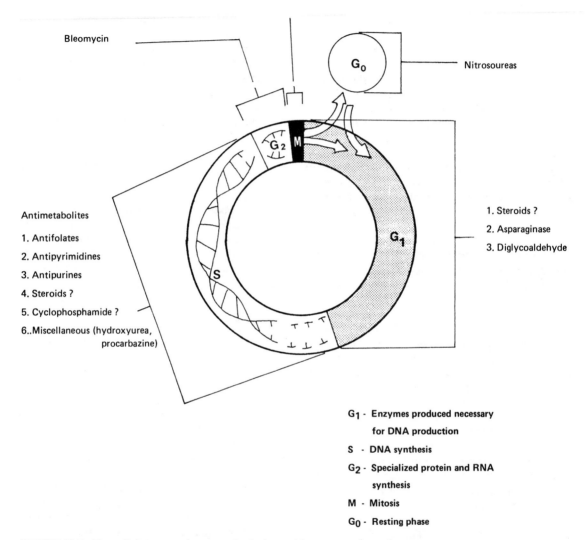

FIGURE 18-7. The cell division cycle proceeds clockwise. The various chemotherapeutic agents act at different points in this cycle. (Adapted from M. L. Pernoll and R. C. Benson, eds., *Current Obstetric and Gynecologic Diagnosis and Treatment.* Norwalk, Conn.: Appleton & Lange, 1987, p. 908.)

state (G_0 phase). The length of the G1 phase is highly variable due to the inclusion of the G_0 phase.

b. Chemotherapeutic agents

Considerable experience has been gained over the past 25 years in the use of chemotherapeutic agents in the treatment of various malignancies. Some tumors with poor vascularity may temporarily be somewhat resistant to the effects of some of the chemotherapeutic agents. In other tumors, if the malignant cells have mutated to a more hardy type of cell, the resistance may be stronger. Both of these effects may occur in bulky tumors.

Chemotherapy is generally withheld from the patient if the white blood cell count is less than 3000/mm³ or if the platelet count is less than 100,000/mm³. The lowest levels of these parameters are usually seen after about 7–14 days of chemotherapeutic treatment. **There are several different categories of chemotherapeutic agents, such as: (1) the alkylating agents, (2) the antimetabolites, (3) the antibiotics, and (4) the plant alkaloids.** Hormonal agents may also be used in specific situations, as may some unclassified agents.

A number of chemotherapeutic agents act at specific phases of the mitotic cycle. The **phase-specific** agents are those drugs that act primarily during one part of the mitotic cycle, such as dactinomycin (Cosmegen) and doxorubicin hydrochloride (Adriamycin RDF), which mainly affect cells in the G1 phase of the cell cycle. Bleomycin primarily affects those in the G2 phase. Furthermore, hydroxyurea and methotrexate primarily affect those cells in the S phase of the cycle. **Cycle-specific** drugs may affect any phase of the cell cycle, including the resting stage; examples of these agents are the alkylating agents and cisplatin (Platinol).

1) Alkylating agents

The members of this group are melphalan (Alkeran), chlorambucil (Leukeran), triethylenethiophosphoramide (Thiotepa), and cyclophosphamide (Cytoxan). These agents cause alkylation of DNA, which prevents DNA replication by forming a cross linkage between the DNA strands. They work best on cells in the S interphase period. These agents are most useful in the treatment of ovarian tumors. Cytoxan is also used in the treatment of germ-cell tumors, squamous carci-

nomas, and sarcomas. Leukeran has also been used in the treatment of tubal carcinomas. Bone marrow depression is a common side effect, and cyclophosphamide also may cause gastrointestinal side effects, hemorrhagic cystitis, sterility, and alopecia.

2) Antimetabolites

The antimetabolite agents consist of methotrexate (Methotrexate) and fluorouracil (Adrucil). These cycle-specific agents have an effect on the cell because they resemble normal compounds; when they are utilized by the cell, they block an essential enzyme. Methotrexate inhibits the enzyme folic acid reductase and thus blocks its conversion to tetrahydrofolate, which is needed for the synthesis of the purine and pyrimidine subunits of nucleic acid. The drug fluorouracil interferes with the thymidine synthetase enzyme, which is essential for DNA synthesis. Methotrexate is the primary agent for the treatment of trophoblastic tumors. The side effects of Methotrexate are bone marrow depression, alopecia, liver failure, renal failure, dermatitis, and gastrointestinal problems. The agent 5-fluorouracil (Efudex) has been used in an ointment formulation in the treatment of vaginal and vulvar intraepithelial neoplastic lesions. Pain and ulceration are common side effects of the topical use of this agent.

3) Antibiotics

The members of this group of antibiotics consist of dactinomycin (Cosmegen), doxorubicin hydrochloride (Adriamycin RDF), mitomycin (Mutamycin), and bleomycin sulfate (Blenoxane). These agents are naturally elaborated chemicals from the Streptomyces bacteria that interfere with RNA and DNA synthesis. Dactinomycin (Cosmegen) is often utilized in the treatment of trophoblastic tumors. Doxorubicin hydrochloride is used to treat endometrial carcinomas, sarcomas, and ovarian carcinomas. Mitomycin is used in the treatment of carcinoma of the cervix, and bleomycin is used to treat squamous carcinomas, choriocarcinomas, and germ-cell tumors. The side effects of these antibiotics consist of bone marrow depression, alopecia, local tissue necrosis, and gastrointestinal problems, all of which occur commonly with the first two agents. Cardiomyopathy and cardiac arrhythmia may occur with doxorubicin hydrochloride. The side effects of bleomycin consist of pneumonitis and pulmonary fibrosis, as well as skin reactions, stomatitis, and alopecia.

4) Plant alkaloids

The chemotherapeutic agents in this category are vinblastine sulfate (Velban), VP-16-213 etoposide (VePesid), and vincristine sulfate (Oncovin). These agents cause metaphase arrest of the tumor cells and prevent replication. They are useful in the treatment of germ-cell tumors, sarcomas of the ovary, and choriocarcinoma. Bone marrow depression and neurotoxicity are the most common side effects of these agents, and vincristine sulfate may also cause gastrointestinal problems.

5) Progestational agents

The progestational agents are used in the treatment of endometrial carcinoma. They include medroxyprogesterone acetate (Depo-Provera), hydroxyprogesterone caproate, and megestrol acetate (Megace). These agents bind to specific tissue receptors to produce their effects. Liver dysfunction and alopecia are possible side effects.

6) Antiestrogenic agents

The primary antiestrogenic drug in this category is tamoxifen citrate (Nolvadox). This agent is used in the treatment of breast cancer, uterine cancer, and ovarian cancer, and its side effects consist of hot flushes, vaginal bleeding, and pruritus.

7) Miscellaneous agents

Cisplatin (Platinol) causes the inhibition of DNA synthesis and can be used in treating all genital malignancies. Its side effects commonly include renal toxicity, ototoxicity, and myelosuppression. Hexamethylmelamine is an agent used in the treatment of ovarian carcinomas; however, its mechanism of action is unknown. Bone marrow depression and neurotoxicity are some of its common side effects.

5. Radiation therapy for malignancy

a. General considerations

Radiation may occur in a number of forms, some of which are harmful while others are helpful to plant and animal life. Electromagnetic radiation consists of: (1) visible light, (2) ultraviolet light, (3) infrared light, (4) radio waves, (5) X-rays, and (6) gamma rays. The latter two radiation modalities are similar in that they are photons of energy that can penetrate tissues to produce ionization. The radiations that occur from the decay of an atomic nucleus (e.g., cobalt 60) are called gamma rays, in contradistinction to those that originate outside of the nucleus (electrons). When a suitable target, such as tungsten, is bombarded by electrons, X-rays are produced. The energy that is imparted to the X-ray photons is the difference in the orbital energies between the inner and outer shells. High-energy electrons are called beta particles and are derived from the decay of certain isotopes (^{32}P). These particles do not penetrate deeply into the tissues.

b. Types of radiation equipment

The various **external radiation** modalities that are used today consist of such equipment as the betatron, the cobalt generator, and the linear accelerator, each of which can produce high-intensity radiation at depth in the tissue. The low-voltage equipment of years past caused extensive skin damage when therapeutic radiation dosages were applied to pelvic tumors. In contrast, the supervoltage-megavoltage equipment of today avoids this complication. Radiation may be classified as: (1) low voltage (superficial) (85–150 keV), (2) medium voltage (orthovoltage) (180–400 keV), (3) supervoltage (500 keV–1 MeV), and (4) megavoltage (more than 1 MeV).

The technique of administering **internal irradiation (brachytherapy)** consists of placing a radiation source into an applicator (e.g., the Fletcher-Suit afterloading applicator) that is then inserted into the uterus and vagina for a period of time. The milligrams of radium (or other radioactive source) in the **intracavitary** applicator is multiplied by the number of hours that it remains in place to give the total number of **milligram-hours** of radiation dosage. Most applicators today are *after-loaded,* which means that the radiation source (radium or cesium) is loaded after the applicator has been properly positioned in the vagina and packed away to prevent any shifting during the 24–48 hours of the treatment period. An X-ray film of the pelvis will allow you to check the applicator's position in relationship to the clinical extent of the tumor so as to obtain the best dosimetry curves.

The **implantation** of radioactive needles or isotope seeds, such as radon (^{222}Rn) and iodine (^{125}I), may be used in superficial accessible tumors. The **intraperitoneal instillation of isotopes,** such as gold (^{198}Au) or phosphate (^{32}P), can be used in the treatment of ovarian carcinomas. Since radioactive phosphate (^{32}P) is a pure beta-electron emitter, it penetrates the tissue only superficially.

c. Terminology

The most commonly used unit of radiation is the **rad (radiation absorbed dose).** One rad is the absorbed dose of ionizing radiation that is equivalent to the absorption of 100 ergs per gram of irradiated material. A **gray (Gy) is equivalent to 100 rads.** A **roentgen (R)** is the internationally accepted unit for radiation quantity, and it is that quantity of radiation that produces one electrostatic unit of charge of either sign in one cubic centimeter of dry air at 0°C and standard atmospheric pressure. An **electron volt (eV)** is the amount of energy required to accelerate an electron through a potential difference of 1 volt. A **kilo electron volt (keV)** is equal to 1,000 electron volts, and a **million electron volt (MeV)** is equivalent to 1 million electron volts.

The term **dosimetry** refers to the measurement of the dose that the patient receives, which is determined by calculating the dose at different distances from the source of radiation. The **inverse square law** states that the intensity of the radiation varies inversely as the square of the distance from the source. Thus, the radiation that is present at 2 cm from the source is $(1/2)^2$, or one-fourth that at 1 cm. At 4 cm from the source, the dose is $(1/4)^2$, or one-sixteenth of that at 1 cm. The **half-life** of a radioactive substance is the time that it takes for half of the radioactivity to disintegrate.

d. Radiation effects on tissue

Irradiation may cause tissue damage in three different ways: (1) the photoelectric effect, (2) the Compton effect (scattering), and (3) pair production. All three of these processes result in the ionization of molecules and the production of free radicals. Free hydrogen ions and hydroxyl radicals are produced from the tissue water. Some of these hydrogen atoms find other hydrogen atoms and form a molecule of hydrogen (H_2). Other hyrogen atoms find hydroxyl radicals and reform water (H_2O). **The hydroxyl radicals (OH) also recombine in like manner to form H_2O_2.**

If there are increased amounts of soluble O_2 present in the tissue, there are even more H_2O_2 molecules (peroxide) formed (oxygen effect). These molecules affect the tissue by oxidizing chemical bonds and disrupting cellular activity. When such damage occurs in the nucleus of a cell, then the cell dies. Large amounts of radiation are required to disrupt the cell membrane (1,000 R) or the cytoplasmic enzymes (1 million rads), whereas the chromosomes of most proliferating cells have been found in tissue culture experiments to be subject to damage by only a few hundred rads.

e. Complications of radiation therapy

The appropriate dosage of radiation to the pelvis is dependent upon how it is administered, the time frame in which it is delivered, and the volume of tissue to be radiated. A total of 5,000 rads could be fractionated over a period of five weeks (of five days each) with good tolerance by the patient, whereas if the same dose were to be given in only one day each week for five weeks, it would not be tolerated, unless the volume of tissue to be irradiated was very small (e.g., 1 sq cm). If the area of tissue to be irradiated is the whole pelvis, then large doses of radiation would not be tolerated.

The bowel has the lowest tolerance for irradiation (i.e., 4,500–5,500 R), and the bladder has slightly more tolerance (i.e., 6,000–7,000 R). *The acute complications of radiation therapy consist of tissue edema and necrosis in the region of treatment.* Acute cystitis, proctitis, gastrointestinal symptoms, and rare cases of bone marrow depression may occur. Intestinal damage may occur if the patient has had intracavitary radiation in the face of pelvic adhesions and the fixation of the bowel in the pelvis. Local damage to the mucosa of the bowel may cause proctitis, ulceration, and eventually scarring and stricture of the rectosigmoid colon. Vesicovaginal or rectovaginal fistulae may also occur. Later, ureteric stenosis with progressive hydronephrosis may suggest a recurrence of the malignancy; however, excessive scarring with the obstruction of the ureter secondary to the radiation treatment may be the true etiology in such instances.

PART III

Normal obstetrics

CHAPTER 19

The diagnosis of pregnancy

. . . .

To know just what has to be done, then to do it, comprises the whole philosophy of practical life.
—*Sir William Osler**

. . . .

1. Symptoms and signs of pregnancy

**Any female patient who is in the reproductive
age group should be considered pregnant until
proven otherwise.** A possible pregnancy should be
a primary consideration regardless of the patient's
complaints, since the course of treatment for other
medical conditions may be hazardous to the fetus, and
in turn may involve you in medicolegal problems. As
a consequence, you should always **think pregnancy**
in your management of the female patient.

a. Presumptive findings of pregnancy

Probably one of the most prominent symptoms of
pregnancy is **undue fatigue.** When properly questioned, almost all patients who are pregnant will admit
to this symptom. **Nausea and/or vomiting, breast
swelling and tenderness, increased frequency
of urination,** and, in patients who have been pregnant before, **"a feeling that she is pregnant"** are all
valuable clues. These have been called the presumptive symptoms of pregnancy.

The presumptive signs of pregnancy also include:

(1) the cessation of menses (amenorrhea or oligomenorrhea), (2) a dusky discoloration of the vaginal
mucosa, **which has been called Jacquemin's sign
(sometimes referred to incorrectly as Jacque-
mier's sign, Kluge's sign, or Chadwick's sign),** at
6–8 weeks' gestation, (3) an increased skin pigmentation (chloasma) or the development of striae on the
breasts, the abdomen, or the thighs, and (4) a developing lordosis. While all of the above findings are
clues to the possible diagnosis of pregnancy, they cannot be used to diagnose pregnancy positively.

b. Probable findings of pregnancy

**The probable signs of pregnancy consist of
uterine enlargement with an accompanying enlargement of the abdomen beyond 4 months'
gestation, changes in the consistency of the cervix and uterus, ballottement rebound, Braxton
Hicks contractions, and positive endocrine assay tests for pregnancy.**

By 6–8 weeks' gestation, the cervix assumes a dusky
blue color and becomes softened. This cervical softening has been termed **Goodell's sign.** A fingertip
softening of the isthmus of the cervix has been called
Ladin's sign. Hegar's sign, described by **Reinl,** is
the softening of the entire isthmus of the uterus transversely at about 6–12 weeks' gestation (Fig. 19-1).
When the cervix may be flexed upon the corpus of the
uterus, **McDonald's sign** is said to be present. On
occasion, vaginal or uterine arterial pulsations may be
detected **(Pargamine's sign or Oslander's sign).**
The uterus becomes softened and assumes a globular
shape at about 6–8 weeks' gestation, but is not yet
enlarged.

Between the 5th and the 7th week of pregnancy, a
localized softening occurs over the site of the

---

*Reprinted with permission from Robert Bennett Bean, *Sir
William Osler: Aphorisms from His Bedside Teachings and
Writings,* William Bennett Bean, ed. Springfield, Ill.: Charles
C Thomas, Publisher, 1968, p. 92.

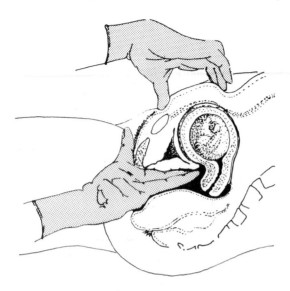

FIGURE 19-1. Hegar's sign.

placenta. **This softening has been called von Braun's sign, or Piskacek's sign, but it should really be attributed to Dickinson** (Fig. 19-2). Beyond 8–9 weeks' gestation, an appreciable change in the size of the uterus can be detected on the bimanual examination, in which the size of the uterus approximates the length of gestation (i.e., at the 12th week of pregnancy, the uterus measures 12 cm from the top of the fundus to the internal examining hand during the bimanual examination). As the uterus rises out of the pelvis beyond the 16th week, the fetus will sometimes bounce away from the examining hand and rebound with a slight tap upon ballottement (ballottement rebound). On occasion, during the examination of the uterus beyond the 20th week, it may be possible to detect irregular mild contractions, or **Braxton Hicks contractions.**

A positive pregnancy test is probable evidence for pregnancy. It should be noted that commercial home pregnancy testing kits have a high rate of false-negative results of the order of 20–25%, but a relatively low false-positive rate (about 5%).

c. Positive findings of pregnancy

The positive diagnosis of pregnancy requires that the fetus itself be identified. In patients who are beyond 16–18 weeks' gestation, you may *detect fetal movements* during the abdominal examination.

In addition, *fetal heart valve movements, or the fetal body itself,* may be detected by ultrasonography. With any of these three findings (i.e., fetal movements, fetal heart valve movements, or fetal body), a definitive positive diagnosis of pregnancy may be made. An ultrasound scan can identify a gestational sac by the 5th or 6th week and will detect fetal heart rate activity by the 6th or 7th week.

2. Tests for pregnancy

Since the discovery of a test for human chorionic gonadotropin (hCG) in 1929 by S. Ascheim and B. Zondek, the detection of this hormone has formed the basis for all chemical tests for pregnancy. By the 1960s, the original biological tests for pregnancy were largely replaced by immunologic techniques because of their increased sensitivity and accuracy. As the sensitivity of these tests increased, however, problems with cross-reactivity with similar compounds began to occur. *Luteinizing hormone (LH) shares the same alpha chain with hCG, but their beta chains are different.* It soon became apparent that

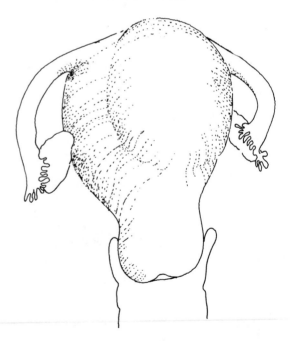

FIGURE 19-2. Dickinson's sign (von Braun's sign, Piskacek's sign).

the pregnancy tests were measuring LH and/or hCG, and that a test that would specifically identify the hCG moiety and not the LH molecule was necessary.

In 1972, a specific radioimmunoassay (RIA) that would identify the beta-subunit of the hCG only was developed. With this test it became possible for the first time to measure hCG with a great amount of sensitivity and specificity.

One of the most popular pregnancy tests today is the enzyme-linked immunosorbent assay (ELISA). This technique utilizes a specific monoclonal antibody. An enzyme identifies the antigen and induces a visible color reaction. The test is simple and is sensitive to 25–50 milli-international units per milliliter (mIU/ml).

The hCG hormone is present in the serum at about 8 days after fertilization, and the value doubles approximately every 29 to 53 hours during the first 30 days after conception has taken place. By about the 60th day of pregnancy, the hCG level peaks at about 100,000 mIU/ml, after which it rapidly decreases to about 5,000 mIU/ml by 100–130 days' gestation, where it remains for the rest of the pregnancy. (Note: The half-life of hCG is about 24–37 hours).

The use of these highly specific tests to detect pregnancy are valuable in the identification of not only an intrauterine pregnancy, but also in the detection of other pregnancy complications. These tests may be used in a quantitative fashion to detect a threatened abortion, or to follow the course of a patient who has trophoblastic disease. The tests that can provide a sensitivity of 50 mIU/ml are satisfactory for diagnostic purposes. Furthermore, those techniques that specifically assay the beta-subunit of the hCG molecule are preferred.

3. Pseudocyesis

Pseudocyesis (i.e., false pregnancy) occurs in about 1:5,000 pregnancies. These patients may present with many of the symptoms of pregnancy. Often they report fetal movements and weight gain associated with amenorrhea. They will often dress in loose clothes that are appropriate to pregnancy and may be quite convincing in their appearance. They may strongly resist any suggestion that they may not be pregnant, even when the β-hCG tests are repeatedly demonstrated to be negative. These patients are usually psychotic (i.e., schizophrenic) and are difficult to manage due to their fixation on their "pregnancy." Psychiatric assistance is often necessary in these cases.

CHAPTER 20

Maternal physiology

1. Cardiovascular system

a. Pregnancy changes

Pregnancy is a kind of stress test for the cardiovascular system. The woman who has a normal heart will readily adapt to the changing workload of the pregnancy without any difficulty; however, the patient who has a diseased heart will frequently decompensate under these stresses. Most of the cardiovascular stresses during pregnancy are secondary to the increase in the plasma volume and the demands for an increased cardiac output.

1) Plasma volume

The total blood volume increases up to 45% during pregnancy. The plasma volume increases during the first trimester to reach approximately 35% more than the nonpregnant levels by the 24th week of pregnancy, and finally up to about 50% more than normal levels between the 33rd week of gestation and term (Fig. 20-1). Multiparous patients will have an increase in their plasma volume of about 300 ml more than will the primigravida. There is also a larger in-

*Reprinted with permission from Robert Bennett Bean, *Sir William Osler: Aphorisms from His Bedside Teachings and Writings,* William Bennett Bean, ed. Springfield, Ill.: Charles C Thomas, Publisher, 1968, p. 92.

PV   multiple gestation > singleton
     multiparous   primigravida

crease in the plasma volume in a multiple gestation than in a singleton pregnancy. These changes generally return to normal by 2–4 weeks' postpartum. ✱

✱ return to ⓝ

2) Red cell volume

The red cell volume progressively increases throughout pregnancy and reaches a value of 20–25% higher than the normal volume, or about 1,800 ml (e.g., the normal nonpregnancy red cell volume is about 1,400 ml). This amount may increase to as much as 2,050 ml with twin gestations, or up to 2,350 ml with triplet pregnancy. These changes usually return to normal by eight weeks' postpartum. ✱ There is a slightly slower expansion of the red cell mass as compared to the plasma volume expansion, which results in a temporary dilutional effect during the second trimester that has been termed the **physiological anemia of pregnancy.** Usually, this effect disappears in the third trimester as the red cell mass catches up to the plasma expansion. It has been found that approximately 500–600 ml of blood is usually lost at delivery, especially if an episiotomy has been performed. The usual blood loss during a cesarean section is of the order of 1,000 to 1,200 ml.

b. Cardiac output

The cardiac output is the product of the heart rate multiplied by the stroke volume. It may be reported in terms of the body surface area, as in the *cardiac index* (i.e., the cardiac index is the cardiac output in liters per minute per square meter of the patient's body surface area), or it may be reported in just liters per minute. The mean cardiac index in normal pregnancy increases by 45% by 20–24 weeks' gestation.

CO/BSA = cardiac index

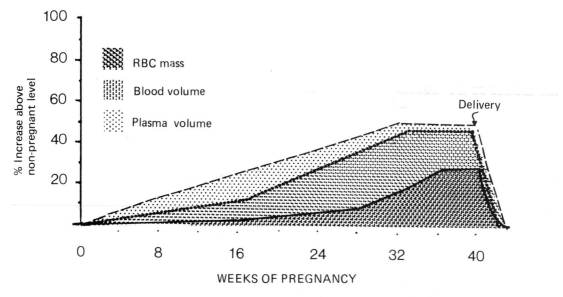

FIGURE 20-1. Percentage changes in blood volume, plasma volume, and red cell mass during pregnancy. (Redrawn with permission from J. Metcalfe, J. H. McAnulty, and K. Ueland, "Cardiovascular Physiology," *Clinical Obstetrics and Gynecology,* 24 (1981), p. 693.)

The cardiac output increases progressively up to about 28–32 weeks of pregnancy, after which it rises more slowly up to term. During labor, *the cardiac output may increase 20–50%* with each contraction. The highest values are usually attained during the first hour postpartum, due to the increased venous return of blood from the contracted uterus and from the lower extremities.

c. Heart rate

The *heart rate increases* throughout pregnancy to reach a value that is *approximately 20% (15 bpm)* higher than the nonpregnant state. During labor, tachycardia may occur secondary to the exertion and pain, which may transiently influence the cardiac output.

d. Stroke volume

The *stroke volume increases* during early pregnancy and is mainly responsible for the increased cardiac output during the first half of gestation. During the last half of gestation, the heart rate increase also contributes to the cardiac output increase. *The stroke volume increases to 25–38% more than the normal volume* (i.e., the normal stroke volume is about 75 ml). In the postpartum period, the stroke volume remains high for about two weeks before returning to normal.

e. Peripheral vascular resistance

The peripheral vascular resistance is directly proportional to the blood pressure and inversely proportional to the cardiac output. *The mean blood pressure and the peripheral vascular resistance decrease during the first and second trimester, while the cardiac output rises.* During the last trimester, there is a slight increase in the peripheral vascular resistance due to the fact that the enlarging uterus tends to compress the inferior vena cava and reduce the venous return to the heart. The pulmonary vascular resistance also decreases somewhat during pregnancy.

It is evident that with all of the cardiovascular changes that occur in pregnancy, the times of greatest cardiovascular stress are primarily during the late second trimester and the immediate postpartum period. If the patient has cardiac disease, it should become symptomatic during these periods.

2. Pulmonary system

a. General considerations

There are three major factors in pregnancy that affect ventilatory mechanisms: (1) there is an upward displacement of the diaphragm of about 4 cm, with an associated flare of the subcostal margins from 68–103 degrees, and an increase in the chest circumference by 6 cm; (2) there is an increase in the progesterone levels, which results in hyperventilation in early pregnancy, occasionally bordering on dyspnea; and (3) there is an increase in the blood volume and blood flow to the lungs to meet the needs of the mother and the fetus.

The entire cardiac output passes through the pulmonary circuit for the purpose of gas exchange. *The pulmonary circuit is a low-pressure, high-capacity system with a relatively low vascular resistance.*

Some of the mechanical aspects of the pulmonary defense system involve the removal of particulate matter. Particles of between 1–5 microns in size are deposited on the mucus and then by means of the ciliated epithelium (*i.e., mucociliary elevator*) are carried from the bronchioles to the trachea, where they are expectorated. Particles of 10 microns in size or larger are removed in the nasopharynx or in the trachea. The **mucociliary elevator** may be altered adversely by high concentrations of oxygen, cigarette smoke, and alcohol. The cough reflex and bronchiole constriction, which are mediated by the vagus, assist in the removal of any particulate matter in the peripheral airways. Histiocytes (fixed tissue macrophages) and alveolar macrophages may ingest some particulate matter. The pulmonary tissue contains both T and B cells. There are, in the upper air passages, a large amount of secretory IgA surface antibodies, whereas in the lower passages, the IgG aids in the opsonification and phagocytosis of the particulate material. IgE is usually only present in patients with allergic pulmonary conditions.

b. Pregnancy changes

There is an increase in the tidal volume (0.1–0.2 l) in pregnancy. There is hyperventilation and a lowering of the blood pCO_2 (i.e., to a pCO_2 of 27–32 mm Hg) with the development of a respiratory alkalosis, which is compensated for by a moderate reduction in the plasma bicarbonate from 26–22 mMoles/l, thus preserving the pH of the blood. The vital capacity (VC) does not change appreciably; however, there is some decrease in both the expiratory reserve volume (ERV) (about minus 15%) and the residual volume (RV) (about minus 20%), which results in a significant reduction in the functional residual capacity (FRC) (about minus 18%). There is an increase in the expiratory capacity (EC) at about seven months' gestation, which appears to compensate for the decreased ERV so that the total lung capacity (TLC) remains unchanged (Fig. 20-2).

3. Renal system

a. Physical changes

During pregnancy, certain changes occur as a result of the hormonal and mechanical effects of the pregnancy. Indeed, *the actual size of the kidneys increases;* they will have lengthened by 1–1.5 cm by term. Most of this increased size is probably due to the increased renal blood flow and the renal vascular volume, as well as to perhaps a slight amount of hypertrophy.

The renal collecting system dilates early in pregnancy and this effect persists until about three months' postpartum. These *physiologic hydroureters,* combined with: (1) the decreased peristalsis of the ureters (i.e., relative stasis of the urine), (2) the increased urine volume in the renal pelvis and ureters, and (3) the presence of glucosuria, all tend to provide conditions that are quite suitable for the development of urinary tract infections (*asymptomatic bacteriuria occurs in from 2–12% of pregnancies*). These changes are due to the increased levels of estrogen and progesterone that are present as well as to the mechanical compression that results from the enlarging uterus. **The ureter on the right side generally dilates more than the one on the left because of the dextrorotation of the uterus and the resultant pressure that is placed upon the right ureter as it crosses the iliac artery at the pelvic brim.** This compression may be demonstrated with an intravenous pyelogram (IVP) as a filling defect in the ureter called the *iliac sign.* The bladder tone decreases during pregnancy and its capacity nearly doubles. There is little change in the mucosa of the bladder, except for the *increased hyperemia* that is common to all of the pelvic organs. At term, *edema of the bladder,* secondary to the pressure of the presenting part, is also

ml

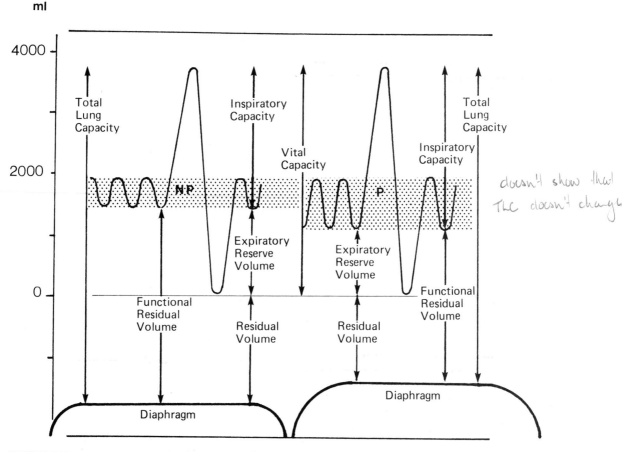

FIGURE 20-2. Lung capacities and volumes. *Left panel:* Nonpregnant (NP). The tidal volume is shaded. *Right panel:* Pregnant (P) (at term). The tidal volume is shaded. Note that the baseline of the residual volume and the functional residual volume is slightly less than in the nonpregnant patient, due to the elevation of the diaphragm. The expiratory reserve volume also decreases.

present. Vesicoureteral reflux occurs in 3.5% of pregnant patients during the last trimester.

b. Functional changes

1) Glomerular filtration rate

The glomerular filtration rate (GFR) and the renal plasma flow (RPF) increase as early as the second month of pregnancy and rise to nearly 50% above normal. This increase persists until the third trimester, when the RPF decreases to the nonpregnant level. As the filtration proceeds from the efferent to the afferent end of the glomerular vessels, the oncotic

pressure increases in the bloodstream owing to the transfer of fluid across the vessel wall. When the glomerular hydrostatic pressure equals the vascular oncotic pressure (i.e., when it reaches filtration equilibrium), then the glomerular filtration ceases.

When the molecular weight of a substance exceeds 70,000, filtration through the glomerulus does not occur. **Essentially all of the filtered water and salts are reabsorbed; otherwise, the urine output would be about 150 liters/day.** Most of the excreted solutes are small molecules that are water soluble and are not protein bound. *Glucosuria occurs in 5–40% of pregnant women owing to the inability of the tubules to reabsorb the increased filtration of*

hypoNa's ↓ bp → renin ↑

glucose. *About 80% of the filtrate is absorbed in the proximal tubules—a process that is not dependent upon hormonal regulation.* **Sodium reabsorption is controlled by aldosterone, while the water concentration is determined by vasopressin, the antidiuretic hormone (ADH) which acts upon the distal tubules.**

The blood urea nitrogen (BUN) and the serum creatinine are both only crude indices of renal function, since over 50% of the renal function must be lost before either becomes greatly abnormal. A plasma creatinine level of greater than 0.8 mg/100 ml, or a BUN of more than 14 mg/100 ml, indicates the possibility of renal disease. The creatinine clearance is a useful test for measuring the GFR in pregnancy and in following patients who have compromised renal function. **The creatinine clearance may be calculated as follows: urine creatinine concentration (mg/ml) times the 24-hour urine volume (ml), divided by the product of the plasma creatinine (mg/100 ml) and 1,440 (minutes/day). The usual creatinine clearance values in pregnancy are of the order of 120–130 ml/min.**

There is a glomerular-tubular balance in pregnancy that allows for an increase in the sodium reabsorption by the tubules to almost equal the increased GFR. Since the normal intake of sodium is about 150–200 mEq/day, it is necessary for the renal tubules to reabsorb 99.5% of the filtered sodium. This glomerular-tubule balance is necessary to maintain the extracellular fluid volume.

2) Hormonal aspects

During pregnancy, there is an increased level of plasma renin activity and aldosterone secretion. **The vascular dilatation and the need for an increased blood volume in pregnancy require that there be an increased retention of sodium and water.** Increased estrogen levels also may be a factor in causing the increase in the extracellular fluid volume. A direct action of estrogen on the renal tubules may account for the increased reabsorption of sodium. Progesterone has an antagonistic action to the salt retention and potassium-losing effects of aldosterone, which may be the reason that hypokalemia does not occur in pregnancy in spite of the high levels of aldosterone.

The elevated progesterone levels in pregnancy result in a mild hyponatremia and in arteriolar vasodila-

tation. **The decreased sodium load that is presented to the macula densa, plus the detection of a hypovolemia by the baroreceptors, act as stimuli to the juxtaglomerular cells for renin production and release.**

The renin glycoprotein substrate (i.e., angiotensinogen) that is produced in the liver is converted by the **renin** into angiotensin I (Fig. 20-3). The **angiotensinogen** production is increased by corticotropin and glucocorticoids, as well as by estrogens. **Angiotensin I** is biologically inactive until it is acted upon in the lung by a converting enzyme to form the biologically active **angiotensin II.** Further degradation of angiotensin II into several smaller peptides, including the biologically less active **angiotensin III,** may then occur.

Angiotensin II, an octapeptide, is the active component of the renin-angiotensin system that causes vasoconstriction and the release of aldosterone and ADH. The ADH causes water retention, while the aldosterone facilitates the salt and water reabsorption. These actions result in a correction of the initial stimulating factors of pregnancy by expanding the blood volume and increasing the sodium retention of the pregnant woman.

Renin is synthesized and stored in a specialized part of the nephron, **the juxtaglomerular apparatus,** a complex of tubular and vascular elements located at the hilus of the glomerulus. The components of the juxtaglomerular apparatus are **the macula densa and the efferent and afferent arterioles. The macula densa is located at the transition from the loop of Henle to the distal tubule.** The afferent arteriole contains the specialized juxtaglomerular cells, which consist of both endocrine and smooth muscle cells that synthesize, store, and release renin. They are innervated by adrenergic nerves.

The rate that renin is secreted is controlled by an intrarenal vascular receptor, the macula densa, the renal nerves, and certain circulating factors, such as epinephrine, potassium, vasopressin, and angiotensin II. The **intrarenal vascular receptor** is a stretch receptor. When there is a **decreased amount of stretch present,** there is an **increase in the renin secretion,** whereas when there is an **increased amount of stretch present,** then there is **a decrease in renin secretion.** As a result, an inverse relationship exists between the renal perfusion pressure and the amount of renin release. **The macula densa causes the renin secretion to increase in**

JG cell have

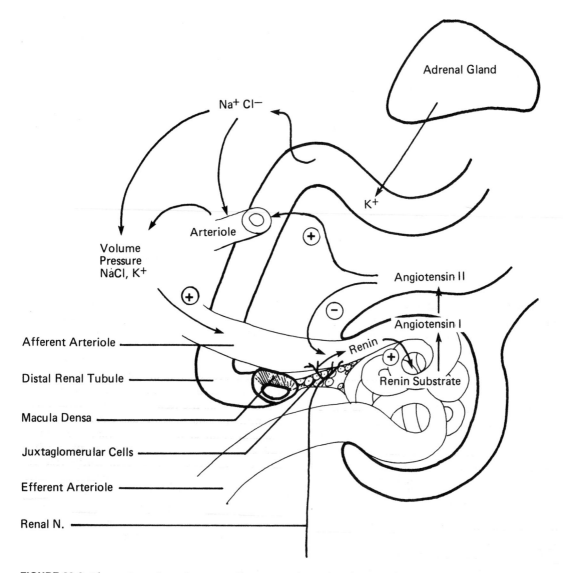

FIGURE 20-3. The renin-angiotensin system. Plus signs indicate stimulation and minus signs indicate inhibition. (Adapted from E. G. Bigieri and J. D. Baxter, in P. Felig, J. D. Baxter, A. E. Broadus, and L. A. Frohman, eds., *Endocrinology and Metabolism.* New York: McGraw-Hill, 1981, p. 556.)

sodium deficiency states and to decrease when sodium intake is high.

The **sympathetic nervous system** is also involved in the control of renin, apparently by the direct stimulation of the beta-adrenergic receptors that are located on the juxtaglomerular cells. Circulating cate-

cholamines will also stimulate the release of renin; however, this function is probably mediated through the extrarenal beta-adrenergic receptors. **Potassium, angiotensin II, and vasopressin inhibit renin secretion.** Hemorrhaging stimulates renin secretion because the reduction in blood volume causes increased renal sympathetic nerve activity, an increase in the circulating catecholamines, and a decrease in the renal perfusion pressure.

Under the influence of angiotensin II, the blood pressure increases without the concomitant bradycardia that is normally seen with other vasoconstrictors (e.g., epinephrine). This increase is apparently due to the central effect of angiotensin II on the vagal tone of the heart.

The renin-angiotensin system, in cooperation with the corticotropin levels and the circulating levels of sodium and potassium, controls the release of **aldosterone** from the zona glomerulosa of the adrenal gland. Those agents that block the secretion of renin or the action of angiotensin II will also result in a decreased secretion of aldosterone. Angiotensin II stimulates the secretion of aldosterone by causing an increased conversion of cholesterol to pregnenolone in the zona glomerulosa cells of the adrenal gland. **Decreased plasma sodium levels result in an increased production of aldosterone.** Angiotensin II stimulates the pituitary, causing an increase in the secretion of corticotropin and vasopressin, which in turn causes an increase in the drinking response.

4. Gastrointestinal system

Due to the elevated progesterone levels in pregnancy, there is a relaxation of the smooth muscle of the intestine, which results in the development of hypomotility of the bowel. This causes a *prolonged gastric emptying time.* Although there is a decreased amount of gastric acid secretion, *pyrosis (heartburn)* is common because of the reduced pressure at the sphincter and the reflux of gastric contents into the distal esophagus. While this effect is largely due to the increased amount of progesterone, the anatomical changes in the esophagogastric angle, due to the enlarging uterus, may also be implicated. The incidence of hiatal hernia is also increased in pregnancy (by 13–22%).

Constipation is relatively common in pregnancy, because of the decreased peristalsis of the bowel. The stasis and prolonged retention of the stool in the lower bowel allows for a greater than normal amount of water to be resorbed, which leads to the development of a firm, hardened stool and difficulty in evacuation. Straining at stool causes an elevation of the venous pressure in the hemorrhoidal

venous system and results in *hemorrhoids,* which are a common cause of intestinal bleeding in pregnancy.

5. Skin

There are some skin changes in pregnancy that occur primarily as a result of the changes in the hormone levels. The melanocyte-stimulating hormone (MSH) is elevated from about the second month of pregnancy to term. This results in an increased amount of pigmentation of the nipples and areolae, the umbilicus, the linea alba (nigra), and the axillary, vulvar, and perianal areas. *Melasma, or chloasma,* is an irregular, splotchy hyperpigmentation of the forehead and cheeks of the pregnant woman, although it may also be seen in women who are taking birth control pills. Nevi and freckles will also darken during pregnancy.

Postpartum hair loss may occur that is similar to the hair loss seen with typhoid fever, scarlet fever, pneumonia, and severe emotional distress. Normal scalp hair development encompasses three stages of growth: anagen, catagen, and telogen. During the **anagen** stage, the hair follicles will actively grow hair. In the **catagen** phase, the hair follicles involute. In the **telogen** stage, the hair follicles enter a resting state. Normally, the scalp hair is asynchronous in its growth and appears to be growing constantly. **Pregnancy has a tendency to cause synergy of the hair growth pattern.** If all of the hair follicles enter the telogen stage, it will appear that the patient is losing her hair, whereas if they all enter the anagen stage, an increased growth of hair may be apparent because of this phenomenon. Occasionally, there may be a considerable increase in the hair growth; however, true hirsutism should suggest the possible presence of a virilizing tumor.

On occasion, the rectus muscles of the abdomen may separate as the uterus enlarges, resulting in *diastasis recti abdominis.* This separation of the rectus muscles may be surgically repaired after the pregnancy has terminated.

The so-called *stretch marks, or striae gravidarum,* that occur across the breasts, the upper arms, the thighs, and the abdomen are apparently the result of the stretching of the skin, plus a "stria factor," which may be an effect of adrenocortical hyperactivity. After a long period of time, the stria will become silver colored. There is no known way to prevent the development of the striae, or to ameliorate their severity once they occur.

Local congestion of the vaginal mucosa occurs early in pregnancy. The proliferation and branching of the arteriolar vessels of the skin will result in the development of spider angiomas in 66% of white women and in 10% of black women. These lesions occur most commonly on the anterior chest, neck, face, and arms. The presence of erythema of the hypothenar eminences and the palmar areas of the hand are due to the elevated estrogen levels. The development of venous varicosities of the legs, vulva, and anus is also common in pregnancy.

6. Musculoskeletal system

During pregnancy there is an accentuation of the lumbar spine lordosis, which causes an upper spine kyphosis as the center of gravity moves backward in the lower spine and forward in the neck region. With the increasing weight gain of pregnancy, the patient's balance becomes even more precarious and the risk of an accidental fall increases. The lordosis occurs quite early in pregnancy and can be observed by an astute physician as the patient walks. This change also predisposes the woman to the development of low backaches. The synchondroses at both the symphyseal and sacroiliac areas separate and become more mobile. **Symphyseal separations** may be as much as 3–7 mm or more; when the separation exceeds 10 mm, the patient may complain of pain and tenderness with radiation down the inner thighs. The sacroiliac mobility frequently results in unilateral low back pain.

Coccydynia, while usually the result of a previous traumatic fracture of the coccyx, can occur in a thin woman when the spinal curvature allows the tip of the coccyx to be directed backward, thus allowing for its compression when the woman sits upon a hard surface.

7. Hematologic system

a. Anemia

It was shown in one study that the hemoglobin concentration at term in pregnant women was about 12.1 grams/dl, as compared to an average of 13.3 grams/dl

in nonpregnant women. In another study, only 6% of patients at term had hemoglobin values below 11 grams/dl. It has generally been accepted that hemoglobin values below 11 grams/dl in late pregnancy probably do represent a state of anemia, which in most cases turns out to be an iron deficiency anemia. **From a practical standpoint, however, a hemoglobin of less than 10 grams/dl, or a hematocrit of less than 30%, has been used in many institutions as the criteria for anemia in pregnancy.**

b. Iron distribution

Iron is distributed in several body compartments as follows: (1) **storage iron** (27%), (2) **hemoglobin iron** (67%), (3) **myoglobin iron** (3.5%), (4) **a labile iron pool** (2.2%), (5) **other tissue iron** (0.2%), and (6) **transport iron** (0.08%). While there is an increase in the amount of iron in each of these compartments during pregnancy, the percentage distribution remains essentially unchanged. **The storage iron accounts for 600–800 mg in the adult woman, whereas the hemoglobin iron averages about 1,700 mg.** When pregnancy occurs, these values increase by 20%. About half of the storage iron is in the ferritin state, with the remainder being hemosiderin. **Since storage iron is always lost first when an anemia develops, its absence is usually the first sign of an iron deficiency anemia.** With further losses, the red blood cell indices decrease and begin to reflect a hypochromic, microcytic anemia.

c. Iron absorption

Iron absorption occurs principally in the duodenum (i.e., the proximal small intestine). Gastric acids convert the various forms of iron that are ingested (i.e., animal hemoglobin, ferric iron from vegetable complexes) to the ferrous form, which becomes more soluble in the alkaline contents of the duodenum. The intestinal mucosal cells of the duodenum and the upper intestine then regulate the amount of iron that may be absorbed. The developing mucosal cells in the basal layer of the crypts of Lieberkühn receive deposits of ferrous iron. The absorbed ferrous iron is then converted to **ferritin** by a chelating agent (i.e., ascorbic acid) and an energy source [i.e., adenosine diphosphate (ADP)], which is then oxidized by ceruloplasmin to convert the iron to the ferric form. **The ferritin acts as a storage depot and is therefore a possible rate-limiting factor in the absorption of iron; the saturation of the cell with ferritin may halt any further absorption of iron from the intestinal lumen.** The ferritin transfers the iron across the cell, where it is then absorbed by the transferrin into the bloodstream. **Transferrin** transports the ferritin to other body sites for subsequent utilization.

d. Iron requirements

The increasing need for iron as the pregnancy advances is reflected in the increasing efficiency of intestinal iron absorption. **The adult nonpregnant human will normally absorb and excrete very little iron.** Only 0.9 mg of iron is excreted each day (i.e., epidermal cell loss and sweat, 0.2 mg; urine, 0.1 mg; the remainder, via the loss of gastrointestinal cells, blood, and bile, 0.6 mg). Iron lost via the menstrual period accounts for about 25–45 ml of blood per month, or if this loss is extrapolated over 30 days, then an additional 0.7–1.4 mg/day of iron may be lost. **Therefore, the normal menstruating female will lose, on the average, about 2.0 mg of iron per day.**

The iron requirements of the entire pregnancy are about 1,000 to 1,200 mg. The recommended dietary allowance (RDA) of iron is 18 mg per day. As the red blood cell mass begins to expand after the 20th week of gestation, the **ordinary dietary iron becomes insufficient** to prevent the loss of the storage iron deposits, because the **normal American diet provides for only about 6 mg of iron per 1,000 calories.** The usual 2,400-calorie diet should therefore provide about 14 mg of iron, of which as much as 25–30% (3.5–4.2 mg/day) may be absorbed in late pregnancy. During the early part of pregnancy, however, the total iron requirements of pregnancy cannot be attained by dietary means alone, since only 10% (1.4 mg/day) may be absorbed in the first trimester, and 25% (3.5 mg/day) in the second trimester. **As a consequence, iron supplementation should be provided for every pregnant woman in order to preserve the storage iron and prevent the development of an iron deficiency anemia.**

The total iron requirements of pregnancy (about 1,200 mg) are accounted for in the following manner: (1) the expansion of the maternal red blood cell mass (400 mg), (2) the transfer of iron to the fetus and placenta (300 mg), (3) the daily loss of iron for the entire pregnancy (200 mg), and (4) the blood loss at the time of delivery (270 mg).

e. Coagulation changes

During pregnancy, there is an increase in the plasma levels of some of the coagulation factors. **Fibrinogen,** which normally averages about 300 mg/dl, may increase by 50% to about 450 mg/dl during pregnancy. **This increase in fibrinogen probably accounts for the increased erythrocyte sedimentation rate (ESR) that has been seen in pregnancy.** Factors VII (proconvertin), VIII (antihemophilic globulin), IX (plasma thromboplastin component, or Christmas factor), and X (Stuart factor), are all increased in pregnancy. Factors XI (plasma thromboplastin antecedent) and XIII (fibrin-stabilizing factor) are decreased in pregnancy. The clotting time of the blood remains normal and the platelet count is not appreciably decreased during pregnancy. The level of maternal plasminogen (profibrinolysin) increases considerably, owing to the increased amounts of circulating estrogens.

8. Endocrine system

There are a number of alterations in the endocrine system during pregnancy, which include: (1) the amount of secretion and excretion of the hormones, (2) the metabolism and degradation of the various hormones, and (3) the amount of protein binding of each of the hormones.

a. Human placental lactogen

Human placental lactogen (hPL) increases throughout pregnancy and contributes to the diabetogenic effect of pregnancy. It may also be involved in the secretion of insulin-like growth factors, which in turn may be associated with fetal growth. The pituitary growth hormone, however, is decreased during pregnancy. With the delivery of the placenta, the hPL decreases immediately, and in women with diabetes, there is a considerable postpartum reduction in the insulin requirements. The secretion of insulin is increased in pregnancy, and due to the antagonism of hPL to the effects of insulin, a hyperinsulinemia develops. The progesterone and cortisone levels may also contribute to these anti-insulin effects.

TABLE 20-1. Thyroid function studies

Test	Normal	Hypothyroidism	Hyperthyroidism	Pregnancy
Measurement of unsaturated serum-binding protein concentration:				
T_3 resin uptake as percentage of uptake (T_3RU)	25–35	Decreased	Increased	Decreased
T_3 resin uptake as percentage of unity (T_3RU%)	0.8–1.2	Decreased	Increased	Decreased
Measurement of circulating thyroid hormones:				
Positively associated with protein concentration				
PBI (μg/dl)	4–8	Decreased	Increased	Increased
T_4 Murphy-Pattee (T_4) (μg/100 ml)	4–11	Decreased	Increased	Increased
T_3 RIA (T_3) (ng/dl)	50–150	Decreased	Increased	Increased
Independent of binding protein concentration				
Free T_4 (μg/dl)	0.6–1.7	Decreased	Increased	
Free T_4 index (ng/dl)	1–3.5	Decreased	Increased	Normal
Measurement of thyrotropin:				
TSH by radioimmunoassay (μU/ml)	0–10	Increased	Decreased	Normal
Measurement of iodine uptake:				
RAI uptake (%)	10–35	Decreased	Increased	Contraindicated

Reprinted with permission from D. N. Danforth and J. R. Scott, eds., *Obstetrics and Gynecology.* Philadelphia: J.B. Lippincott Company, 1986, p. 142.

b. Prolactin

Prolactin increases in the mother throughout pregnancy to levels that may be 10 times higher than normal. There is a concomitant increase in the plasma prolactin levels in the fetus, which may be of fetal pituitary origin rather than being transferred from the mother. While the etiology of the increased levels of prolactin is unknown, it is possible that the elevated estrogen levels may stimulate the secretion of prolactin and that progesterone may inhibit lactalbumin synthesis until after delivery, when the progesterone influence is removed. The prolactin levels in the amniotic fluid decrease after 24 weeks' gestation.

c. Endorphins

During pregnancy, there is an increase in the precursor beta-lipotropin, from which *beta-endorphin* is derived (see Chapter 4). The beta-endorphin level increases throughout pregnancy. Lower levels are found, however, in patients who deliver under epidural anesthesia than in those who deliver without anesthesia. It has been suggested that, in certain stressful deliveries, the fetus may be delivered in a depressed condition, secondary to the increased levels of fetal endogenous opioids (i.e., beta-endorphins).

d. Thyroid

The thyroid gland enlarges during pregnancy and there is an increase in the basal metabolic rate (BMR) by about 25%. This increase in the BMR may be accounted for by the products of conception. *The thyroxine (T_4) levels increase as early as the second month, as do the triiodothyronine (T_3) levels; however, due to the elevated levels of thyroxine-binding globulin (TBG) proteins (alpha globulins), the amount of free hormone is essentially the same (i.e., as much as 85% of the T_4 is bound to TBG). The triiodothyronine resin uptake is decreased.* The cholesterol level is increased (Table 20-1). The placenta produces a chorionic thyrotropin, but its role in the production of a hyperthyroid state in pregnancy is unclear. The thyroid hormones do not cross the placenta.

e. Parathyroid

The level of parathyroid hormone has been variously reported to be increased, normal, or decreased in pregnancy, and it is regulated by the blood calcium levels. The calcitonin levels are considerably increased, as are the plasma vitamin D values, in pregnancy.

f. Adrenal

The adrenocorticotropic hormone (ACTH) is increased during the second and third trimesters. Cortisol is also increased in pregnancy and is bound to a cortisol-binding globulin (i.e., transcortin); however, the free cortisol is increased only slightly. In contrast, deoxycorticosterone (DOC) may be increased considerably during the last trimester of pregnancy. Since there are significant levels of DOC in the amniotic fluid and in the fetal plasma, it has been suggested that the maternal plasma levels may be derived from the fetus. The conversion of progesterone to DOC has also been suggested. Aldosterone secretion increases early in pregnancy, and the renin substrate and angiotensin levels may increase up to tenfold. The natriuretic effect of progesterone is antagonized by the aldosterone. The testosterone and the androstenedione plasma levels are increased in pregnancy and are probably derived from the ovary.

9. Genital system

The changes in the genital system during pregnancy are considerable. The success of the pregnancy resides in large part in the capability of the uterus to accommodate the rapidly enlarging products of conception.

a. Vagina and cervix

The initial congestion of the pelvis during pregnancy is amply demonstrated by the velvety, dusky blue or violaceous color of the mucous membranes of the vagina and cervix, which appears at about the time of the first missed period and intensifies over the next few weeks. The cervix also undergoes softening, due to the edema present, and the endocervical glands develop hypertrophy and hyperplasia. The cervical mucus forms a **plug (i.e., operculum),** which is finally expelled nine months later as the **bloody show** just prior to the onset of labor (i.e., usually within 72 hours).

b. Uterus

The uterus enlarges from a weight of about 50–70 grams in the nonpregnant state to about 1,000–1,100 grams at term by means of hypertrophy. Its capacity increases by 500–1,000 times over normal to accommodate as much as 10 liters or more, although the average volume of the conceptus will only be of the order of about 5 liters. The uterine muscle accomplishes this tremendous change entirely through the stretching and the hypertrophy of the myometrial cells, rather than by the development of new cells. The individual muscle cells may increase their length from 50–500 microns. During the first 12–14 weeks, the uterine enlargement is primarily due to the hormonal effects of the estrogen and the progesterone. **It is at this point in time (i.e., 14–16 weeks' gestation) that the uterine cavity is finally obliterated as the developing conceptus completely fills the uterine cavity space.** From about the fourth month onward, the uterus stretches and distends according to the demands of the products of conception and becomes an abdominal organ. This growth pressure is also exerted upon the cervix, so if there is an incompetent cervix present, then a second trimester loss may occur.

Due to the presence of the rectosigmoid colon, with its continual passage of firm stool, the uterus will usually rotate to the right. This *dextrorotation,* along with the enlargement of the uterus, places tension upon the broad ligaments and the round ligaments. This tension and stretching may result in round ligament pains.

The uterine wall consists of layers of interlacing muscular fibers that produce a sphincter-like effect upon the penetrating blood vessels. After delivery, this constriction of the vessels by the contracted uterus acts to prevent the development of a postpartum hemorrhage. From early pregnancy onward, the patient may feel periodic mild irregular contractions of the uterine muscle (i.e., Braxton Hicks contractions).

The hormone **relaxin** is produced by the corpus luteum in small amounts throughout pregnancy. This hormone's function has not been completely defined; however, it does seem to be involved in the softening, or "ripening" effect, of the cervix near term.

During pregnancy there is an increase in the size and the number of the blood vessels and the lymphatics, and there is also a hypertrophy of the nerves supplying the uterus. **The uterine blood flow is of the order of 500–750 ml per minute at term.** Although the initial amount of uterine blood flow increases throughout pregnancy, the blood flow per gram of tissue seems to remain somewhat constant. The uterine blood flow is divided into that flow which supplies the intervillous space (approximately 90%) and that flow which supplies the myometrium (about 10%). Some of the studies in animals have shown that the uterine vascular bed is almost completely dilated, perhaps secondary to the estrogen levels. However, the administration of estradiol-17β to sheep in late pregnancy has been shown to increase the placental blood flow by as much as 25%.

c. Tubes and ovaries

With the onset of pregnancy, the ovarian corpus luteum is stimulated by chorionic gonadotropin to produce progesterone to maintain the pregnancy during the first seven weeks, after which time steroid-ogenesis in the placenta is well established. At the time of a cesarean section, small, elevated patches of papillary excrescences that bleed easily may be found on the ovaries, uterus, and the fallopian tubes. This *decidual reaction* is secondary to the hormonal stimulation of the pregnancy.

10. Metabolism

During pregnancy, profound changes take place in the maternal metabolism, especially those concerned with the increasing blood volume, the increasing mass of the uterus and the breasts, and the rapidly growing products of conception. **A woman's weight will usually increase by at least 24 lbs throughout the pregnancy, with approximately a 2-lb weight gain in the first trimester, an 11-lb gain in the second trimester, and another 11-lb gain in the third trimester.** It is recommended that the patient gain between 20 and 27 lbs during a normal pregnancy. This weight gain is partially accomplished by the retention of about 6.5 liters of water; of this amount, about 3.5 liters are present in the products of conception and the remainder are due to the maternal blood volume expansion and the increased size of the uterus and breasts. There is also a gain of about 1,000 grams of protein during pregnancy, with about 500 grams being found in the placenta and the fetus and the remainder in the maternal tissues (i.e., the uterine muscle, the glandular tissue of the breasts, the red blood cells, and the plasma proteins).

There does not seem to be a clear definition of maternal obesity during pregnancy. Some studies have used a value of more than 120 or 150% of the patient's standard weight, with a height adjustment. Others have utilized the value of more than 198 or 250 lbs while pregnant as a measure of obesity; however, this method does not take into account the patient's height, and certainly the height would have a significant effect upon the determination of weight excess. If the patient's normal nonpregnant weight for height is exceeded by 20%, plus the 27 lbs due to the pregnancy, then this might be one way to define obesity. From a practical viewpoint, a weight of more than 200 lbs should make you suspect the presence of gestational diabetes in the patient. Other diseases, such as hypertension, toxemia, and dysfunctional labor, are also more common in obese patients. Indeed, nearly two-thirds of women who weigh more than 250 lbs in pregnancy will develop an obstetric complication.

In normal-sized women, the weight gain during pregnancy is directly related to the resulting fetal weight. If there has been only a minimal weight gain, then the infant may be small at birth. If there has been an adequate weight gain in the normal patient, then the infant will be of average size. The obese woman, however, should not diet during pregnancy, and her total weight gain should be at least 20 lbs or more.

The recommended daily allowances (RDA) for the various vitamins and minerals during pregnancy are as follows: (1) Vitamin A = 5,000 IU, (2) Vitamin D = 400 IU, (3) Vitamin E = 15 IU, (4) Vitamin C = 60–80 mg, (5) Vitamin B_1 (thiamine) = 1.5 mg, (6) Vitamin B_2 (riboflavin) = 1.6 mg, (7) Vitamin B_3 (niacin) = 15–18 mg, (8) Vitamin B_6 (pyridoxine) = 2.5 mg, (9) Vitamin B_{12} = 4.0 μg, (10) folate = 0.8 mg, (11) zinc = 20 mg, (12) magnesium = 450 mg, (13) iodine = 125–175 μg, and (14) calcium = 1,200 mg.

Pregnancy has been described as a *diabetogenic event*. The interplay of the placental lactogen, estrogen, progesterone, and perhaps the corticosteroids seems to have a deleterious influence on the maternal metabolism to bring this situation about. Placental lactogen causes an increase in the plasma free fatty acids, ketones, and triglycerides through its lipolytic action. The increased secretion of insulin in response to glucose ingestion (i.e., the relative insulin resistance) appears to be secondary to both progesterone and estrogen. Due to the utilization of glucose by the fetus, the fasting maternal glucose levels are usually lower than normal in spite of the fact that glucose production increases. Glucose is transported across the placenta to the fetus by facilitated diffusion, but **insulin does not cross the placenta.** Due to the increased insulin resistance in pregnancy, the mother's plasma glucose concentration may show an exaggerated increase following the ingestion of glucose (i.e., abnormal glucose tolerance test). These levels return to normal following pregnancy. If there is an inherited or an acquired defect in the pancreatic beta cell function, the demands of pregnancy may precipitate the development of overt diabetes mellitus.

In pregnancy, there is an elevation in total lipids, total cholesterol, phospholipids, free fatty acids, ketones, and triglycerides. Due to these elevated levels, starvation during pregnancy results in an exaggerated response with the development of a more intense ketosis than in nonpregnant individuals. **In at least one study, it was noted that the infants of mothers who experienced ketosis had a lower intelligence quotient (I.Q.)** than those born to other women.

11. Immunologic considerations

a. Maternal-fetal allograft

Pregnancy is a unique situation immunologically in that the fetus represents an allograft on the maternal organism. Several theories have been advanced to account for the fact that the fetus is not immediately rejected by the maternal host tissues. It has been suggested that: (1) there is a maternal-fetal barrier due to poorly expressed alloantigens or to blocking antibodies that affect antigen expression; (2) masking of the surface antigens by a sialomucin coating or by blocking antibodies may occur; (3) suppressor factors may be synthesized by the maternal, fetal, or placental systems; (4) the maternal antibodies are ingested and digested by cells through pinocytosis; or (5) there is a separation of the maternal vascular and lymphatic systems. While each of these proposed mechanisms is attractive, it is unknown at the present time whether any of these explanations is correct.

b. Maternal immunologic system

The maternal organism is capable of responding to infections in pregnancy. IgG is the only immunoglobulin that may cross the placenta and provide a passive immunity for the fetus; the IgM, IgA, IgD, and IgE immunoglobulins do not cross the placenta.

CHAPTER 21

Fetoplacental physiology

To carefully observe the phenomena of life in all its phases, normal and perverted, to make perfect that most difficult of all arts, the art of observation, to call to aid the science of experimentation, to cultivate the reasoning faculty, so as to be able to know the true from the false—these are our methods.

—*Sir William Osler**

1. Placental development

a. Implantation

On the 6th day following fertilization, the blastocyst attaches itself to the endometrium with the inner cell mass adjacent to the endometrial surface. Apparently, the trophoblastic tissue releases a substance that destroys the surface epithelial cells, which thus allows the blastocyst to burrow into the endometrium (**implantation**), following which the endometrium then grows over the invasion site (Fig. 21-1). **As the invasion proceeds, the maternal venous blood vessels are tapped to form lakes of blood, which in turn coalesce between the solid trophoblastic columns to form the primitive intervillous space. Chorionic villi can be identified by about 12 days after fertilization.** While the maternal venous blood vessels are tapped early, the arterial blood vessels are not involved until after the 15th day, and **by the 17th day, a functioning placental circulation is established.**

*Reprinted with permission from Robert Bennett Bean, *Sir William Osler: Aphorisms from His Bedside Teachings and Writings,* William Bennett Bean, ed. Springfield, Ill.: Charles C Thomas, Publisher, 1968, p. 61.

chorion vs amnion

trophoblastic → *cytotrophoblast* → *syncitiotrophoblast*

b. Early placental development

The cytotrophoblastic columns are anchored to the decidua at the basal plate—which consists of cytotrophoblastic tissue from the columns plus the syncytium from the trophoblastic base—to form the floor of the **intervillous space (IVS).** As the zygote grows, the villi proliferate into tree-like structures classified as **primary, secondary, and tertiary.** These villi hang down from the chorionic plate into the IVS. The roof of the IVS consists of trophoblastic tissue and fibrous mesoderm. True cotyledons develop at about the 7th week.

The overlying endometrium that covers the conceptus is called the **decidua capsularis,** while the decidual tissue lying between the blastocyst and the myometrium is termed the **decidua basalis** (Fig. 21-2). The villi that lie on the decidua basalis develop a leafy appearance and are called **chorion frondosum.** The decidua of the remainder of the endometrial cavity is called the **decidua vera.** By about the 3rd or 4th month, a large part of the chorion in the area of the decidua capsularis loses its villi and becomes known as the **chorion laeve (or "bald" chorion). The trophoblastic tissue is divided into the cytotrophoblast, which consists of individual cells, and the syncytiotrophoblast, in which the nuclei share a common cytoplasm (i.e., a syncytium).**

c. The placenta

The human placenta is classified as a hemochorial placenta because it has three layers of fetal tissue interposed between the maternal and the fetal circulations (i.e., trophoblast, mesenchyme, and fetal capillary endothelium). In some species, the maternal endothelium, connective

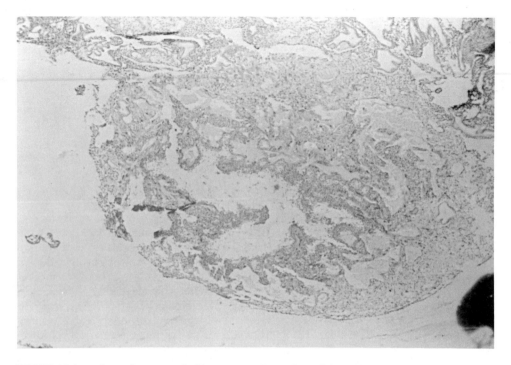

FIGURE 21-1. Early implantation of a blastocyst on the surface of the endometrium. (Courtesy of Soheir Nawas, M.D.)

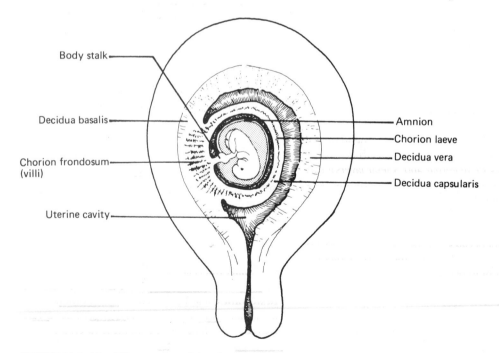

FIGURE 21-2. The different types of decidua in early pregnancy.

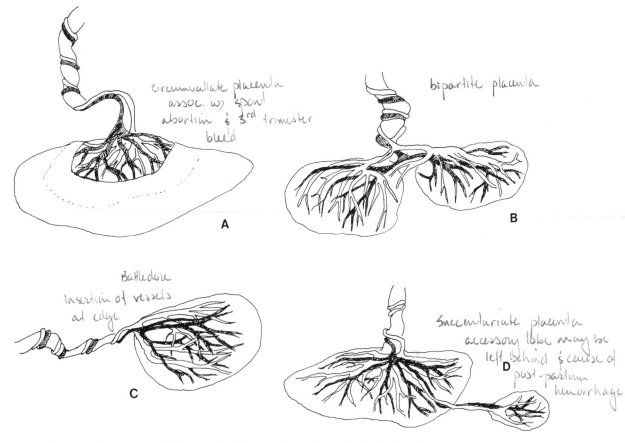

circumvallate placenta assoc. w/ spont abortion & 3rd trimester bleed

bipartite placenta

A

B

Battledore insertion of vessels at edge

Succenturiate placenta accessory lobe may be left behind & cause of post-partum hemorrhage

C

D

FIGURE 21-3. Different types of placentas. (A) Circumvallate placenta. (B) Bipartite placenta. (C) Battledore placenta. (D) Succenturiate lobe.

tissue, and epithelium are interposed between the fetal trophoblast, connective tissue, and fetal endothelium in a variety of layer combinations. While such a classification has been useful in defining the placentas of pigs (3 maternal and 3 fetal layers); sheep, cows, and goats (2 maternal and 3 fetal layers); cats and dogs (1 maternal and 3 fetal layers); rhesus monkeys and humans (0 maternal and 3 fetal layers), and rabbits, rats, mice, and guinea pigs (0 maternal and 1–2 fetal layers), it has not been very useful from a physiologic viewpoint because the transfer of substances is not necessarily impeded when there are additional layers, nor is it unimpeded with fewer layers.

d. Types of placentas

There are a number of morphologic variations in the anatomy of the placenta. In 3% of patients, a small accessory lobe may be present **(i.e., succenturiate lobe),** which may be left behind at the time of delivery and become a cause of postpartum hemorrhage. **A bilobed placenta, or placenta bipartita,** occurs in 1:350 deliveries. **A ring-shaped placenta** occurs in 1:6,000 deliveries. An overgrowth and an infolding of the chorion may produce an edge of whitened tissue about the placenta; this type is called a **circumvallate placenta.** This particular placental malformation has been associated with abortion and with third-trimester vaginal bleeding. If the umbilical cord inserts into the edge of the placenta, it is called a **battledore placenta** (Fig. 21-3).

A **velamentous insertion of the cord into the membranes** may also occur; if this portion of the membranes presents at the cervical os, then a **vasa previa** is said to be present. In these cases, the blood vessels may rupture—with or without the concomi-

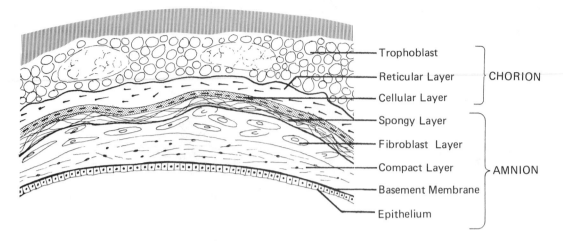

Trophoblast
Reticular Layer   } CHORION
Cellular Layer

Spongy Layer
Fibroblast Layer
Compact Layer   } AMNION
Basement Membrane
Epithelium

FIGURE 21-4. Composite diagram showing the relationships of the layers of amnion and chorion.

tant rupture of the membranes—which may result in the exsanguination of the fetus. Another rare type of placentation involves the persistence of the villi of the chorion laeve, which results in a large, thin placenta that is part of the fetal membranes (**i.e., placenta membranacea**).

The normal term placenta is a circular, plate-like structure that weighs about 500 grams, or about 14% of the fetal weight. It usually measures 15–20 cm in diameter and 2–3 cm in thickness. The chorionic and amniotic membranes contain the amniotic fluid, which provides for the development of the fetus. These thin membranes have several layers (Fig. 21-4, Fig. 21-5).

The **umbilical cord** usually measures from 50–70 cm in length but may be as short as 20 cm or as long as 150 cm. It consists of a small amount of connective tissue and a gelatinous substance (i.e., Wharton's jelly) in a cord-like structure surrounded by amnion and contains two umbilical arteries and one umbilical vein. The cord is somewhat erectile and is not easily compressed if the blood flow and pressure are normal. The vessels tend to coil about each other, especially the vein, which may result in false knots, or even true knots, if the cord is knotted upon itself. This latter complication usually occurs with longer cords in which the infant has maneuvered itself through a loop. The blood pressure is about 60 mm Hg (systolic) and 30 mm Hg (diastolic) in the arteries and about 12–20 mm Hg in the umbilical vein.

The ductus venosus is under nervous control and

may function as a regulator of the blood flow to the liver and to the inferior vena cava; it may also regulate the umbilical vein pressure.

e. Placental circulation

The uteroplacental blood flow is estimated to be about 500–750 ml/minute at term, with the majority of the blood flow going to the placental circulation. The placental circulatory bed is usually maximally dilated. On the fetal side, more than 90% of the umbilical blood flow is to the cotyledonary villus vessels.

The maternal circulation of the placenta is derived from the uterine artery, which traverses the uterine muscle to the basal layer of the endometrium. Studies by **Elizabeth Ramsey** and her coworkers in 1963 using radiopaque dye demonstrated the mechanism of the placental circulation. According to these studies, the circulation of the placenta is as follows: (1) the spiral arteries (the terminal branches of the uterine arterial system) enter the basal plate of the placenta where they open into the floor of the intervillous space (IVS); (2) the spiral artery blood spurts into the IVS of the cotyledon, where it then fountains up through the hollow center of the IVS toward the chorionic plate; and (3) the blood then drains down past the tree-like fronds of the fetal villous branches to the maternal veins in the basal plate, and thence to the veins that drain the uterus (Fig. 21-6). There are perhaps 36–60 cotyledons in the placenta, of which only

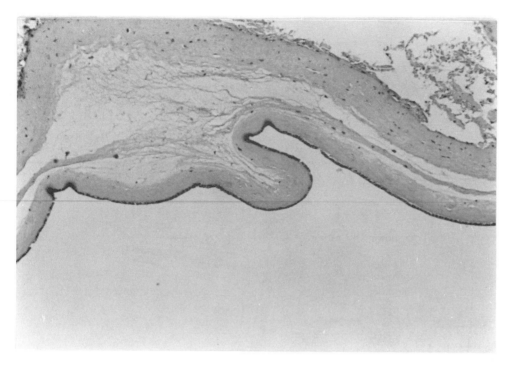

FIGURE 21-5. Amnion and chorion (lower to upper surfaces). The amniotic epithelium is on the lower surface. Immediately above it is the thin compact layer. Above the fibroblast layer is the looser spongy layer. The reticular area above these layers lies just below the trophoblastic tissue, which is somewhat fragmented. (Courtesy of Remi Gomila, M.D.)

about 12–15 may be fully developed. Since the spiral arteries of the cotyledons and their accompanying veins traverse the myometrium of the uterus, uterine contractions temporarily shut off the arterial and venous blood flow to the IVS. (Note: This fact provides the basis for the contraction stress test of fetal status.)

f. Placental endocrine functions

One of the first placental hormones produced by the developing early trophoblastic tissue is the **human chorionic gonadotropin (hCG).** This hormone is present in the maternal serum by the 9th day after ovulation and fertilization have taken place. The titers increase to a maximum level by about 60–80 days' gestation, after which they decrease to low levels by about the 120th day. This glycoprotein hormone has a molecular weight of about 38,000 and has a high carbohydrate content (30%). It is made up of an alpha- and a beta-subunit, which are divided into two different moieties. The α-subunits of all human glycoproteins are similar, whereas the β-subunits are separate and distinct. This difference allows for the detection of hCG by testing for its β-subunit (see Chapter 19). This hormone is produced in the **syncytiotrophoblastic tissue** rather than in the cytotrophoblastic cells. Its primary function is to maintain the production of progesterone in the corpus luteum during the first 40 days or so of pregnancy until the placenta can produce enough progesterone by itself. The higher levels of hCG at 8–10 weeks' gestation may further serve to shut down the production of progesterone in the corpus luteum of the ovary. It has been suggested that the peak production of hCG may also assist the male testicular production of testosterone, which is essential for male sexual differentiation, since it may act as a substitute LH when the fetal pituitary is not fully developed.

Human placental lactogen (hPL) is a polypeptide hormone (M.W. 22,000) that has both lactogenic and growth hormone activities. This hormone can be detected very early in pregnancy (6 weeks postfertili-

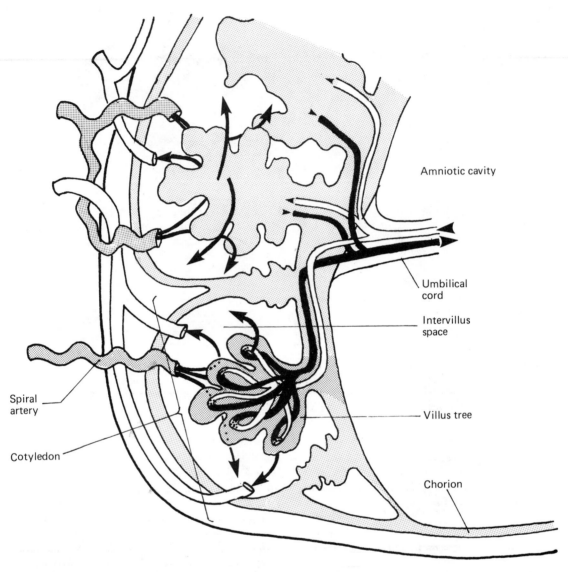

FIGURE 21-6. The fetal and maternal placental circulation.

zation), after which it increases throughout pregnancy. It disappears immediately after delivery with the removal of the placenta. This hormone seems to be concerned with the diabetogenic and anti-insulin effects of pregnancy, which in turn cause an increase in protein synthesis. This increased supply of amino acids is beneficial to the fetus. Human placental lactogen (hPL), however, does not seem to be essential for the continuation of a normal pregnancy.

Human chorionic thyrotropin (hCT) (M.W. 28,000) is a glycoprotein that is thought to be produced by the placenta. Its function in pregnancy is unknown.

Adrenocorticotropic hormone (ACTH) is also thought to be produced by the placenta, perhaps in the chorionic tissue. Chemically it may be somewhat different from normal pituitary ACTH, since it is not suppressed by dexamethasone. The role of placental ACTH is unknown in pregnancy.

Antibodies against the serum of pregnant women that have been developed in animals have allowed the identification of antigens that seem to be specific for pregnancy. It is unknown whether these **pregnancy-specific** compounds have a role in pregnancy.

Estrogens are produced in the placenta by the conversion of dehydroisoandrosterone sulfate to estrone and estradiol-17β; by the 7th week more than 50% of the estrogens in the maternal serum are derived from the placenta. In the third trimester, the dehydroisoandrosterone sulfate, which is derived from the adrenal gland of both the mother and the fetus, is converted by the liver into 16α-hydroxydehydroisoandrosterone sulfate. This compound is then transferred to the placenta, where the placental sulfatase enzyme cleaves the sulfate from the molecule. It is then aromatized and converted to **estriol,** after which it is transferred to the maternal bloodstream for excretion. About 90% of the estriol produced during pregnancy is derived from fetal precursors.

Progesterone is produced in the placenta from lipoprotein cholesterol early in pregnancy and increases gradually throughout pregnancy to reach a level of about 250 mg/day near term. Beyond about the 6th or 7th week of gestation, the removal of the ovaries has no effect on the conceptus or on progesterone levels.

2. Placental transfer mechanisms

a. Early zygote development

The initial development of the zygote following fertilization is as follows: **(1) 0–24 hours, the one-cell stage; (2) 24–36 hours, the two-cell stage; (3) 36–48 hours, the four-cell stage; (4) 48–72 hours, the eight-cell stage; and (5) 72–96 hours, the sixteen-cell stage.** Between 72 and 120 hours after fertilization, a solid ball of cells called the **morula** is formed and enters the uterine cavity, where it is transformed into a fluid-filled **blastocyst. On day 6, the blastocyst implants in the endometrium, with the embryonic pole in contact with the endometrial surface. The embryonic period (i.e., the period of organogenesis)** then **extends from about day 13 to day 56 after fertilization (i.e., organogenesis extends from about day 31 to 71 after the last menstrual period). Organogenesis is followed by the fetal period,** **which encompasses the remainder of the pregnancy (i.e., day 71 to day 280).**

On the 7th or 8th day, the inner cell mass develops at one end of the blastocyst. From this mass of cells are derived the embryo, the yolk sac, and the amnion. **This embryonic disk consists of a plate of primitive ectoderm with its overlying endoderm layer** (Fig. 21-7). The amniotic cavity develops and becomes lined by the contiguous ectoderm from the embryonic disk. Superficial to the embryonic disk is a space (i.e., the blastocoele) that becomes lined by the contiguous endoderm to form the primitive yolk sac. The areas of the blastocyst between the *ectoderm* and the *endoderm* are filled with primary *mesoderm.* **From these three germ layers (i.e., ectoderm, mesoderm, and endoderm), all of the fetal tissues and organs are ultimately derived** (Fig. 21-8).

As the amniotic membrane and the amniotic space develop, they eventually envelop the embryo and come into contact with the inner side of the chorion by the end of the first trimester. There are no blood vessels, nerves, or lymphatic channels in the amnion, but both the amnion and the chorion have extensive endocrine capabilities.

b. Transfer mechanisms

The transfer mechanisms of the placenta involve the following: (1) simple diffusion, (2) facilitated diffusion, (3) active transport, (4) pinocytosis, and (5) solvent drag. The physiochemical characteristics that significantly increase the transfer of a chemical across the placental membrane are: (1) the concentration gradient (i.e., from a high concentration to a low one), (2) the molecular size of the substance (i.e., less than 700 daltons), (3) the electric charge (i.e., un-ionized), (4) the protein binding (i.e., unbound), and (5) the lipid solubility (i.e., soluble).

The increase in the plasma volume and the decrease in the amount of plasma albumin during pregnancy affects the placental transfer of substances. It is obvious that when substances are highly protein bound, or in low concentrations in the maternal plasma, there is minimal transfer of the substance across the placenta to the fetus. With decreased protein binding more of a substance is free, allowing for a greater transfer across the placenta. The amount of uterine blood flow and the villus exchange area that is

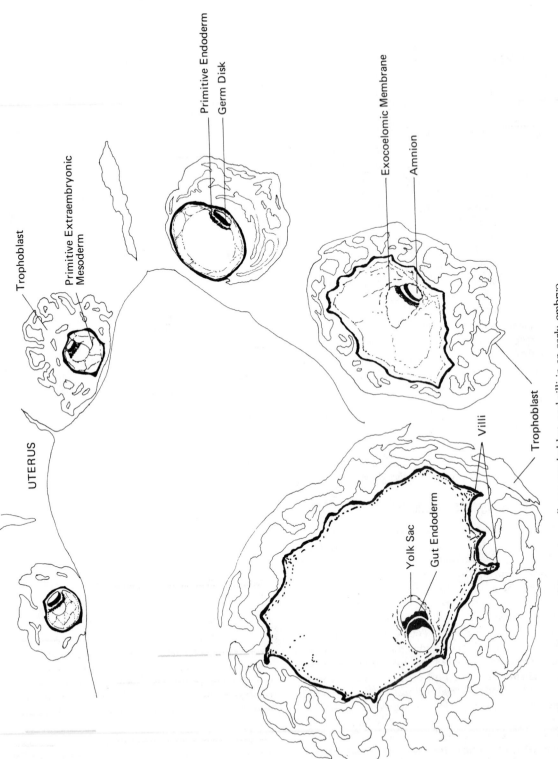

FIGURE 21-7. The development of the amnion, yolk sac, trophoblast, and villi in an early embryo.

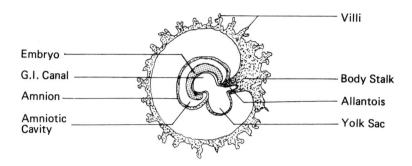

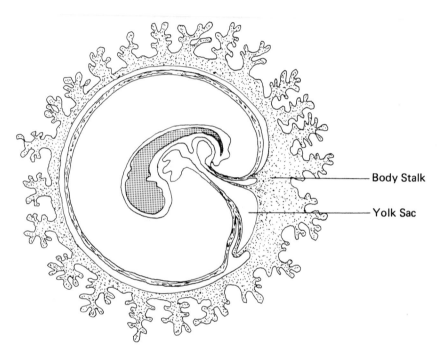

FIGURE 21-8. The further development of the amniotic cavity, yolk sac, allantois, and umbilical cord.

involved are also important factors in the transfer of materials. Uncharged particles cross more rapidly, as do molecules that are lipid soluble. Furthermore, the physical and chemical properties of the three tissue barriers certainly may affect the mechanism of diffusion or, as in the case of active transport, may limit the amount of expendable energy needed for transport.

Oxygen, carbon dioxide, and univalent ions are usually transported across the placenta by **simple diffusion.** Glucose and divalent ions such as calcium,

iron, and phosphorus are transported by **facilitated diffusion. Active transport,** which requires the expenditure of energy, is the mechanism for the transport of amino acids and vitamins. **Pinocytosis** requires that the cell envelop a large molecule in a vacuole in order to transport them across to the other side. In situations in which there is a mass flow from one membrane compartment to another, substances may be dragged along with the fluid **(i.e., solvent drag).**

3. Amniotic fluid

The amniotic fluid is involved in the exchange of substances between the mother and the fetus in ways that are largely unknown. *Substances are circulated and recirculated in this changing pool of fluid.* **The half-life of amniotic fluid has been estimated to be about 90 minutes. The amniotic fluid provides: (1) a cushion for the fetus, (2) a constant temperature buffer, (3) a waste deposit area for fetal urine, (4) a source of fluid for fetal swallowing, (5) a reservoir for protein (i.e., 0.8 grams of protein per day) and minerals, (6) fluid for respiratory activity, (7) fluid for muscular exercise of the limbs and trunk, (8) protection of the skin from drying out, and (9) prevention of deformation of fetal parts (e.g., skull). It may also serve many other functions that have yet to be defined** (see Chapter 26). In some cases, there may be an excess of fluid *(i.e., hydramnios),* of the order of about 2,000 ml instead of the normal 800–1,000 ml, or a lack of fluid *(i.e., oligohydramnios).* Oligohydramnios has been variously defined as a volume of fluid that is "less than normal," or as less than 500 ml, or as less than a pocket of fluid that measures 1 (or 2) cm in a vertical plane on an ultrasound examination. A less than normal amount of fluid may be found in patients who are postdates or who have a fetus with renal agenesis or intrauterine growth retardation (60%). It has been suggested that if the largest amniotic fluid pocket is measured in each of the four quadrants of the abdomen and these amounts are summed to produce an *amniotic fluid index,* then a more accurate evaluation of oligohydramnios may be determined. If this amniotic index was less than 5.0 cm, then, at least according to one study, there was a greater incidence of nonreactive nonstress test results (30%), fetal heart rate decelerations (44%), meconium staining (54%), and low five-minute Apgar scores (23%).

The amniotic fluid contains variable amounts of particulate matter, such as scalp hair, lanugo, fetal cells, and vernix caseosa. In addition, uric acid, creatinine, bilirubin, and various other solutes are also present. The volume of the amniotic fluid is about 50 ml at 12 weeks' gestation, 500 ml at 24 weeks, and 1,000 ml at 38 weeks, after which it gradually decreases. Fetal urine is increasingly added from midpregnancy onward, so that at term the fetus may excrete 600–700 ml per day of hypotonic urine. Fetal

swallowing and the exchange of amniotic fluid by fetal breathing movements also increases as pregnancy advances.

4. Fetal growth and development

a. Cardiovascular system development

The two heart tubes join together to form a single heart tube by the 20th day (Fig. 21-9). Shortly thereafter the four primitive chambers of the heart become defined (i.e., the sinus venosus, the atrium, the ventricle, and the bulbus cordis). The primitive tubular heart bends upon itself so that the atrium and the sinus venosus become more dorsal to the truncus arteriosus and the bulbus cordis. *By the 28th day, the atria are formed as the septum primum descends toward the atrioventricular cushion. The bulbus cordis forms the right ventricle and the primitive ventricle forms the left ventricle, with the wall between them becoming the interventricular septum. Cushions of tissue appear at the atrioventricular ring and become the mitral and tricuspid valves.* The septum primum unites with the atrioventricular cushions; however, a foramen secundum remains, which connects the two atria. By the end of the 7th week, a portion of the septum secundum that lies alongside the septum primum *(i.e., the crista dividens)* extends cranially down over the foramen secundum (i.e., foramen ovale) in the right atrium. A part of the septum primum in the left atrium forms a valve, which allows the blood to only flow through the intra-atrial opening *(i.e., foramen ovale)* from the right atrium to the left atrium.

By the 22nd day, early contractions of the primitive heart begin; however, they do not become effective until about the 28th day. With the use of ultrasound, the fetal heartbeat can be detected as early as the 44th day.

In the fetus, the *ventricles of the heart act in parallel* instead of in the serial configuration that is seen in the adult. Of the total cardiac output (in sheep), about 67% is derived from the right ventricle and only 33% from the left ventricle. This difference in output is due to the shunting of blood through the foramen ovale and the ductus arteriosus. The systemic arterial pressure and the pulmonary artery pressure in the fetus are the same, averaging about 55 mm of Hg. To ensure a right-to-left shunt of the blood in the heart at the

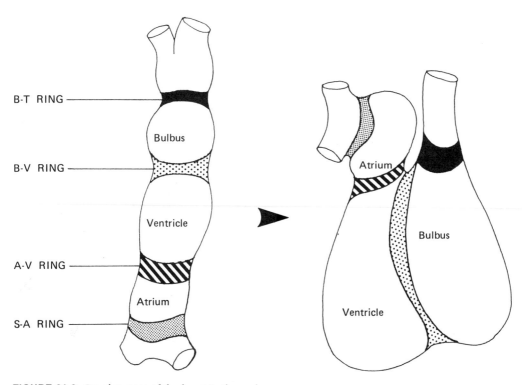

FIGURE 21-9. Development of the heart in the embryo.

foramen ovale, there is a slightly higher pressure in the right atrium (3 mm Hg) than in the left atrium (2 mm Hg). The average fetal heart rate at 5 months is about 155 bpm, after which it gradually declines to about 140 bpm at term. During the last trimester, the heart rate is controlled by the sympathetic and parasympathetic (vagus) nervous system. Vagal fibers impinge on the sino-auricular node (SA node) and the atrioventricular node (AV node) and are responsible for the slowing of the heart as well as for the beat-to-beat baseline variability of the heart rate. Sympathetic nerves are widely distributed to the heart and, when stimulated, cause an increase in the heart rate as well as an increase in the strength of the cardiac contractions.

The umbilical venous blood returning from the placenta flows at an average of 175 ml/kg/min with a pressure of about 12 mm Hg (Fig. 21-10). The fetus requires a continuous supply of oxygen at a level of about 7 ml/kg of body weight. The blood has an oxygen saturation of about 80–85%, and **the fetal scalp blood pO$_2$ is of the order of about 28–30 mm Hg.** Upon reaching the liver, about half of the blood perfuses the hepatic circuit through the **portal sinus branch** of the umbilical vein, while the other half is shunted through the **ductus venosus branch** to the inferior vena cava. This highly oxygenated blood then passes to the right atrium, where it meets with superior vena cava blood flow, which contains relatively unoxygenated blood. The **crista dividens** shunts the inferior vena cava blood flow across the **foramen ovale** into the left atrium and down into the left ventricle, where it is ejected out the ascending aorta. The oxygen saturation of the ascending aorta will have decreased to about 65%; however, it is to be noted that the liver, the heart, and the brain generally receive the most oxygenated blood. The superior vena cava blood flow, with an oxygen saturation of only about 40%, is deflected first into the right atrium by the crista dividens and then into the right ventricle, where it is ejected out the pulmonary artery. Most of this pulmonary artery blood flow (65–90%) goes across the **ductus arteriosus** into the descending aorta (with an oxygen saturation about 60%), and the

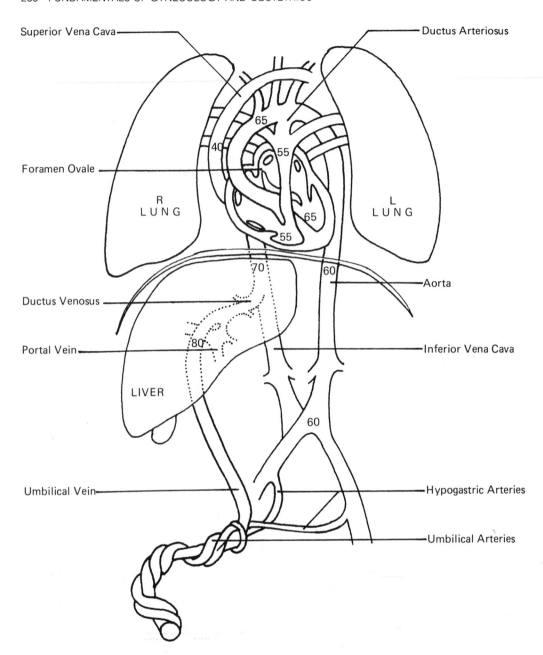

FIGURE 21-10. The fetal circulation. (Redrawn with permission of J. J. Sciarra, D. A. Eschenbach, and R. Depp, *Gynecology and Obstetrics,* vol. 3. Philadelphia: Harper & Row, 1987, p. 2.)

remainder passes through the pulmonary circuit. **The vascular resistance in the placental circuit is very low and the system is widely dilated, whereas in the pulmonary circuit, there is a very high vascular resistance, which accounts for the low blood flow in the latter organ during intrauterine existence.** The combined blood flows then pass down the aorta to the common iliac arteries, the hypogastric arteries, and finally back to the placenta through the terminal umbilical arteries. Recently, ultrasound blood flow studies using the Doppler effect have shown that there are lower fetal aortic blood flow velocities in fetuses who pass meconium in utero in prolonged pregnancies and in those associated with intrauterine growth retardation (IUGR).

b. Fetal pulmonary system development

1) Breathing movements

In a high percentage of cases, by the time the fetus has obtained a gestational age of 28 weeks (about 1,000 grams in weight), the pulmonary system will have matured sufficiently to allow the fetus to survive if delivery should take place. While the presence of *intrauterine breathing movements* were noted as far back as 1888, respiratory-like movements of the chest wall of the in-utero human fetus have only recently been demonstrated to occur as early as *11 weeks' gestation.*

It has been shown that there are two types of in-utero respiration in the lamb fetus. The **first** is a rapid, shallow, irregular pattern that occurs in 90% of the fetal breathing movements (FBM). An association of this pattern with the occurrence of rapid-eye-movement sleep (REM) has been noted. The **second** pattern occurs in only about 5% of the FBM and consists of a slow, deep respiration that occurs at a rate of about 1–4 breaths per minute. Fetal coughing, hiccupping, and gasping have all been associated with pressure fluctuations that occur independently of the amniotic fluid changes. The tracheal fluid movement tends to be low in the early morning and high in the early evening (diurnal variation), and this pattern has been shown to correlate with the times when the fetal breathing movements also wax and wane. It has been noted that when the maternal blood glucose concentrations are low, the fetal breathing movements disappear. Hypoxia has a similar effect, unless the pCO$_2$ is increased as well (in sheep), in which case the fetal

breathing movements increase, as does the tracheal fluid exchange. It has also been noted that fetal breathing movements decrease several days prior to the onset of labor. **Under normal conditions, fetal breathing movements may occur between 30 and 90% of the time, with a frequency of 30–70 movements per minute.** Interestingly, there is an increase in the fetal heart rate variability (measured by electronic fetal monitoring) during periods of gross fetal body movements and fetal breathing movements. Substances that are central nervous system (CNS) *stimulants* (e.g., epinephrine, isoproterenol, caffeine, etc.) also cause an increase in fetal breathing movements, whereas those that are *CNS depressants* (e.g., meperidine, diazepam, nicotine, general anesthetics, barbiturates, etc.) result in a decrease in the fetal breathing movements. One study noted that when fetal breathing movements were present for less than 50% of the time, especially in the presence of deep and prolonged respiratory movements, fetal death occurred in 8% of these cases. In addition, fetal distress, secondary to uteroplacental insufficiency, was noted in 84% of these cases.

2) Lung development

During the period of lung development, amniotic fluid is present in the lung under pressure, which apparently aids in maintaining the patency of the developing tubules and alveoli. By the 34th week of pregnancy, lecithin and phosphatidylglycerol, which are produced by the type II pneumocytes of the lungs, begin to be produced in large quantities (Fig. 21-11). The presence of these surface-active materials in the lung of the newborn infant prevents the collapse of the alveoli with each expiration by reducing the surface tension. *In the absence of this surfactant system, the newborn would, in many instances, suffer from respiratory distress syndrome (RDS) and would probably die* (see Chapter 26).

c. Renal development

The pronephros and the mesonephros, the first two primitive kidneys, are gradually replaced by the metanephros, which begins to form as a cap of metanephric tissue (i.e., the metanephric blastema) over the mesonephric buds. By about 12–14 weeks' gestation, the nephrons have begun to have some function; however, the urine that is formed in fetal life

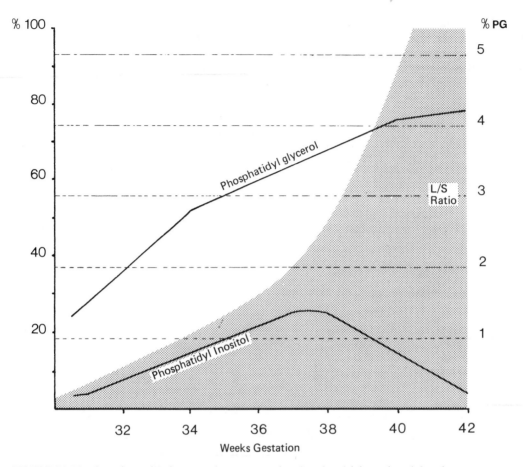

FIGURE 21-11. The relationship between the L/S ratio, the phosphatidylglycerol, and the phosphatidylinositol levels in late pregnancy. The L/S ratio levels (1:0, 2:0, 3:0, and 4:0) and phosphatidylglycerol values (1%, 2%, 3%, and 4%) are depicted on the right value scale, whereas the phosphatidylinositol value in percent is shown on the left.

is hypotonic, indicating the fetal kidney's lack of concentrating ability. **Ultrasonic studies have shown that at 30 weeks' gestation, the fetal urine production is about 10 ml per hour. This urine excretion increases to 27 ml per hour, or 650 ml per day, at term.** The urine produced by the fetal kidneys is a significant contribution to the amniotic fluid, and in its absence, **oligohydramnios** will result.

d. Gastrointestinal system development

By the end of the first trimester, the fetal intestine has developed the capability of peristalsis, **and by the 16th week, the fetus begins to swallow amniotic fluid. Near term, as much as 450 ml of amniotic fluid may be ingested per day.** If this function is interfered with, **hydramnios** will occur. The contents of the lower bowel consist of a greenish-black sticky material called **meconium,** which consists of biliverdin (the green pigment) and various excretory products. **The evacuation of meconium by the fetus may occur as the result of a vagal stimulation or, perhaps more commonly, as the result of hypoxia.** The mechanism involved may be the release of arginine vasopressin from the pituitary with its resultant stimulation of the smooth muscle of the colon.

The biliverdin that is found in the bowel comes from the <u>small amount</u> of <u>bilirubin conjugation</u> <u>and</u> <u>excretion</u> that is <u>performed by the fetus.</u> The large amount of <u>unconjugated bilirubin</u> that is produced by the breakdown of the fetal erythrocytes is <u>cleared by</u> the <u>placenta from the fetal circulation to the maternal liver</u>, where it is conjugated and excreted. The fetal hepatic enzymatic functions gradually develop over the course of pregnancy; however, even <u>at birth, many</u> of the <u>fetal enzymes</u> may <u>not be fully developed</u>. **This incomplete development is particularly evident in the immature infant, who has a diminished ability to convert bilirubin and subsequently develops jaundice.**

e. Central nervous system development

Electrical activity in the subcortical areas of the brain has been detected as early as 6 weeks' gestation. The central nervous system of the fetus is developed enough by 7½ weeks of gestation to allow the fetus to flex the neck and trunk following perioral stimulation. Toward the end of the third month, it is possible to evoke widespread body movements by facial stimulation. *By the 10th week, the fetus begins to make spontaneous movements* and responds to specific stimuli to evoke the opening of the mouth, cause plantar flexion of the toes, instigate squinting, and invoke partial finger closure, the latter of which becomes complete by the 16th week. *Sucking movements* are present by the 3rd and 4th months. **Respiration and swallowing are present by the 16th week. The eyelids grow over the eye at about the 8th week and remain fused until about the 24th week.** *It is thought that by the 7th month, the fetal eye is capable of responding to light.* **Between the 24th and the 26th week of gestation, the fetus is capable of hearing sound in utero.** Although taste buds are apparently present by the 3rd month, taste is probably not established until the 7th month. While the olfactory epithelium is present by the 7th week, the sense of smell is probably not present until about the 7th month and is still quite poor at birth. There are free nerve endings (i.e., to detect pain and temperature), lamellated corpuscles (i.e., deep pressure), tactile corpuscles, and neuromuscular spindles present in the fetus by the 4th month.

At about 18–20 weeks, fetal eye movements begin to appear, and clusters of eye movements begin to occur at about 24 weeks' gestation. *Low-frequency eye movements* (i.e., an average of 1–10 per minute over a 5-minute period) may be seen in the fetus between weeks 18 and 21 and continue up to week 38, when they decrease abruptly. *Moderate-frequency eye movements* (i.e., 11–20 per minute) begin to increase around the 22nd to the 25th week of gestation and continue to increase up to 30–33 weeks, when they tend to stabilize. *High-frequency eye movements* (i.e., 21–35 per minute) begin at 30–33 weeks and are the most common eye movements present at term. Rapid eye movement may be defined as more than 20 movements per minute, and its appearance seems to correlate with the FHR patterns that are related to the rest-activity cycles (i.e., rapid eye movement and non–rapid eye movement sleep) seen in the fetus beyond 34 weeks' gestation.

f. Hematologic development

1) Red blood cells

At the beginning of the 3rd week, blood cells begin to appear in the mesenchymal tissue near the yolk sac and the allantois. The blood cells are derived from hemocytoblasts, which in turn come from the undifferentiated mesenchyme. These early blood cells are nucleated, but they gradually lose their nuclei and acquire hemoglobin to become first reticulocytes, and then erythrocytes. **These red cells constitute two distinct lines:** (1) large erythrocytes, which are primitive, and (2) small erythrocytes, which are mature. The primitive erythrocytes disappear by the end of the first trimester. *The globin moiety is primitive in these early forms of hemoglobin, which have been classified as Gower-1 and Gower-2 hemoglobin.* In Gower-1 hemoglobin, there are four epsilon-peptide chains per molecule of protein, whereas in the Gower-2 hemoglobin there are two alpha and two epsilon chains per molecule of protein.

From the 4th to the 6th month, <u>hematopoiesis occurs mainly in the mesenchyme of the liver and spleen.</u> <u>By the time of birth</u>, the <u>bone marrow and lymph nodes become the only sites of blood formation.</u> **Hemoglobin F (HbF), or fetal hemoglobin, has a great affinity for oxygen and a greater ability to release carbon dioxide than is the case with adult hemoglobin (HbA).** This difference may be explained by the fact that HbF has a pair of α-peptide chains and a pair of γ-chains per molecule of hemoglobin. Furthermore, two types of γ-chains have been identified in HbF. HbA, on the other hand, has a pair of α-chains and a pair of β-chains per molecule of hemoglobin. In addition, another normal adult hemoglobin, HbA$_2$, has a pair of α-chains and a pair of δ-chains. This type of hemoglobin is only present in very small amounts at term, although it increases thereafter.

The life span of the fetal erythrocyte is approximately 80 days, as opposed to the 120-day life span of the erythrocyte of the adult. The fetal blood volume is about 78 ml/kg, excluding the placental blood volume, or 125 ml/kg if this is included.

2) The oxygen dissociation curve

HbF has the unique ability of being able to bind more oxygen than HbA at any given pH and oxygen tension. This means that HbF may become saturated with oxygen at pO$_2$ levels that will only saturate a small percentage of the maternal hemoglobin. The hemoglobin of the fetus increases to about 15.0 g/dl by mid-pregnancy, and to even higher levels at term. **About 75% of the fetal hemoglobin at term is of the HbF variety, although this percentage falls off rapidly during the first year of life.**

3) Leukocytes and platelets

Lymphoblasts, the precursors of the large and small lymphocytes, are present in the mesenchyme at 8 weeks' gestation and in the lymph nodes by the 12th week. In early embryonic life, megakaryocytes appear in the liver and spleen, and adult levels of platelets are present in the fetus near term.

g. Endocrine development
1) Insulin and IFS

The endocrine function of the pancreas appears very early in the fetus, and *insulin* can be detected in the plasma by 12 weeks' gestation. The levels of insulin are dependent upon the amount of plasma glucose present, and are elevated in the fetuses of diabetic mothers. **Insulin does not cross the placenta.**

Insulin-like growth factors (IGF), or insulin-like fetal somatotropin **(IFS)** hormones **(somatomedins),** are low–molecular weight single-chain polypeptides that are similar to insulin and are present in both the maternal and fetal plasma. Little is known as to their role. The IGFs have been divided into two separate groups: the basic group (IGF-I) and the neutral group (IGF-II). The basic IGFs include human IGF-I (Sm-C/IGF-I), which seems to be identical to somatomedin-C (Sm-C). It is a 70–amino acid peptide whose gene is located on the number 12 chromosome. Since this Sm-C/IGF-I increases at the time of puberty, it has been suspected that it might be involved in the linear growth of bones. The neutral IGFs include IGF-II, a 67–amino acid protein whose gene is on the short arm of chromosome number 11, near the gene for insulin. Many tissues possess separate receptors for these agents (i.e., type I and type II receptors) and for insulin. It has been postulated that there may be a link between the IGF hormones and placental lactogen, since both the IGF and the placental lactogen levels increase in a parallel manner throughout pregnancy and then decrease rapidly after the delivery, following the removal of the placenta. It is not known, however, whether these hormones are involved in the growth of the fetus.

2) Pituitary hormones

There is evidence of high cord levels of *pituitary growth hormone* in the fetus, but little is known as to its role. The fetal pituitary also releases β-endorphin. Other pituitary hormones, such as *the adrenocorticotropic hormone (ACTH), the follicle-stimulating hormone (FSH), the luteinizing hormone (LH), and prolactin* have all been identified in the fetal pituitary by 10 weeks' gestation.

3) Thyroid and parathyroid hormones

The fetal thyroid is functioning by the end of the first trimester of pregnancy. During the last two trimesters, iodide is concentrated by the gland with increasing avidity. By the middle of the second trimester, there is an increased secretion of thyroid-stimulating hormone (TSH) and thyroid hormones. **While TSH does not cross the placenta in appreciable amounts, the long-acting thyroid stimulators (LATS), LATS protector, and thyroid-stimulating IgG immunoglobulins, if in a high enough concentration in the maternal plasma, may cross over into the fetus.** The fetal *parathyroid glands* are functional by the end of the first trimester.

4) Adrenal gland

The large fetal adrenal gland has a central cortical zone (i.e., fetal zone) that is not present in the adult gland. Among the functions of the fetal adrenal gland is the role that it plays in the production of placental estrogen precursors (i.e., dehydroisoandrosterone sulfate, or DHAS), in the maturation of the fetal lung, and finally, in the initiation of labor. During pregnancy, 90% of the estriol secretion is derived from the fetal DHAS. At 28 weeks' gestation, the adrenal gland is about the size of the fetal kidney. The growth of the fetal adrenal gland is most rapid during the last 6 weeks of intrauterine life. Cortisol secretion, which is under the regulation of the pituitary gland's adrenocorticotropic hormone (ACTH), may play at least a permissive role in parturition. *In an anencephalic fetus, there is a delay in the onset of labor, which has been thought to be secondary to the low levels of ACTH, DHAS, and estrogen production, due to an atrophic adrenal gland.* It has been suggested that 50–75% of the steroids that are secreted by the fetal adrenal gland are derived from the cholesterol of low-density lipoprotein (LDL), which appears to be supplied by the liver.

h. Genital system development

1) Undifferentiated gonad

The first primordial germ cells appear in the wall of the yolk sac at 24 days' gestation, and by the 6th week of development they will have migrated to the genital ridge. Between days 21 and 30, the pronephros has been formed, has disappeared, and has been replaced by the mesonephros, which contains many nephric vesicles, some of which connect with the pronephric duct (i.e., mesonephric, or wolffian duct). The mesonephros is attached to the urogenital ridge in the 5th week by a ureteric bud, which grows from each mesonephric duct into a ridge. A cap of metanephric tissue (i.e., the metanephric blastema), along with numerous nephric vesicles, forms and becomes the metanephros, or definitive kidney. *During this same period, a gonad appears medially to the mesonephros* (Fig. 21-12).

At about the 6th week (44–48 days), an outpouching of the peritoneum near the upper end of the mesonephric duct occurs and extends caudalward to become the paramesonephric duct (i.e., müllerian duct). In both sexes, the primordial germ cells migrate to the developing undifferentiated gonad at about six weeks' gestation, where they intermingle with the advancing sex cords. If a male develops, the gonad is distinguishable as being a male testis by the 7th week; if a female gonad develops, then it is not evident until about the 10th week.

2) Male gonad

The male gonad develops the seminiferous tubules and rete testis from the medullary sex cords, and the cortical germinal epithelium disappears. Leydig cells (i.e., interstitial cells) arise from the mesenchyme and ultimately produce testosterone. At puberty, the rete testis and the seminiferous tubules become patent, while the germ cells within them develop into spermatogonia for the production of spermatozoa. **The germinal epithelium develops into sustentacular cells (i.e., Sertoli cells), which assist in the process of spermatogenesis. Medullary cells (i.e., early Leydig cells) produce testosterone, which assists in the development of the wolffian ducts into the vas deferens, the epididymis, the seminal vesicles, and, by the 8th to 9th week postfertilization, the penis and the scrotum.** The testosterone is converted to **dihydrotestosterone (DHT)** by 5α-reductase at the cellular level. While some of the mesonephric tubules disappear or go to form the paradidymis, part of the tubules form the vasa efferentia. The mesonephric duct becomes the epididymal duct, the vas deferens, and the ejaculatory duct, and the outpouching of its terminal end becomes the seminal vesicles by the 13th week. The paramesonephric ducts (müllerian) atrophy in the male under the stimulus of the **müllerian inhibiting factor (MIF),** except for their upper and lower ends, which become, respectively, the appendix testes and the prostatic utricle. Cells in the urogenital sinus contribute to the formation of the prostate, the urethral glands, and the bulbourethral glands (Cowper's glands).

3) Female gonad

The female gonad is formed by the invasion of the mesenchyme of the gonad by the sex cords of the germinal epithelium. The primordial follicles develop

Text continues on p. 296

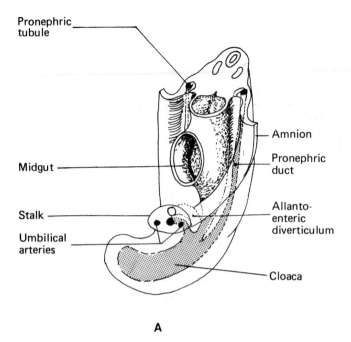

A

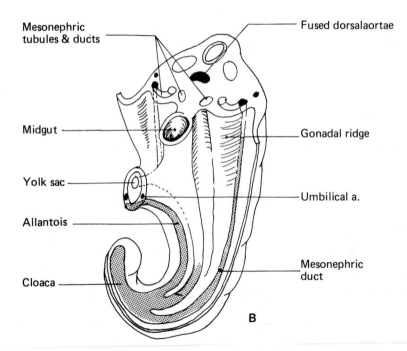

B

FIGURE 21-12. Development of the female reproductive organs in early embryogenesis. (A) Fourth week (with 18 to 24 somites). (B) Fifth week. The gonadal ridges may be noted medial to the mesonephric ducts. The differentiation of the gonad into a testis does not occur until about the sixth week. (C) and (D) show the further development of the genital tubercle, the cloaca, and the urogenital sinus, along with the concomitant development of the mesonephric ducts into the metanephric ducts and finally the permanent kidneys.

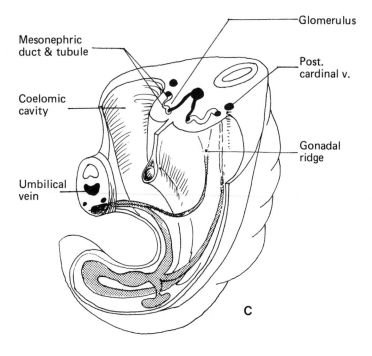

C

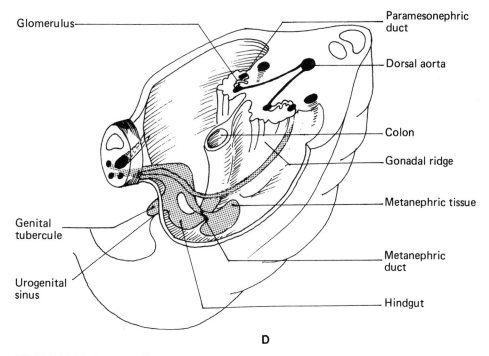

D

FIGURE 21-12. *(continued)*

when the primary ovocyte is surrounded by the germinal epithelial pregranulosal cells. The cortical germinal epithelium remains. Interstitial cells (Leydig cells) are present in the hilar region of the gonad; however, they do not proliferate as they do in the testes.

By the 5th month of intrauterine life, a peak population of germ cells is reached **(variously estimated to be between 5 and 7 million)** and the decline in ovogonia will have begun. **By the 7th month, the last of the ovogonia will have entered meiosis.** Further cellular division will not occur thereafter until puberty, when ovulation (when it enters the second meiotic division) and fertilization occurs (when it completes meiotic division, with the formation of the second polar body).

By the 9th or 10th week, the paramesonephric (müllerian) ducts fuse caudally to form the uterovaginal canal (from which the uterus and the vagina develop). The lower end of this canal becomes the müllerian tubercle, which appears on the dorsal wall of the urogenital sinus (Fig. 21-13). A vaginal plate develops about the 9th week between the uterovaginal canal and the urogenital sinus. By the 20th week, the canal has elongated and has been canalized to form the vagina. The hymen remains as the residual block of tissue between the vagina and the urogenital sinus. The source of the vaginal epithelium has been in dispute, but it has been variously attributed to: (1) the endodermal urogenital sinus (the most likely source), (2) the mesodermal mesonephric and paranephric ducts, or (3) various combinations of these structures. Although the vagina initially is in contact with the urogenital sinus (future urethra), it later separates from it and opens directly into the vestibule. In the female, the mesonephric (wolffian) ducts disappear, except for some remnants, such as the epoophoron, the paroophoron, and Gartner's duct. The end of the mesonephric duct also gives rise to the appendix of the broad ligament.

4) External genitalia

During the 6th week, the cloaca, which is the terminal end of the hindgut, is divided by the urorectal septum into the primitive urogenital sinus and the anorectal canal. **The genital tubercle and the genital folds develop into the clitoris and the labia majora, respectively.** The labia minora develop from the urethal folds, which arise from the thickenings on the medial aspect of the genital folds (Fig. 21-14).

In the male, the genital tubercle becomes the penis and the genital folds fuse in the midline to form the scrotum. The urogenital sinus penetrates the genital tubercle to form the urethra, which by the 14th week opens at the junction of the shaft and the glans. A cord of epithelial cells on the shaft of the penis shifts the meatal opening to the tip of the penis, and the earlier opening closes. The skin then folds about the glans to form the prepuce.

i. Fetal metabolism

The metabolism of the fetus depends almost entirely upon the nutritional substrates that are presented to it by the mother. The following basic elements are required: (1) an adequate nutritional intake by the mother, (2) an adequate maternal plasma concentration of each nutrient, (3) a sufficient maternal blood supply to the placental intervillus space, (4) an adequate placentation with sufficient fetal chorionic villi, and (5) an adequate fetal vascularity to supply the villi.

In the early part of gestation, the fetus is composed primarily of water with a minimal amount of fat tissue being present. In the middle of the second trimester,

FIGURE 21-13. Further development of the paramesonephric (müllerian) ducts. *From upper left in a clockwise direction:* The early development of the müllerian ducts. The cranial ends develop first and remain open to become the fimbriated ends of the fallopian tube. The ducts grow caudally and cross the mesonephric (wolffian) ducts medially, where they fuse with each other to form the uterovaginal canal. The mesonephric ducts degenerate and remain as vestigial remnants along the uterus and upper vagina. The lower end of the uterovaginal canal joins with the urogenital sinus to form the urogenital tubercle. The upper portions of the fused müllerian tubes form the uterus and cervix, and with the urogenital sinus, they also form the vagina. The upper unfused ends of the müllerian ducts become the fallopian tubes. The uterovaginal canal gradually cannulates to form the uterine cavity and the vagina.

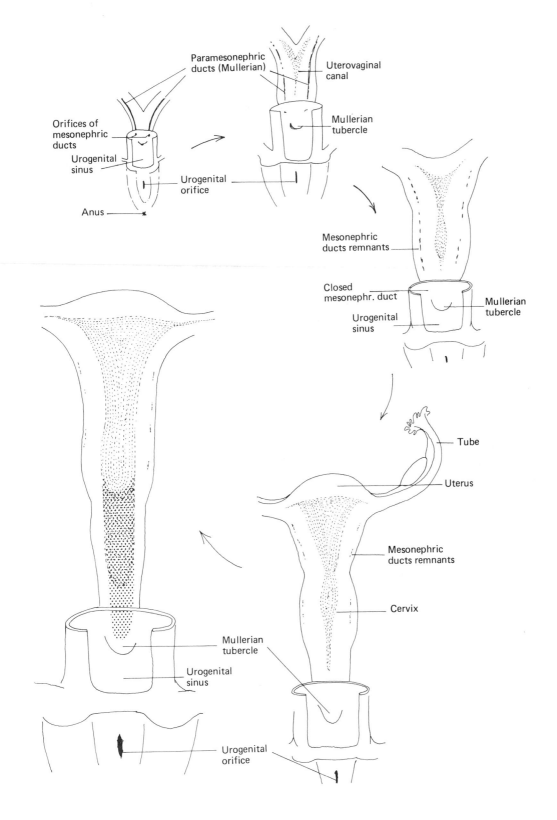

Paramesonephric ducts (Mullerian)

Uterovaginal canal

Orifices of mesonephric ducts

Urogenital sinus

Urogenital orifice

Mullerian tubercle

Anus

Mesonephric ducts remnants

Closed mesonephr. duct

Urogenital sinus

Mullerian tubercle

Tube

Uterus

Mesonephric ducts remnants

Cervix

Mullerian tubercle

Urogenital sinus

Urogenital orifice

297

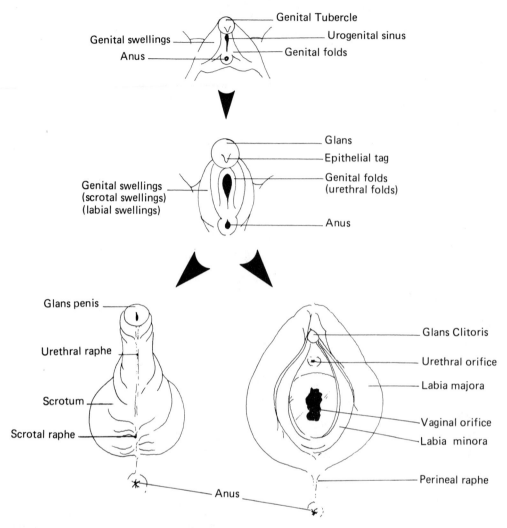

FIGURE 21-14. The differentiation of the external genitalia of both sexes. *Top:* The undifferentiated stage of the development of the external genitalia. *Middle:* The intermediate stage of development of both sexes at about 10 weeks' gestation. *Lower:* The final development of the external genitalia in both sexes. The genital folds have closed to form the male urethra and the genital swellings have fused to form the scrotum. In the female the genital folds remain open to form the labia minora, while the genital swellings form the labia majora.

this relationship reverses so that fatty tissue becomes increasingly more prominent near term. **Indeed, most of the fat that is acquired by the fetus is obtained beyond the 33rd week of gestation.**

Glucose provides the major energy nutrient for the fetus and an adequate supply is necessary for normal growth. An excess of glucose leads to macrosomia, whereas a relative lack of glucose results in fetal growth retardation. Glucose is transferred across the placenta by facilitated diffusion. The role of insulin-like somatotropins in fetal growth is not fully understood at this time.

The essential amino acids necessary for fetal growth are leucine, threonine, valine, tryptophan, phenylalanine, lysine, methionine, cystine, isoleucine, and histidine. Amino acids are transported by active transport. Fatty acids and glycerol will also cross the placenta.

The development of **intrauterine growth retardation (IUGR)** may either involve a summation of a number of the factors that may interfere with fetal nutrition or may result from any one factor, if its effect is sufficiently great. Clinically, inadequate uterine blood flow and placental perfusion has been commonly seen with the type of IUGR that occurs in association with hypertension and toxemia. While the association of nutritional deprivation and IUGR has been difficult to define with accuracy, an extreme lack of maternal weight gain (i.e., less than 11 lbs) during pregnancy is commonly seen in association with this problem.

j. Fetal immune system

Although it was formerly thought that the fetus was immunologically incompetent, it has since been found that the fetal immune system develops quite early in pregnancy. Lymphocytes may be present by the 7th week, and the ability to recognize an antigen may be present by the 12th week (only IgA is missing by the 12th week). By term, the fetus has a well-developed immune system.

CHAPTER 22

Genetics

The important thing is to make the lesson of each case tell on your education. The value of experience is not in seeing much, but in seeing wisely.

—*Sir William Osler**

1. Basic concepts

a. DNA

Prior to 1950, although little was known about the nucleic acids, it was recognized that nucleic acid extracted from the thymus gland contained adenine, guanine, cytosine, thymine, deoxyribose (a sugar), and phosphoric acid. This compound was called **deoxyribonucleic acid (DNA)** and was found to be concentrated mainly in the cell nucleus. **DNA is a substance that stores genetic information; it remains constant within a species unless a mutation occurs.**

In 1953, **J. D. Watson and F. H. C. Crick** suggested that the structure of DNA consisted of two very long, thin, polymeric chains twisted about each other in a **double helix formation** (Fig. 22-1). The backbone of the polynucleotide chain consists of alternating sugar and phosphate residues. The 5' position of one pentose ring is connected to the 3' position of the next pentose ring via a phosphate group. The two polynucleotide chains in the double helix are associated by hydrogen bonding between the nitrogenous

*Reprinted with permission from Robert Bennett Bean, *Sir William Osler: Aphorisms from His Bedside Teachings and Writings,* William Bennett Bean, ed. Springfield, Ill.: Charles C Thomas, Publisher, 1968, p. 41.

bases. The only arrangements possible for DNA involve the pairing of adenine (A) with thymine (T), and guanine (G) with cytosine (C). **Thus, the pairing of a purine (A or G) with a pyrimidine (T or C), called "base pairing," provides the only sequence possible to maintain the double helix formation.** The double helix strands separate during replication (i.e., the "S" phase), and each chain then becomes a template for the formation of complementary molecules (Fig. 22-2). The enzyme DNA polymerase, as well as several other enzymes, aid in this process.

The human nucleus is approximately 0.06 μm in diameter. The 46 chromosomes contain double-stranded DNA, which is about 1.8 m in length and contains 6×10^6 K bases. However, since the nucleus is only 10 μm in diameter, it becomes obvious that the DNA must have to be packaged in a more compact unit. This packaging involves the use of **histones.** There are several types of histones, H1, H2A, H2B, H3, and H4. Two molecules of histones (i.e., two each of either H2A, H2B, H3, or H4) unite to form a core **nucleosome** cylindrical structure (6×11 nm). The 140 base pairs of DNA wind about this structure in two coils. H1 assists in another segment of 60 base pairs to connect the adjacent nucleosomes. Thus, every 1,000 base pairs of DNA have five nucleosomes [i.e., $5 \times (140 + 60) = 1,000$], which are then linked to other nucleosomes to form a cylinder, which in turn forms a **chromatin fiber.** When many of these chromatin fibers aggregate, they form a **chromatin band,** which, when combined with other chromatin bands, then forms a **chromosome.**

Since 1969, **banding** techniques have been developed to identify different regions of the chromosome. One of the original banding procedures utilized quinacrine dihydrochloride fluorescent staining followed

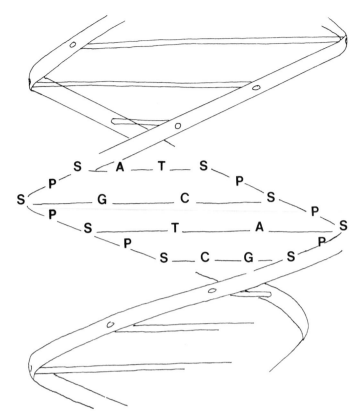

FIGURE 22-1. The Watson-Crick double helix model of DNA. The sugar (S) and phosphate (P) groups alternate. Each sugar is attached to a nitrogenous base, which may be of four different types: adenine (A), thymine (T), guanine (G), and cytosine (C).

by fluorescent microscopy to identify the fluorescent positive bands and the nonfluorescent negative bands **(Q-bands).** All of the banding techniques produce darkly stained positive bands and lightly stained negative bands. Later staining techniques identified the **G-bands.** The G-bands and the Q-bands are usually located in the same areas; they are thought to represent a concentration of adenine-thymine (A-T) nucleotide pairs. The **R-bands** are usually negative bands. The X chromosome may be studied using the Q-, G-, or R-banding techniques. The **C-banding** procedure stains the centromeric regions and the distal two-thirds of the long arm (Y_q) of the Y chromosome. The positive C-bands apparently represent concentrations of repetitive DNA. Thus both the X and the Y chromosomes can be identified by banding techniques.

Coding sequences, or **exons,** of DNA are separated by intervening noncoding sequences, or **introns,** on the genome. The coding sequences may be "unique," coding for a specific RNA, or they may be "moderately repetitious" or "highly repetitious." These different

DNA types can be demonstrated on the chromosome by some banding techniques. For example, positive R-bands and negative G-bands or Q-bands are believed to generally represent a unique sequence of DNA. Positive C-bands represent highly repetitious DNA, and positive G- and Q-bands apparently may represent either moderately repetitious or highly repetitious DNA.

b. RNA

Nucleic acids that have uracil instead of thymine, and a ribose instead of deoxyribose, are called **ribonucleic acids (RNA).** RNA is primarily concentrated in the cytoplasm of the cell, and is a molecule that contains four nucleotides joined together by 3'–5' phosphodiester bonds. When the DNA strands separate and act as templates for replication during the cell cycle, complementary deoxyribonucleotides are attracted to form another double helix. During the DNA synthesis, or phase S of the cell cycle, DNA is effec-

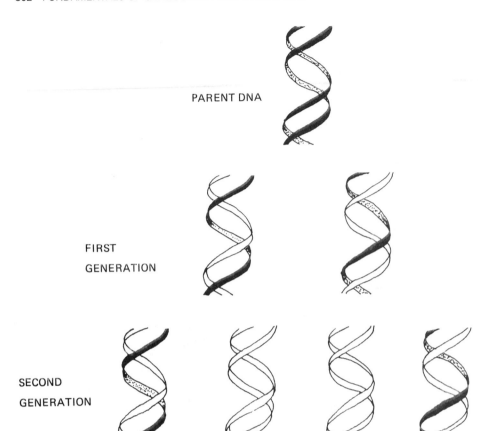

PARENT DNA

FIRST GENERATION

SECOND GENERATION

FIGURE 22-2. Replication of DNA.

tively doubled. RNA synthesis primarily occurs during the cell cycle at times other than the S phase. **Transcription** occurs when the genetic information contained in the DNA is produced in the complementary sequence of bases in the RNA. This process is catalyzed by the enzyme RNA polymerase. There are apparently three forms of this enzyme, and each transcribes a different RNA: (1) polymerase I makes the large ribosomal RNA (rRNA), (2) polymerase II transcribes messenger RNA (mRNA), which transcribes most of the cell's proteins, and (3) polymerase III produces transfer RNA (tRNA) and the small ribosomal RNA (rRNA).

c. Messenger RNA

Messenger RNA (mRNA) is separate from transfer RNA (tRNA) and ribosomal RNA (rRNA) and has a

rapid turnover, with a half-life of 2–4 minutes. Apparently the ribosomes receive genetic information from the gene by means of mRNA. The hereditary information is transferred from the 5′ unique-sequence region through the repetitive intervening sequences to the 3′ region. After the mRNA has received the genetic information, it then moves to the cytoplasm, where it associates with the ribosomes and begins the process of **translation.**

d. Ribosomal RNA

The ribosomes are particles in the endoplasmic reticulum involved in incorporating the amino acids into the growing polypeptide chain. The composition of a ribosome is that of a protein and a high–molecular weight r-RNA, and it works with mRNA in synthesizing protein. There are two classes of rRNA,

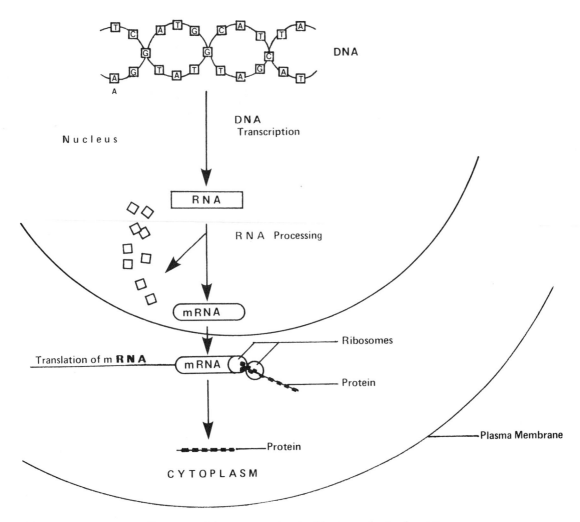

FIGURE 22-3. Schematic illustration of the processes involved in the synthesis of protein. (Adapted from D. N. Danforth and J. R. Scott, eds. *Obstetrics and Gynecology,* 5th ed. Philadelphia: J. B. Lippincott Company, 1986, p. 24.)

one of which has a molecular weight of 500,000 and the other a molecular weight of 1,000,000. Since the rRNA is transcribed from a certain DNA segment, or **codon** (i.e., a sequence of three bases representing 1 of the 20 amino acids or ones which have regulatory functions), it actually is complementary. However, rRNA does not have the RNA polymerase–binding sites that are required for translation.

e. Transfer RNA

Transfer RNA (tRNA), or soluble RNA (sRNA), is also located in the cytoplasm and functions as an agent in

transferring activated amino acids to a ribosomal complex. Initially, the amino acid is activated by adenosine triphosphate (ATP) in the presence of an aminoacyl-RNA synthetase, which is specific for each amino acid. The next step is the combination of aminoacyl-adenate with a specific tRNA to form an aminoacyl-tRNA complex. This complex is then aligned by the mRNA-ribosome complex and the amino acid is added to the developing complementary polypeptide chain. RNA separation then occurs when the protein synthesis is complete (Fig. 22-3). This formation of the polypeptide chain through the use of genetic information carried in the messenger RNA to align the amino acid sequence in a specific way is called **translation.** Sometimes, the portion of the mRNA that has already been translated is degraded prior to the completion of the translation. The various RNAs are then free to repeat the process again to synthesize additional polypeptides.

f. Chromosomal analysis

In 1956, J. H. Tjio and A. Levan, using human tissue culture techniques, were able to show that the chromosome count in humans is 46, of which 44 are autosomes and 2 are sex chromosomes. This contribution marked an important advance, since all of the previous studies had noted that the human chromosomal count was 48.

It has recently been noted that **a single chromosome is present in the cytoplasmic mitochondria,** which has the capability of protein synthesis. The chromosome is circular with an inner L strand and an outer H strand, the latter of which contains almost all of the coded information. **The female contributes almost all of the cytoplasm to the zygote, whereas the male contributes only to the nucleus.** Any mitochondrial diseases or special attributes may be transmitted (i.e., through mitochondrial inheritance) to either males or females of the next generation, but they could only be transmitted into the following generation through the female line, since the female would provide the cytoplasm for the next generation zygote. These mitochondrial genes were first discovered in the 1960s. More recently, some anthropologists and geneticists have been able to trace this mitochondrial DNA to a **single woman,** or perhaps a group of women with the same mitochondrial DNA, who lived about 200,000 years ago in Africa (or perhaps in Asia). This time frame was calculated by assuming that over the course of a million years there should have been about a 2–4% spontaneous mutation rate occurring in the mitochondrial DNA components. The importance of these findings is that all of the different races of humankind on this earth are closely related genetically, with only very minor differences being present. Recently, the science of molecular genetics has been able to utilize specific restriction enzymes on the DNA of cells obtained by amniocentesis or chorionic villus sampling to detect specific genetic defects in the fetus. A radioactive DNA probe can distinguish sickle cell trait, sickle cell anemia, and normal hemoglobin. This

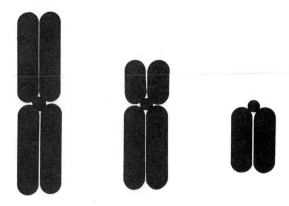

FIGURE 22-4. Diagrammatic representation of the three types of chromosomes based on the position of the centromere. *From left to right:* Metacentric, submetacentric, and acrocentric.

technique has not yet proven to be effective in detecting other genetic defects, since the specific restriction enzyme must be known in order to cleave the DNA where the point mutation that causes the disorder occurs.

Recent techniques of gene mapping, or DNA sequencing, may be useful in detecting the identity of individuals involved in patrimony and criminal activities. Each individual appears to have a unique genetic "fingerprint" that contains elements from both parents.

The nomenclature for describing cytogenetic abnormalities consists of: (1) the number of chromosomes, (2) followed by a comma, (3) the sex chromosomes present, (4) followed by a comma, and (5) the type of chromosomal anomaly. For example, monosomy X (Turner's syndrome) would be recorded as 45,X, and Down's syndrome as 47,XY,+21. Other abbreviations used in noting chromosomal anomalies are: centromere (cen), short arm (p), long arm (q), isochromosome (i), deletion (del), mosaicism (mos), duplication (dup), inversion (inv), reciprocal translocation (rcp), translocation (t), chimerism (chi), ring (r), break (:), and break and reunion (: :). In addition, a question mark (?) may be used whenever doubt exists; diagonal slashes (/) may be used to separate mosaics; and plus (+) or minus (−) signs may be used to indicate that the entire autosome is extra or missing. The chromosomes may be described according to the position of the centromere as: (1) metacentric, (2) submetacentric, or (3) acrocentric (Fig. 22-4).

1) Technique

If human cells are grown in a culture and then stimulated to grow with phytohemagglutinin, the exposure of the cells to colchicine will arrest the cellular growth in the **metaphase** condition. When these cells are exposed to a hypotonic solution, they will swell and disperse the chromosomes. An air-dried preparation of these cells can then be made and the chromosomes stained, photographed, and cut out to be displayed as a **karotype.** Peripheral blood lymphocytes require growth in a nutrient media for 48–72 hours, whereas bone marrow only requires 3–4 hours. In contrast, the tissue culture of chorionic villi (3–7 days) and amniotic fluid cells (14–21 days) require a much longer growth period.

A karyotype classification was developed in an attempt to standardize the nomenclature. The 44 autosomes, when displayed from the largest to the smallest chromosome, results in seven groups as follows: **Group A (1–3), Group B (4–5), Group C (6–12), Group D (13–15), Group E (16–18), Group F (19–20), and Group G (21–22). The Y chromosome is similar to the chromosomes of Group G (i.e., 21–22) and is thus included with this group. The X chromosome, which is similar to those chromosomes in Group C (6–12), is therefore included in that group** (Fig. 22-5).

g. Cell division

The germ cells undergo two major types of cellular division before fertilization may take place. The first is **mitosis** in which the daughter cells receive an identical amount of genetic material as was present in the parental cell, and the second is **meiosis,** in which the genetic material is reduced by half (forming two haploid cells).

1) Cell cycle

The longest part of the cell cycle is the accumulation of amino acids, nucleotides, proteins, and other substances needed to enable the chromosomal DNA to duplicate itself. This part of the cycle is called the **G1 phase.** During the synthesis **(S)** stage of the cycle, these elements double the content of the DNA. After the S phase, a **G2 phase** occurs, following which the cell then enters mitosis. **Mitosis is divided into four stages: prophase, metaphase, anaphase, and telophase.**

During the **prophase** of mitosis, the chromosome consists of two sister chromatids. Near the end of prophase, the centrioles migrate to each pole and become the two daughter centrioles. The **metaphase** begins with the formation of spindle fibers between the two centrioles and the centromeres of the chromosomes. Also, the integrity of the nuclear membrane weakens during this phase. The chromosomes then split at the centromere with the sister chromatids moving toward opposite poles. The **anaphase** encompasses the time it takes for the sister chromatids to move to the opposite poles. The **telophase** begins when the sister chromatids reach the opposite poles; in this stage, a new nuclear membrane forms for each of them to produce two new complete cells. The total cell cycle takes about 12–24 hours in the human, with DNA synthesis taking about 7–7.5 hours.

2) Meiosis

Prior to the union of the sperm and the ovum, each gamete must reduce its total complement of genetic material by half (forming haploid cells) so that the resulting zygote will contain contributions from both the father and the mother. Meiosis provides this **reductional division** and, in addition, allows for **the recombination of the genetic material from each parent,** providing an exchange of genetic information.

There are two divisions in meiosis: **meiosis I,** reductional division; and **meiosis II,** the production of two additional haploid cells.

a) Meiosis I

During **meiosis I** there are four stages, as in mitosis, only the **prophase stage** is much more complicated. **The subdivisions of the prophase of meiosis I are leptotene, zygotene, pachytene, diplotene, and diakinesis.** During the initial leptotene phase, long thin strands of chromosomes are present. **In the zygotene phase, the homologous chromosomes pair off with each other and exchange chromatin material in synapsis (i.e., the exchange of genetic information).** The X and Y chromosomes undergo end-to-end synapsis with their short arms, whereas the autosomes join in a side-to-side synapsis. Tetrads of the sister chromatids occur in the **pachytene** stage. During the **diplotene** stage, the homologous chromosomes move apart and the chiasmata be-

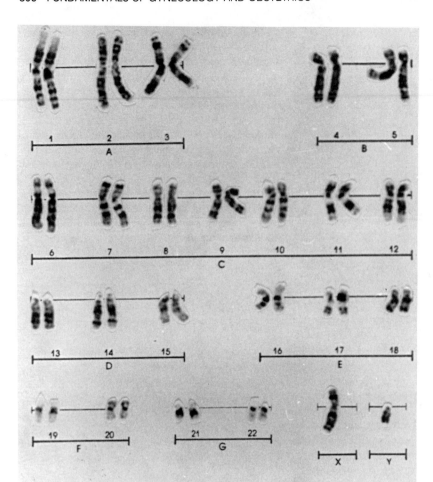

FIGURE 22-5. Human metaphase chromosomes arranged in the standard classification known as a karyotype. This is a normal male karyotype from a G-banded metaphase, with 46,XY chromosomal constitution. It was prepared in the Cytogenetics Laboratory, Section of Genetics/Pediatrics, LSU Medical Center, in Shreveport, Louisiana. (Courtesy of Theodore C. Thurmon, M.D., Chief, Section of Genetics, LSU School of Medicine, Shreveport, Louisiana.)

come visible. The final stage of the meiotic I prophase, **diakinesis,** is characterized by the chromosomes becoming more condensed.

In the **metaphase stage,** the nuclear membrane disappears, and the equatorial spindle develops. During the **anaphase stage,** the chromosomes begin to move toward the poles. **The telophase stage results in the production of two haploid cells. The net result of meiosis I is that the total chromo-** **somal content is reduced by one-half in the resulting haploid cells.**

b) Meiosis II

The mechanism of meiosis II is the same as that of mitosis; the cellular division merely creates more haploid cells. Usually four haploid cells are produced, of which no two cells will be identical in genetic complement because of **the recombination of the genetic material that took place during synapsis.**

3) Chromosomal aberrations: definitions

Aneuploidy results when there is a loss or gain of a chromosome. Nondisjunction and anaphase lag will result in aneuploidy.

Polyploidy involves the addition of one or two extra haploid sets of chromosomes. If the first or second polar body is not cast off and fertilization occurs, there will be one paternal and two maternal haploid sets of chromosomes, or triploidy. Double fertilization of a single ovum will result in triploidy with one maternal and two paternal haploid sets of chromosomes. Tetraploidy may occur if there is replication without an intervening mitosis—a condition seen in spontaneous abortions.

Homozygous and heterozygous classifications involve whether or not the genetic material is the same at a given site. Genes are present in pairs in all somatic cells. The two homologous genes may not always be the same, but may be alternative forms, or alleles. If the two genes at the same locus of the homologous chromosomes are the same, then they are said to be **homozygous.** If they are different, then they are **heterozygous.**

Nondisjunction is the process during cell division in which the chromatids of a tetrad or a homologous pair go to only one daughter cell, with no chromatids going to the other daughter cell.

Translocations are interchanges between both homologous and nonhomologous chromosomes. If the individual is normal, then it is assumed that no genetic material has been lost and that a **balanced translocation** exists. If the translocation between two chromosomes does not involve their centromeres, then it is called a **reciprocal translocation.** If acrocentric chromosomes join at the centromere, a **Robertsonian translocation** is said to be present.

Deletions are the result of breaks in a chromosome in which an intervening or terminal fragment is lost.

Mosaicism is the occurrence of two or more chromosomal patterns in the tissues of an individual. In other words, two or more cell lines of different genetic or chromosomal constitution were both derived from the same zygote. This condition usually occurs

secondary to nondisjunction during the first zygotic division, subsequent to the cleavage following fertilization, or it may be due to an anaphase lag which resulted in the survival of at least two cell lines with different complements. Nondisjunction during meiosis I results in the production of trisomic and monosomic gametes. If one of these cells is fertilized by a normal gamete, the resulting embryo may be either trisomic or monosomic, but it will not be mosaic.

Chimerism occurs in an individual with two or more genotypes, each derived from different zygotes, which subsequently fuse.

Spontaneous mutation may be induced by ultraviolet light, radiation, and chemical substances. These mutations occur at some locus on the X chromosome in about $1:1,000$ (0.1%).

Inversions occur when there are two breaks in a chromosome along with a 180-degree inversion of the segment.

Duplications occur when there is a translocation between homologous chromosomes or a transfer of material between sister chromatids.

Isochromosome formation results when the cell division splits the chromosome transversely instead of longitudinally. In this situation, one daughter cell receives both short arms, while the other receives both long arms of the chromosome.

The **ring** chromosome occurs when the chromosome suffers breaks in both the short and the long arms, which then connect to form a ring. The resulting acentric fragment is usually lost during the following anaphase.

A **dicentric** chromosome results from chromosomal interchange during the G1 phase of the cell cycle when there are two breaks. The acentric fragment is lost and the sister chromosomes join. The dicentric chromosome has two centromeres (dicentric), which result in mitotic instability since they may migrate to opposite poles during telophase. Secondary rearrangements of chromosomal material may occur.

2. Clinical genetics

a. Indications for genetic counseling

While the most common reason for genetic amniocentesis is for the detection of Down's syndrome in the mother who is over 35 years of age, there are other reasons for instituting a genetic evaluation. They are: (1) a family history of a genetic defect in either the parents or the siblings (i.e., aneuploidy, balanced translocation carrier, mosaicism), (2) a previous abnormal child in which the genetic diagnosis has not been made, (3) a history of an X-linked chromosomal disorder in the family, or (4) a patient who has had three or more spontaneous abortions.

1) Down's syndrome

A cytogenetic evaluation should be performed if the maternal age will be 35 years or older at the time of delivery. The usual incidence of trisomy-21 is 1:800 liveborn infants; however, this amount doubles in women who give birth over age of 35. Women younger than 35 who request amniocentesis for cytogenetic culture and evaluation must be managed on an individual basis, and the relative risks and benefits involved should be thoroughly discussed with them. The risk of Down's syndrome at the age of 35 is 1:378; at the age of 40, 1:106; and at the age of 45, 1:30. **An increase in the incidence of Down's syndrome may also be associated with an advanced paternal age (i.e., the incidence doubles after the paternal age of 55 years).**

Not only is the incidence of trisomy-21 increased with increasing age, but so also is the incidence of other autosomal trisomies and some X chromosomal polysomies (e.g., 47,XXY; 47,XXX). The estimated incidence of all chromosomal abnormalities shows an increase with age similar to that of Down's syndrome. The risk at age 35 is 1:204; at age 40, 1:65; and at age 45, 1:20.

2) History of previous anomaly

A cytogenetic evaluation should be performed if the patient has previously given birth to a child with either an autosomal trisomy or a sex chromosomal problem. If the mother was less than 24 years of age when she had a child with Down's syndrome, then she would have an increased risk of having another child with trisomy-21 (i.e., a 0.7% incidence). With regard to abnormalities other than trisomy-21, the risk would be 1.7%. As a consequence, couples with such histories should be offered antenatal genetic studies. Parents who have a numerical chromosomal abnormality (i.e., aneuploidy) are probably also at risk, since it has been recorded that

20–30% of the offspring of individuals with 45,X/46,XY, and 15–20% of offspring of patients with 47,XXX or 45,X/47,XXY, are chromosomally abnormal.

3) Balanced translocation

The presence of a balanced translocation in a parent is an indication for genetic counseling. It has been noted that in about 25% of individuals with Down's syndrome as a result of a translocation, one of the parents will have the same translocation chromosome. If the father alone has the translocation chromosome, the risk is only 2–3%, in contrast to a risk of 10% when the mother carries it. It should be noted, however, that other Robertsonian translocations do not carry similar risks.

4) Chromosomal inversions

Chromosomal inversions change the sequence of a gene but not the number; as a consequence, such individuals are phenotypically normal. Unbalanced gametes can occur if there is a recombination or a crossing over within the inverted segment during meiosis. These gametes show a loss of some genes and a duplication of others. If the mother has an inversion, evidence indicates that there is a 10–15% risk of having an abnormal infant, in contrast to only about 2–5% when the father has an inversion. **In couples who have repeated spontaneous abortions, a genetic assessment for the presence of translocations and inversions should be carried out.**

5) Environmental disorders

Environmental or chemically related fetal disorders do not lend themselves to genetic evaluation. While chromosomal breakage or rearrangements may be looked for after a maternal exposure to irradiation, it is impossible to precisely predict gene mutations and fetal abnormalities in such cases.

6) X-linked disorders

Affected individuals with X-linked recessive disorders, such as hemophilia and muscular dystrophy, or sex-limited autosomal dominant disorders, are usually male (46,XY). In such situations, it may be important to determine the sex of the fetus by karyotype analysis. X-chromatin (Barr body) and Y-chromatin analysis (fluorescent Y) are not reliable tests for definitive sex determination.

The likelihood of another fetus being affected when a couple has already had one child with an autosomal dominant disorder is 50% if one parent is heterozygous and 100% if one parent is homozygous. The probability of a second affected child in patients with an autosomal recessive disorder would be 25%. In X-linked disorders in which the mother is a carrier (i.e., heterozygous), half of the male offspring will theoretically display an abnormal phenotype. **There are about 1,906 Mendelian disorders, of which 124 are X-linked disorders, 1,172 are autosomal dominant disorders, and 610 are autosomal recessive disorders.** Relatively few of these genetic problems can be diagnosed antenatally.

3. Intrauterine diagnosis

a. Amniotic fluid genetic analysis

The evaluation of the fetal somatic cells present in the amniotic fluid has been used extensively to detect certain genetic anomalies of the fetus. The fetal cells collected by amniocentesis are cultured and then a chromosomal analysis is carried out to determine the presence of any abnormal chromosomes. This procedure is usually performed at between 15 and 18 weeks' gestation in order to allow for enough time to complete the cell cultures (i.e., 2–3 weeks) in case pregnancy intervention is decided upon.

It is generally accepted that the risk of amniocentesis to the mother is of the order of 1:1,000. The risks include infection, Rh isoimmunization, and hemorrhage. Similarly, the fetal risk is also very low and consists of hemorrhage, infection, injury, abortion, or death. In addition, fetal skin scarring and dimpling is a common enough complication that it should be mentioned when counseling the patient. **The overall risk of amniocentesis is probably less than 0.5%.**

The technique of amniocentesis is relatively simple. A pocket of amniotic fluid is located away from the fetus and the placenta by ultrasonography. Usually, the best locations are either on the side of the fetal small parts, behind the nape of the neck, or beneath the presenting part, which may be elevated by one hand just over the pubis prior to the insertion of the needle. The overlying skin is surgically prepped, draped, and anesthetized with local anesthetic solution down to the peritoneal surface of the abdominal wall. A 20- to 22-gauge long spinal needle is inserted into the amniotic sac, and approximately 30 ml of amniotic fluid is then withdrawn. The fetal heart tones are monitored before and after the procedure.

The fetal sex can be determined by chromosomal analysis. **The use of maternal serum and amniotic fluid α-fetoprotein levels, in patients who have had a previous infant with a neural tube defect, may be beneficial in defining that particular diagnosis.** There are many enzyme tests of the amniotic fluid that can be utilized to detect certain inborn errors of metabolism (i.e., Tay-Sach's disease, Fabry's disease, Lesch-Nyhan syndrome, Gaucher's disease, Niemann-Pick disease, and perhaps another 75 chromosomally related conditions).

b. Chorionic villus sampling

While amniocentesis is the most common technique currently being used in the detection of prenatal genetic disorders, it cannot safely be utilized prior to about 15 weeks' gestation because of technical problems. As a consequence, the diagnosis of chromosomal or biochemical abnormalities has usually been delayed until the 18th week or beyond, which then may require a second-trimester abortion with its additional risks.

In 1973, the first attempts to obtain fetal tissue by transcervical **chorionic villus sampling (CVS)** were carried out in patients who were undergoing elective abortions. Since that time, this procedure has been performed on hundreds of patients at between 6 and 12 weeks' gestation. The technique consists of inserting a small bore (1.5 or 2.4 mm) plastic catheter through the cervix under continuous ultrasonic guidance until the chorionic villi are reached, at which point the villus material is aspirated into a syringe containing a special media. Chromosome preparations can be made immediately from these villi or cells, or the cells may be cultured for 5–7 days to provide a greater number of cells for cytogenetic analysis.

The complete safety of this procedure has not yet been determined; however, it would appear that it is a safe technique (i.e., having less than 4–5% fetal losses worldwide) that could be quite valuable in the diagnosis of prenatal genetic disorders, since it can provide information much earlier in pregnancy. The experience of the operator, and of the cytogenetic laboratory in handling the chorionic tissue, is critical in obtaining good results. The preliminary findings on the rate of complications are as follows: spontaneous abortion, 3.8%; chorioamnionitis, 0.6%; delayed rupture of the membranes and/or oligohydramnios, 0.8%; and a discrepancy between the karyotype of the villi and that of the fetus, 1.7% (usually due to mosaicism). Maternal septic shock with renal failure has been reported with this procedure with the survival of the patient after a hysterectomy and a bilateral salpingo-oophorectomy. The success of obtaining a successful biopsy, according to one study, was of the order of 95%, with 56.9% being obtained on the first catheter pass, 23.9% on the second pass, and 13.8% in those who require multiple passes.

4. Principles of genetic counseling

a. Counseling in Down's syndrome

In recent years, it has been possible to diagnose many congenital anomalies prior to birth. As a consequence, genetic counseling has become the responsibility of the practicing physician. Patients have also become more knowledgeable concerning congenital abnormalities and expect that you will guide them and provide them with the knowledge of the relative risks involved in common anomalies. There is a 2–3% risk of congenital abnormalities in the general population.

The most common congenital abnormality is Down's syndrome. Depending upon her age, your patient's risk may range from 1:378 at the age of 35 to 1:106 at the age of 40, and finally, 1:30 at the age of 45. If a distant relative of the husband has Down's syndrome, there is usually no increased risk; however, should the husband's brother be so afflicted as a result of a translocation, then the risk is increased. About 2–3% of Down's syndrome cases involve a translocation. If one of the parents has a balanced translocation, the theoretic risk of a phenotypically normal child having the same balanced translocation is about 50%. The children of an individual carrying a balanced translocation involving one chromosome member 21 would have a 1–2% empiric risk of having Down's syndrome.

b. Counseling in other conditions

1) Autosomal dominant anomalies

If the effects of a specific gene are produced when it is present on only one of the chromosomes, then the gene is said to be dominant. In contrast, a recessive gene must be present on both chromosomes in order to produce its effect. Usually, the dominant genes carry through from one generation to the next. There is a 50% risk of involvement of a particular gene in each child of the affected heterozygous individual.

A dominant gene may not always be expressed in the individual's appearance. **The percent of the population in which the dominant gene is expressed is referred to as the amount of "penetrance."** Furthermore, different people may show a variety of expressions, from total absence to a completely manifested condition, with a variety of phenotypic conditions in between. **This degree of involvement in an individual has been termed the gene's "expressivity."** The **genotype** of an individual refers to that person's genetic makeup, whereas the **phenotype** of the individual refers to their physical appearance.

One of the most common autosomal dominant disorders is achondroplasia. The parents of an achondroplastic child may be phenotypically normal as the result of nonpenetrance, or they may have a mildly expressed form of the disease. If they are completely normal, then the achondroplasia must be assumed to be due to a new mutation. New mutations are said to occur on the order of 10^{-5} to 10^{-6} per locus per gamete per generation.

2) Autosomal recessive anomalies

Autosomal recessive diseases are often more severe than autosomal dominant conditions. Usually in these cases, the parents are normal and are carriers (i.e., heterozygous) for a specific gene. There is a 25% risk of involvement of the children of the affected couple. **Almost all inherited enzyme defects (i.e., inborn errors of metabolism) are due to recessive inheritance in which both chromosomes contain the gene (i.e., homozygous condition).** In some instances, the woman and her husband may be related (i.e., consanguinity), which increases the chance that the recessive genes will come together in the homozygous condition. The *Hardy-Weinberg equilibrium* is often used to determine the probability that a parent is heterozygous. If a population follows the Hardy-Weinberg equilibrium, then the measurement of the gene frequency in one generation will allow for a description of the expected genotype frequencies in subsequent generations. That is, the square of the sum of gene frequencies is equal to the next generation's genotypic frequencies [i.e., $(p + q)^2 = p^2 + 2pq + q^2$]. Thus, if the two alleles (p and q) are assumed to be possible at a single locus in a diploid organism, then the frequency of the three possible genotypes (i.e., homozygous p^2, heterozygous $2pq$, and homozygous q^2) are related to each other by the equation $p^2 + 2pq + q^2 = 1$. It should be remembered that there are many more heterozygotes for a specific allele than there are homozygotes in the population. As a consequence, p and q refer to gene or allelic frequencies [e.g., gene "A" (normal allele) = 0.7, gene "a" (mutant allele) = 0.3]. The homozygous condition is AA (p^2) and aa (q^2), and the heterozygote condition is Aa ($2pq$). For example, let us say that a certain condition has an incidence of 1 in 20,000 individuals. Thus, the q^2 (aa) = 1/20,000, and therefore q = 1/141 and p = 1 − (141), or 140/141, since p = (1 − q). The formula therefore predicts the number of individuals that carry gene "a" as follows: $2pq + q^2$ [or $2 \times 140/141 \times 1/141 + (1/141)^2 = 1/70$]. This indicates that 1 person out of 70 will carry the recessive gene, and that 1 out of 20,000 will actually have the disease.

3) X-linked dominant inheritance

In X-linked dominant disorders, there are no male-to-male transmissions. While both males and females are affected, the males often show more severe effects (e.g., vitamin D–resistant rickets). Since the males only transmit to their daughters and not to their sons, and the females transmit the trait to 50% of both their sons and daughters, there are twice as many females affected as there are males affected. Other examples of these disorders are some types of hereditary hematuria and the Xg^a blood group.

4) X-linked recessive inheritance

The majority of X-linked recessive disorders are found in males. A carrier female transmits the disorder to 50% of her male children, and 50% of the daughters will be carriers like the mother. If the unaffected female carrier marries an affected male, then an affected female child could result, due to her homozygous condition. About one-third of the X-linked disorders that appear spontaneously in a family will be due to a new mutation. Examples of X-linked recessive disorders include: (1) color blindness, (2) hemophilia A and B, (3) glucose 6-phosphate dehydrogenase deficiency, (4) Duchenne type pseudohypertrophic muscular dystrophy, (5) Lesch-Nyhan syndrome, and (6) agammaglobulinemia.

5) Multifactorial or polygenic inheritance

Most genetic conditions involve multiple factors and therefore a defect cannot be traced to a single dominant or recessive gene. Conditions such as spina bifida, cleft lip, and congenital heart defects are examples of **multifactorial inheritances** in which many environmental factors interact with the genes to produce an anomaly. The usual incidence of a child having a cleft palate is 0.1%. This risk increases to 4% after one affected offspring and up to 10% after two affected offspring.

CHAPTER 23

Antepartum care

Care more particularly for the individual patient than for the special features of the disease.

—*Sir William Osler**

1. The identification of the high-risk patient

Although **preconceptional counseling** is the best method of ensuring a quality pregnancy, many of your patients will not seek medical attention until the pregnancy is already an accomplished fact. It is important, therefore, that you **teach your patients** the necessity for counseling ahead of time, so that you may be able to identify and prevent any potential hazards to maternal and fetal well-being. One eminent obstetrician, Dr. Frank R. Lock, has stated, "Yet we live in a country which professes that health is the inalienable birthright of all of its citizens—and this surely includes the right to be well born."[1]

Ideally, the prenatal care of a woman should be started prior to the actual onset of the pregnancy. Any young girl who becomes sexually active, or any woman who is contemplating a pregnancy, should be considered as a candidate for preconceptional counseling. This approach to

prenatal care requires that a complete history and physical examination, basic laboratory studies, and a frank discussion of sex, nutrition, the impact of social habits (e.g., alcohol, smoking, drug abuse), and physical condition (e.g., overweight, underweight, medications, exercise, and occupational hazards), should be carried out with an emphasis on the effect these factors can have upon the outcome of a pregnancy. Medical conditions should be brought under control or cured. Hazardous social habits should be reduced to a minimum or eliminated entirely, and appropriate amounts of sleep, exercise, and diet should be recommended.

a. Age

The **patient's age** is an important factor. Young mothers (i.e., less than 20 years old) generally have more **premature births and infants of low birth weight,** which is probably secondary to their generally poor diet. In contrast, women over the age of 35 are associated with an increased incidence of **Down's syndrome** as well as other congenital abnormalities. In addition, there is a striking increase in the maternal mortality rate with increasing age (i.e., $13.1:100,000$ at 20–24 years of age, as contrasted with $119.3:100,000$ at 40–44 years of age). Placental abruption in women over 40 years of age is about double that of women who are under 30.

b. Parity

There is an increased risk of placenta previa and placenta acreta in women who are of advanced parity (i.e., five or more children), which is possibly due to endometrial scarring secondary to repeated childbearing. Postpartum hemorrhage and uterine rupture

---

*Reprinted with permission from Robert Bennett Bean, *Sir William Osler: Aphorisms from His Bedside Teachings and Writings,* William Bennett Bean, ed. Springfield, Ill.: Charles C Thomas, Publisher, 1968, p. 97.
[1] Reprinted with permission from Frank R. Lock, "The Right to Be Well Born: Quality versus Quantity in Obstetrics and Gynecology," *American Journal of Obstetrics and Gynecology* 105 (1969), pp. 651–658.

are also more common, as are other complications such as cephalopelvic disproportion, abnormal presentations, and poor labor.

c. Height

Patients of *small stature* (i.e., less than 5 feet tall), generally have a small pelvis, even though it may be of gynecoid configuration; thus they are at greater risk for cephalopelvic disproportion and may require delivery by cesarean section.

d. Pregnancy weight

It has been noted that if the initial prepregnancy weight is less than 120 lbs, and if it is coupled with a pregnancy weight gain of less than 11 lbs, then there is an increased incidence of low–birth weight infants, who will have an increased neonatal mortality rate. If the initial prepregnancy weight is more than 20% above the standard weight for height measurement, and the pregnancy weight gain is excessive, there may be an increased incidence of dystocia and birth trauma secondary to a large-for-gestational-age (LGA) infant. Patients who weigh more than 200 lbs seem to also have an increased risk of developing diabetes and hypertension.

e. Diabetes

About 3–12% of women will become diabetic during pregnancy. If the blood sugars are not maintained in the euglycemic range, it is thought that there is an increased incidence of macrosomia and congenital abnormalities. Glucosuria occurs in normal pregnant women in about 5–40% of cases (see Chapter 34).

f. Hypertension and renal disease

Patients with chronic renal disease, and/or hypertension are at greater risk for fetal intrauterine growth retardation, abruptio placentae, premature labor, and superimposed toxemia. In the presence of severe renal disease, pregnancy may be contraindicated (see Chapter 33).

g. Hemoglobinopathy

There are five types of hemoglobinopathy that commonly occur in the United States: (1) sickle cell trait (SA), (2) sickle cell anemia (SS), (3) sickle cell–hemoglobin C disease (SC), (4) sickle cell–thalassemia (STh), and (5) hemoglobin C disease (CC) (see Chapter 35).

h. Isoimmunization

Patients who have Rh negative blood should be monitored throughout pregnancy to detect any evidence of Rh_o (D) sensitization. The presence of irregular antibodies, such as Kell, Duffy, or Kidd, should also be followed carefully. The administration of anti-Rh_o (D) antibody at 28 weeks' gestation and again within 72 hours following delivery in a nonsensitized Rh negative patient (who has an Rh positive infant) is currently being recommended (see Chapter 37).

[handwritten margin note: ABO IgM doesn't cross placenta / IgA & IgG cross placenta / IgM in breast milk?]

i. Previous prematurity

A history of previous premature deliveries should alert you to the possible presence of an incompetent cervix or other uterine abnormalities (i.e., diethylstilbestrol congenital anomaly, septate uterus, uterus bicornis, or leiomyomas) (see Chapter 14).

j. Employment

Since 51% of women are employed today outside of the home, there is a higher risk than in the past of pregnant women being exposed to a wide variety of hazardous chemicals and toxic agents that could endanger the fetus. **The patient's employment environment should be thoroughly assessed to detect any problems that might affect the outcome of the pregnancy.** In many industries, the patient is exposed to hazardous working conditions and subjected to lethal toxins, mutagenic substances, dangerous chemicals, and irradiation. It is important for you to understand the types of major industries in your community and the various jobs that your patients may be involved in during their work days. Many industrial plants will provide tours through their facilities and will cooperate with you in assessing the risks and hazards in the workplace, since they are also interested in providing healthful jobs for their employees.

If a medical condition, an obstetric condition, or a job-related condition occurs during pregnancy, then it is essential that you make a decision as to whether the patient may continue to work. Such decisions may take the following forms: (1) the **patient may continue to work** without danger or discomfort, (2) the patient may continue to work, but certain **desirable modifications** in her working conditions may be suggested for her comfort, (3) the patient may continue to work, but only if specific **necessary modifications** are made in her working conditions for safety and comfort, or (4) the **patient may not continue to work at all.** Such information may be conveyed to the employer **only** with the patient's express written permission. **All such decisions must be time-limited and require reassessment at periodic intervals.** Normal pregnancy is not a disease, nor is it a disability; a woman with a normal pregnancy can continue to work at a job that has no greater hazards than are present in the community in which she lives until she goes into labor (see Chapter 4).

2. Gestational age determination

Perhaps one of the most pressing problems in obstetrics today is the determination of the gestational age of the fetus. When the condition of the patient or of the fetus warrants consideration of an early delivery, the gestational age determination becomes quite critical (see Chapter 26).

a. Last menstrual period (LMP)

If you take the date of the last menstrual period (LMP) and subtract 3 months and add 7 days, you will arrive at the determination of the estimated date of confinement (EDC) by Nägele's rule. Alternately, you may add 280 days to the first day of the last menstrual period, or you can add 9 months and 7 days to the LMP to arrive at the same EDC. The calculation of the EDC in this manner will provide an accuracy in determining the true delivery date of about ±3 weeks.

The use of the ovulation/fertilization date instead of the LMP has been used by some authors as the reference date for gestational age determination. The date of ovulation/fertilization, however, is highly variable. The use of birth control pills just prior to the onset of pregnancy also interferes with the gestational age calculation, due to the frequency of amenorrheic episodes following the cessation of oral contraceptive therapy.

b. The initial pelvic examination

The patient's first pelvic examination will often aid in determining the number of weeks of gestation (see Chapters 4 and 19). At about 6 weeks' gestation, a soft spot may be noted at the junction of the cervix and the fundus, and by the 8th week, this softness extends across the entire width of the cervix. Between the 7th and 8th weeks, the uterus becomes more globular and is noticeably softened. In some instances, a slightly more prominent bulge may be noted on one side of the uterus over the implantation site. **By the 8th week, the uterus begins to enlarge, and by the 10th week, the examiner may find that the superior-inferior diameter of the uterus is about 10 cm.** This measurement will correlate fairly well with the number of weeks of gestation as the uterus rises out of the pelvis and becomes an abdominal organ. After 16 weeks, the superior-inferior diameter of the uterus (i.e., the fundal measurement) will equal the number of weeks of gestation until about 34 weeks' gestation, after which the measurements will fail to correlate (Fig. 23-1).

c. The fetal heartbeat

The fetal heartbeat may be detected with an ultrasonic scan at week 6 or 7, with an ultrasonic Doppler at about week 9, or with the Hillis-DeLee fetoscope at about 17 to 20 weeks' gestation.

d. Fetal movements

The patient may detect fetal movements (i.e., quickening) between weeks 16 and 20. A multiparous patient will typically feel fetal movements by 17.5 weeks, whereas the primigravida patient will not notice fetal movements until about 19.5 weeks. If you instruct your patient to be alert for fetal movements between weeks 16 and 20, she may notice them somewhat earlier (i.e., between weeks 16 and 18) (see Chapter 19).

e. Ultrasound

The use of ultrasound has been of considerable assistance in determining the gestational age of the fetus. **A gestational sac or "ring" may be identified in the uterus by sonography at about 5 weeks' gestation.** The length of the embryo (i.e., crown-rump

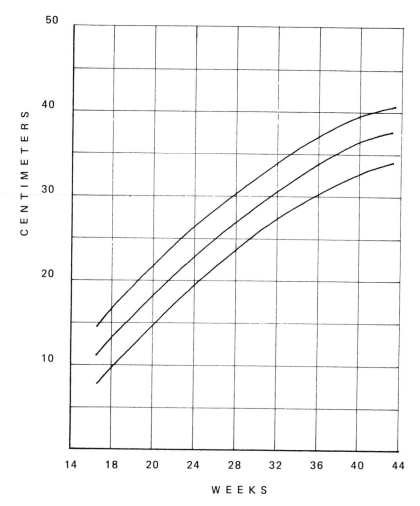

FIGURE 23-1. Uterine fundal height chart that can be placed in the prenatal record. If the measurement from the symphysis pubis over the uterus to its top falls below the 10th percentile line at any week, the pregnancy becomes at risk for IUGR, and other diagnostic tests can be done. (Redrawn with permission from D. N. Danforth and J. R. Scott, eds., *Obstetrics and Gynecology,* 5th ed. Philadelphia: J. B. Lippincott Company, 1986, p. 469.)

length) at about 10 to 12 weeks' gestation may be quite accurate in determining the fetal gestational age. **By the 6th or 7th week, the fetal heart action may be detected, and by the 14th week the fetal head and chest can be defined.** Between the 16th and 26th weeks, the accuracy of the fetal biparietal diameter in predicting gestational age will be accurate ±11 days. After 30 weeks' gestation, the accuracy of the biparietal diameter of the fetal head in gestational dating decreases to about ±3 weeks; thus, the bi-

parietal diameter should not be utilized to determine fetal gestational age after 30 weeks' gestation. Other sonographic parameters, such as the **femur length** and the fetal **weight determination,** are also of value. The **continuing growth of the fetal biparietal diameter** in the third trimester as measured by ultrasound may also be evaluated in order to diagnose the presence of intrauterine growth retardation. If all of the above parameters are plotted on a gestational assessment graph, it becomes possible to at least visualize the most likely date for the EDC and to more rationally calculate the gestational age of the fetus (Fig. 23-2).

3. Continuing prenatal assessment

Continuing normal prenatal care should be carried out at monthly intervals during the first 28 weeks, at two-week intervals from weeks 28 to 36, and then at weekly intervals until delivery. If complications should occur, these visits should be increased in frequency as necessary. The establishment of weekly visits from weeks 16 to 20 will assist you in determining the time of quickening and will allow you to detect the first time that the fetal heart tones may be heard by the fetoscope, which will be of considerable value in dating the pregnancy.

The early identification of high-risk maternity patients allows for an orderly transfer of the patient to a secondary or a tertiary medical center, where the obstetric expertise and the pediatric intensive care nurseries required to manage such patients are available. The **perinatal regionalization networks** that have been developed over the past few years have had a considerable impact on improving the salvage of low–birth weight (LBW) infants.

a. Periodic examinations

You should measure the patient's **weight** and calculate her overall weight gain for the pregnancy on each visit. In addition, the **blood pressure** and the results of **urine sugar and protein tests** should be obtained. Your examination of the patient should consist of detecting the **fetal heart sounds** and measuring the **height of the uterine fundus in centimeters.** In later gestation (i.e., after 26 weeks), **Leopold's maneuvers** should be performed and the **fetal lie defined** on each visit. The presence of dependent peripheral **edema** of the legs should be noted. In addition, any complaints or concerns that the patient may have concerning her pregnancy should be recorded and discussed.

b. Laboratory examinations

1) Routine tests

A complete blood count, blood type and Rh with an antibody screen, urinalysis, urine culture, gonorrheal culture, serological test for syphilis (RPR, VDRL) and a Papanicolaou smear should be obtained initially. The hemoglobin and hematocrit values should be obtained initially and then at monthly intervals after 24 weeks. **Periodic laboratory tests** should be obtained in order to detect Rh sensitization and other potential problems. The RPR and a gonorrheal culture should be repeated at 36 weeks' gestation. In black patients, a hemoglobin electrophoresis should be obtained to detect sickle cell disease. An evaluation of the serum levels of α-fetoprotein should be considered between 15 and 19 weeks' gestation.

2) Diabetes mellitus

If the patient gives a history of having had: (1) a previous large infant (i.e., more than 4,000 grams); (2) a previous unexplained stillbirth; (3) a neonatal death or abortion; (4) a previous fetal abnormality; (5) current glucosuria; (6) a history of diabetes in her parents or siblings; or (7) is obese (i.e., more than 200 lbs), then the possibility that the patient may have diabetes mellitus should be considered. Due to the fact that diabetes can have such a devastating effect upon the pregnancy, it is now recommended that all pregnant patients should also be routinely screened for diabetes at 26–28 weeks' gestation (see Chapter 34).

c. Evaluation of weight gain

The patient's diet during pregnancy is very important, and if there is a lack of appropriate weight gain, then nutritional counseling is in order. The patient should gain between *20 and 27 lbs* during pregnancy, almost all of which should be gained in the last two trimesters (Fig. 23-3). The total projected minimal weight gain by trimester that some investigators have recommended is: 0.65 kg (1.5 lbs) in the first trimester; a total of 7.0 kg (15.5 lbs) by the end of the second trimester; and 11 kg (24 lbs) by the end of the third trimester.

The **nutrition** of the pregnant patient should be carefully evaluated. **Most women require about 2,100 to 2,400 Kcal/day during the reproductive years. With the advent of pregnancy, an additional 300 Kcal/day should be taken in to supply the needs of the growing fetus, according to the recommendations of the National Research Council.** The protein requirements are normally 45

Text continues on p. 319

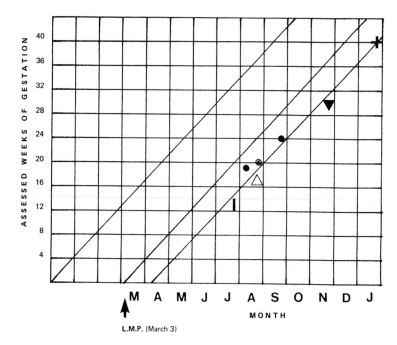

L.M.P. (March 3)

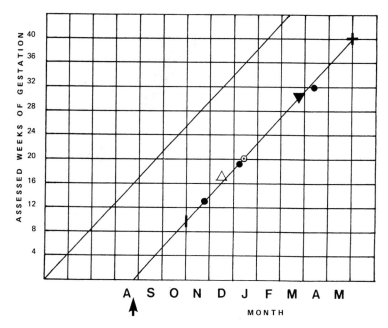

L.M.P. (August 21)

FIGURE 23-2. Generic graph for plotting gestational age. *Upper:* Graph for a 23-year-old woman, gravida 2 para 1, unsure LMP = March 3. Line to the right extrapolated from clinical data projects true EDC. (Legend: + EDC; • fundal height; ⊙ fetal heart tones first heard; △ quickening (primigravida, 19 weeks; multigravida, 17 weeks); ▌ first examination; ▼ ultrasound.) *Lower:* Graph for a 22-year-old woman, gravida 1, para 0, class D diabetic. Line to the right indicates that the EDC is probably correct. (Legend: + EDC; • fundal height; ⊙ fetal heart tones first heard; △ quickening (primigravida, 19 weeks; multigravida, 17 weeks); ▌ first examination; ▼ ultrasound; ◇ X-ray; ★ positive HCG). (Redrawn with permission from T. R. Johnson and B. A. Work, Jr., "A Dynamic Graph for Documentation of Gestational Age," *Obstetrics and Gynecology* 54 (1979), pp. 115–116.)

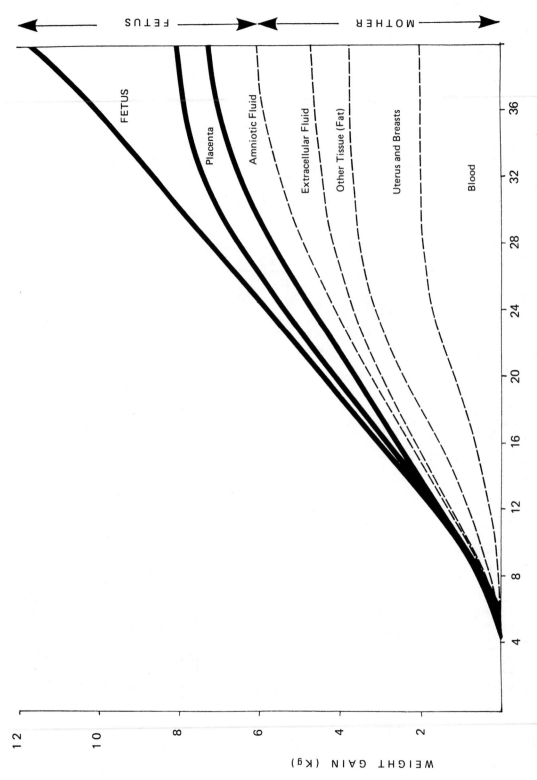

FIGURE 23-3. Pattern and components of weight gain during pregnancy. (Redrawn with permission from R. M. Pitkin, "Nutritional Support in Obstetrics and Gynecology," *Clinical Obstetrics and Gynecology* 19 (1976), pp. 489–513.)

grams/day for the mature nonpregnant woman; however, pregnancy places an additional requirement of 30 grams/day, for a total of 75 grams/day. In the teenager, this amount of protein may need to be even greater (i.e., 1.5–1.7 grams of protein per kilogram of pregnant weight).

All pregnant patients should receive iron supplementation. The routine administration of multivitamins to pregnant women has been controversial; however, if the dietary intake of vitamins is adequate, then vitamin supplementation will probably not be required. The requirement for folic acid is increased during pregnancy, so this is one vitamin that should perhaps be administered routinely. **The administration of 1 mg/day of folic acid will provide ample prophylaxis against megaloblastic anemia.** While this treatment may mask an undiagnosed pernicious anemia and allow for the development of neurologic sequelae, the risk of such occurrence is of the order of 2:10,000. **Vitamin B_{12} occurs only in foods of animal origin, and therefore in patients who are strict vegetarians, there is an increased risk of giving birth to a vitamin B_{12}–deficient infant.**

The recommended weight gain in pregnancy is 20–27 lbs. Much of this gain can be accounted for by the requirements of the fetus and the pregnancy as follows: fetus, 7.5 lbs; placenta, 1.5 lbs; amniotic fluid, 2 lbs; uterine weight, 2.5 lbs; blood volume expansion, 3.5 lbs; breasts, 2 lbs; and dependent edema, 2 lbs—for a total of 21 lbs.** It has been found that the fetal weight tends to parallel the maternal weight gain. The prepregnancy nutritional status of the patient should also be considered in counseling the patient. **For the patient who is already 20% above the recommended weight for her height, the projected weight gain should perhaps be of the order of about 20 lbs.** In addition, close scrutiny of the amount of protein, carbohydrates, and fat in the diet should be carried out. In patients who are underweight at the beginning of pregnancy, an attempt should be made to increase the caloric intake while maintaining a well-balanced diet.

d. Evaluation of social habits

The patient's social habits are of considerable significance in regard to the outcome of the pregnancy. **Smoking** in pregnancy may result in an infant who weighs 200 grams less than the normal infant. This effect has been explained as being secondary to the vasoconstrictive action of the nicotine on the uterine vasculature, as well as to the inactivation of the hemoglobin by carbon monoxide. In addition, smokers commonly experience a loss of appetite and often fail to gain weight in pregnancy. There is also a decreased plasma volume in patients who smoke, which has been associated with fetal growth retardation.

If the mother consumes an excessive amount of alcohol during pregnancy (e.g., 6 oz/day), then the **fetal alcohol syndrome** may develop. This condition consists of craniofacial defects, growth retardation, and cardiovascular and limb deformities. The perinatal mortality rate of infants with fetal alcohol syndrome is about 17%.

The use of over-the-counter (OTC) medications by the patient should be discouraged. Drug interactions may account for about 2–3% of all congenital abnormalities (see Chapter 28).

e. Coitus

Coitus during pregnancy should be avoided in women who are threatening to abort or who have had episodes of premature labor. In these instances, the sexual excitement, as well as the prostaglandins that are present in the semen, may cause uterine contractions and may aggravate an already irritable uterus. Coitus in the presence of ruptured membranes may result in infection. Douching after coitus, or at any time, either during pregnancy or otherwise, should be avoided.

f. Travel

Many patients will ask your advice concerning travel during pregnancy. If the patient's pregnancy is entirely normal, then you should consider some of the general risks that may be involved. Prolonged sitting in a car or on an airplane may predispose the patient to thrombophlebitis and pulmonary embolism. Travel often involves long hours and a hectic pace, which may overly fatigue the patient. Frequently, during travel the patient may be remote from proper medical care facilities, which could be a serious problem if a complication should develop or if premature labor should occur. The exposure of the patient to parasites and infectious agents that may be endemic in a foreign country may also result in serious problems.

Commercial airliners pressurize their cabins at about 7,000 feet above sea level. An accidental cabin decompression at high altitudes (e.g., 30,000 feet) could cause problems with nitrogen retention in both the mother and the fetus. Scuba diving should not be performed in pregnancy for the same reason. The fetus apparently does not eliminate the nitrogen from its bloodstream as well as the mother, even if the mother follows the recommended decompression times in the "dive tables" in returning to the surface. This is especially true if the mother flies in a commercial airplane within 24 hours of scuba diving, due to the added risk of both the mother and fetus developing the "bends" because of the decreased atmospheric pressures in the cabin and the residual nitrogen remaining in the bloodstream from scuba diving.

g. Exercise

The recommendation that a woman should exercise in pregnancy is a recent development. Indeed, there is still no evidence to show that regular exercise will improve the outcome of pregnancy. **Earlier studies had seemed to indicate that there was a diversion of the blood flow away from the uterus during exercise to support the actively working muscles, perhaps to the detriment of the fetus.**

It has been noted that exercise does increase the **core body temperature** dramatically. Strenuous exercise in the nonpregnant woman for 30–60 minutes will increase the temperature to 39° C, whereas the same type of exercise for 15 minutes will not elevate the temperature above 38° C. There are no comparable data in pregnant women. **In animal studies, there is apparently an increase in fetal abnormalities, especially neural tube defects, when the core temperature exceeds 38° C** (i.e., the critical temperature is apparently about 38.9° C, or 102° F), and it is suspected that the same may be true in humans.

The safety of the mother and infant must be the goal of any exercise program developed for the pregnant woman. Due to the fact that little is known about the ultimate effects of exercise in pregnancy, a conservative approach should be utilized until more information becomes available. The exercise program should encompass a number of different activities, such as walking, swimming, dancing, calisthenics, and other sports that the patient wishes to pursue.

According to the **Guidelines of the American College of Obstetricians and Gynecologists (ACOG)** the patient who exercises during pregnancy

should: (1) exercise at least three times per week to maintain a training effect, (2) not engage in exercise in which there are ballistic movements, deep flexion movements, or excessive stretching, and (3) have a warm-up period before starting exercise and a cooling-off period at the end of the exercise. The patient's heart rate should not exceed 140 bpm, the exercise should not exceed 15 minutes, supine exercises and those involving Valsalva's maneuver should be avoided, and the patient should not allow her core body temperature to exceed 38° C. Adequate liquids should be taken to prevent dehydration, and an adequate number of calories should be added to the diet to cover the needs of the exercise.

It has been suggested that the pregnant woman who has not been athletically active prior to pregnancy should probably not undertake an exercise training program during the pregnancy. In these women, there is probably not a sufficient amount of *collateral circulation* to the muscles as might be expected in a woman who was athletically active prior to her pregnancy. As a conseqence, in order for the body to supply the actively working muscles during exercise in the nonathletic woman, a major diversion of blood flow would have to occur, with the blood being directed away from other nonessential organs, such as the uterus.

If the athletically active woman should elect to exercise during pregnancy, then she should endeavor to follow the guidelines that have been issued by the ACOG. Following the exercise period, the pregnant woman should assume the left lateral decubitus position and rest for at least 10 minutes. While **exercise in pregnancy** has been a controversial subject, the present available evidence would seem to indicate that, if the recommended guidelines are followed, then exercise may be permissible in the athletically active normal pregnant women.

Pregnant women with medical complications, such as hypertension, diabetes, thyroid disease, anemia, or cardiac arrhythmia, should probably not exercise at all in pregnancy. Very thin or very obese women, as well as sedentary unathletic women, should not exercise during pregnancy. Patients with obstetric complications, such as a breech presentation, intrauterine growth retardation, a history of premature labor, a history of bleeding, an incompetent cervix, or a multiple gestation, should also avoid exercise.

4. Patient education

a. Patients at high risk

During pregnancy, special care should be given to patients who are at high risk, such as: (1) those who are under 16 years of age, or over 35 years of age, (2) those who are financially underprivileged, (3) those who have a history of three or more pregnancies within a period of three years, (4) those who have a history of poor reproductive performance, (5) those who are on a special medical diet, (6) those who follow a fad diet, (7) those who smoke, drink, or abuse drugs, (8) those who are appreciably underweight at the beginning of pregnancy, (9) those who have a hemoglobin of less than 11 grams/dl, and finally (10) those whose monthly weight gain beyond 12 weeks' gestation is less than 2 lbs.

It has been shown that there are **four general phases of tissue growth:** (1) **hyperplasia,** in which there is an increase in the number of the cells, (2) **hyperplasia and hypertrophy,** in which there is both an increase in the number of the cells as well as in the size of the cells, (3) **hypertrophy,** in which there is an increase in the cellular size without a change in the number of cells, and (4) **maturity,** when all of the growth of the cells is completed. It is evident that nutritional deprivation may have different effects upon the cells of specific tissues depending upon the growth phase that the specific tissue is undergoing at the time of the insult. If the hyperplasia phase is interrupted, the tissue will ultimately have fewer cells, and no amount of refeeding at a later time will replace them. On the other hand, an interruption of the growth during the hypertrophy phase will merely produce smaller cells, an effect that later refeeding may completely reverse.

b. Home childbirth

Modern obstetrics has resulted in an unprecedented decrease in both the perinatal and maternal mortality rates. In the past few years, however, there has been a trend in childbearing which suggests that the birth process should occur in a more "natural setting," such as the home, where the family members can provide support for the laboring mother. Furthermore, there has been an estrangement between some patients and the established medical profession. These patients have come to believe that the physicians of today are actually causing complications in pregnancy care by the use of the new medical technology. In other instances, some religious groups have failed to accept any medical care at all. As a consequence, there has been a resurgence in the interest in having home births, often with little or no prenatal care.

In one reported study, the perinatal mortality rate between 1975 and 1982 in an Indiana religious group was estimated to be **48:1,000** births, as compared to **18:1,000** in the remainder of the state. The maternal mortality rate in this group during this same period was estimated to be of the order of **872:100,000** live births as compared to **9:100,000** live births for the rest of the state. These high mortality statistics are unacceptable in modern medicine and reflect what one would expect to find in a Third World country where there is minimal or no medical care available. **(For example, in Bangladesh during the period 1968–1970, the maternal mortality rate was 570:100,000 live births).**

Patients should be educated as to the risks involved in "fad" practices such as home delivery. Indeed, many hospitals have introduced the **birthing room** concept, in which the patient's husband, and sometimes even her children, are allowed to be present in the labor room with her throughout the labor and delivery process. Some physicians prefer to call this approach **family-centered care (FCC), single-room maternity care (SRM), labor-delivery-recovery room care (LDR), or labor-delivery-recovery postpartum care (LDRP).** A special attempt is made to make the room as home-like as possible, with drapes, lamps, and other furnishings that one might expect to find in a master bedroom in the home. The medical equipment, including a portable anesthesia machine, is camouflaged as furniture or placed behind screens, and the bed breaks down into a delivery table at the time of delivery so that the patient does not have to be moved into the sterile atmosphere of the delivery room. This approach makes much more sense than a home delivery because the facilities needed in case of a serious emergency are immediately available.

CHAPTER 24

Labor and delivery

. . . .

Don't touch the patient—state first what you see; cultivate your powers of observation.

—*Sir William Osler**

. . . .

1. False vs. true labor

Labor has been divided into two phases: the latent phase and the active phase. The distinction between the latent phase of labor and "false labor" is difficult if not impossible to determine. **False labor usually ceases prior to the onset of the active phase of labor and therefore can only be recognized in retrospect.** In actual fact, false labor and the latent phase of labor are the same thing in a functional sense, because effacement of the cervix occurs with either type.

a. Cervical effacement

The cervix is made up of connective tissue consisting of collagen and a ground substance containing elastin and proteoglycans. *The amount of collagen present in the cervix is closely related to the rate of cervical dilatation.* **Patients who have a high concentration of collagen seem to have more prolonged labors than those with a lower concentration.** During pregnancy there is a dynamic and continuous breakdown of the collagen in the cervix, so that by term, there is less than one-third of the amount pres-

---

*Reprinted with permission from Robert Bennett Bean, *Sir William Osler: Aphorisms from His Bedside Teachings and Writings,* William Bennett Bean, ed. Springfield, Ill.: Charles C Thomas, Publisher, 1968, p. 37.

ent as there was in the nonpregnant cervix. This decreased amount of collagen has been cited as the cause of the softness or *ripeness* of the cervix that is seen in the last few days or weeks of pregnancy. Certain agents, such as prostaglandin E_2 (PGE_2), will cause collagen breakdown also, which might account for this drug's striking ability to soften or ripen the cervix. The regulators of the synthesis and catabolism of the cervical connective tissue are thought to be relaxin, estrogen, progesterone, prostaglandins, leukotriens, and catabolin. It is possible that the estrogens sensitize the cervix to the effect of prostaglandins, which then initiate a high degree of proteolytic activity to degrade the collagen and other connective tissues in order to produce the clinical "ripening." Some of the more prominent enzymes that appear to be involved in this process are collaginase and granulocyte elastase, in addition to other proteolytic enzymes.

b. Latent labor

The distinction between latent (or false) labor and active labor is often difficult; however, certain considerations may assist you in making this distinction. **Latent labor is characterized by its irregularity.** The contractions usually are greater than five minutes apart and are irregular in interval, strength, and duration. **The cervix is less than 90% effaced and less than 3 cm dilated in the latent phase of labor. The main effect of latent labor seems to be the preparation of the cervix, which gradually effaces completely and dilates up to 3 cm, which appears to be the baseline dilatation from which active labor begins** (Fig. 24-1). **This latent phase of labor may take up to seven hours in a primigravida and five hours in a multigravida although these times may be highly variable.**

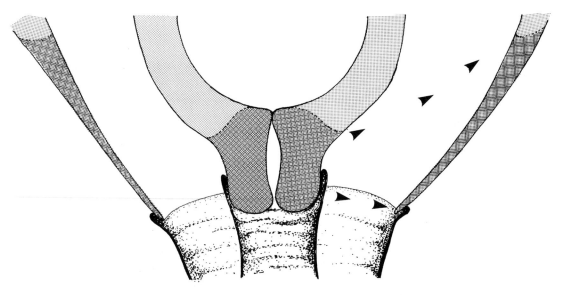

FIGURE 24-1. Effacement and dilatation of the cervix in the primigravida in early labor. Cervical shortening occurs first with gradual thinning of the cervical tissue. Dilatation progresses to about 3 cm by the time that the effacement is essentially complete and the active phase of labor is ready to begin. With the onset of active labor, the cervix continues to dilate as the tissue retracts and thins out in the lower uterine segment. The arrows signify the direction of the cervical dilatation and the "taking-up" of the tissues of the lower uterine segment as the labor progresses.

Moreover, in the case of false labor, the contractions may often start and stop. This should not be confused with dystocia or failure to progress and lead you to perform an unnecessary cesarean section, since true labor (i.e., active labor) has actually not even begun in this situation.

c. True labor

True labor, or the active phase of labor, is characterized by its **regularity.** The interval between contractions is almost always less than five minutes (usually 3 minutes) and the contractions are regular. The contractions are consistently strong, lasting 45–60 seconds from the beginning to the peak of the contraction, and may be somewhat painful, depending upon the patient's tolerance for pain. **The cervix will always be effaced at least 90–100% and will be dilated to about 3 cm. Further, the cervix will dilate rapidly from this point onward** (Fig. 24-2). A failure of the cervix to progressively dilate beyond 6–7 cm should be considered as evidence of a secondary arrest of labor.

1) First stage of labor

According to E. A. Friedman's data, the minimal progress that should occur in labor is a cervical dilatation of **no less than 1.2 cm/hr in the primigravida and 1.5 cm/hr in the multigravida. Based upon this data, the dilatation from 3–10 cm should require no more than 5.8 hours in the primigravida and 4.6 hours in the multigravida.**

2) Second stage of labor

The length of the *second stage of labor,* from complete dilatation to the delivery of the infant, is of the order of 45 minutes in the primigravida, and anywhere from zero to three contractions (i.e., 0–10 minutes) in the **multigravida. The second stage usually should not be allowed to extend beyond two hours, since the risk of uterine rupture increases considerably thereafter.** In addition, there is an increased risk of hemorrhage and infection beyond this time limit. While this "two-hour rule" is not absolute, any prolongation of the second stage be-

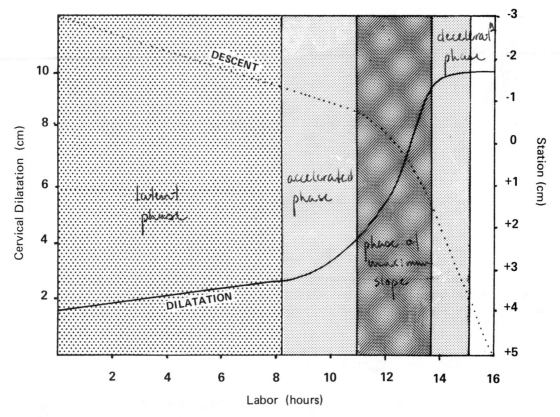

FIGURE 24-2. Labor curves showing the relationship between the cervical dilatation and the descent of the fetal head. The initial period of about eight hours encompasses the *latent* period. As the cervix becomes dilated to about 3–4 cm, the onset of true labor occurs with first the *accelerated phase,* then the *phase of maximum slope,* then followed by the *deceleration phase* as the cervix becomes completely dilated. The second stage of labor then begins and lasts until the fetus is delivered. The descent of the fetal head accelerates primarily during the phase of maximum slope and the deceleration phase of active labor. (Adapted from E. A. Friedman, "Dysfunctional Labor," in A. B. Gerbie and J. J. Sciarra, eds., *Gynecology and Obstetrics,* vol. 2. Philadelphia: Harper & Row, 1984, Chapter 72, p. 4.)

yond this point should alert you to the fact that serious consequences may result.

3) Third stage of labor

The third stage of labor (i.e., from the delivery of the baby to the delivery of the placenta) usually lasts about 10–15 minutes. If the placenta has not delivered by 30–60 minutes, or if undue hemorrhage becomes a problem, then manual removal of the placenta should be accomplished.

4) Fourth stage of labor

Some older physicians will list a *fourth stage of labor,* which encompasses the first hour or so following delivery, in which bleeding, shock, or other complications may make their first appearance. It is often worthwhile to remain in the hospital and observe the patient closely during this period.

d. Labor contractions

Active phase labor contractions usually occur at three-minute intervals, reach an intensity of

about 40–60 mm Hg, and last about 45–60 seconds from the beginning to the peak of the contraction. The upper segment of the uterus is the contractile portion, and the lower portion is passive. With each contraction, there is a retraction, or a taking up of the uterine muscle, and a thinning out of the tissue of the lower uterine segment as the upper segment becomes thicker. **In between contractions, the baseline resting tonus of the uterus should be about 8–12 mm Hg.**

e. Station

During the first stage of labor, the primary goal of the labor contractions is to overcome the **obstruction of the cervical ring,** whereas during the second stage, it is mostly the **soft tissue obstruction of the pelvis** that must be overcome as the fetal presenting part descends further into the pelvis. According to the classic labor curve, the fetal presenting part essentially descends in an inverse manner to the curve of the dilatation of the cervix; by the time the cervix is completely dilated, the presenting part should have descended to at least about a +1 or a +2 station. The *station of the fetal presenting part* has traditionally been based upon an arbitrary division of the pelvic canal into 5 cm levels above the level of the ischial spines (i.e., zero station) and 5 cm levels below the spines. Thus, a −5 station indicates that the presenting part is "floating"; a 0 station is said to be present when the fetal head is engaged; and a +5 station exists when the fetal head is on the perineum ready for delivery. **A more practical and simpler classification based upon an arbitrary division of the pelvis into thirds, both above and below the ischial spines, is frequently used clinically** (Fig. 24-3). Thus, if the presenting part presents at the pelvic inlet, the presenting part is said to be **floating,** or at a −3 station. When the head is **dipping** into the pelvis and is no longer easily displaced with the abdominal hand, then it is at a −2 station. When the head is not easily displaced and presents just short of the 0 station, then it is at a −1 station. When the head is **engaged,** the biparietal diameter of the fetal head will have passed through the pelvic inlet and the foremost tip will be at the spines, or at the 0 station. When the presenting part has descended to the perineum and is visible at the introitus, it is said to be at the +3 station. The in-between thirds below 0 station are +1 and +2. Confusion as to the actual station

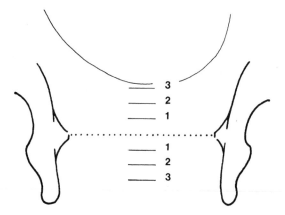

FIGURE 24-3. Stations of the fetal head.

of the presenting part may occur if there is excessive *fetal head molding (i.e., compression of the fetal skull)* or especially in the presence of *caput succedaneum (i.e., edema of the scalp).*

f. Presentation of the fetus

The "lie" of the fetus is based upon a comparison of the long axis of the fetus with that of the mother. If the fetus lies transversely, then a **shoulder (acromion)** will be the presenting part. If the fetus lies longitudinally, then either the head **(vertex)** or the buttocks **(breech)** will present. **Leopold's maneuvers are important techniques used in defining the fetal "presentation," or presenting part. The part of the fetus (i.e., breech, vertex, or shoulder) that overlies the pelvic inlet is the presenting part.**

In the vertex presentation, it is also important to know whether the head is flexed or extended. A midposition presentation of the head (sinciput or large fontanelle) will usually convert during the course of labor to either a flexed position (i.e., vertex or occiput anterior) or to an extended position (i.e., brow, or when fully extended, a face presentation). Thus, the **attitude of the fetus** (i.e., the relationship of the head to the thorax, such as flexion or hyperextension) must be detected. The **military attitude** (i.e., when the head is erect upon the body with no flexion or hyperextension), a **face presentation** (i.e., hyperextension of the fetal head) or the normal vertex position (i.e., the head flexed) may be detected by performing Leopold's fourth maneuver and then may be confirmed by noting the findings on the vaginal examination. In the breech presentation, whether the head is flexed upon the chest or hyperextended with the occiput toward the back should be determined, since a breech presentation with a hyperextended head should be delivered by cesarean section (see Chapter 38).

The **position** of the fetus is often more specifically defined as the relationship of the fetal presenting part to the four quadrants of the pelvis, such as a left occiput anterior (LOA), a right occiput anterior (ROA), a left occiput posterior (LOP), a right occiput posterior (ROP), a left occiput transverse (LOT), a right occiput transverse (ROT), or a left sacrum anterior (LSA), to name but a few of these positions. **Often, an occiput posterior presentation may be predicted when the infant is lying on the right side in an anthropoid pelvis.**

Finally, the **station** of the presenting part of the fetus is usually defined as the level of the fetal presenting part in relation to the ischial spines.

If the head tilts so that the *anterior parietal bone* of the fetal head (in an occiput transverse position) descends first, with the sagittal suture tilted back toward the sacrum (i.e., the sagittal suture is "smiling"), **an anterior asynclitism** is said to be present. This position may occur in a woman with a pendulous abdomen. If, on the other hand, the *posterior parietal bone* descends first, with the sagittal suture up anteriorly near the symphysis (i.e., the sagittal suture is "frowning"), then a **posterior asynclitism** is present. If the sagittal suture is in the mid-position, then **normal synclitism** is present.

g. Mechanism of labor

The mechanism of labor, or the cardinal movements of labor in a vertex presentation (i.e., LOA or ROA) are as follows: (1) engagement, (2) descent, (3) flexion, (4) internal rotation, (5) extension, (6) external restitution of the head, and (7) expulsion.** An easy way for you to remember these movements is by the use of the mnemonic device "**E**very **D**ecent **F**amily **I**n **E**urope **E**ats **E**ggs" (Fig. 24-4). In this presentation, the fetal head enters the inlet in an *occiput transverse/oblique* position and moves down the "Lazy S"–shaped curve of the pelvis by *flexion* of the head and *internal rotation,* which moves it into the occiput anterior position so that the head rests upon the shoulder as it descends over the promontory of the sacrum. When the head descends to the levator ani sling, it begins to *extend* as it moves upward toward the introitus. With the delivery of the head, which had been in an occiput anterior position at delivery, there is a restitution of the head back to the normal frontal position, following which the shoulders and the rest of the infant are *expelled* from the vagina. To some degree, the shoulders and the hips also undergo these same cardinal movements that the head has undergone during the birth process.

2. The onset of labor

a. Progesterone withdrawal theory

For many years, attempts have been made to explain the onset of labor by a variety of theories. *At the present time, no one theory has totally explained all of the events that occur in labor, and yet, each hypothesis has certain aspects that are attractive.*

One method of classifying certain species in regard to parturition is according to the *source of progesterone* beyond the early part of pregnancy. For example, the source of progesterone continues to be the corpus luteum in rats, rabbits, pigs, and goats, whereas it is produced by the placenta in humans and the other primates, guinea pigs, sheep, and cows. Furthermore,

FIGURE 24-4. Mechanism of labor in a left occiput anterior position. (A) The fetal head is floating. (B) The fetal head *engages* in the occiput oblique or transverse position. (C) The fetal head *descends* into the pelvis as it begins to *flex and internally rotate* to the occiput anterior position. (D) The fetal head *extends* as it reaches the pelvic floor and moves up toward the introitus. (E) The fetal head undergoes *external restitution* with the head moving from the position of looking over the shoulder to the normal front facing position. (F) The fetal shoulder stems under the symphysis pubis and then is delivered as the infant is directed downward slightly. (G) With the delivery of the anterior shoulder, the remainder of the infant is *expelled* rapidly.

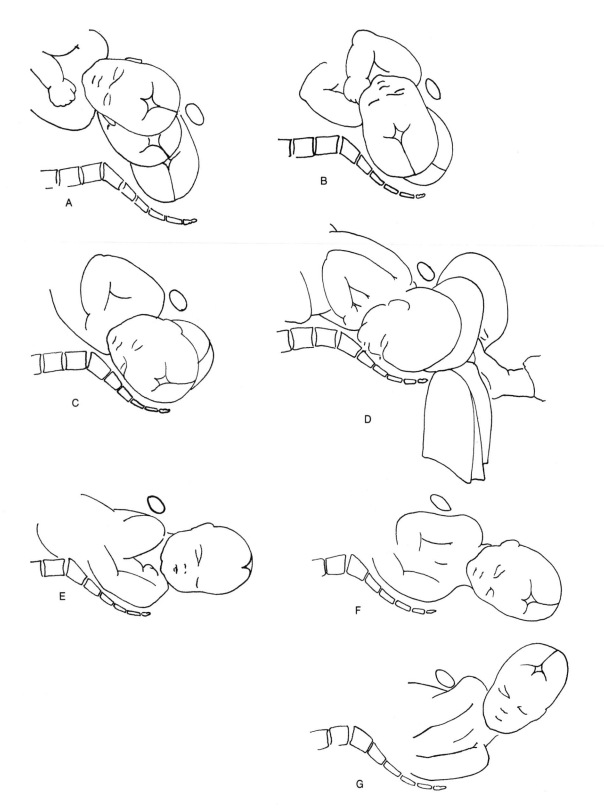

A

B

C

D

E

F

G

the onset of labor is dependent upon the withdrawal of progesterone in those animals that are dependent upon its production by the corpus luteum, by and large, and also by some of those that are dependent upon the placenta; however, this is not the case with humans.

b. 17-Alpha-hydroxylase

A theory that may explain the mechanism of labor in ruminants such as sheep and cows may help to explain the mechanism in humans. This theory involves the presence or absence of the placental enzyme *17-alpha-hydroxylase,* which converts progesterone to pregnenolone and then to estrogen in these animals. This enzyme is increased in late pregnancy by the increasing cortisol levels, and these increased 17-alpha-hydroxylase levels in turn cause an increasing production of estrogen and a decreasing amount of progesterone. **The change in the estrogen: progesterone ratio stimulates the synthesis of prostaglandins.** This enzyme sequence does not occur in the primate placenta. While the human placenta does not have this 17-alpha-hydroxylase enzyme, it does have an abundance of **aromatizing enzymes,** which can produce estrogens by the conversion of androgens, such as dehydroisoandrosterone (DHA), from the adrenal cortex fetal zone. **Thus, the primate placenta can regulate the estrogen:progesterone ratio by this means.**

Unfortunately, the progesterone withdrawal theory does not appear to be the answer in humans, since the maternal blood progesterone levels do not decrease prior to the onset of labor. Whether this process contributes to the onset of labor remains to be seen. It is possible that a relative decrease in the local tissue progesterone concentration may occur, since it has been demonstrated that there are a decreased number of myometrial progesterone receptors in the uterus near term (i.e., after 38 weeks) as opposed to the nonpregnant uterus.

c. Oxytocin theory

Oxytocin has long been considered to play a role in the instigation of labor contractions. Certainly, the role of oxytocin in ensuring that there is an adequate contraction of the uterine muscle in the postpartum phase of labor to reduce the amount of blood loss cannot be denied. *In fact, an increase in oxytocin*

levels has only been demonstrated "at the end of labor" during the expulsion of the fetus, and not before. Furthermore, patients who have posterior pituitary lesions with diabetes insipidus do not have a prolonged gestation time. Also, animals that have been hypophysectomized have a normal onset of labor. In addition, oxytocin does not increase the development of gap junctions in the myometrial cells. The role of oxytocin in the initiation of labor is not completely known, but it may have an adjunctive role, rather than a primary one, in the initiation of labor.

d. Organ communication system

An attractive hypothesis is that of the "organ communication system," in which it is postulated that the fetus communicates with the mother and signals when it is ready to be delivered. This theory presupposes that there may be a fetal organ system that, after maturing to a certain point, releases a specific chemical signal to the maternal organism to initiate the onset of labor. **In W. S. Playfair's *A Treatise on the Science and Practice of Midwifery,* published in 1880, the following statement was made: "The former is the opinion which was held by the older accoucheurs, who assigned to the foetus some active influence in effecting its own expulsion."**[1] It would seem from this observation that the organ communication system hypothesis is not a new one, but rather, one that has been suspected for more than 100 years.

It has also been known for some time that patients who had an anencephalic fetus were subject to having a prolonged gestation. This delay in the onset of labor is not due to the loss of the pituitary gland per se, but is probably secondary to the associated adrenal hypoplasia, especially of the fetal zone.

The studies involving parturition in sheep, while not exactly applicable to the human, have shown many similar events. **To begin with, it appears that a functional fetal hypothalamus, pituitary gland, and adrenal gland are necessary if labor is to occur at the appropriate time.** One of the initiating events in labor appears to be **an increase in fetal cortisol,** which may in turn act upon the

---

[1] W. S. Playfair, *A Treatise on the Science and Practice of Midwifery,* third American ed. Philadelphia: Henry C. Lea (now Lea & Febiger), Publisher, 1880, p. 248.

placenta to increase the production of estrogens. **Cortisol may have an effect upon the aromatization enzymes in the placenta that convert the androgens to estrogens.** This **cortisol hypothesis,** while attractive as a theory, does not in itself seem to provide a full explanation of the onset of labor.

The **increase in estrogens, however, does seem to have an effect upon the synthesis and release of prostaglandins.** It has been found that prostaglandin E_2 (PGE$_2$) and prostaglandin $F_{2\alpha}$ (PGF$_{2\alpha}$) will stimulate uterine contractions at any time during pregnancy; they have also been found to be capable of softening or ripening the cervix and of causing effacement. **The obligatory precursor to the synthesis of the 2-series prostaglandins (i.e., PGE$_2$ and PGF$_{2\alpha}$) is arachidonic acid** (Fig. 24-5). If this compound is given intravenously to pregnant rabbits, then labor will ensue. If inhibitors of prostaglandin synthetase (i.e., arachidonic acid cyclooxygenase) are administered, the gestation will be prolonged, or if preterm labor is present, then it will be stopped.

One site of the production of PGE$_2$ is the *amnion,* but PGE$_2$ cannot be metabolized there because there is no 15-hydroxyprostaglandin dehydrogenase present. In contrast, the PGE$_2$ that is produced in the *chorion laeve* may be catabolized because in this instance, the 15-hydroxyprostaglandin dehydrogenase enzyme is present. Both PGE$_2$ and PGF$_{2\alpha}$ are synthesized in the *decidua vera.* **There is a large amount of arachidonic acid in the glycerophospholipids of the amnion and chorion. The enzyme phospholipase A_2 from the amnionic membranes releases arachidonic acid from phosphatidylethanolamine.** Some of the other enzymes in the amnion and chorion that are involved are phosphatidylinositol-specific phospholipase C, diacylglycerol lipase, and monoacylglycerol lipase.

In summary, it is thought that the **onset of labor** requires the transmission of some chemical signal, **perhaps a heat-stable proteinaceous material in the fetal urine** that is produced in the fetal kidney and secreted into the amniotic fluid. The amniotic fluid occupies a large area in the uterine cavity and communicates directly with the amnion, the chorion laeve, the uterine decidua vera, and indirectly, with the mother. This fetal chemical signal may serve **to stimulate the release of arachidonic acid** by means of phospholipase A_2 and other enzymes in the membranes. Apparently, the amount of available cal-

cium may be a rate-limiting step in the release of arachidonic acid. As the immediate precursor for the prostaglandins, the arachidonic acid also serves to regulate prostaglandin production. **Once the prostaglandins are released, they initiate uterine contractions, and then labor ensues.** While this theory is very attractive and seems to explain many of the molecular events of the process of parturition, it still has not been fully defined at the present time.

It is of interest that intracervical or intrauterine microorganisms may cause inflammation of the membranes with the release of proteases and phospholipase A_2 and C. The phospholipases can then cause the release of prostaglandins, which soften the cervix and stimulate premature labor contractions. The proteases may cause the premature rupture of the membranes.

3. Uterine contractions

The myometrial protein that is important in the development of a muscular contraction is the **myosin** molecule. The interaction of myosin and **actin** in the myometrial cells takes place after the phosphorylation of the myosin light-chain. This phosphorylation takes place by means of the *myosin light-chain kinase,* which is activated by **calcium** (Ca^{++}). Another compound, **calmodulin,** a calcium-dependent regulatory protein, is necessary for the expression of the **light-chain kinase enzyme** and the initiation of the contraction. This flux of calcium, essential for the initiation of a contraction, is sequestered in the sarcoplasmic reticulum in the intracellular vesicles. While this calcium storage is occurring, the muscle is in a state of relaxation. **An inhibition of this calcium storage in the sarcoplasmic reticulum of the uterine smooth muscle allows the release of the calcium into the cell, directly stimulating the uterine myofibrils to produce a contraction.** The reverse of this process includes the dephosphorylation of the myosin light-chain by means of the **myosin light-chain phosphatase,** which then results in muscular relaxation. This process is assisted by the cAMP-dependent protein kinase.

The mechanism of action of hormones, such as oxytocin and prostaglandin, in initiating contractions of the uterine smooth muscle may be mediated by means of a "second messenger" (e.g., cyclic adenosine monophosphate, or cAMP); however, the particular messenger in this instance has not been defined.

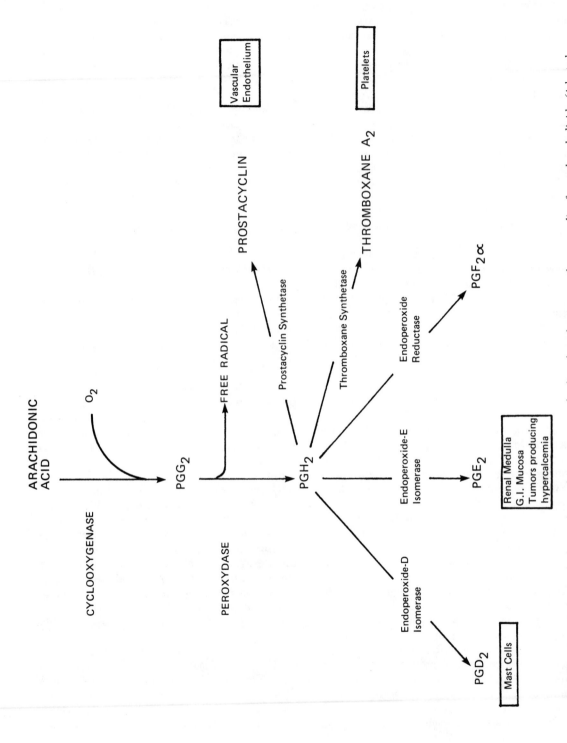

FIGURE 24-5. Pathway for the biosynthesis of primary prostaglandins, thromboxanes, and prostacyclins from phospholipids. (Adapted from J. B. Wyngaarden and L. H. Smith, Jr., eds., *Cecil Textbook of Medicine*, 17th ed. Philadelphia: W. B. Saunders Company, 1985, p. 1238.)

Conceivably, a guanine 5'-triphosphate (GTP) binding protein may modify the cAMP second messenger in some way to produce this reaction.

During pregnancy, the myometrial cells are enmeshed in a collagenous extracellular matrix that aids in the transmission of the contractile stimuli. Of more importance, however, is the development of the **gap junctions,** which connect the myometrial cells for either an electrical or a metabolic coupling. The gap junctions act as low-resistance contacts to ensure a smooth propagation of electrical impulses between the cells and throughout the myometrium, which results in synchronous uterine contractions. These gap junctions become more prominent in the myometrium at term, increase throughout labor, and then decrease within the first 24 hours' postpartum. **It would appear that the gap junctions are important for the initiation and maintenance of labor. Prostaglandins and estrogens increase the formation of gap junctions, whereas progesterone and prostacyclin inhibit them.** Oxytocin does not cause any increase in the gap junctions.

4. Patient assessment

Upon admission to the hospital, the pregnant woman in labor may be filled with fear and concern about both the status of her baby and her abilities to survive the pain and hazards of childbirth. You should take the time to make the patient feel comfortable and to reassure her that she will receive adequate pain relief consistent with her safety and that of the baby. It has been demonstrated that the maternal emotional response (i.e., alarm reaction) to labor may have a significant effect on the uterine contractions. As the cortisol levels and the plasma epinephrine values increase, the uterine contractions may decrease (see Chapter 5).

a. Basic studies

During the initial examination of the patient in the labor room you should determine whether the patient is indeed in labor, and if so, how far along the labor has progressed. The patient's history should be reviewed and the physical examination carried out to determine if there are any general medical problems that might influence the labor and delivery. The initial hospital laboratory studies should routinely include the determination of the *hemoglo-*

bin and hematocrit values, since the blood loss at delivery could be sufficient in a person with a severe anemia to result in hemorrhagic shock or even death. Routine serology, and the collection of a tube of blood to send to the blood bank on a type-and-hold or type-and-screen request, should be carried out. A routine urinalysis should also be performed. **Using a large bore needle you should administer a balanced salt solution, such as lactated Ringer's solution (125 ml/hr), so as to maintain an open intravenous site in case a blood transfusion becomes necessary intrapartum.**

In checking the vital signs, you should keep in mind that during labor there is a significant increase in the heart rate (20%) and in the cardiac output of the patient (50%) with contractions. The cardiac output may increase by as much as 80% in the third stage of labor. The blood pressure may increase by 15–20 mm Hg during labor, with an additional 10% increase during each contraction. Due to the hyperventilation that occurs during labor, the patient's pH may become alkalotic (i.e., 7.55); however, during the third stage of labor the blood pH may become more acidotic (i.e., 7.37) due to the anaerobic myometrial metabolism.

b. Status of membranes

The status of the amniotic membranes is important; if they are reported to be ruptured, a careful *sterile examination* of the vaginal vault secretions should be performed. If the vaginal secretions show an alkaline pH (nitrazene test), evidence of ferning, or the presence of fetal squames or lanugo hairs, this diagnosis may be confirmed. In addition, the presence of an occult umbilical cord prolapse should be sought by an immediate sterile bimanual examination after an *obvious rupture* of the fetal membranes has occurred. The presence of meconium staining may also be associated with a cord prolapse.

If there is a question of prematurity, and the patient has not had recent intercourse, a sample of the amniotic fluid in the vaginal vault should be obtained for a phosphatidylglycerol (PG) determination.

Artificial rupture of the membranes (AROM) will often assist in the induction of labor; however, it should not be performed if the fetal presenting part is not fully "seated" in the pelvis or if the cervix has an unfavorable Bishop score for induction (see Chapter 38).

c. Effacement

The amount of cervical effacement should be carefully assessed. **The presence of prostaglandins and the decrease in progesterone is thought to cause a softening or ripening of the cervix.** This softening is due to the separation of the collagenous fibers by increased amounts of the various glycosaminoglycans. **The cervical thickness at the beginning of true labor in a primigravida will be much thinner (i.e., effaced) than in a multiparous patient. The concept of "completely effaced" should be modified in the multiparous patient, since the cervix will be considerably thicker in the multipara than in the primigravida when fully effaced.** Once the patient's cervix has begun to rapidly dilate beyond 3–4 cm, the cervix should be considered to be 100% effaced for all practical purposes.

Since effacement is, for the most part, an arbitrary determination of thickness, it is essential that the cervical dilatation be carefully evaluated as corroborative evidence. **The cervical os should not be stretched by separating your examining fingers as it is being measured, since this may increase the measurement considerably and lead to a false assessment as to the presence of true labor.** The examining finger tip should be "walked" across the area between the edges of the cervix to determine the cervical dilatation. The assessment of the amount of cervical dilatation should be standardized, since the actual centimeter measurements may vary somewhat from one patient to the next. A practical clinical assessment is as follows: (1) complete dilatation—no cervix palpable, (2) 9 cm—anterior lip only is palpable, (3) 8 cm—anterior lip and one side are palpable, (4) 7 cm—anterior lip and both sides are palpable, and (5) cervical dilatation from 1–6 cm can be measured by the palpable estimation of the cervical opening. *During the evaluation of the cervix, the position of the fetal sagittal suture should also be determined, which, when correlated with the results of Leopold's maneuvers, will assist in defining the fetal position.*

d. Fundal height

The abdominal examination should include the fundal height measurement. At term, you should become concerned about the size of the fetus when the fundal measurement is greater than 38 cm. **As the measurement approaches 40 cm or greater, the risk of having a baby that weighs more than 8 lbs be-** comes more likely, and problems such as cephalopelvic disproportion or shoulder dystocia become increasingly more common.

5. Labor assessment

a. The four "P's"

The classic "three P's" of labor assessment should be modified to include the "patient." Thus, you should assess the conduct of labor by the status of these **"four P's": (1) the passage, (2) the passenger, (3) the powers, and (4) the patient.** The **first** evaluation concerns your assessment of *the clinical pelvic measurements—the passage.* This information, coupled with the information that has been collected from the *Leopold's maneuvers, the fundal measurement, and the vaginal assessment of the fetal position,* will provide you with the required knowledge concerning the **second** of the four P's—*the passenger.* The **third** P concerns the *powers,* or the *uterine contractions.* Problems involving these three factors are the principal reasons for dystocia, or the failure to progress in labor. The **fourth** P concerns the condition of the *patient,* whose status may have some effect upon the course of labor, especially when dehydration, fatigue, or excessive sedation is found to be present.

The older physicians might add a fifth P, which is the *aggressive physician*—who might be tempted to engage in active intervention before it might be necessary—or a sixth P, the *procrastinating physician*—who does not take appropriate action in a timely fashion. Certainly, patience is truly a virtue in managing the obstetric patient; however, there is a fine line between "aggressive medical management" and "procrastination." The conscientious physician will constantly keep these aspects of the case in mind. It has been truly stated that **"all things obstetric should be timed."**

b. Status of X-ray pelvimetry

In the past, the presence or potential of encountering dystocia was an indication for the physician to obtain X-ray pelvimetry. Unfortunately, due to the limitations of the radiologic techniques, little was gained by knowing the pelvic measurements, since such knowledge usually did not really change the clinical course of treatment. In almost every case, the patient was allowed a trial of labor. **Clearly, unless the information that is to be gained by X-ray pelvimetry will potentially change the management of the problem, then this technique should not be utilized.** There is only a slight risk that the exposure of the fetus to diagnostic X-rays may lead to the subsequent development of leukemia; however, in spite of this, X-rays should not be used unless there is a valid reason. Currently, the use of X-ray pelvimetry is almost completely limited to specific problems, such as: (1) a possible pelvic bony contraction, due to injury or disease, and (2) a possible vaginal delivery in a breech presentation.

6. Progress of labor

a. Length of labor

Throughout pregnancy, the patient may periodically experience small, painless, irregular contractions (Braxton Hicks contractions). Near term, the interval between these contractions decreases, although the contractions still remain irregular and may resemble episodes of mild false labor. Just prior to the onset of true labor (up to about 72 hours), the mucus plug (i.e., the operculum) in the cervix is usually shed, resulting in a **bloody show,** which is mostly cervical mucus with a few streaks of associated blood. Not infrequently, false labor will progress directly into **true labor,** which by definition consists of **a series of regular contractions that results in progressive cervical dilatation that eventually leads to the expulsion of the fetus from the uterus.**

1) Primigravida

In the primigravida, when the uterine contractions become effective (i.e., intensity of 40–60 mm Hg; interval of 3–4 minutes) and the cervix is dilated to 3 cm and is completely effaced, the accelerated phase of the active stage of labor begins. The primigravida should progress a minimum of 1.2 cm/hr to be considered as having a normal labor. The phase of maximal slope then occurs as the cervix dilates from 3 cm to 10 cm; this phase lasts for about 5.8 hours (i.e., five hours and 48 minutes). The second stage of labor then begins and lasts for about 45 minutes before the fetus is delivered. During the second stage, the intrauterine pressures may be of the order of 50–70 mm of Hg, and the high pressure spikes of 80–100 mm Hg that appear on the electronic fetal monitoring strip chart near the end of labor reveal the patient's attempts to "push." **For a primigravida to progress from 3 cm to complete dilatation (5 hours and 48 minutes), and then from complete dilatation to delivery (45 minutes), results in a total length of labor of about 6 hours and 33 minutes.** This is the usual **maximal** time sequence that may be seen in the normal primigravida patient. **In my experience, the average time sequence in many instances will be of the order of 4 hours and 45 minutes in the primigravida.**

2) Multipara

The multiparous patient will maximally require about 4.6 hours (i.e., 4 hours and 36 minutes) to progress from 3 cm to 10 cm (at a rate of 1.5 cm/hr) and from 0–10 minutes to progress from complete dilatation to delivery. In my experience, this time interval is usually closer to about 2 hours and 10 minutes in the normal multiparous patient. While these times are approximations only, they do provide a crude index of what should be considered the **maximal length of time for normal labor and delivery.** As such, they provide an **early warning system.** You should be aware of any deviations from these "maximal" values and should evaluate any variations in the patient's labor pattern from these norms. In such a manner, problems with dystocia become more easily detected. The use of Friedman's labor curve is very helpful in this regard. In addition, you should also pay attention to the rate of descent of the fetal presenting part. You should periodically assess the labor contractions manually by palpating at least three contractions and comparing them to the output of the electronic fetal monitoring strip chart. **It is helpful to enter these data onto the labor curve record. The shorthand notation for "contractions every 3 minutes and 50 seconds duration, and of good quality," for example, would be "3/50/G." Alternatively, the contractions may only be of poor quality (P), or of fair quality (F).**

b. Electronic fetal monitoring

The use of electronic fetal monitoring has been a major advance in obstetrics in this century

and has allowed the physician to continuously monitor the fetal status throughout labor (see Chapter 37). Since the fetal heart tones are difficult to hear with the stethoscope during a contraction, the traditional practice was to only listen in the interval between contractions. This method has been shown to be incorrect, since the major changes in the fetal heart rate (FHR) occur transiently during the contraction. Since late decelerations frequently are within the normal range of FHR values (i.e., 120–160 bpm), they would be missed using a stethoscope.

c. Electronic fetal monitoring— is it cost effective?

While there is still controversy regarding the routine use of electronic fetal monitoring in all pregnancies, it would seem to be cost effective to do so, since if only one child could be prevented from developing neurological damage, then it would be well worth the cost. Variable decelerations (due to cord compression) are the most common abnormal patterns that are seen in electronic fetal monitoring. Although cord compression patterns (or combined patterns) do not commonly lead to fetal damage, unless they are prolonged and unrecognized, the potential is nonetheless present in the unmonitored patient. In view of this, it would seem that the monitoring of almost all laboring patients would be worthwhile. A test has recently been proposed in which the presence of a **nuchal cord** may be detected by applying pressure over the neck region of the monitored fetus and then looking for accelerations or decelerations on the monitor strip. This technique may provide a way to identify most cases of cord compression due to a nuchal cord prior to labor; however, it would not detect the occult cord prolapse.

While extensive nursing care utilizing periodic FHR monitoring with a Doppler instrument has been recommended in lieu of continuous electronic fetal heart rate monitoring, this approach is not practical in most hospitals because of the shortage of private nursing personnel for each laboring patient. Furthermore, the lack of continuous FHR data and a proper visual interpretation of the changes in the fetal heart rate would be a drawback in interpreting the results of the audible FHR monitoring technique.

Hazards do exist in the use of fetal heart monitoring. The physician may read "too much" or "too little" into the FHR tracing and make a wrong decision based upon such information. In addition, there is a legal hazard involved, as the "medical experts" in a malpractice action may make various interpretations of the FHR tracings. Nevertheless, the fact still remains that the intelligent use of the FHR monitor provides a considerable degree of assurance as to the fetal status in most instances. The fact that it can be misused, or that it is not 100% accurate, should not be an indication that fetal heart rate monitoring should be abandoned, as some groups have suggested.

d. Analgesia
1) General considerations

The terms analgesia and anesthesia share essentially the same definition, which is "the loss of the sensation of pain." Practically speaking, analgesia in obstetrics usually involves those simple medications that only partially ameliorate pain, whereas anesthesia implies the complete relief of the pain.

James Young Simpson (1811–1870) of Edinburgh, Scotland, was instrumental in introducing anesthesia into obstetrics when, on January 19, 1847, he administered ether to a laboring patient on whom he performed a version and extraction of a child who did not survive. On November 8, 1847, he successfully delivered the child of Dr. and Mrs. Carstairs of Edinburgh with the patient under chloroform anesthesia. The child was named "Anaesthesia" to commemorate the event. The controversy that then ensued was based upon the scriptural injunction that "In sorrow thou shalt bring forth children" (Gen. 3:16). The use of anesthesia seemed to contravene the biblical injunction and was therefore considered to be evil. It was not until 1853, when **Dr. John Snow** administered chloroform to **Queen Victoria** during the birth of Prince Leopold, that the use of anesthesia finally became acceptable. Dr. Simpson was later made a baronet and the inscription on his coat of arms reflected his contribution to obstetrics in reading "Victo Dolore" (pain conquered).

In regard to analgesia, you should be cognizant of the value of "TLC" (i.e., tender loving care) in the management of the obstetric patient. **When you take the time to instruct your patient and to psychologically prepare her as to what to expect during labor and delivery, and to reassure her that adequate pain-relief measures will be taken, then your patient will often develop sufficient confidence in you, and in the obstetric person-**

nel, as to require very little analgesia during the labor. Your presence in the vicinity of the patient during labor is important in this regard, and you should make every effort to visit your patient frequently during the labor process. Fear is a prominent part of the patient's appreciation of pain and the relief of such fear is very important. Your calm reassurance and presence will often eliminate the patient's fear and provide her with a measure of relaxation and relief of her pain.

The ideal agent or procedure used to alleviate pain during labor would be perfectly safe for both the mother and fetus as well as simple in its application. Although there are no ideal analgesics available today, a number of approaches have been utilized effectively in selected circumstances.

2) Psychoprophylaxis

The association of psychological factors and the degree of pain experienced with labor was perhaps first clinically recognized by Grantly Dick-Read in 1942. It was his belief that fear accentuated the pain of labor and childbirth, and that the increased pain, in turn, caused the patient to become tense and even more fearful, which then led to a **"fear-pain-fear" sequence.** If the fear could be relieved, he postulated, the patient would experience less pain. **This concept of "natural childbirth," or perhaps more appropriately termed "prepared childbirth," has become well accepted by the lay public in recent years.** The basic approach to relieving the patient's pain involves education coupled with psychological assistance and support from the physician or the woman's male partner, and perhaps the use of a distraction technique (e.g., Lamaze method) to take the patient's mind off of her discomfort. Such an approach has proven to be an effective "analgesic," providing pain relief during labor.

3) Hypnosis

One of the oldest and safest analgesic techniques is hypnosis. While only 9% of patients are natural somnambulists (i.e., individuals who are capable of being hypnotized to anesthetic depths without training), probably 90% of all patients can be hypnotized to some degree. Indeed, the Egyptian "temple sleep," which was practiced centuries before the time of Christ, was probably a form of hypnosis. In 1776,

Franz Anton Mesmer of Vienna wrote a thesis on this subject; the technique of "mesmerism" became fashionable for a time but then later fell into disrepute for many years. It remained for **James Braid,** a Manchester surgeon in the nineteenth century, to revive an interest in this procedure, which he called *hypnosis.* The main disadvantage to the use of hypnosis in obstetrics is the amount of time that is required of the physician to train most patients in the technique in order to allow them to attain a sufficient degree of pain relief in labor. In specific problem cases, however, it still is an excellent form of analgesia/anesthesia.

4) Analgesic agents

Almost all drugs cross the placenta and enter the fetal circulatory system. The primary goal of maternal drug therapy in labor is to relieve pain, with maternal sedation or tranquilization being perhaps a secondary goal in anxious or agitated patients. Care must be taken in administering meperidine or any other narcotic too early in labor. *In general, these drugs should not be given prior to about 5 cm of cervical dilatation, so as to avoid a prolongation of the latent phase of labor.*

The most common analgesic used today is meperidine hydrochloride (Demerol). If given intramuscularly, its absorption is maximal in about one or two hours and its duration in the fetus is prolonged. **In contrast, when meperidine is given intravenously, it peaks in about six minutes in the baby and then rapidly leaves the fetal circulation.** The usual intravenous dose should not exceed 50 mg, and it should not be necessary to repeat this dose more than once throughout the entire course of the labor. Usually, single-drug therapy is more effective and predictable than a combination of drugs; however, some physicians prefer to add promethazine hydrochloride (Phenergan), 25 mg, to the meperidine therapy in order to obtain additional sedation. The use of this drug not only provides some tranquilization but also takes the "edge" off of the meperidine effect, which may cause uncomfortable nausea or irritableness in some patients when used alone. Vistaril (hydroxyzine hydrochloride), 50 mg q4-6h I.M., may also be used. Do not use barbiturates with meperidine, since they are antagonistic, not synergistic, in their effects. Due to the fact that the respiratory function of the newborn infant may be suppressed by meperidine, excessive sedation of the infant at birth may cause difficulty in initiating respiration. Excessive doses of this agent are those of more than 150–200 mg. The administration of naloxone hydrochloride (Narcan), 0.01 mg/kg body weight I.V., I.M., or S.C., will reverse the effects of meperidine without causing any additional fetal sedation.

e. Anesthesia for delivery

1) Sensory innervation of the genital tract

The sensory innervation of the uterus, the cervix, and the upper vagina is mediated through nerves that go through Frankenhäuser's ganglion to the middle and superior hypogastric plexuses and thence along the lumbar and lower thoracic sympathetic fibers to the spinal cord at T10, T11, T12, and the upper two lumbar segments of the cord (Fig. 24-6). **The sensory innervation of the lower vagina and pelvic floor derives from the ventral branches of S2, S3, and S4, which constitutes the pudendal nerve.** The pudendal nerve passes posteriorly to the place where the sacrospinous ligament attaches to the ischial spine (i.e., Alcock's canal), after which it swings anteriorly and superiorly to supply the perineal region as the inferior hemorrhoidal nerve, the labial nerve, and the dorsal nerve of the clitoris (Fig. 24-7).

2) Local anesthetic blocks

When toxic reactions occur in the use of local anesthetics in the perineal region, they are almost always due to **the inadvertent administration of the agent intravascularly** to produce high levels of the drug in the circulation. *The patient may complain of dizziness, nausea and vomiting, tinnitus, peri-oral numbness, or a metallic taste in her mouth and may suddenly develop slurred speech just prior to becoming comatose or developing generalized convulsions.* The immediate control of the convulsions and the institution of supportive care of the respiration and blood pressure (i.e., to prevent hypotension and cardiac arrest) should be carried out. To protect the fetus, the patient should be placed in the left lateral recumbent position, and adequate fluids and oxygen should be administered.

a) Local block

Regional anesthetic procedures consist of local block, pudendal block, paracervical block, caudal block,

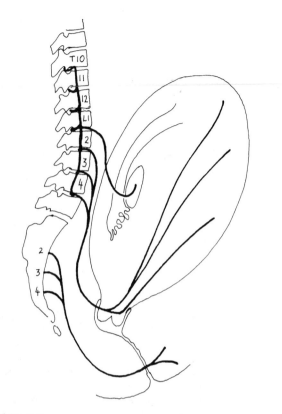

FIGURE 24-6. The pain pathways during parturition. The uterus is supplied with sensory pain fibers that go from the uterus to the spinal cord by accompanying the sympathetic nerves. They go from the uterine, cervical, and pelvic plexuses to the hypogastric nerve, the superior hypogastric plexus, the lumbar and lower thoracic sympathetic chain, and then finally through the white rami communicantes and posterior roots to enter the spinal cord primarily at T11 and T12, and secondarily at T10 and L1. The pain pathways from the perineum travel through the pudendal nerve to S2, S3, and S4.

epidural block, and spinal block (Fig. 24-8). The **local infiltration** of the perineal areas with 8–10 ml of a 1% lidocaine anesthetic solution at the point where the episiotomy will be made must be done at least five minutes prior the delivery to allow for adequate anesthesia to develop. Chloroprocaine hydrochloride (Nesacaine), 5–10 ml of a 2% solution, may also be used. This technique is also effective in the repair of lacerations of the perineal tissues following delivery. The maximal dosage of the various local anesthetic agents should not be exceeded.

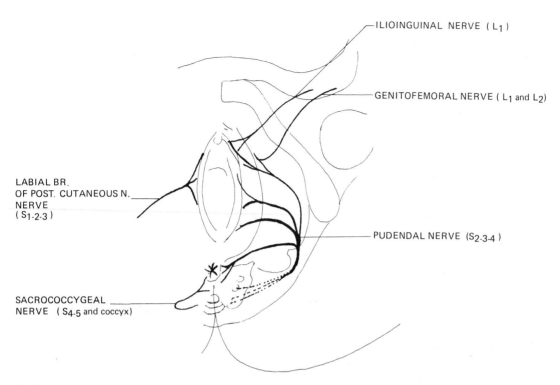

ILIOINGUINAL NERVE (L₁)

GENITOFEMORAL NERVE (L₁ and L₂)

LABIAL BR.
OF POST. CUTANEOUS N.
NERVE
(S₁₋₂₋₃)

PUDENDAL NERVE (S₂₋₃₋₄)

SACROCOCCYGEAL
NERVE (S₄₋₅ and coccyx)

FIGURE 24-7. Nerve supply to the perineal region.

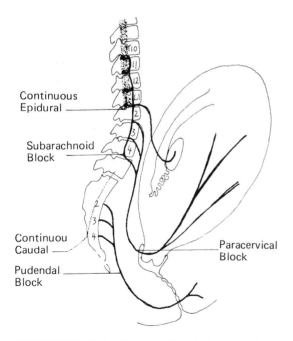

Continuous
Epidural

Subarachnoid
Block

Continuou
Caudal

Pudendal
Block

Paracervical
Block

FIGURE 24-8. Regional anesthesia techniques used in obstetrics.

b) Pudendal block

The **pudendal block** technique involves the placement of the anesthetic solution at the point where the pudendal nerve emerges from beneath the sacrospinous ligament to supply the perineum. This procedure is performed by placing a long 22-gauge spinal needle, with or without a needle guide, inside the vagina over the sacrospinous ligament. A small amount of local anesthetic solution may be placed in the vaginal mucosa, followed by the insertion of the needle 1.0–1.5 cm into the sacrospinous ligament and beyond into Alcock's canal, where the pudendal nerve lies (Fig. 24-9). *Aspiration of the needle to be certain that a vascular channel has not been entered must always be done prior to any infiltration of an anesthetic solution.* Both chloroprocaine and lidocaine may be used in the same manner for the pudendal block as in the local block.

c) Paracervical block

The discomfort of uterine contractions during labor cannot be relieved by local or pudendal block anesthesia; however, another technique that partially

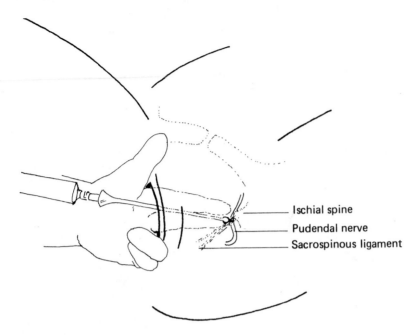

Ischial spine
Pudendal nerve
Sacrospinous ligament

FIGURE 24-9. Pudendal block technique.

produces this result is the **paracervical block** (i.e., uterosacral block), in which the local anesthetic solution is placed at the 4 and 8 o'clock positions in the vaginal fornices. An amide anesthetic, such as 8–10 ml of a 1% lidocaine (Xylocaine) solution, will provide a block for 60–90 minutes. Although this procedure is quite effective in relieving pain, it is associated with rather severe fetal bradycardia in a considerable number of cases (10–25%). If bradycardia occurs, it generally begins about 6–8 minutes following the injection of the anesthetic solution and lasts for 6–10 minutes. This condition has been attributed to uterine vascular constriction and increased myometrial tonus in the mother, with a resultant decrease in the perfusion of the intervillous space. *This anesthetic technique is contraindicated in patients who may already have fetal compromise.*

3) Regional anesthetic blocks

a) Epidural/caudal block

To obtain almost complete relief of the discomfort of uterine contractions during labor, a regional anesthetic, such as an epidural block or a caudal block, may be used with good success during the **active phase** of labor. An epidural block is placed at the L2,

L3, or L4 interspace, either as a single injection, or by means of a catheter that is inserted through an 18-gauge needle into the epidural space as a continuous block. A caudal block is placed through the sacral hiatus in the sacrum and is often administered continuously by means of a catheter.

The risks involved in epidural or caudal blocks consist of: (1) inadvertent spinal anesthesia, (2) hypotension, (3) systemic toxicity, and (4) a delaying effect on labor. If the dura mater is punctured during the performance of an epidural block, a total *spinal anesthetic blockade* may occur with resultant hypotension, and possibly cardiorespiratory arrest and death. When an epidural block is administered, the sympathetic blockade and vasodilatation of the splanchnic bed, combined with compression of the inferior vena cava by the uterus, may result in *hypotension*, unless the patient has had **a rapid infusion of a balanced salt solution (500–1,000 ml) prior to the placement of the block** and is placed in a left lateral decubitus position to relieve the pressure of the uterus on the inferior vena cava.

The engorged internal vertebral venous plexuses that are encountered during the performance of an epidural block (or those along the base of the sacral hiatus in the case of the caudal anesthesia) are vulnerable to perforation, which could allow the injection of the anesthetic solution directly into the circulation. If this occurs, *systemic toxic symptoms* such as coma and convulsions may occur. Convulsions may be controlled by the administration of thiopental sodium (Pentothal), 75–125 mg I.V., or diazepam (Valium), 5–10 mg I.V.

Epidural anesthesia may not always result in equal effects bilaterally. In addition, when an epidural or caudal anesthesia is effective, it *removes the patient's voluntary expulsive efforts* in the second stage of labor and often results in a delay in the fetal descent and rotation. Delivery in such cases may require a midforceps rotation.

b) Spinal block

Although spinal anesthesia provides for pain relief at the time of delivery, this technique cannot be used during the process of labor, since it will decrease the strength of the labor contractions. It is ideal for cesarean section, provided that the surgery does not become prolonged beyond the effectiveness of the anesthetic solution. It may be used in primigravidas, or in patients who require difficult forceps deliveries, but it is probably not necessary for most multiparous patients. Preanesthetic loading with a balanced salt solution will assist in preventing hypotension. A spinal block is performed in a manner similar to that of an epidural block, except that the spinal needle is inserted through the dura mater into the spinal canal and spinal fluid is obtained prior to the administration of the hyperbaric anesthetic solution. **The patient should be placed in a reverse Trendelenburg's position to prevent the initial cephalad migration of the anesthetic agent.** Having the patient remain in this position for 30–60 seconds tends to "fix the level" of the block. If a longer period is used, the block will tend to settle even lower and will cover only the lower abdomen and perineum (i.e., the saddle area), and as such, has been termed a *saddle block.*

The complications of spinal anesthesia are essentially the same as those that occur with an epidural block, and in addition, the problem of *postspinal headache* may occur in a small percentage of patients (less than 2%). This complication is thought to be due to the leakage of spinal fluid from the needle hole in the dura mater. This problem seems to occur much less frequently when a small gauge needle is utilized

and when a minimum number of attempts are needed to perform the spinal tap. The placement of a few milliliters of the patient's blood in the epidural area, so as to produce a clot to cover the hole *(i.e., blood patch),* has often been successful. Bed rest and hydration have also been helpful in providing symptomatic relief.

4) General anesthesia

It is essential that only trained anesthesia personnel administer general anesthetic agents to patients. Moreover, it is essential to place an endotracheal tube in all pregnant patients who are undergoing general anesthesia, since the risk of aspiration pneumonitis, secondary to the inhalation of the gastric contents, is a significant one (see Chapter 31). The use of a clear antacid solution, such as a 0.3 molar solution of sodium citrate (30 ml), within 30 minutes of the performance of surgery is currently recommended. Particulate suspension antacids have been less effective because, while these agents may combat the acid effect of the gastric contents, the particulate matter of the antacid itself may become a significant problem if aspiration pneumonitis should occur.

Recently, the diagnosis of **malignant hyperthermia** has been recognized as a major complication of anesthesia. Apparently, the "triggering" anesthetic agent causes a blockage of the calcium reentry into the sarcoplasmic reticulum. As a consequence, with each neuronal stimulus, more and more calcium ions are released that will not be reabsorbed. This process results in a state of hypermetabolism, with a depolarization of the cell membranes and a leakage of potassium, magnesium, and phosphate ions into the plasma. In addition, myoglobin is released, which may obstruct the renal tubules and cause kidney failure. The elevated potassium may cause cardiac arrythmia, and Factor VIII and fibrinogen decrease, resulting in widespread bleeding.

This syndrome usually begins with a tachycardia and muscular rigidity, followed by increasing blood pressure, increasing temperature, and flushing. As events unfold, the coagulation becomes impaired, the temperature may reach 44° C (113° F) or higher, and pulmonary edema may occur. Eventually, hypotension, hypothermia, bradycardia, and cardiac arrest occur. The use of **dantrolene,** a muscle relaxant, will reverse the syndrome if it is administered before the syndrome becomes full-blown. Its action consists of blocking the outward flow of calcium from the sarcoplasmic reticulum. The patient should be hyperventilated with oxygen (100%), given sodium bicarbonate, 1–2 mEq/kg, and administered dantrolene sodium (Dantrium), 1 mg/kg I.V. push (up to a maximum of 10 mg/kg). Body cooling techniques should be utilized. Intravenous insulin should be given to combat the hyperkalemia. Procainamide hydrochloride (Pronestyl), 200 mg, may be used for life-threatening cardiac arrhythmias.

The detection of the patient who might be a candidate for malignant hyperthermia is difficult. Patients with heavy musculature, scoliosis, or the Duchenne type of muscular dystrophy may have an incidence of malignant hyperthermia that is as high as 50%. Since this condition is hereditary, if it is present in one family member, it may be present in all of the members of the family. A *muscle biopsy* may define the patient who is at risk for this syndrome. The assay of the *creatine kinase* (CK) levels has also been used to screen patients. Elevated levels signify muscle-cell destruction. Another sign that is positive in 50% of patients susceptible to malignant hyperthermia involves the occurrence of *masseter muscle spasms* shortly after the administration of succinylcholine chloride prior to the intubation of the patient at the time of surgery.

7. Spontaneous delivery

a. Delivery

1) When to move the patient to the delivery room

As the patient nears the end of her labor, she will begin to actively "push" (i.e., bear down) during contractions and become much more active and vocal. **In patients who have not been given tranquilizing or antinausea agents during labor, a brief period of nausea, and occasionally vomiting, may occur when the cervix nears complete dilatation.** In *multiparous* patients, it is wise to anticipate this point in labor by a few minutes (i.e., when the cervix is dilated about 8–9 cm) and take the patient to the delivery room before she has a precipitate delivery in the labor bed. If the fetal descent does not proceed as rapidly as anticipated, then the patient should remain out of stirrups for as long as possible,

so as to avoid any leg vein compression and thrombophlebitic problems in the postpartum period. In the *primigravida,* the second stage of labor is of the order of 45 minutes or more, so there will almost always be plenty of time to move the patient to the delivery room area.

The patient should have had the lower portion of the pubic hair (i.e., at the site of the possible episiotomy) shaved upon admission. When the patient is placed on the delivery table, and her legs strapped into the stirrups, the buttocks should just barely extend over the end of the table. If, on one hand, she moves up on the delivery table, then there may be some difficulty in delivering the baby. On the other hand, should the buttocks extend too far over the end of the table, a low back injury may occur. The patient is then prepped and draped for the delivery.

As the fetal head extends in its passage through the birth canal and begins to approach the vaginal introitus, the perineum and the perianal area will begin to bulge outward somewhat with each contraction. As the fetal scalp begins to be seen between the labial folds with each contraction, there may be an expression of fluid or feces from the protuberant anus. *Although the term "crowning" is frequently used when about 3–4 cm of fetal scalp can be seen between contractions, the classical definition of crowning is defined as "when the vaginal outlet encircles the largest diameter of the fetal head."* Usually, by the time the vaginal introitus has reached this degree of dilatation, however, the fetal head is within seconds of delivery.

2) Timing of the episiotomy

If an **episiotomy** is to be performed, it should be carried out after there is at least 4–5 cm of vaginal dilatation, but before the point of complete crowning (see Chapter 26). **If the episiotomy incision is performed too early, excessive blood loss and often additional lacerations, or an extension of the incision, will occur.** If it is performed too late, then most of the deep fascial lacerations beneath the mucosa will have already occurred and one of the purposes of the episiotomy incision will have been defeated.

3) Controlling the fetal head

After identifying the position of the fetal head by locating the anterior and posterior fontanels and the

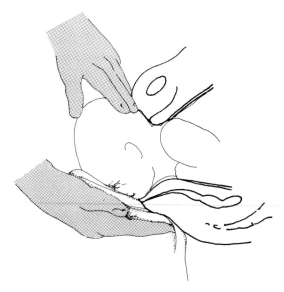

FIGURE 24-10. The Ritgen maneuver in delivering the fetal head.

connecting sagittal suture (i.e., usually an occiput anterior position), the physician should place the flat of one hand over the fetal head to guide its expulsion in a slow and graduated manner. The physician's other hand, with the fingers extended and wrapped in a sterile towel, should be inserted into the region of the perineal body near the anus in an effort to lift the infant's chin gently over the posterior perineum (i.e., Ritgen maneuver) (Fig. 24-10). The fetal head should then be guided millimeter-by-millimeter over the perineum so that a rapid expulsion and possible "expansion effect" on the fetal skull does not occur. Such rapid reexpansion of the fetal head could be hazardous, especially in the premature or hypoxic infant.

4) Nuchal cord

Following the delivery of the fetal head, the face and nares should be immediately wiped free of mucus and blood. **The nares and pharynx should be thoroughly suctioned with a bulb syringe or with a DeLee suction trap prior to the infant's first breath.** A finger is then swept across the fetal neck to detect the presence of one or more loops of nuchal umbilical cord. A nuchal cord occurs in 25% of cases. If a loop is found, it should either be pulled over the fetal head to release it, or it should be doubly clamped

and cut in order to free the neck. The remainder of the delivery of the fetal body should then be carried out immediately.

5) Delivery of the fetal shoulders

After the delivery of the fetal head, it will undergo restitution to the frontal position (i.e., external rotation) and will turn to face one of the mother's thighs. If it looks at the mother's right inner thigh, then the initial position was probably a left occiput anterior position (LOA). If it looks at the left thigh, then the position was most likely a right occiput anterior position (ROA). If it delivers looking upward at the ceiling, then the infant is in an occiput posterior position (OP). The fetal head will drop posteriorly as the shoulder stems beneath the symphysis pubis. Subsequent downward and then upward traction will usually deliver first one shoulder, and then the other, followed by the remainder of the fetal body. **Care should always be taken that the fetal head is not flexed upon the body, since this flexion can result in excessive stretching of the brachial plexus, which may cause neurological injury.** The head and shoulders should be manipulated together by placing traction and pressure on the fetal shoulders themselves, rather than by twisting or pulling on the fetal head alone. After delivery, the infant may then be held in the left hand with the thumb in one axilla and the little finger in the other to support the back, while the middle three fingers support the head and prevent it from rotating. The infant's body should be cradled in the crook of the left arm, leaving the right hand free to work on the infant (Fig. 24-11).

b. The management of the third stage of labor

1) Delivery of the placenta

The third stage of labor begins with the delivery of the infant and ends with the expulsion of the placenta. If excessive bleeding is not encountered, you can wait for 30–60 minutes for the delivery of the placenta. **The signs of placental separation** are: *(1) the rising up of the uterus in the lower abdomen as the placenta moves into the lower part of the uterus, (2) a gush of blood from the vagina, and (3) the advancement of the umbilical cord as it lengthens.* Usually, the pulsations of the umbilical cord will have

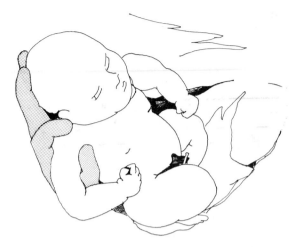

FIGURE 24-11. Holding the baby at delivery. If you are right handed, then you should hold the baby in the crook of your left arm with your thumb and little finger in the axillae and the middle three fingers supporting the infant's neck and head. This technique allows you to use your right hand to suction the infant and clamp and cut the cord.

ceased by this time. The uterus is then grasped firmly with one hand placed on the patient's abdomen while at the same time slight traction is applied on the umbilical cord with the other hand. If the placenta has completely separated from the uterus and has dropped into the vagina, it will be delivered easily into a waiting basin. If difficulty is encountered, however, it may be possible to elevate the uterine body with one hand, while applying gentle traction on the umbilical cord with the other hand to further dislodge the placenta from the uterus (Brandt-Andrews maneuver) (Fig. 24-12). If these maneuvers fail, you may have to insert one hand into the vagina to locate and assist in the removal of the placenta. **If the removal requires the insertion of the hand up into the uterine cavity, then the procedure is termed a "manual removal of the placenta."** This procedure often requires adequate anesthesia in order to perform it safely and with comfort to the patient. If a manual removal of the placenta becomes necessary, it is essential to thoroughly explore the uterine cavity after the placenta has been removed to be certain that there are no remaining fragments of the placenta present and to be sure that there has been no perforation of the uterus secondary to the procedure.

2) Examination of the placenta

The placenta should be examined closely to be sure that all of the cotyledons and membranes are intact, that there is no evidence of infarction, and that there are two umbilical arteries and one umbilical vein present. If there have been clinical signs of possible abruptio placentae, you should look for the presence of an organized clot on the maternal surface of the placenta. The type of placentation should also be noted (e.g., battledore, circumvallate, etc.) and the placenta should be weighed. **In infants who have a low Apgar score, you should obtain a specimen of arterial blood from the placenta for pH and/or other acid-base parameters. This sample can be taken from the cord, or, if a cord blood arterial sample is not possible, then it can be taken from the arteries that overlie the veins on the placental surface.**

3) Examination of the vagina, cervix, and uterus

Immediately following the delivery of the placenta, the vagina and cervix should be visualized using a retractor or a speculum in order to detect the presence of any lacerations. If it is difficult to see using this method, then it is possible to locate any lacerations by palpating the walls of the vagina. The placement of sponge forceps on the cervix at the 3 and 9 o'clock positions will often bring the cervix into view. If the cervix still cannot be seen, then you should palpate for cervical lacerations by placing one finger within the cervical os and the second finger outside of the cervix. It will be then possible to sweep the fingers around the cervix circumferentially to detect any cervical lacerations, since the fingers will come together if a laceration is present (Fig. 24-13).

Lacerations of the vagina are classified as follows: (1) a **first-degree laceration** involves the surface epithelium, but not the underlying tissues, (2) a **second-degree laceration** involves both the superficial as well as the deep tissues, but not the rectal sphincter, (3) a **third-degree laceration** involves the superficial and deep tissues, and also the rectal sphincter, and (4) a **fourth-degree laceration** involves superficial and deep tissues, the rectal sphincter, and the rectal mucosa. **Neither cervical lacerations nor episiotomy incisions are classified according to the degree of the incision.**

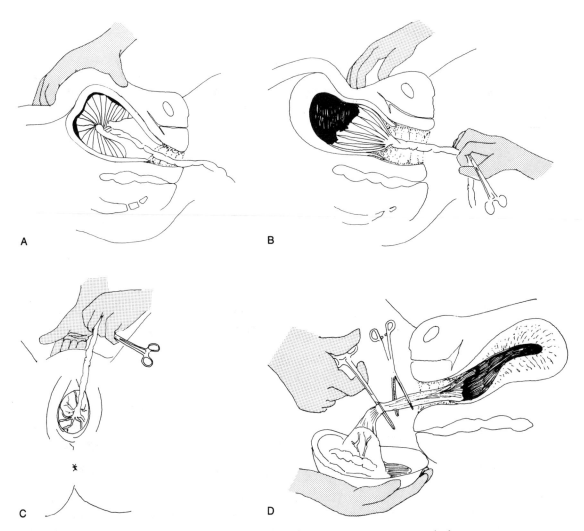

FIGURE 24-12. Delivery of the placenta. (A) The Brandt-Andrews maneuver is instituted when the uterus assumes a globular shape and rises up in the lower abdomen. (B) The uterus is grasped and alternately squeezed and kneaded while applying *gentle* traction on the umbilical cord. (C) The placenta releases and is extruded first into the vagina and then out through the introitus. (D) The last panel demonstrates the care that must be taken as the main placenta is delivered in order to tease all of the remaining membranes out of the uterus. This may be done by alternately grasping the membranes with hemostatic forceps, all the while advancing the tenuous strands of membranes out of the vagina.

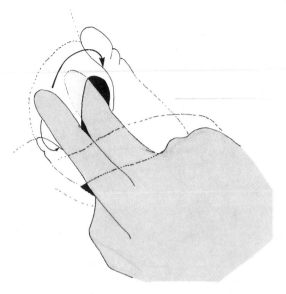

FIGURE 24-13. The detection of a cervical laceration by palpation. The index finger is placed on the outside of the cervix and the midde finger inside the cervix. The fingers are then swept around the full 360 degrees of the opening. If a laceration is present, the fingers will meet at the site of the laceration.

You should always check the fundal height during the repair of the laceration or the episiotomy, especially if you use a vaginal sponge for hemostasis to provide a better visualization of the incisional line. It is important to be aware that the patient could bleed behind such a pack, and in rare instances, a patient may actually exsanguinate into her uterus and die during the time that it takes for the physician to repair the episiotomy.

When the last suture has been placed and the vaginal pack has been removed from the vagina, you should insert two fingers into the cervix and sweep out any clots that may be present while gently massaging the uterus *(i.e., Credé's maneuver)* before sending the patient to the recovery room. By removing the clots that have accumulated in the uterus during the episiotomy repair, you will allow the uterus to clamp down to prevent any further bleeding. If this is not done, the patient may later pass a large number of clots in the recovery room and will appear to have begun to bleed again. This unnecessary complication may require you to take the patient back to the delivery room for a reexamination.

4) The "fourth stage" of labor

Some older physicians speak of a **fourth stage of labor,** which consists of the first 1–2 hours after delivery. Due to the striking increase in the patient's cardiac output during the first hour after delivery, cardiac patients should be watched very closely for cardiac decompensation during this period. It is usually during this time period that atony of the uterus and postpartum hemorrhage may occur. Blood loss will be at a minimum if the uterus is able to contract down upon the spiral arteries in the placental site, and thus produce hemostasis. On occasion, conditions may be such that the uterus cannot perform this function effectively (e.g., due to multiple gestation, hydramnios, prolonged labor, chorioamnionitis). In situations involving extensive vaginal bleeding, it may be necessary to utilize ecbolic agents, such as oxytocin, methylergonovine maleate (Methergine), or prostaglandins, to control the bleeding. If an episiotomy hematoma occurs, it will often develop during this initial period of postpartum observation. Close observation of the patient during the first 1–2 hours postpartum may allow for prevention or amelioration of some of these complications (see Chapter 39).

c. Blood loss with delivery

It is important to monitor blood loss throughout the delivery process. The average delivery without an episiotomy probably involves about 339–490 ml of blood loss. With an episiotomy, the blood loss may be increased by a further 154–225 ml. In view of the archaic definition of "postpartum hemorrhage" (i.e., more than 500 ml at delivery and during the first 24 hours), it would seem reasonable to utilize the value of 1,000 ml of blood loss before making this diagnosis. A careful examination of the vagina and the cervix should always be performed at the time of delivery to detect any lacerations. Generally, all lacerations of a second degree or greater should be repaired.

d. Immediate care of the newborn

1) The initiation of respiration

The transition from a fetal placental system to the neonatal respiratory system is dependent in large part upon the successful initiation of breathing at birth. A number of factors are involved in this important milestone. Certainly, there is a degree of *thoracic expan-*

sion at the moment of birth as the chest rebounds from the compression experienced in the birth canal. In addition, the *infant will have been massaged* by the uterine contractions throughout the labor and delivery process. At the moment of delivery, the *tactile stimulation* of the infant by the physician may also stimulate respiration. **It has been demonstrated that changes in the blood gases, such as a decrease in the pO_2 and/or an increase in the pCO_2, as well as variations in the ambient temperature, may stimulate the fetal respiratory center.**

The newborn infant is an obligatory nose-breather and thus it is important to clear the nares as well as the pharynx of blood and mucus as soon as possible after the head has been delivered. This procedure is especially important if there has been any meconium staining present, since the aspiration of the meconium may lead to respiratory distress, pulmonary hypertension, hypoxia, and possible fetal death. *Recent evidence indicates that the fetus may aspirate meconium in utero and that it is not always possible to prevent meconium aspiration by scrupulous pulmonary toilet at birth.*

a) Establishment of respiration

The lungs of the neonate are at about $1–2$ cm H_2O subatmospheric pressure at the pleural surface during the initiation of respiration, which involves the descent of the diaphragm and expansion of the thoracic cage. Expiration is more passive than inhalation and is due primarily to the elastic recoil of the lung. This lung elasticity is related to changes in the surface active materials. **The presence of pulmonary surfactant provides surface tension at the air-liquid interface and assists in decreasing the elastic recoil effect and preventing the alveoli from collapsing at the end of each expiration.** If there is a deficiency in pulmonary surfactant, the decreased lung compliance and functional residual capacity will require high ventilatory pressures and an increased respiratory rate to achieve adequate volume exchange in the lungs.

b) Surfactant

While surfactant may be found in very small infants (i.e., $500–700$ grams), it is generally not until 28 weeks' gestation and beyond that it is found in any quantity. As a consequence, when a deficiency of sur-

factant in association with a very compliant thorax is found in a premature infant, there is a nearly total collapse and expansion of the lungs with each breath. As a result, so much pressure is required to move air into the lungs that the soft tissues of the thorax are sucked inwards with each breath *(i.e., retraction).*

The most common surfactant lipid is phosphatidylcholine (lecithin), which constitutes $80–90\%$ of the lipid component. Of this, dipalmitoylphosphatidylcholine accounts for more than 50% of the total **lecithin** fraction. Two other surface active acidic phospholipids have been described: phosphatidylinositol (PI) and phosphatidylglycerol (PG). These two components are essential because of their ability to stabilize the lecithin in the surfactant layer. Another lipid that has surface active properties is sphingomyelin, but since this lipid changes little as term approaches, it serves as a reference baseline for evaluating the increases in the lecithin fraction (ie., the lecithin/sphingomyelin ratio) (L/S ratio).

Surface active lecithin appears in the amniotic fluid as early as $24–26$ weeks' gestation; however, it is not until about the $34–35$th week that there is a significant increase. When lecithin is compared to sphingomyelin (L/S ratio), a value of $2:1$ is generally compatible with functional pulmonary maturity. This ratio may vary, however, from one laboratory to another and depending on which detection technique is used. **Phosphatidylglycerol (PG) initially appears at about the 35th week of gestation and signifies final surfactant maturity.** It has been noted that PG is absent in infants who develop respiratory distress syndrome (RDS). Conversely, if PG is present at a level of 3% or greater, then RDS will not occur. It also appears earlier in patients with diabetes mellitus (classes F and R), in patients with severe hypertension and proteinuria, and in patients with prolonged rupture of membranes.

c) Respiratory distress syndrome

Hyaline membrane disease, or the **respiratory distress syndrome (RDS),** has been recognized for more than 80 years; however, it has only been during the past 40 years that the magnitude of the problem has been appreciated. Its rate of occurrence is inversely related to the maturity of the fetus, and it requires at least an hour of breathing after birth before the pathologic picture becomes fully manifest. Fetuses of small size may not live sufficiently long enough for the full clinical picture to develop. **Clinically, cyanosis and respiratory distress, with chest retractions that begin shortly after birth, are the most prominent symptoms seen, and death generally occurs within 72 hours of birth.** The lungs at autopsy usually show variable degrees of atelectasis, with *hyaline-like membranes* lining the terminal bronchioles along with cellular debris, fibrin, and plasma transudate. Due to the deficiency of the surfactant and the mechanical problems inherent in attempts to expand the lungs, there remain many areas of atelectasis, which may be only partially perfused. Other areas that are well expanded may then be over-perfused, which leads to membrane formation. The treatment of the infant with continuous positive end-expiratory pressure ventilation seems to be of benefit, since it tends to prevent atelectasis.

2) Circulatory adjustments

a) Cardiovascular changes at birth

In utero, the pulmonary vascular resistance is high and the blood flow through the lungs is low. Studies of sheep fetuses have shown that with the first breath of the fetus at delivery, the pO_2 rapidly increases. **With a pO_2 of 37 mm Hg and above, the pulmonary vascular resistance begins to fall. When the pO_2 reaches 53 mm, the ductus arteriosus functionally closes (in sheep).** The decrease in the level of prostaglandins is also involved in the closure of the ductus arteriosus. When the umbilical cord is clamped, the peripheral systemic vascular resistance increases, which causes a reversal of the pressure gradient across the foramen ovale. Due to the decrease in the pulmonary vascular resistance, this increasing systemic peripheral vascular resistance then forces the closure of the foramen ovale. As a consequence of all of these changes, the fetal circulation makes the transition to that of a neonate. *When this transition occurs, the two ventricles begin to work in series and have equal outputs. The pulmonary circuit opens up and becomes a low-resistance circuit, replacing the placenta as the organ of respiration.*

b) Pulmonary hypertension

In certain situations, the pulmonary vascular resistance may remain high (pulmonary hypertension secondary to hypoxia, meconium aspiration, etc.), which causes a reversal of the changes that normally occur at birth. This *persistent fetal circulation* (i.e., pulmonary hypertension) may be lethal to the fetus.

3) The Apgar score and asphyxia

In the Apgar score, which is used to assess the infant at the time of birth, two sets of values are usually recorded; the first assessment is recorded at one minute after birth, and the second assessment is noted at five minutes. The scoring is based upon five physical findings of the infant at birth: (1) the heart rate, (2) the muscle tone, (3) the respiratory effort, (4) the reflex irritability, and (5) the color (Table 24-1).

An Apgar score of 7–10 is considered to be

TABLE 24-1. The Apgar score*

Rating	0	1	2
Appearance	Pale or Blue	Body Pink, extremities blue	Pink all over
Pulse	Absent	< 100	> 100
Grimace	None	Grimace	Cry
Activity (tone)	Limp	Some flexion	Spontaneous movement
Respiration	Absent	Hypoventilation, gasping	Vigorous crying

*To be performed exactly 1 and 5 minutes after complete birth of the infant.

Reprinted with permission from D. Cavanagh, R. E. Woods, T.C.F. O'Connor, and R. A. Knupple, *Obstetric Emergencies,* 3rd ed. Philadelphia: J. B. Lippincott Company, 1978, p. 316.

normal. **An Apgar score of 4–6 may be considered to represent mild to moderate depression, whereas an Apgar score of 0–3 is indicative of severe depression.** The 1-minute score is representative of the events that have occurred during labor and especially during the delivery process. Low scores at this point should alert you to the fact that you should begin immediate resuscitation measures, since these infants are obviously in distress at delivery; however, the score has no long-term prognostic significance. **The 5-minute Apgar score is more prognostic of later infant mortality or morbidity.** Occasionally, a 10-minute score will be listed, if the infant has required a significant amount of resuscitation. Surprisingly, an Apgar score of 1–3 at the 5-minute evaluation at birth is associated with seriously damaged infants in only about 6% of cases. **It has been noted that the incidence of cerebral palsy does not seem to be related to the Apgar scores at birth, since in retrospective analysis of 55% of such children in one study, the Apgar score was 7–10 at one minute, and in 73%, the Apgar score was 7–10 at five minutes.** The finding of an umbilical cord arterial blood pH value that is indicative of acidosis (i.e., pH < 7.20) may be a valuable technique in the assessment of those infants who have had abnormal fetal heart rate tracings prior to delivery or who have a low Apgar score at birth. The normal acid-base **umbilical cord arterial blood values** are: pH = 7.25–7.35; pO_2 = 18 mm Hg; and pCO_2 = 40–48 mm Hg. The **normal umbilical cord venous blood values** are: pH = 7.35–7.38; pO_2 = 28–30 mm Hg; and pCO_2 = 38–40 mm Hg. The umbilical cord arterial blood values reflect the fetal tissue levels since the blood is coming from the fetus and going to the placenta.

It should be remembered that the presence of maternal acidosis may lead to low umbilical cord pH values in the presence of adequate oxygenation in the fetus. Patients who have had vomiting, dehydration, heavy sedation, infection, or cyanotic heart disease should also have a maternal pH blood value drawn at the same time as the cord specimens are obtained. Furthermore, the infant's tone, color, and reflex irritability may be somewhat dependent upon the level of fetal physiologic maturity, and a *low value in the premature infant* may not be a valid indication of an anoxic insult or cerebral depression. The infant's tone and responsiveness are also dependent upon the amount of maternal sedation, and thus may not truly

reflect the infant's actual condition. The Apgar score is a crude index of perinatal events and should not be considered to be a precise indicator of the fetal condition or prognosis. The infant's Apgar score should not be considered to be sufficient evidence to predict the occurrence of cerebral palsy unless the Apgar score is 0–3 at 10 minutes, the infant remains hypotonic for several hours after birth, and the infant has seizures in the immediate neonatal period. The presence of a significant acidosis in the cord blood specimen at the time of delivery has perhaps a greater prognostic significance in predicting the infant's eventual outcome than does the Apgar score.

4) Resuscitative measures

Fortunately, only 0.5–1.0% of neonates will require extensive resuscitation at birth for more than a minute. Perhaps the most important element in infant resuscitation is that you *anticipate* that you may have a problem before the delivery and that you prepare the team to handle any asphyxia problems before they occur. This approach allows time for you to check all of the equipment and to be sure that the oxygen masks, the infant laryngoscopes, and the endotracheal tubes are ready and available. During labor, there may be certain risk factors that may alert you to the fact that problems may occur at delivery. Such conditions as toxemia, third-trimester bleeding, diabetes, prematurity, postmaturity, dysfunctional labor, cephalopelvic disproportion, or documented fetal distress are all factors that should alert you to the possibility that the fetus may be compromised.

It should be immediately apparent at birth whether or not the infant will require resuscitative measures (Fig. 24-14, Fig. 24-15, Fig. 24-16). The infant who requires such resuscitation will be limp, pale, or bluish-tinged, with ragged or absent breathing and minimal to no spontaneous activity. The Apgar score will be low (i.e., less than 6 at the 1-minute evaluation). The more depressed the infant, the more intensive the resuscitative efforts will have to be.

The "ABC's" of infant resuscitation should be employed in infants who have a low initial Apgar score. **The "A" represents the anticipation of the problem, and the assessment of the fetal status and the condition of the airway.** Airway suctioning, followed by positive pressure ventilation with 100% oxygen, should be instituted immediately in any infant with a heart rate of less than 100 bpm. **The "B"**

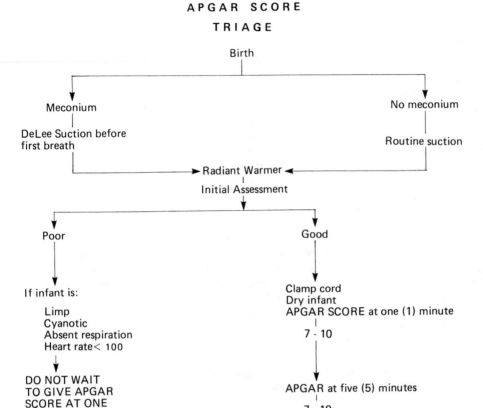

FIGURE 24-14. The initial triage evaluation of the neonate. (Courtesy of Dennis Smith, M.D.)

is concerned with the infant's breathing. You should auscultate the breath sounds high in the axillae on each side to determine whether sufficient air exchange is occurring. **The "C" is concerned about the infant's circulation.** If enough oxygen is being delivered to the infant, then the heart rate should improve rapidly. If not enough oxygen is being delivered to the lungs, then endotracheal intubation and suctioning should be accomplished by using a size 0 laryngoscope blade to visualize the vocal cords and then inserting an endotracheal tube (ET), size 2.5 mm for an infant weighing 1,000 gms; 3.0 mm for a weight of 1,000–2,000 gms; 3.5 mm for a weight of 2,000–3,000 gms; or 4.0 mm for a weight of more than 3,000 gms. The initial ventilatory efforts should be directed toward inflation of the lungs gradually over 3–5 seconds to a peak pressure of 20–30 cm of water. This effort should be continued at a rate of about 50 breaths per minute until the infant begins to demonstrate adequate spontaneous respirations on its own.

Once the trachea has been cleared and adequate amounts of oxygen are being delivered to the baby, the heart rate should increase to more than 100 bpm within 60 seconds. If the heart rate does not respond, then cardiac massage should be started. The hands should be placed about the chest with the thumbs over the midsternum, and compressions should be carried out at 120 times per minute.

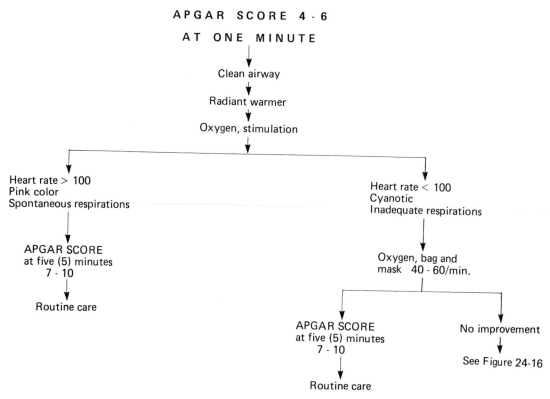

APGAR SCORE 4 - 6
AT ONE MINUTE

Clean airway

Radiant warmer

Oxygen, stimulation

Heart rate > 100
Pink color
Spontaneous respirations

Heart rate < 100
Cyanotic
Inadequate respirations

APGAR SCORE
at five (5) minutes
7 - 10

Routine care

Oxygen, bag and
mask 40 - 60/min.

APGAR SCORE
at five (5) minutes
7 - 10

No improvement

See Figure 24-16

Routine care

FIGURE 24-15. The management of infants with Apgar scores of between 4 and 6 at one minute. (Courtesy of Dennis Smith, M.D.)

The **"D" (drugs) and "E" (extras and evaluation)** of the resuscitation scheme should be considered by the pediatrician or the neonatal subspecialist. If the fetus should require more extensive therapy, such as volume expanders, sodium bicarbonate, or other medications, expert neonatal care should be utilized. As a consequence, whenever you anticipate prior to delivery that the fetus may be in severe distress, it is always wise to ask for a pediatrician to be present at the delivery to manage the infant.

Since the infant may lose as much as 4.5° C of body heat within one minute in the relatively cold room air, it is essential that the newborn infant be placed in a warmer as soon as possible following delivery to prevent **hypothermia.** If the infant is placed under a radiant heater immediately after the delivery, the loss of body heat will be reduced to about 1.5° C.

Every newborn infant should receive 0.5–1.0 mg of Vitamin K (phytonadione) within one hour of birth.

e. The initial physical examination

1) The initial evaluation of the infant

At the time of the delivery, the infant should be cradled on your left forearm (if you are right handed) with a thumb and little finger resting in each axilla and the middle three fingers supporting the fetal neck and head. This will leave the right hand free to suction the infant and to clamp and cut the umbilical cord. The umbilical cord and placenta contain between 100 and 140 ml of blood. If the infant has a blood volume of about 78 ml/kg (approximately 234 ml total blood volume in an infant weighing 3,000 gms), then the infusion of 100–140 ml, or nearly 43–60% of the infant's total blood volume, by stripping the cord, would seem to be an excessive amount of blood to administer to the baby. While the infant almost always tolerates this infusion, it does increase the risk of neonatal jaundice. At the same time, the extra blood provides for an

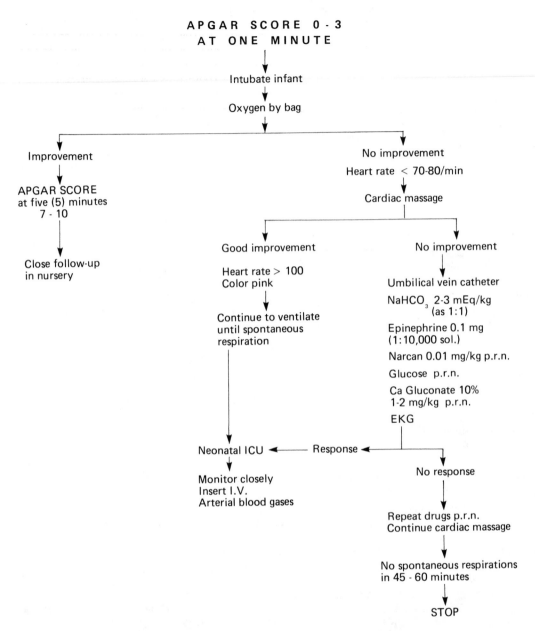

FIGURE 24-16. The management of severely depressed infants with Apgar scores of 0 to 3 at one minute. (Courtesy of Dennis Smith, M.D.)

increased amount of iron stores for the fetus. The placement of the infant at the same level as the mother at delivery, and the avoidance of such an unnecessary transfusion, would seem to be the best approach.

The prime consideration at birth is to immediately establish an adequate airway and regular respirations in the infant. The cord may then be clamped and the infant placed in a warmer to maintain its body temperature and to avoid hypothermia. Usually, a 1% silver nitrate solution is placed in the infant's eyes to prophylactically treat the infant for possible gonorrheal ophthalmia. Recent studies have indicated that erythromycin ointment may be of value in preventing neonatal conjunctivitis resulting from Chlamydia trachomatis.

The umbilical cord should be inspected for the presence of two arteries and one vein. The incidence of finding only one umbilical cord artery is about 0.85% of singleton deliveries. About 30% of these babies will have associated congenital abnormalities of the cardiac or renal systems.

The infant should be systematically examined from head to toe to detect any abnormalities. The head should be palpated to detect the presence of a cephalohematoma, or other abnormalities. The palate should be inspected and palpated. The placement of the ears (normal or low) should be determined. The neck should be examined for masses or webbing. The chest should be inspected and the location of the point of maximal cardiac impulse determined. The abdomen should be palpated to determine the size of the liver and the spleen and to detect the presence of any masses. The genitalia should be inspected to be sure that both testicles are in the scrotum in the male and that there is no ambiguity of the external sexual organs. The legs should be "frog-legged" to detect a congenital hip dislocation, and the anus should be inspected for patency. The infant is then rolled onto its stomach so that the spine can be palpated and inspected for any abnormalities. This entire brief examination takes only a few seconds. This cursory physical examination is then followed up in the nursery with a complete examination in which the infant is evaluated in detail.

CHAPTER 25

Puerperium

We are constantly misled by the ease with which our minds fall into the ruts of one or two experiences.
—*Sir William Osler**

1. Daily postpartum care

a. Immediate care

Just prior to removing the sterile drapes and sending the patient to the recovery room, you should inspect the vagina for vaginal packs and probe the cervix for any clots, while massaging the uterus to be certain that it has clamped down tightly and that the *bleeding has been controlled*. The patient's perineum should be washed with soap and water, dried with towels, and a clean sterile perineal pad should be placed over the vulva. The patient should then be covered with a warm blanket.

During the first few hours after delivery, you should pay special attention to the status of the uterus and the amount of vaginal bleeding. The uterine size and consistency should be checked frequently to detect any relaxation of the uterus. When the uterus is found to be soft and boggy, it should be massaged until it is firm. In some instances there may be very little evidence of any external bleeding because of the accumulation of blood in the uterus. If the amount of external bleeding is evaluated without an evaluation of the uterus, severe *hidden hemorrhage* may go unrecognized. Another source of hidden hemorrhage is

*Reprinted with permission from Robert Bennett Bean, *Sir William Osler: Aphorisms from His Bedside Teachings and Writings,* William Bennett Bean, ed. Springfield, Ill.: Charles C Thomas, Publisher, 1968, p. 54.

bleeding into a *hematoma* of an episiotomy incision, or into the retroperitoneal spaces of the broad ligament or paracolic gutters. Excessive complaints on the part of the patient of severe pelvic or episiotomy pain immediately postpartum should alert you to this possibility (see Chapter 39). Vital signs should be obtained every 15 minutes during the first 1–2 hours, and if they are stable, then they should be taken at 2–4-hour intervals for the first 6–12 hours.

The urine output should also be closely monitored during the first 6–12 hours. Urinary retention may occur secondary to the trauma of the delivery, or it may be due to the use of regional anesthesia; however, most women will void within four hours of delivery and will continue to do so at regular intervals thereafter. If the patient is unable to void within 4–6 hours, then catheterization should be carried out. Urinary retention also may be associated with uterine atony and postpartum hemorrhage.

b. Continued care

The patient should be encouraged to ambulate as soon as she leaves the recovery room and is returned to her room, unless she has had a regional anesthetic for delivery, in which case ambulation should be delayed until she has completely recovered from the anesthesia. The early ambulation of patients has been shown to hasten recovery and to aid in the prevention of thrombophlebitis and pulmonary embolism in the postpartum period.

A perineal heat lamp or wet perineal care performed three times each day will often provide the patient with a measure of comfort if she has had an episiotomy performed. The use of an anesthetic spray on the episiotomy site is also helpful in providing pain relief.

"discharge"

The initial vaginal lochia consists of red blood cells, decidual tissue, and bacteria. **In the first 3–4 days, the bleeding from the uterus will be sufficient to color the lochia red (lochia rubra).** As the bleeding decreases over the next week, the lochia will become paler **(lochia serosa),** and after 10 days, the lochia will be primarily yellowish-white **(lochia alba)** due to the presence of leukocytes as the tissues begin to heal. If there is a prolongation of the reddish lochia beyond two weeks, then retained placental fragments or subinvolution of the uterus may be present. The development of a **foul odor to the lochia,** especially if it is associated with a fever, indicates the possibility of a postpartum **endometritis.**

Uterine cramps *(i.e., afterpains)* are commonly seen in multiparas, especially during nursing. Fortunately, they last for only a few days and the administration of an analgesic for a day or so will usually provide relief.

Vascular and lymphatic engorgement of the breasts occurs on about the third day postpartum. The nursing woman should be taught to care for her breasts and nipples. Cleanliness and the use of nipple shields for fissures or irritation are both effective measures. A supportive nursing brassiere should also be utilized. In the past, the presence of a fever was always attributed to breast engorgement; however, a cause-and-effect relationship between these two events has never been satisfactorily proven. In general, a fever should be considered to be indicative of an infection until proven otherwise (see Chapter 16).

If the patient does not desire to breast-feed, then you may wish to suppress lactation. The patient should avoid any stimulation of her breasts and use a breast binder and ice packs for a few days. If a lactation suppression medication is to be used, then bromocriptine (Parlodel) is both safe and effective. A dosage regimen of 2.5 mg p.o. b.i.d. for two weeks has been used to inhibit prolactin secretion.

The bowels will generally move within the first 48 hours following delivery; however, stool softeners are often helpful, especially in the patient who has had an episiotomy incision.

2. Maternal-infant bonding

In recent years, there has been considerable concern expressed over the **maternal-infant bonding** relationship between the newborn infant and the mother. This relationship has been likened to the **imprinting process** that has been described in animals, wherein the newborn becomes attracted and then emotionally attached to its mother or to a substitute maternal figure in the early neonatal period. Indeed, in goslings, the imprinting occurs immediately and the gosling will follow and emotionally attach itself to the first moving object that it sees. This process in the human has been termed **bonding;** however, there is some controversy as to whether this is an immediate process or whether it may extend over perhaps the first year of life.

Those who believe that bonding occurs immediately have advocated that the infant be handled by the mother as soon as possible following birth. Some mothers may forego analgesia during labor in the belief that if it is used, then the infant will be too sedated to participate in the bonding event. The **Lamaze method** of having the patient concentrate on breathing techniques and having a partner to coach her throughout the labor and delivery process has been effective in eliminating the need for analgesics in some patients. Grantly Dick-Read's **prepared-childbirth** approach, in which the patient is instructed as to what to expect at each stage of her pregnancy and throughout the labor and delivery process, by a concerned and compassionate physician who is willing to sit with his patient during the labor and provide her with tender loving care, has also been shown to diminish the need for analgesics. Another method that may encourage maternal-infant bonding involves the concept of "gentle birth," in which the delivery of the infant is carried out in quiet surroundings, with soft music and dimmed lights, and the infant is then placed in warm water, where it is stroked immediately after birth **(Leboyer method).** The mother then handles the infant immediately after it has stabilized. The circumcision (if it is to be done at all), is delayed until a later time, so that there is nothing to interfere with this bonding process.

Both prolactin and opioids are elevated in the blood of mothers who have just delivered, as it is in women who are runners, secondary to the stress of these activities. The opioid hormone present following delivery has been identified as the one that may be extracted from the pancreas, and it appears to be 2–4 times more potent than β-endorphin and 50 times stronger than morphine. It has been suggested by one author that from a teleologic viewpoint, the release of the opioid hormone may: (1) stimulate the release of prolactin for milk production, (2) provide a pleasurable feeling of contentment and well-being that may reinforce the birth process and provide conditioning for the future proliferation of the species, (3) be related to the release of glucose from the pancreatic cells, which is necessary to fuel the effort of delivering a baby, and finally (4) produce an emotional state in the mother that facilitates the bonds of maternal love and affection. The maternally derived opioids in the breast milk may provide the fetus who is nursing a basic degree of security and contentment that may have a long-range effect on the infant's subsequent behavioral development.

Other investigators have taken the stance that "bonding" is a series of interrelated events that occur in the prenatal, neonatal, and postnatal periods, and that the immediate neonatal period may not be as important as others have thought. It is possible that the fetus in utero may develop some degree of comfort and attachment to the mother and the environment. The fetus's senses of hearing, sight, and smell at birth may allow it to distinguish the mother's voice and smell from that of the attendants. Shortly following birth, it seems evident that the child can distinguish the mother (or primary caretaker) from others. It is also possible that the use of sedative analgesic drugs in labor may possibly interfere with this process.

Some follow-up studies have indicated that children who have had the opportunity to fully participate in the bonding process seem to be better adjusted than other children. However, these differences in adjustment perhaps illustrate not only the differences in the bonding approach, but also perhaps the differences in the genetic makeup. Also, the fact that parents who are concerned about the bonding process may also be more concerned about environmental influences, and would therefore probably supply a better environment for their children than other parents, must be taken into consideration. The studies conducted thus far seem to confound rather than illuminate the problem; however, it would be very difficult to obtain appropriate controls to study this matter.

Older studies indicate that the child does not define itself as a separate entity from other objects until about seven months of age. It is at that time that the attachment to the mother appears to become fixed. If the infant is separated from its mother at this time, it will result in "protesting behavior" on the part of the infant. In light of such information, the immediacy of the bonding process may be in

some doubt. Further studies need to be done to elucidate the importance and the value of the maternal-infant bonding process.

3. Breast-feeding

During pregnancy, the breasts are prepared by placental lactogen, estrogen, progesterone, prolactin, cortisone, and insulin to develop the milk production capability. Following delivery, the first three of these hormones decrease dramatically. The manipulation of the cervix and uterus during delivery probably triggers the **Ferguson reflex,** which, along with the repeated nursing episodes immediately postpartum, causes a release of oxytocin from the neurohypophysis and a decrease in the prolactin inhibiting factor (PIF) in the hypothalamus. These events result in an elevation of prolactin levels and the **"letdown" of the milk.**

Human milk contains proteins, lactose, fat, and water. Some proteins synthesized by the breast are unique to human milk and are not found in cow's milk, including casein, alpha-lactalbumin, lactoferrin, and lysozyme. In addition, lactose and fatty acids are also synthesized in the breast. The mother's bloodstream supplies the essential amino acids, and the breast synthesizes some of the nonessential amino acids. All of the vitamins are represented, with the single exception of vitamin K. The most predominant immunoglobulin in milk is secretory IgA, which is probably protective for the infant, especially against Escherichia coli bacteria. As a consequence, human milk is the best food for the infant during the first 4–6 months of life.

It should be recognized that nearly all of the medications that are given to the mother will be secreted in the milk (generally about 1%) and may also affect the infant. The passage of a drug into the milk is dependent upon its lipid solubility, its degree of ionization, and its protein-binding properties. In addition, the rate of the breast blood flow and the concentration of the drug in the mother's bloodstream, to some extent determines the concentration of a drug in the milk. The concentration of a given drug in the milk will peak about 30–120 minutes after administration. The pH of breast milk is normally 7.1. Weak bases such as narcotics, antihistamines, and theophylline easily pass into the milk. In contrast, weak acids, such as penicillin, sulfonamides, diuretics, and barbiturates, do not pass into the milk as readily. Certain other drugs, such as monoamine oxidase inhibitors, bromocriptine, and levodopa, interfere with prolactin secretion and thus decrease milk production. Thiazides also suppress lactation. The drugs that are contraindicated in a patient who is breast-feeding include thiouracil, ergotamine, methotrexate, cimetidine, bromocriptine, gold salts, and clemastine.

For patients who have inverted nipples, the technique of stretching the tissues about the nipple each day during pregnancy will often evert them sufficiently to allow nursing to take place. A frank discussion of breast-feeding and your supportive interest in getting the new mother off to a good start will frequently result in a satisfactory breast-feeding experience. The economy, the portability, the ease of preparation for nursing, and the psychological benefits of breast-feeding, not to mention the superb nutritional aspects for the fetus, make this the procedure of choice for most newborns. The breasts do not require any special care while nursing other than the normal cleansing procedures. Soap or other drying agents should not be used on the nipples. Also, the nipples and the surrounding skin may be protected from skin breaks by having the mother insert her finger in the infant's mouth to break the suction at the end of each nursing episode.

4. Circumcision

Circumcision is one of the oldest surgical procedures on record, having been practiced by the ancient Egyptians centuries prior to the use of the procedure by the Hebrews, who utilized it as part of their covenant with God. In 1975, the American Academy of Pediatrics stated that there was no absolute medical indication for the routine use of this procedure. As a consequence, the performance of the circumcision operation has decreased considerably. In spite of this, however, statistics have shown that perhaps as many as 1 million or more circumcisions were performed out of the 3.7 million births that took place in the United States in 1982.

Several instruments have been devised to make the procedure of circumcision safe and easy to perform. A metallic cap is placed over the glans penis with the prepuce being stretched around the outside of the cap. A clamp is then placed so as to crush the tissues at the base of the prepuce where it joins the glans. The

excision of the excess prepuce tissue completes the circumcision. On rare occasions, a fine absorbable catgut suture may be needed to control persistent bleeding. The use of a Bacitracin ointment–infiltrated gauze dressing about the glans area following the circumcision provides some postoperative protection for the sensitive tissues. Complications occur in 1.5–5% of cases. The excessive removal of the prepuce skin is the most common complication, while hemorrhage and infection are quite rare.

The decision as to whether neonatal circumcision should be performed should reside with the parents. The benefits of the procedure are that phimosis and balanitis are eliminated and that it is much easier for the individual to maintain adequate penile hygiene.

5. Postpartum involutional changes

a. Psychological changes

In ancient times, Hippocrates noted that many women underwent emotional changes following the delivery of the baby. Later, Galen (131–210 A.D.) and others attributed these psychological manifestations to black bile and other "humors." While depression and psychiatric disturbances are probably no different in the postpartum state than in nonpregnant individuals, certainly pregnancy includes a number of factors that may trigger an emotional disorder. If **postpartum blues** (i.e., depression) occurs, it usually begins about 1–4 days following delivery and consists of emotional lability, crying, insomnia, mood changes, irritability, and a sense of vulnerability. This syndrome occurs in perhaps as many as 50–80% of patients. Since patients now frequently leave the hospital within the first 48 hours following delivery, this problem is not often seen by the hospital staff. The emotional and psychological letdown following delivery, the fatigue, and the uncertainties of the mother's newfound responsibilities all combine to produce this depression. Many young women have very little inner ego strength to assist them in coping with their environment throughout the pregnancy, during childbirth, or in the early postpartum period. This is especially the case with unmarried teenagers who manifest the failure syndrome: They have failed in their relationships with their parents, they have failed in school, they have failed in their relationships with males, and finally, they have set themselves up for continued failure over the rest of their lives due to their lack of education, their unmarried state, and the burdens and responsibilities of early parenthood. When this type of background is combined with a fear for the normalcy of the infant, and the possibility of adverse responses and rejection by the consort, it becomes a considerable burden that may overwhelm the patient's ability to cope, with the result being emotional depression. Some of the hormonal changes that occur postpartum also add to these problems. For example, the presence of decreased levels of progesterone have been shown to be associated with depression. Fortunately, postpartum depression is usually a transient phenomenon and usually clears up rapidly as the new mother becomes involved in the care of her infant and develops confidence in her abilities. The patient, however, should be warned ahead of time of the possible occurrence of these mood changes, and also should be reassured that they will be only transitory in nature.

Chronic depressive disorders are thought to occur in the postpartum state in from 30–200 out of 1,000 patients. The symptoms of this vaguely defined syndrome involve guilt feelings, anxiety, fatigue, and feelings of inadequacy.

About 1 : 1,000 patients develop **postpartum psychosis.** This disorder is associated with confusion, agitation, mood alterations, fatigue, feelings of hopelessness, hyperactivity, delusions, and hallucinations. It often develops during the first two weeks following delivery, but might not develop until up to three months' postpartum.

It may be possible at times to anticipate which patients might experience postpartum depression. A history of a previous emotional disorder, or a current severe marital problem, should alert you to this possibility. The physician who is **empathetic** will usually receive emotional and psychological satisfaction from the care of his patients. If you fail to have a "good feeling" in dealing with a particular patient, this might be a clue that the patient is so stressed by her efforts to cope with her psychiatric or emotional state that she cannot give you whatever it is that "satisfies" the ego of the physician. It has been said that 75% of the treatment is for the patient and 25% is for the doctor. Perhaps the empathetic physician's 25% has to do with the "sensing" of the patient's psychological dimension—in this case, her ability or inability to cope. Stress also tends to bring out other neurotic behavior in patients, especially in those who are obsessive compulsive. Excess concern for orderliness or cleanliness may be a subtle manifestation of this condition, and the subsequent frustration may lead to depression. An outright rejection of the infant by the mother may bode ill for the child, in that infanticide or child abuse may be the end result. If severe depression is present, or if the patient has a psychotic break accompanied by hallucinations and a loss of contact with reality, then psychiatric consultation should be obtained and alternative plans made for the baby's care.

b. Genital involutional changes

The uterus decreases in size considerably immediately following delivery, but it does not return to the nonpregnant size for about six weeks. Immediately after delivery, the uterus will be about 20 weeks' gestational size; however, it will decrease to 12–14 weeks' size by the 4th day and to about 10 weeks' size at the end of the second week postpartum. The uterine endometrium will have regenerated within the first 7–10 days, except for the placental site. The placental site initially contains many thrombosed vessels and the basal layer of the endometrium (i.e., decidua basalis). The endometrium regenerates under the placental site and lifts up the thrombosed blood vessels and necrotic stroma so that they are gradually exfoliated by the new endometrium. It may take up to six weeks or more for this process to completely regenerate the placental site.

During the course of pregnancy, the vessels of the uterus become greatly enlarged in order to supply enough blood to the uterus; however, in the postpartum period they become obliterated by intimal proliferation. In the interim between pregnancies, these vessels are recannulated. If elastic stains are used on the myometrial tissue and the blood vessels of a hysterectomy specimen, the number of elastic "rings" in the blood vessels represent the number of pregnancies. "open distended"

The cervix will be patulous immediately after delivery but will become essentially closed by the end of the first week, although the external os will remain more dilated. When the cervix heals, there may be stellate scarring present, further defining this patulous external os as being quite different from the clean, smooth cervix of the nullipara.

The appearance of the postpartum vagina is similar to that of a postmenopausal woman with its thin walls without rugae (i.e., due to lack of estrogenic stimulation) up until about the third week, when the rugae again may be seen.

6. Postpartum instructions

It is essential that you properly instruct your patient when she is discharged from the hospital following delivery. **The patient should be informed as to when to return for her checkup, which is generally in about six weeks.** The selection of the time period of six weeks may have originally been based upon Judaic beliefs about "uncleanliness" following delivery. When Yahweh spoke to Moses, he said, "Speak to the sons of Israel and say: If a woman conceives and gives birth to a boy, she is to be unclean for seven days, just as she is unclean during her monthly periods. On the eighth day the child's foreskin must be circumcised, and she must wait another thirty-three days for her blood to be purified" (Leviticus 12:1–5). Thus, 40 days, or about 6 weeks, was the necessary time that had to pass before the woman was considered clean, if she gave birth to a male infant. In the case of the birth of a female infant, she had to wait 14 days plus 66 days (for a total of 80 days) in order to be considered clean.

Usually, by 6 weeks' postpartum, almost all of the changes of pregnancy will have returned to normal, with an exception being the ureters, which require up to 12 weeks to return to their normal size. As an important precaution, the patient should be told that if fever or excess bleeding should occur, she should return to see you immediately.

The patient's medications should be recorded and she should be instructed as to how to take them. Any effects of the medications in the patient who is breast-feeding should be taken into account. Any possible adverse effect of the medicines employed should be pointed out to the patient, and she should be advised to contact you if any problems should occur. The patient should continue taking her iron supplements at least during the first two months' postpartum in order to reestablish her iron stores.

The patient should be instructed to remain well rested during the first 6 weeks following delivery, or perhaps as long as 2–3 months after a cesarean section, and she should take at least 4–6 weeks to gradually resume performing full housework chores and other physical activities. During the first 2 weeks, she should avoid going out among crowds of people and should not have a lot of visitors, so as to avoid exposing both herself and the baby to different bacteria and viruses. The patient should be careful in going up and down stairs, since her balance may still be precarious. The same is true with regard to the taking of baths, since the patient may be more prone to accidents at this time. Intercourse or douches should be avoided for the first 4–6 weeks in order to avoid the possibility of introducing infection into the healing tissues of the uterus and/or the episiotomy site. When coitus is resumed, gentleness is important. The patient should be warned that she may still get pregnant, even if she is breast-feeding. In patients who have received bromocriptine, ovulation may occur within 2 weeks. If the patient is breast-feeding, ovulation may occur in about 10 weeks. If she is not breast-feeding, then ovulation may occur within 4 weeks. The resumption of other activities should be based upon the patient's overall condition and her desires. Each patient is different and the instructions should be tailored somewhat to the individual patient's desires and needs.

CHAPTER 26

Obstetric procedures

The first actual removal of the uterus and ovaries at the time of cesarean section to avoid the ravages of hemorrhage and infection was on July 21, 1869, by Professor Horatio R. Storer, an American gynecologist in Boston, Massachusetts. On May 21, 1876, Edoardo Porro of Pavia, Italy, performed the same operation, and later performed it 25 times with 10 survivors. His name was attached to this operation (Porro's cesarean section).

—D. R. Dunnihoo

1. Amniocentesis

In the early 1950s, the technique of amniocentesis was utilized by **D. C. A. Bevis** in England as a method of determining the degree of fetal involvement in Rh-sensitized mothers. Since that time, the technique has been used for Rh assessment, genetic evaluations, and gestational age determination.

The technique consists of inserting a 20–22-gauge long spinal needle, under sonographic control, through the abdominal wall and into the amniotic cavity under local anesthesia. The needle should be directed at the side of the fetal small parts, the nape of the neck, or in front of the presenting part as one hand elevates it out of the pelvis (Fig. 26-1). The maternal risks primarily involve infection and hemorrhage, but in actual practice these problems are very rare. **The overall risk to the fetus with this procedure is less than 0.5%, unless it is used for genetic purposes, in which case the risk is 0.6–0.9%.** The fetal risks include hemorrhage, infection, fetal trauma or death, rupture of the membranes, and premature labor.

Amniocentesis may be used to obtain amniotic fluid for the determination of (1) α-fetoprotein to detect fetal neural tube defects, (2) the lecithin/sphingomyelin ratio (L/S) and the phosphatidlylglycerol level (PG) for functional fetal lung maturity, (3) the bilirubin level for Rh isoimmunization, (4) the creatinine, osmolality, and lipid-staining cells (i.e., fat cells) for gestational age determination (no longer used), and (5) the amniotic fluid determination of genetic disorders.

Alpha-fetoprotein (AFP) determinations may be performed using either the amniotic fluid or the maternal serum. *The incidence of neural tube defects (NTD) is about 1–2 per 1,000 live births in the United States. If a couple has had one child with an NTD, then they have a risk of about 2% with subsequent children. If there have been two previous affected children, then the risk increases to about 6%. If the father, or more especially the mother, has an NTD, the initial risk of having a child with an NTD is approximately 5 and 10%, respectively.* It was previously thought that patients who had a prior history of NTD, as well as any patient who was concerned about these anomalies, should be offered maternal AFP serum testing between 16 and 18 weeks' gestation. But since about 90–95% of all cases of NTD arise in patients with no prior history of this problem, it is now thought that probably all patients should be offered the opportunity for such screening.

The evaluation of the AFP levels is considered in terms of multiples of the median (MOM) value in order to eliminate as many false-positive and false-negative results as possible. Ultrasonic dating of the pregnancy is necessary to interpret the results appropriately. If two maternal serum AFP screening results are positive, then an amniotic fluid AFP and an acetylcholinesterase level should be obtained to further define the diagnosis. The presence of *low levels of*

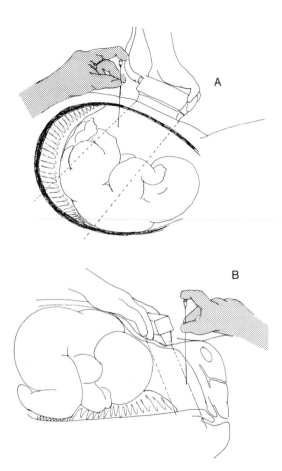

FIGURE 26-1. Amniocentesis may be performed at the following locations: (A) on the side of the small parts, (B) in front of the fetal head. Note the use of the ultrasound to locate a clear pocket of amniotic fluid away from the placenta or the fetus.

AFP have been noted to occur in fetal chromosomal conditions, such as Down's syndrome.

2. Antepartum fetal heart rate monitoring

Dr. E. H. Hon and Dr. R. Wohzgemuth, in 1961, were the first to suggest antepartum fetal assessment with the *maternal exercise test*. In 1972, **Dr. M. Ray** and his colleagues published their clinical experience with the oxytocin challenge test. The *oxytocin challenge test (OCT), or the contraction stress test (CST),* is

based upon the premise that a fetus with a low fetal reserve will manifest a fetal distress pattern (i.e., late decelerations, loss of fetal heart rate variability, or reactivity) if the placental respiratory function is interfered with by uterine contractions. A recent innovation to this test is the *nipple stimulation test,* which requires that the patient stimulate one or both nipples at one-minute intervals for 5–10 minutes to produce uterine contractions. Another assessment test that has been advocated is the *nonstress test,* which was suggested by **Dr. K. Hammacher** in 1969. Hammacher noted that if there were accelerations of the fetal heart rate in association with fetal movements, then the fetus was in good condition.

An increasing interest in the welfare of the fetus has prompted the development of other techniques to assess the fetal condition during the antepartum period. Advances in intrapartum fetal monitoring techniques have provided the practitioner with **central monitoring** equipment that allows the patient's tracings to be transmitted to a central location in the nursing station. This technique has even been extended to **ambulatory monitoring,** where an antepartum **telemetry** monitor worn by the patient transmits signals to a receiver in the labor unit, and finally, to the use of **telecommunications,** whereby a computer and a modem are used to transmit the FHR record over the telephone from the patient's home to the physician's office or to the hospital. These records can also be transmitted by **telecopier** from a physician in a rural area to an urban specialist for consultation purposes. In the past, the storage of FHR records was cumbersome at best. The use of archiving computers in the near future will allow the storage of the patient's FHR records, the history, the findings of the physical examination, the medications administered, and any other pertinent data. If needed later, these data could be reproduced and printed out for teaching or for legal purposes.

a. Oxytocin challenge test (OCT)

The contraction stress test (CST), or the oxytocin challenge test (OCT), is based upon the concept that the fetus is "stressed" by the uterine contractions because they interfere with uterine blood flow to the intervillus space. If the fetus has a good *fetal reserve* (i.e., is in good condition), then such a transient deprivation of oxygen should not result in too much stress for the fetus. On the other hand, if the fetus does not have any respiratory reserve (i.e., is in poor condition), then *late decelerations* of the fetal heart rate (FHR) should occur under this type of stress. In patients who have oligohydramnios, the relative lack of amniotic fluid may cause cord compression patterns to occur (see Chapter 37).

This test requires that the patient be placed in a left lateral decubitus position with the external electronic fetal monitoring equipment applied. Intravenous oxytocin should then be administered, beginning at 0.5 mU/minute and then increasing the dose at 30-minute intervals until three contractions occur, each lasting 40–60 seconds, within a 10-minute period. **If there are no late decelerations (i.e., periodic decreases in the FHR) during the 10-minute "window" containing the three contractions, then the test is considered to be negative.** If *accelerations (i.e., transient increases in the periodic FHR)* occur during the test (termed a *reactive test*), some studies suggest that there is little risk of an intrauterine fetal death within the subsequent week (i.e., fetal mortality 0.4 : 1,000). **A positive test is one that shows persistent late decelerations in more than 50% of the uterine contractions.** The occurrence of an occasional late deceleration that is not persistent should be considered to be a *suspicious* test and warrants further testing within the same week. If less than three contractions per 10-minute window are achieved, then the test should be considered *unsatisfactory*. In those tests in which there are more than three contractions per 10-minute window (e.g., less than 2 minutes apart), or when the contractions last for longer than 90 seconds, uterine hypertonus secondary to hyperstimulation must be considered to be present. The occurrence of late decelerations in this circumstance would not necessarily be indicative of a low fetal reserve or of fetal jeopardy.

b. Nonstress test (NST)

A nonstress test (NST) does not involve the application of stress to the fetus but is merely a recording of the fetal heart rate over a period of time to determine whether there are any accelerations associated with the movements of the fetus. The fetus is most active during rapid eye movement (REM) sleep and at about 1–2 hours after the mother has ingested a meal. The patient is placed in a left lateral decubitus position and the maternal blood

pressure and baseline FHR tracing is obtained, as in the CST procedure. The occurrence of at least two episodes of FHR accelerations within a 20-minute period, that show an increase of 15 bpm and that last for at least 15 seconds, has been termed a *reactive NST test*. Some studies have shown that the antenatal mortality rate in these cases was 3.2 : 1,000. A nonreactive NST shows no FHR accelerations or shows accelerations that do not meet the above criteria. The reactive test should be repeated *twice a week* in postdate or diabetic patients. The occurrence of variable decelerations during a nonstress test may be due to umbilical cord compression secondary to nuchal cord or oligohydramnios. Oligohydramnios may occur in fetal intrauterine growth retardation or in postterm pregnancies. It has been shown that patients who have these patterns present on nonstress testing have a higher incidence of fetal distress in labor, decreased Apgar scores, and nuchal cord involvement.

c. Nipple stimulation test

The breast stimulation or nipple stimulation test is based upon the concept that the stimulation of the breasts causes the release of oxytocin from the posterior pituitary gland, which in turn may cause uterine contractions. The patient is monitored, as in the contraction stress test (CST), while she stimulates her nipples with her fingers for about two minutes, or until a contraction begins. The stimulation is then repeated in five minutes if the contractions do not occur. The goal is to have three contractions of 40–60 seconds each within a 10-minute window. In contrast to the CST, the degree of nipple stimulation and amount of uterine activity cannot be controlled in this test, and thus, the occurrence of hyperstimulation may be more frequent. The criteria that is used to interpret the test, however, is the same as with the CST.

d. Effectiveness of these tests

These tests have been used in the third trimester of pregnancy to detect evidence of a compromise in the fetal reserve, which could cause fetal jeopardy or death. A number of approaches have been suggested with regard to the frequency and type of testing, depending upon the patient's underlying condition (e.g., diabetes, hypertension, postdates, possible IUGR, oligohydramnios, isoimmunization, chronic renal disease, heart disease, hemoglobinopathy, decreased fetal movement, or multiple gestation). It has been suggested that the testing should be conducted either weekly or twice weekly in certain situations. The patient may be tested by means of an NST alone, a CST alone, or with a combination of these two tests.

It should be recognized that there may be considerable error associated with these tests. **The false-positive rate of the CST may be as high as 50%. The absence of reactivity (i.e., accelerations) seems to have a more ominous meaning. The NST has a lower false-positive rate than the CST, and therefore greater reliance may be placed in a nonreactive NST that the fetus may indeed be compromised. The false-negative rate of the CST is between 2.2:1,000 and 10:1,000, whereas the false-negative rate of the NST is about 10:1,000.** If a cord compression pattern *(i.e., variable decelerations)* is present during testing, oligohydramnios may be present. This condition is more commonly seen in the *postterm patient* than in others. If a *sinusoidal wave* pattern (i.e., a smooth undulating wave) is present, then fetal anemia may be present, which in most instances results in a fetal survival rate of the order of 50%. **When the NST results are nonreactive (i.e., abnormal), a CST should also be performed.** If the NST is abnormal and the CST is normal, then repeat testing should be accomplished in several days. If the results of both tests are normal, the fetal respiratory function and reserve should be normal. If the NST results are normal and the CST results are abnormal, then the fetus probably has a decreased fetal reserve. If both the NST and the CST results are abnormal, then the fetus is probably compromised and delivery should be considered.

e. Combination of tests (Biophysical profile score)

One approach to determining the **status of the fetus** is the utilization of the biophysical profile score (BPS), which involves the evaluation of: (1) the fetal breathing movements, (2) the gross body movements, (3) the fetal tone, (4) a reactive FHR, and (5) the quantification of the amniotic fluid volume.

1) Fetal breathing movements

Experiments in fetal lambs have shown that there is a decrease in the fetal breathing movements (FBM) with as little as only an 8 torr change in the pO_2. The ultra-

sonic observation of the fetal diaphragm in the sagittal, coronal, or longitudinal plane **over about a 30-minute period should detect at least one episode of FBM that is of at least 60 seconds duration** (score 2). If there is at least one episode of fetal breathing that lasts for 30–60 seconds within 30 minutes, the score is one. If no fetal breathing movements occur, the score is zero.

2) Gross body movements

Hypoxia will cause a gradual loss of the fetal body movements, which usually follows upon the disappearance of the fetal breathing movements (FBM). **During a 30-minute observation period, there should be at least three discrete body-limb movements (score 2).** A score of one is given if there are only one or two body movements within 30 minutes. Those complexes of multiple movements that occur at the same time are considered as a single movement.

It has been noted that there are about 86 fetal body movements every 12 hours (i.e., an average of 7 movements/hr) at 24 weeks' gestation and that this amount increases to about 132 movements every 12 hours (i.e., an average of 11 movements/hr) by the 32nd week. This level of activity then decreases to 107 movements every 12 hours (i.e., an average of 9 movements/hr) by the 40th week.

Since a sudden decrease or cessation of fetal movements has been viewed as an ominous development, attempts have been made to have the patient monitor the activity of her fetus. If the low-risk patient at 27 weeks' gestation counts the fetal movement over a 30-minute period two times per day and notes at least 5–6 movements during each time period, then the fetus is considered to be in good condition. *If only three movements are detected, then an additional 30 minutes of counting should be carried out.* If the patient does not detect: (1) at least 10 movements in a 12-hour period, (2) at least 1 movement in the morning, or (3) at least 3 movements in an 8-hour period, then she should contact her physician. If the patient becomes concerned about a lack of fetal movement prior to obtaining the above criteria, the physician should conduct a further assessment of the fetus. If there is an **abrupt change in the frequency of the fetal movements,** then this has been considered to be a definite indication that further evaluation of the fetal status is needed and that such tests as the nonstress test (NST) or the oxytocin challenge test (OCT) should be carried out.

3) Fetal tone

The tone of the fetus may be assessed by ultrasonic observation of the fetal hand. **If the fingers or the entire hand open and close, then this can be considered to provide evidence of good tone.** Another sign of good tone is the extension and flexion of the fetal limbs or trunk. **There should be at least one episode of flexion and extension of the extremities, and one episode of flexion and extension of the spine, during a 30-minute observation period** (score 2). A score of one is given if there is only one episode of flexion and extension of either the spine or extremities.

4) Reactive FHR

There should be at least five or more episodes of FHR acceleration with fetal movements during a nonstress test, each of which last at least 15 seconds, and which increase by at least 15 bpm during the 20-minute observation period (score 2). A score of one is given if there are 2–4 FHR accelerations of at least 15 bpm and of at least 15 seconds duration during the 20-minute observation period.

5) Amniotic fluid volume

A search in the four quadrants of the uterine volume should provide evidence of the largest pocket of amniotic fluid. **The two largest perpendicular planes of this pocket should be at least 1–2 cm. Another technique utilizes the vertical diameter of the largest pocket of amniotic fluid in each of four quadrants of the amniotic fluid volume, which, when added up, should be about 12.9 ± 4.6 cm in the normal patient at term.** This sum of the four quadrant measurements has been termed the **amniotic fluid index.** Studies are under way to determine the normal amniotic fluid index at other stages of pregnancy.

6) Interpretation of BPS scores

A +2 score is allowed for a positive finding, a +1 score for a partial response, and a 0 score if
it is abnormal, for each of the five parameters.** A biophysical profile score (BPS) of 8–10 may be considered to be normal and indicates that the infant is not at risk. These tests should be repeated at weekly intervals in the average patient, but twice a week in diabetic or postdate patients. **If oligohydramnios occurs at any time, delivery of the fetus should be strongly considered.** A score of 4–6 should alert you to the fact that the infant may be in jeopardy and may be suffering from chronic asphyxia. In such a situation, the test should be repeated in 4–6 hours, and if the gestation is at least the 36th week, or if oligohydramnios is present, then you should consider delivery. In patients who are at less than 36 weeks' gestation, with a nonmature L/S ratio (less than 2.0), a repeat test should be performed in 24 hours. If the repeat test score is 4 or less, then delivery is indicated.

In patients who have a BPS score of 0–3, then the testing time should be extended to 120 minutes. If the score remains below 4, then delivery is indicated, even in patients who are premature.

7) Results of BPS testing

In the Manitoba prospective study, the crude perinatal mortality rate was 7.37:1,000 and the corrected perinatal mortality rate was 1.9:1,000 when BPS testing was utilized. In contrast, the same data for the general population of Manitoba during 1979–1982 was 14.1:1,000 and 8.81:1,000, respectively. With regard to **the importance of the amniotic fluid volume,** this study noted the following corrected perinatal mortality rates: 2.58:1,000 (normal amount of fluid); 44:1,000 (marginal amount of fluid), and 111.1:1,000 (decreased amniotic fluid volume). It would seem that the biophysical profile scoring technique may be an effective means of assessing the status of the fetus and in improving fetal salvage rates.

3. Episiotomy

The episiotomy is one of the most common operations in obstetrics. Its purpose is to prevent undue **pelvic lacerations,** both overt and obscure, which eventually result in the development of pelvic relaxation. In addition, the widening of the vaginal outlet prevents the unnecessary **constriction of the fetal skull** and a resultant "expansion effect" upon the delivery of the head. Tentorial lacerations with bleeding

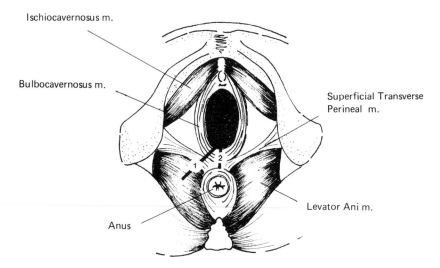

Ischiocavernosus m.

Bulbocavernosus m.

Superficial Transverse
Perineal m.

Levator Ani m.

Anus

FIGURE 26-2. Muscles of the pelvic floor and perineum. (1) The right mediolateral episiotomy cuts across the superficial transverse perineal muscle and into the levator ani muscle. (2) The median episiotomy cuts into the perineal body (central perineal tendon).

into the fetal central nervous system may occur in such a situation. The episiotomy incision involves the perineal muscles and/or perineal body (Fig. 26-2).

The timing of the episiotomy is important. The incision should be carried out when about 4–5 cm of the fetal scalp is visible between contractions. **The decision as to whether to use a median or a mediolateral episiotomy should be based upon the amount of room needed to deliver the baby.** If the perineal body is large and it is anticipated that only a little additional room will be necessary for the delivery, then a median episiotomy should be performed. If the perineal body is small and the delivery will require considerable additional room, then a mediolateral episiotomy should be utilized. It was shown in one study that there was an increased number of third- and fourth-degree laceration extensions when the median episiotomy was utilized, attesting to the fact that this approach was used inappropriately in many instances.

a. Technique of episiotomy repair

1) Median episiotomy

The **median episiotomy** should be closed in the following manner: (1) the vaginal mucous membrane should be closed with a continuous locking suture of

(2-0 or 3-0 chromic or Vicryl suture) *beginning above the apex of the vaginal incision* and continuing down to the caruncula myrtiformes, (2) the **coronal suture** should be placed at the upper level of the perineal body, parallel with the vaginal floor, to avoid a **"dash-boarding"** effect, (3) the remainder of the deep tissues of the perineal body should be closed with interrupted sutures, and finally, (4) the perineal skin should be closed with a subcuticular suture to provide for a good cosmetic closure (Fig. 26-3).

If the **anal sphincter** has been cut, the closure must include the reapproximation of the ends of the sphincter prior to the closure of the perineal body. If the **rectal mucosa** has been cut, then it should be closed with an inverting continuous locking suture or with interrupted inverting sutures before the tissues of the rectovaginal septum are closed over it (Fig. 26-4).

2) Mediolateral episiotomy

The closure of a **mediolateral episiotomy** is performed in much the same manner as the midline episiotomy, except that the sphincter muscles and rectal mucosa are not involved. The vaginal mucosa is closed from above the apex of the incision to the caruncula myrtiformes with a continuous locking 2-0

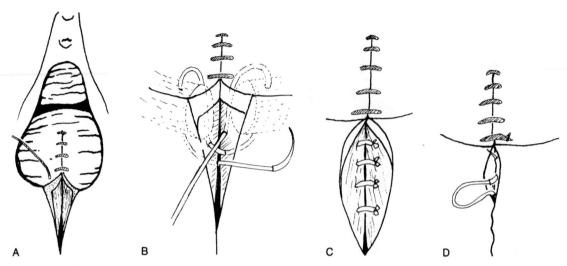

A   B   C   D

FIGURE 26-3. The repair of a midline (median) episiotomy. (A) The vaginal mucosa is closed with a locking suture down to the carunculae myrtiformes. (B) The coronal suture restores the floor of the vagina and prevents "dashboarding." (C) Interrupted deep sutures are placed. (D) The perineum is closed with a subcuticular suture. Note the coronal suture (B) and the subcuticular closure of the perineal portion of the incision.

or 3-0 chromic suture. If the incision is deep, then a few interrupted sutures may be required to close the "dead space" in the depths of the incision. A lateral coronal suture is placed to restore the integrity of the inferolateral vaginal wall (Fig. 26-5). The deep perineal tissues are then closed with interrupted sutures. The skin should be closed with a continuous subcuticular suture. **It is important in laying in the subcuticular suture to always enter the opposite side of the skin edge at the same place as where the previous suture exited in order to avoid a "wrinkling" effect of the incision line and a bad cosmetic closure.** Furthermore, you should not "follow the suture" and place back tension on this suture as it is being placed, since this also will add to the wrinkling effect of the suture line.

4. Obstetric forceps delivery

a. Historical aspects

Although forceps were used in ancient times and were described by Hippocrates and later by Soranus in the second century A.D., they were only used for the extraction of a dead infant at that time. Hakim ibn-e-Sina (Avicenna) (980–1037 A.D.), who wrote the great "Canon of Medicine," which ranked equally with the medical treatises by Galen (131–210 A.D.), is reputed to have been the first to suggest that forceps might be useful in delivering a live baby.

The Chamberlen family is generally credited with the introduction of obstetric forceps. This family kept the secret of the forceps through three generations. **William Chamberlen,** the founder of the family, was a French Huguenot physician who fled France to escape persecution by Catherine de Médici. He set up practice as a barber-surgeon in Southampton, England, in 1569. Two of his sons, **Peter the elder** and **Peter the younger,** also practiced in London. Peter the younger died in 1626 leaving a son named Peter, who, to distinguish himself from both his father and his uncle, became known as **Dr. Peter.** Dr. Peter died in 1683 at Molden, Essex, leaving three sons, Hugh, Paul, and John, who also became physicians. **Hugh Chamberlen,** due to political reasons, was forced to leave England and go to France. In Paris, he attempted to sell the family's secret forceps to

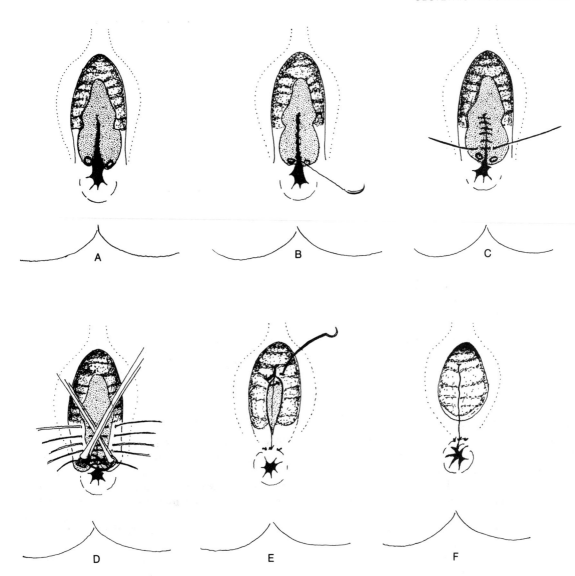

FIGURE 26-4. The repair technique of a fourth-degree laceration. (A) Laceration of the sphincter ani and the anterior wall of the rectum. (B) The rectal wall is closed. (C) The rectal wall is inverted with a second row of sutures to cover the first line of sutures. (D) The tissues between the rectum and vagina are closed with interrupted sutures and the ends of the rectal sphincter are identified and grasped with Allis forceps. (E) After suturing the rectal sphincter ends together with figure-of-eight sutures, the vaginal mucous membrane is closed from the apex down to the carunculae myrtiformes. (F) The closure of the perineal body completes the repair.

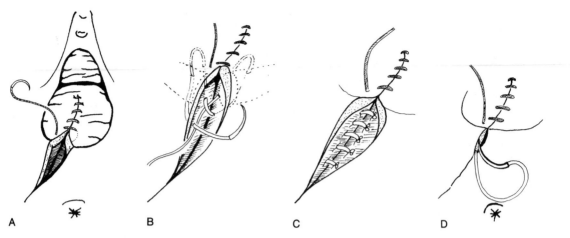

FIGURE 26-5. The repair of a right mediolateral episiotomy. (A) The vaginal mucosa is closed down to the carunculae myrtiformes. (B) Placement of the coronal suture. (C) The deep tissues are closed with interrupted sutures. (D) The perineal incision is closed with a subcuticular suture.

Mauriceau for 10,000 livres. As a condition of the sale, he was supposed to deliver a rachitic dwarf that F. Mauriceau had been unable to deliver; however, Chamberlen also was unsuccessful, the patient died, and the sale fell through. A few years later, the forceps were sold to **Roger van Roonhuyze** in Holland, who in turn sold the invention to licensed physicians in exchange for large sums of money and an oath of secrecy. It was not until later, when the forceps were made public, that it was noted that only one forceps blade, instead of two, had been released. In later years (1813), it was discovered that Dr. Peter Chamberlen was not the inventor of the forceps, as had been previously thought, but rather it was an invention of **Peter the elder,** who had passed them down through the family with modifications.

Since that time, J. Palfyn (1723), A. Levret (1747), and W. Smellie (1751) added further modifications to the forceps, especially the pelvic curve. **Etienne S. Tarnier** (1828–1897) of France developed the "Tarnier forceps" and added the intrinsic axis traction bar that enabled the operator to apply traction in the direction of the anatomical axis of the pelvis. **A. H. Bill's axis traction bar,** which may be used with any forceps, is a variation on this development. **Christian Kielland** (1871–1941) of Norway introduced his straight forceps in 1910 for the delivery of infants who were arrested in an occiput transverse or occiput posterior position. **Edmund Brown Piper** (1881–1935)

was an American physician from Williamsport, Pennsylvania, who practiced in Philadelphia. He introduced his version of the forceps in 1924 for the delivery of the aftercoming fetal head in a breech delivery.

b. Forceps construction

The classical forceps consist of two pieces of metal, connected at the lock, each consisting of a blade, a shank, a lock, and a handle. The tip of the blade is called the toe, whereas the part of the blade next to the shank is called the heel. The blade may be fenestrated (e.g., Simpson's forceps), pseudo-fenestrated (e.g., Luikart forceps), or solid (e.g., Tucker-McLean forceps). The fenestrated blades provide a firmer hold on the baby's head and require less compressive force. The solid and pseudo-fenestrated blades prevent undue friction and damage to the maternal vaginal tissues (Fig. 26-6).

While the original Chamberlen forceps did not have a pelvic curve, modern forceps do have a **pelvic curve** that matches the curve of the pelvic axis (Carus' curve), as well as a **cephalic curve** to fit around the fetal head. The **lock,** if present, is usually at the junction of the shank and the handle of the forceps. It may be an *English lock* (e.g., as in Simpson or Elliot forceps), or a *sliding lock* (e.g., as in Kielland or Barton forceps). An entirely different type of sliding lock is used on divergent forceps, called a *pivot lock*, which

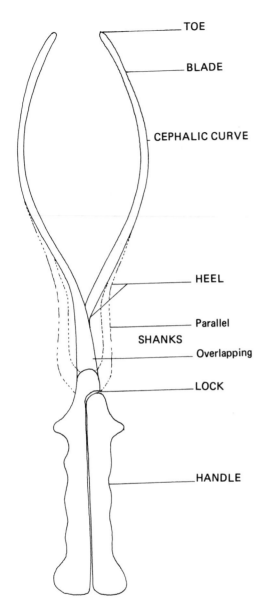

TOE

BLADE

CEPHALIC CURVE

HEEL

Parallel

SHANKS

Overlapping

LOCK

HANDLE

FIGURE 26-6. The anatomy of the Elliot and Simpson obstetric forceps.

consists of a sliding pivot joint at the extreme end of the handles. The *French lock* consists of an eye-bolt on one shank that matches a notch on the other. When the notch is articulated to the eye-bolt, a threaded bolt is screwed down tightly to prevent the separation of the forceps. The *German lock* is illustrated by Tarnier

forceps, in which a notch and bolt arrangement is augmented by a latch-type cross-bolt, which, when latched and screwed down, forces the two blades together on the fetal head (Fig. 26-7). *Axis traction bars* (e.g., Bill's axis traction bar) may be attached to the handles of most types of forceps to provide for a proper pull along the axis of the pelvis (Fig. 26-8).

c. Types of forceps

While literally hundreds of different types of forceps have been manufactured, from a functional point of view there are only three basic types used in obstetrics. The vast majority of forceps are of the **low-forceps** type (e.g., Simpson, Elliot, Tucker-McLean, etc.). The second type of forceps is that of the **"rotating" forceps,** of which the only representatives are the Kielland, the Tarnier, and the specialized Barton forceps. The third type is the **after-coming-head forceps,** of which the Piper forceps is the only example (Fig. 26-9).

d. Classification of forceps operations

The classification of forceps as to their application involves the station of the fetal head at the time that the forceps are applied. In 1974, the American College of Obstetricians and Gynecologists (ACOG) published a classification of forceps operations; this system was modified in 1988 by the ACOG Committee on Obstetrics: Maternal and Fetal Medicine as follows:

1. **Outlet forceps operation:** An outlet forceps operation is the application of obstetric forceps to the fetal skull when: (1) the scalp is visible at the introitus without separation of the labia by the physician, (2) the skull has reached the pelvic floor, (3) the sagittal suture is in the anteroposterior diameter of the outlet of the pelvis, or in the right or left occiput anterior or posterior position (or does not require rotation more than 45° from this position), and (4) the fetal head is at or on the perineum.

2. **Low forceps operation:** This operation requires the following: (1) that the leading point of the fetal skull is at the +2 station or below, and (2) that two subcategories be documented to indicate whether (a) the rotation of the fetal skull does *not* exceed 45°, or (b) the rotation of the fetal skull *does* exceed 45°.

3. **Midforceps operation:** A midforceps opera-

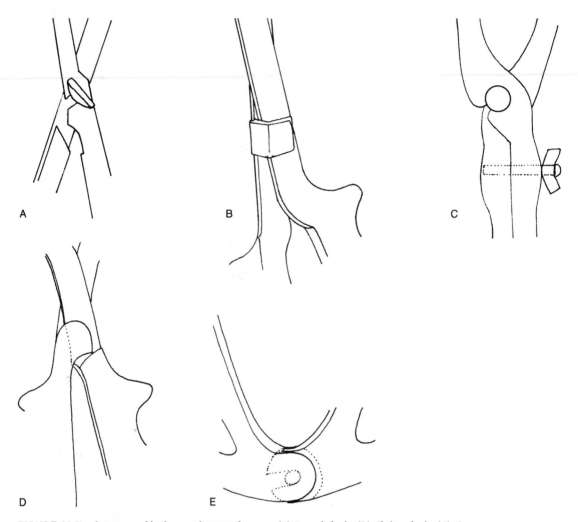

FIGURE 26-7. The types of locks on obstetric forceps. (A) French lock. (B) Sliding lock. (C) German lock. (D) English lock. (E) Pivot lock.

tion is the application of obstetric forceps to the fetal skull after the head is engaged (i.e., below 0 station), but when the conditions for low forceps have not been met (i.e., at +2 station or below).

4. **High forceps operation:** A high forceps operation is the application of obstetric forceps at any time before engagement of the fetal head (i.e., before the 0 station has been reached). This operation is mentioned only to be condemned.

5. **Vacuum extraction operation:** A vacuum extraction procedure is an operation for the extraction of the fetal head by the use of the vacuum extractor cup, which is applied to the fetal scalp. Vacuum extraction operations are classified in relation to the station of the fetal skull (i.e., low or mid) (Fig. 26-10).

The Committee on Obstetrics: Maternal and Fetal Medicine recommended the following indications for the use of forceps operations:

1. Outlet forceps may be utilized to shorten the second stage of labor.
2. Outlet forceps may be utilized in the primigravida if the second stage of labor exceeds three hours with a regional anesthetic, or ex-

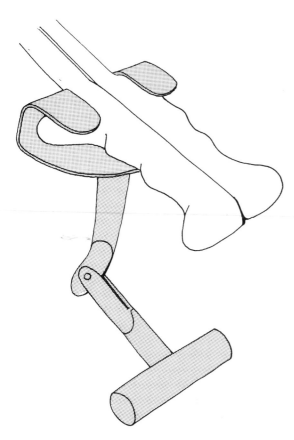

FIGURE 26-8. Bill's axis traction bar allows proper directional pull on the obstetric forceps.

ceeds two hours without such anesthesia. Forceps delivery may be utilized in the multigravida in a similar circumstance if there is a prolongation of the second stage of labor for more than two hours with a regional anesthetic, or for more than one hour without anesthesia.

3. Outlet forceps may be utilized in cases of fetal distress.

4. Outlet forceps may be utilized because of maternal conditions such as cardiac disease and exhaustion.

e. Prerequisites for the use of forceps

Certain prerequisites must be satisfied before you should attempt to apply forceps to deliver a baby. Perhaps the first and most important prerequi-

site is that you must first have **training** in the use of forceps, or be supervised by a physician who does have such training and experience (Fig. 26-11). Other required factors include the following: (1) the fetal head should be fully engaged and well below the spines (it is essential that the amount of fetal head molding and caput formation be taken into account in this evaluation), (2) the fetal head should be presenting and its position should be known, (3) the cervix should be fully dilated and the membranes ruptured, (4) there should be good clinical evidence that there is no cephalopelvic disproportion (e.g., through the Müller-Hillis maneuver, clinical pelvimetry, or fundal measurement), and finally, (5) the patient should be properly prepared for a forceps operation by having her bladder emptied and by having adequate anesthesia available. In addition, if the forceps attempt at delivery requires excessive force or appears to be too difficult to accomplish without fetal trauma, then the procedure should be abandoned and a cesarean section carried out.

While there has been a thrust in some quarters to eliminate the use of forceps operations entirely, it should be fairly stated that there is still a place for the proper use of rotating forceps and low forceps procedures. Physicians who are properly trained in the use of forceps, however, may become a rarity in the future, due to the current litigious atmosphere in our society and the total condemnation of the use of forceps by some leading physicians. As a consequence, these procedures may be lost in the future, and the loss of physicians trained in these procedures could further increase the number of cesarean sections performed in the future.

The use of the Malmstrom vacuum extractor has not enjoyed extensive use, in spite of the fact that a Silastic pliable cup has been utilized in recent times. This latter technique has had a failure rate of 2–3 times that of the original metal extractor cup or of forceps. While there are those who are strongly in favor of the use of the vacuum extractor technique, it has not been proven to be superior to the use of forceps in most instances.

5. Cerclage

In those patients who have an incompetent cervix, a surgical procedure called "cerclage" may be per-

Text continues on p. 372

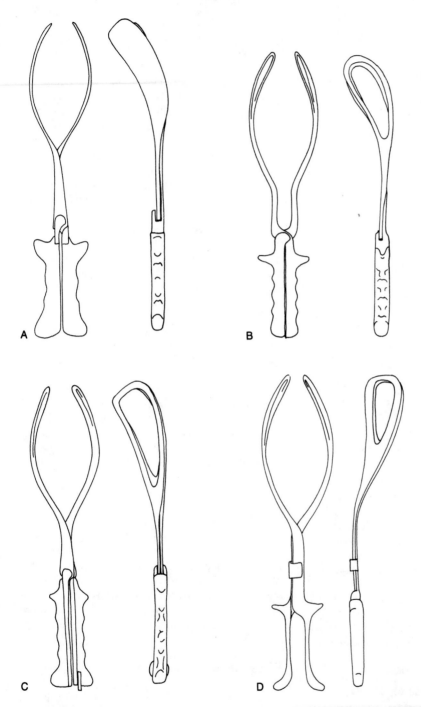

FIGURE 26-9. Commonly used obstetric forceps. (A) Tucker-McLean forceps. (B) Simpson forceps. (C) Elliot forceps. (D) Kielland rotating forceps. (E) Barton rotating forceps. (F) Piper aftercoming-head forceps.

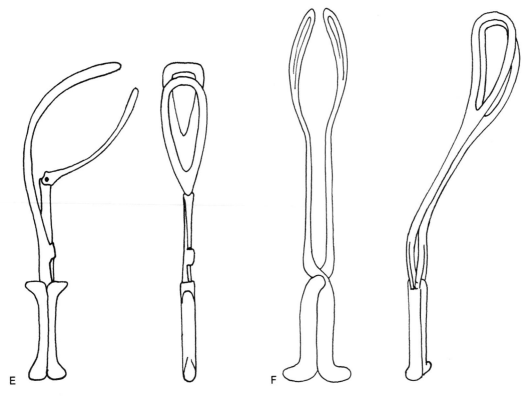

E   F

FIGURE 26-9. *(continued)*

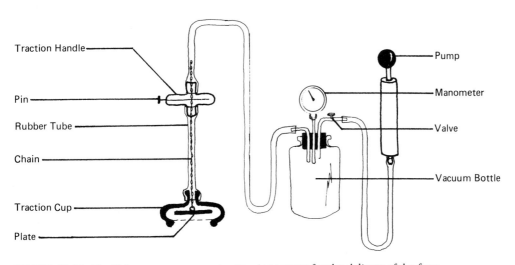

Traction Handle

Pin

Rubber Tube

Chain

Traction Cup

Plate

Pump

Manometer

Valve

Vacuum Bottle

FIGURE 26-10. The Malmstrom vacuum extraction instrument for the delivery of the fetus.

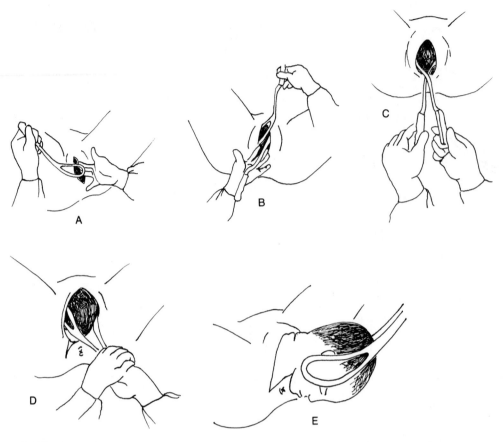

FIGURE 26-11. The technique of performing a low forceps delivery. (A) The placement of the right blade of the forceps. (B) The placement of the left blade of the forceps. (C) If the forceps are in proper position with the fetal sagittal suture in the vertical midline between the blades, then the forceps will easily engage. (D) A downward and then upward "paddle-like" motion should deliver the fetal head easily without force. (E) The proper placement of the forceps blades in front of the fetal ears along the cheek area.

formed to restore the competency of the cervix. The most common procedure used in this situation is the McDonald cerclage procedure, although the Wurm and the Shirodkar procedures have also been used occasionally (Fig. 26-12).

A **McDonald cerclage** is performed under anesthesia in the hospital by placing a continuous suture of no. 2 Prolene in four equal bites beginning at the 12–9 o'clock, 9–6 o'clock, 6–3 o'clock, and finally, the 3–12 o'clock positions at the level of the internal cervical os. The suture is then tightened so that the internal cervical os is reduced to a fingertip in diameter, after which the suture is tied. At the time of deliv-

ery, the suture may be cut and a vaginal delivery carried out. The **Wurm procedure** consists of two perpendicular sutures that are placed at the 12 and 9 o'clock positions that penetrate through both sides of the cervix. The **Shirodkar procedure** is a more permanent operation in which a Mersilene band or umbilical tape is placed at the 12 o'clock position and carried submucosally around the cervix to its origination point. An anchoring suture is then placed submucosally at the 6 and 12 o'clock positions to keep the tape from slipping off of the cervix. An abdominal approach to the cerclage procedure may be utilized on rare occasions.

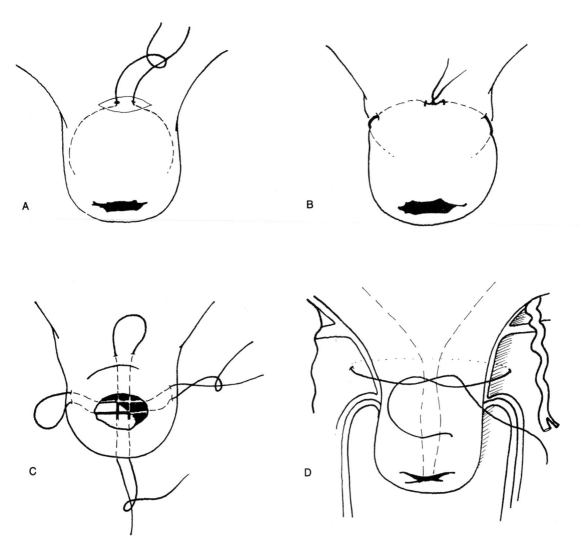

FIGURE 26-12. Cervical cerclage procedures. (A) Shirodkar technique. After elevating the bladder, a permanent submucosal suture is placed at the level of the internal cervical os. (B) McDonald techique. Four equal suture bites are circumferentially placed and tied at the 12 o'clock position in the midline. (C) Wurm technique. Two mattress sutures are placed perpendicular to each other. (D) Transabdominal approach in which a suture is placed at the level of the internal os.

6. Cesarean section

a. Historical aspects

Historically, the term cesarean section has been attributed to the supposed operative birth of Julius Caesar; however, since his mother lived for a number of years after his birth, this story would seem to be an unlikely explanation. In the eighth century B.C., the Roman ruler Numa Pompilius decreed that if a pregnant woman died undelivered, then she should be delivered by the surgical approach. This law, known as the **Lex regia,** was continued by the later emperors and became known as the **Lex caesarea.** This is a more likely explanation of the origin of the concept of "cesarean section." The actual term "cesarean" was applied at least as early as the Middle Ages and was supposedly derived from the Latin verb *caedere,* meaning "to cut." In its early history in the United States, the operation was fatal to most women who were subjected to it, and in 1878, a mortality rate of 52.5% was recorded in the 80 procedures that had been performed up to that time. In 1880 there were 50 cases reported of cesarean hysterectomy from seven countries with an overall maternal mortality rate of 58% and a fetal survival rate of 86%. The primary risks involved were **infection** and **hemorrhage.** In 1852, silver wire sutures were introduced by **Dr. Frank E. Polin,** a surgeon in Springfield, Kentucky, and it turned out that these sutures were much safer to use than the silk threads that had been used initially. In 1882, **Dr. Max Sänger** of the University of Leipzig popularized uterine sutures in cesarean section to arrest hemorrhage, and in his published monograph he emphasized the necessity of closing the edges of the uterine incision. Dr. Sänger also introduced the "classical cesarean section incision." Although the **Porro operation** (i.e., cesarean section with a supracervical hysterectomy and the marsupialization of the cervix to the abdominal wall) was performed before this time in an attempt to solve these two surgical hazards, the reduced risk of infection (and the preservation of the uterus) was further advanced by the extraperitoneal cesarean approach, which was first performed by **Dr. F. Frank** in 1907. Others **(W. Latzko, E. G. Waters)** introduced modifications of this approach that were used up until the time that antibiotics were well established in the 1950s.

With the advent of antibiotics in the 1940s (i.e., sulfa drugs, penicillin), the development of adequate blood-banking facilities in the 1940s and 1950s, and the advances in both obstetric and anesthesia training programs during the past 30 years, the risk of dying from a cesarean section operation has been reduced to less than 2:1,000. The major risks, however, have remained much the same: **hemorrhage, infection, and thromboembolism. Pulmonary embolism is the leading cause of maternal death today, and in 1983, it accounted for 25% of all maternal deaths.**

The incidence of cesarean section (C/S) has increased from about 5% in the 1950s to as high as 25–30% in large referral centers today. A recent report estimated that the average cesarean section rate in U.S. hospitals is about 22%. These increases have paralleled the national obstetric concern that fetal morbidity and mortality should be reduced. Current efforts in the profession have been directed toward reducing the number of cesarean sections performed to a lower level that is still consistent with a high rate of fetal salvage. This level is probably somewhere between 10 and 15%. The threat of litigation in obstetrics has been cited as a possible cause for the increased cesarean section rate seen in recent years.

b. Types of incisions

The abdominal skin incision for a cesarean section may be either a vertical incision or a Pfannenstiel incision (see Chapter 18). While many physicians favor the latter type, it does take a little longer to deliver the baby with this approach and, in addition, it is more difficult and time-consuming for the next physician to do an emergency cesarean section on a subsequent pregnancy if fetal distress is present. Upon excising the fascial tissues down to the level of the peritoneum, the peritoneum should be tented with thumb forceps, checked for any underlying bowel, and then incised. Upon entering the abdominal cavity, a moist laparotomy cloth should be placed in each of the paracolic gutters to absorb the amniotic fluid and blood from the opening of the uterus. This precaution will also decrease some of the ileus that may occur in the patient postoperatively. The peritoneal bladder flap should then be rapidly identified and incised in a "smiling" manner to allow the bladder to be reflected inferiorly off of the lower uterine segment. *There are two basic types of uterine cesarean section incisions.* The first type involves the lower uterine segment and may consist of either a **vertical incision,** or more commonly, a **transverse incision** in the lower uterine segment (Fig. 26-13). The second type of incision is a vertical incision in the upper or contractile portion of the uterus, called a **classical incision** (Fig. 26-14).

Once the uterine incision is begun, it should be extended transversely or vertically, depending on which incision is used, with bandage scissors. The technique of tearing the lower transverse incision should be abandoned, since tears into the lateral uterine vessels may cause excessive blood loss. The incision should be extended in a "smiling" manner with two fingers of one hand inside of the incision line to protect the fetus as the incision is carried out.

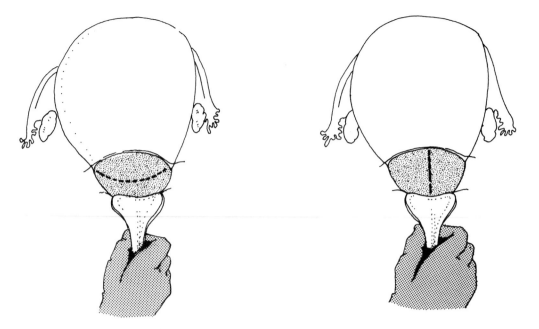

FIGURE 26-13. Incisions in the lower portion of the uterus. *Left:* Kerr incision. *Right:* Selheim incision.

The fetal head is cupped by the physician's hand and lifted out of the uterine incision, where the infant is suctioned, the umbilical cord clamped and cut, and the baby handed off to the waiting pediatric attendant for further care. The edges of the uterine incision may be grasped with Pennington clamps and the suture closure carried out using a continuous 0 chromic suture. You should be careful not to include the endometrial lining of the uterus in the closure. Indeed, the wound edges should be inverted by the closure, since it would appear from some studies that this procedure may be of value in making a stronger scar. A second layer of continuous horizontal Lembert sutures will usually accomplish an adequate closure of the uterine incision. The bladder peritoneum should be replaced and closed with 2-0 chromic catgut (Fig. 26-15, Fig. 26-

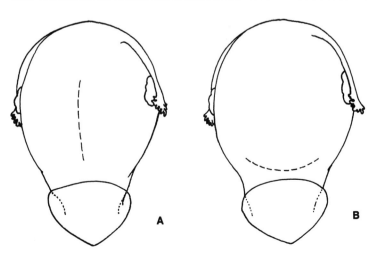

FIGURE 26-14. Incisions in the upper (active) uterine segment. (A) Classic incision. (B) Kerr incision.

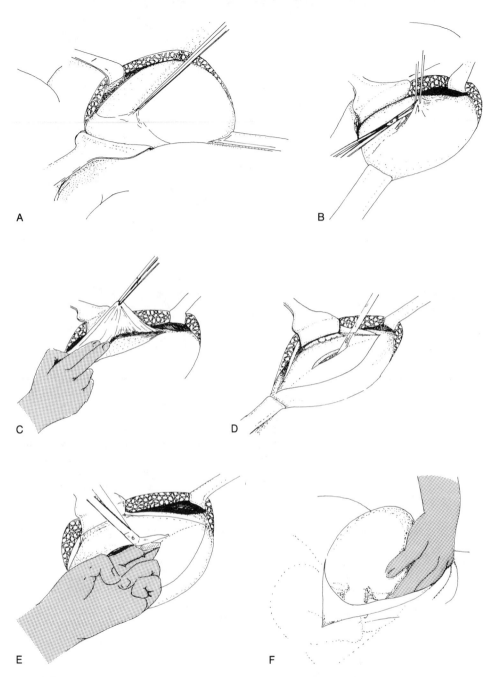

FIGURE 26-15. The technique of performing a cesarean section. (A) The bladder reflection of the peritoneum is identified. (B) The peritoneum is incised to reveal the lower uterine segment. (C) The bladder is reflected inferiorly under the bladder retractor. (D) The uterus is incised transversely with a knife about 2–3 cm below the peritoneal incision. (E) The uterus has been opened and the membranes ruptured. The two fingers of one hand are inserted to prevent the bandage scissors from cutting the fetus and the incision is extended in a curvilinear fashion. (F) A hand is inserted in front of the fetal head to release the suction and then to elevate the head into the incision for delivery.

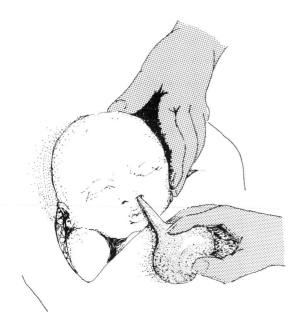

FIGURE 26-16. Infant suctioning at cesarean section.

16, Fig. 26-17). Care should be taken that this flap is not advanced superiorly on the body of the uterus, since this would complicate any future cesarean sections.

The lower segment uterine incision has been favored because the risk of a subsequent rupture with the lower transverse cervical incision is only about 0.5%, with perhaps two-thirds of these ruptures being of the *silent dehiscence,* or "window separation" type, which is found incidentally at sur-

gery and does not constitute much of a risk to either the mother or her baby. **In contrast, the incidence of uterine rupture in the classical incision is of the order of about 2%.**

Uterine ruptures that are unrelated to the scarring of the uterus, such as those that occur spontaneously during labor or those that result from trauma, may be catastrophic, with severe hemorrhage and a high fetal and maternal mortality rate. This type of rupture is in contrast to the rupture of a previously scarred uterus, which usually is much less severe.

The concept of "once a cesarean section, always a cesarean section" that was promulgated by Dr. E. B. Cragin in 1916 has been the rule in obstetrics until just recently. Today, this dictum has come under considerable criticism, since there has been almost no evidence presented in the literature to support such an approach. Currently, selected patients who have had a previous cesarean section may be delivered safely by the vaginal route under certain conditions.

c. Reasons for cesarean section

The indications for a primary cesarean section may involve either maternal and/or fetal conditions, including such problems as cephalopelvic disproportion, abnormal presentations, uterine dystocia, placenta previa, abruptio placentae, toxemia, diabetes, and fetal distress. According to one study, the usual indications for cesarean section in 1984 were dystocia (35%), fetal distress (20%), breech presentation (15%), and other (30%).

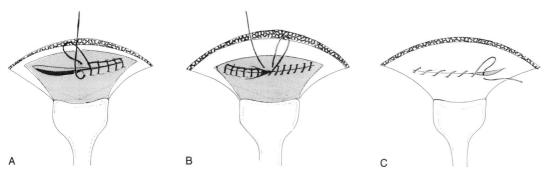

A   B   C

FIGURE 26-17. Closure of the uterine wound. (A) The first layer of the uterine incision is closed with a continuous inverting locking suture for hemostasis, being careful not to include the endometrium in each bite. (B) A second layer consisting of a continuous inverting Lembert suture is placed. (C) The peritoneum is loosely approximated. It is important not to advance the peritoneum further up the uterine body with this peritoneal closure.

The increase in the number of cesarean sections performed over the past few years has mainly been due to the more widespread use of cesarean section for the primigravida breech and premature breech presentations, and to a more liberal approach in the management of fetal distress owing to sophisticated electronic fetal monitoring techniques that now identify the fetus-at-risk with more accuracy than ever before. The frank breech presentation with a fetus that does not have a hyperextended head and is of average size, in a multiparous patient with an adequate pelvis, however, is still a candidate for a vaginal delivery. While the use of *external cephalic version* has again received attention as a method of preventing a breech presentation and a subsequent cesarean section, its acceptance has been somewhat limited in practice due to complications such as fetal bruising, abruptio placentae, and fetal distress.

d. Morbidity

The infection rate in patients who have a cesarean section is of the order of 25–30% or more, depending upon the population group, the presence of prolonged rupture of the membranes, and the presence of prolonged labor. Cultures, and especially Gram-stained smears, of the uterine cavity and of the fetal membranes at the time of surgery are of benefit in identifying the predominant organisms that may be involved. The use of prophylactic antibiotics is justified; however, they should be administered intraoperatively after the umbilical cord has been cut in order to prevent the fetus from being treated unnecessarily, which may interfere with the pediatric evaluation of the infant.

If postpartum endometritis occurs, then a combination of ampicillin and an aminoglycoside, or an aminoglycoside and clindamycin, may be administered to cover the polymicrobial infection until the offending organisms have been recovered and identified by culture methods.

e. Vaginal delivery of a previous C/S patient?

Although the concept of always doing a cesarean section in patients who have previously had one was disputed by some physicians more than twenty years ago, it was not until the early 1980s that the profession as a whole began to question the risks involved in delivering selected patients with uterine scarring by the vaginal route **(VBAC stands for "vaginal birth after cesarean").** Part of this concern was generated by the tremendous increase in the cesarean section rate, which was addressed by the National Institutes of Health in September of 1980. At the present time, more and more physicians have elected to deliver their patients with a previous scar of the uterus vaginally, after the patient has been fully apprised of the risks involved and has requested such a delivery. **In 1982, the American College of Obstetricians and Gynecologists (ACOG) established guidelines to assist the physician in selecting patients for this approach.** These guidelines include the following as factors in determining whether VBAC is appropriate: (1) only one unextended previous low-segment cesarean section, (2) a vertex presentation, (3) an average-sized infant (i.e., no larger than 3,600 grams), (4) the availability of continuous electronic fetal monitoring, (5) a nonrecurrent indication for the cesarean section (e.g., no significant cephalopelvic disproportion), and perhaps of most importance, (6) **the presence of an adequate blood bank, 24-hour anesthesia coverage, and an obstetrician (and supporting pediatrician) in the hospital, with the ability to perform a cesarean section within 30 minutes.** While not all previous cesarean section patients will be delivered vaginally in the future, enough of them will be managed in this manner to perhaps decrease the morbidity and mortality of childbearing even further. In recent studies of more than 8,000 operative deliveries of cesarean section patients, the incidence of uterine rupture and dehiscence of the scar was 1.8%, whereas the incidence of rupture was only 0.5% in patients undergoing vaginal delivery. These statistics would seem to confirm the safety of vaginal delivery in these women. In one small animal study using rabbits, in which cesarean section scars were submitted to a tearing tension, it was shown that in about 86% of these uterine scars, the tears occurred in the muscle rather than in the scar itself. While the results of such a study cannot be compared directly with the events in the human uterine muscle, they do provide information that seems to support the concept of VBAC.

7. Cesarean section hysterectomy

A cesarean hysterectomy may be indicated in a number of situations, such as a grossly defec-

tive uterine scar, a severely damaged uterus from trauma, significant dysplasia or carcinoma-in-situ of the cervix, multiple leiomyomas, placenta acreta, increta, or percreta, or uterine atony with severe uterine hemorrhage.

Although a cesarean hysterectomy has been viewed with some trepidation by physicians in the past, in actual fact it is a much easier procedure than hysterectomy in the normal nonpregnant individual if care is taken to maintain scrupulous hemostasis (since the increased vascularization of the tissues may lead to a greater blood loss than usual). Due to the edema of the tissues, the skeletonization of the uterine vessels and the dissection of other tissue planes becomes much easier. The only minimally difficult portion of the procedure is the identification of the cervix; however, with a doubly gloved hand in the intrauterine cavity, it is easy to ascertain the delineation of the cervix and the vagina. The basic principles of surgery, such as the maintenance of the **tissues on constant tension,** and the placement of all **clamps in close proximity to the uterus and cervix,** will assist in the safe removal of the uterus. In rare cases in which the patient's condition is unstable and potentially fatal, it may be necessary to perform a supracervical hysterectomy in order to complete the surgery rapidly and finish the operation, so that the patient's condition can be stabilized more effectively.

8. Assessment of fetal well-being

a. Amniotic fluid

1) Amount present

There is a slight decrease in the amniotic fluid from about 38 weeks' gestation until term, and in the postdate pregnancy (i.e., more than 42 weeks), there may be a marked decrease in the amount of amniotic fluid present. Fetal renal agenesis also leads to a diminished amount of amniotic fluid (i.e., oligohydramnios) due to the fact that the fetus cannot excrete urine. In contrast, the presence of an esophageal atresia prevents the fetus from swallowing amniotic fluid, and in these cases an excess of amniotic fluid may develop (i.e., hydramnios).

2) Fetal lung maturity

During the past 30 years, a number of tests have been developed to determine the well-being of the fetus.

To determine the *maturity of the fetal lungs,* several tests of the amniotic fluid have been developed that are based upon the presence of the surface-active phospholipids, which are produced by the type II pneumocytes that line the alveoli. These substances lower the surface tension of the alveoli so that the alveoli do not completely collapse with each breath. **These surfactants are primarily glycerophospholipids, of which 50% are dipalmitoylphosphatidylcholine (i.e., lecithin). This substance increases rapidly after 34 weeks' gestation in comparison to another phospholipid called sphingomyelin. The difference between the concentrations of these two lipids forms the basis for the lecithin/sphingomyelin ratio (L/S ratio) determination.** If a value of more than 2.0–2.5 is present, then the chance of the infant developing the respiratory distress syndrome (RDS) after delivery is minimal. **A similar surfactant, phosphatidylglycerol (PG), is a stabilization factor for the surface-active layer; when this surfactant is also present, it adds considerable confidence to the prediction that RDS will not occur following the delivery of the infant.** The analysis of these surfactants by thin-layer chromatography requires precise laboratory procedures. Some of the other less demanding tests that have been developed are based upon the ability of the surfactant to stabilize a foam air-liquid interface, such as the foam stability test (Shake test), or the absorbance of light (i.e., optical density) at 650 nm wavelength in a spectrophotometer.

3) Other maturity tests

Other amniotic fluid indicators of possible fetal maturity are: (1) a bilirubin value (i.e., Δ O.D. 450) that approaches 0.010 or less indicates a gestational age of about 36–38 weeks; (2) an amniotic fluid creatinine value of 2 mg/dl or greater indicates fetal "maturity"; (3) an amniotic fluid osmolality below 300 mOsm/l reflects the level of maturity, since from about the 20th week of pregnancy onward, the osmolality of the amniotic fluid decreases by 1 mOsm/l per week; and (4) the number of fetal epithelial cells in the amniotic fluid that stain with Nile blue sulfate to produce orange-stained bodies, indicating the maturity of the sebaceous glands (i.e., the presence of more than 20% of "fat cells" indicates fetal maturity). The impreciseness of these tests, plus the development of more accurate procedures (i.e., ultrasound gestational dating techniques), has reduced the usefulness of these procedures in determining the maturity of the fetus. As a consequence, these tests are no longer used.

b. Biophysical tests

1) Ultrasonography

a) The physics of ultrasound

The use of diagnostic ultrasound in gynecology was first introduced by Dr. I. Donald and his colleagues in 1958. The generation of sound waves above 20,000 cycles/second (hertz), produces ultrasound, which exceeds the range of human hearing. In general, the transducers that are used clinically have a frequency of **1.5–5 megahertz (MHz).** The ultrasonic beam is transmitted through the tissues and is reflected back by the different tissue densities. The sound wave is initially derived from a piezoelectric crystal, which has been stimulated by electrical energy. The average speed of sound in the tissue is *1,540 meters per second* (m/s). **Low-frequency ultrasonic beams allow for a deep penetration of the tissues, whereas high-frequency ultrasonic beams have a shorter wavelength and do not penetrate as deeply.** As a consequence, the low-frequency beams have poor resolution, while the high-frequency beams have good resolution.

Several different modes of ultrasonic imaging have been utilized. The **A mode** (amplitude mode) produces vertical spikes along a continuum of a horizontal field of an oscilloscope, so that amplitude versus distance is displayed. This technique was the first one used to measure the biparietal diameter of the fetal head. A series of three spikes were recorded on the oscillographic screen, which represented the outer table of the fetal skull on one side, the midline area between the cerebral hemispheres in the middle, and the outer table of the skull bone on the opposite side.

The **B mode,** or brightness mode, produces dots of light across a vertical field. When the dots coalesce, a two-dimensional image results. A change in the brightness of the echos received by the transducer represents the amplitude of the returning signal and produces a cross-sectional image of the body when gray-scale processing is used. When the B scan produces multiple cross-sectional scans, it can then display them as moving structures **(i.e., real-time scan).**

The **M mode** (motion mode) is generated by a slowly sweeping B-mode trace. This technique is used in echocardiography to visualize the motion of the valves and the walls of the heart.

Mechanical scanners use the beam of a single rotating or oscillating crystal to produce the scan. Usually, there are three transducers on a wheel, which rotates about 10 revolutions per second to produce the multiple sequential scans, which are then displayed. If four or more fixed transducers are pulsed to produce a B-mode scan, it is called a **linear array** type of scanner. A **phased array** (or electronic sector) scanner has an array of transducer elements whose sonic beams are focused electronically by small time delays between the pulses. The advantages of phased arrays over the sequential arrays derive from their smaller-sized transducer assembly and their ability to be focused more accurately.

A transducer may operate on one of two modes: pulsed or continuous. In the *pulsed mode,* it produces a short burst of energy and then listens for the returning echos to the same transducer during the silent period. A *continuous mode* is sent through one crystal and received by another one.

Doppler ultrasound equipment utilizes the Doppler effect to measure the characteristics of blood flow and fetal heart motion. The Doppler effect involves the shift in the frequency of the perceived sound waves whenever there is a change in the relative motion between the sound source and the receiver.

Special transducers have been developed that contain a detachable, reusable **needle guide** for performing special procedures, such as amniocentesis and umbilical vessel blood sampling.

Recently, **transvaginal transducers** have been developed for investigators who are conducting infertility studies in which it is necessary to detect the time of ovulation. These transducers have also been useful for other purposes, since the close approximation of the transducer to the pelvic organs will allow for a better evaluation of ectopic pregnancies, ovarian cysts, and other pelvic pathology.

b) Safety of ultrasound

Since its first introduction into medicine more than 25 years ago, a lingering doubt has remained that perhaps this truly fantastic technique that has opened a window upon the fetus in utero may also be a time bomb in terms of fetal and maternal safety. In-vitro studies of cell suspensions have had conflicting results. Some studies have reported sister chromatid exchange, alterations in the surface charges, changes in the membrane permeability, and a failure of the cells to grow and to survive, whereas other reports have not been able to confirm these findings. In animal studies (i.e., mice and rats), fetal weight reduction has been observed by a number of investigators. A statement issued by the American Institute of Ultrasound in Medicine (AIUM) in March 1983 indicated that there had been no reported adverse biological effects on either patients or instrument operators due to exposure at intensities and in conditions typically used in present diagnostic and examination practices. Furthermore, it was noted that no hazards had been identified that would prohibit the prudent and conservative use of diagnostic ultrasound.

The indications for the use of ultrasound should have a firm medical basis. This technique should not be used for frivolous reasons, such as to satisfy the mother's curiosity or to obtain a picture for the baby's scrapbook. **Guidelines for the use of ultrasound in antepartum obstetric patients were published in the September 1986 issue of the *Ultrasound in Medicine and Biology* journal.** It was recommended that a frequency of 3–5 MHz should be used. A real-time scanner should generally be used. All ultrasonogram examinations should be *documented in the patient's chart.* Further recommended guidelines included the use of ultrasound for the determination of the following data in each trimester: (A) During the **first trimester,** (1) the gestational sac may be identified, (2) the crown-rump measurement may be obtained, (3) the fetal cardiac activity may be detected, (4) the fetal number may be determined, and (5) the anatomy of the uterus may be evaluated; and (B) during the **second and third trimesters,** (1) the presence of fetal life, fetal position, and number may be identified, (2) an estimate of the amount of amniotic fluid may be made, (3) the location of the placenta may be determined, (4) the gestational age of the fetus may be further assessed with determination of the biparietal diameter of the fetal head and the femur length, and in addition, the fetal growth may be assessed with the measurement of the abdominal circumference, (5) the uterus and the adnexal organs may be evaluated, and finally (6) cer-

tain aspects of the fetal anatomical development, such as the cerebral ventricles, the spine, the kidneys, the stomach, the urinary bladder, the abdominal wall, and the umbilical cord, to name but a few, may be evaluated.

2) Use of ultrasound

One of the first uses of ultrasound in obstetrics was to determine the gestational age. The date of **the last menstrual period (LMP)** can be used to predict the estimated date of confinement (EDC) with a 90% certainty within about (±) 3 weeks. The period from the time of *quickening* to delivery is about 22 weeks, and the time period from when audible *fetal heart tones* can be heard by a fetoscope to delivery is about 19.5 weeks. About 7–10% of patients will deliver before 38 weeks' gestation, and 6–10% will deliver after 42 weeks' gestation, with the remainder delivering between 38 and 42 weeks (i.e., at term). The correlation of the ultrasonic gestational age determinations with these clinical findings will often provide a much more accurate dating of the gestation.

Ultrasonography has many uses other than the dating of a pregnancy. When bleeding occurs in early pregnancy, it is often of value to determine the status of the conceptus. A *blighted ovum* can be diagnosed by an ultrasonogram after nine weeks' gestation, because there will be no fetal tissues present within the gestational sac, and more important, because there will be no fetal heart motion, which normally should be present beyond eight weeks' gestation. The appearance of the sac may also be helpful when bleeding occurs in early pregnancy, since the sac may lose its regular outline in an impending abortion. Depending upon the length of time since the demise of the fetus, the fetal outline may also become disrupted sonographically.

When the sonogram reveals a honeycombed appearance throughout the uterine cavity, a *hydatidiform mole* may be diagnosed. Occasionally, bilateral theca-lutein cysts of the ovaries may also be noted in such cases.

The appearance of the uterine contents is also an important clue in diagnosing an ectopic pregnancy. In an early intrauterine pregnancy (i.e., prior to 12–14 weeks), if there is a true sac present, then a *double ring* should be evident sonographically on one side of the sac. This double ring is indicative of the separation between the decidua capsularis of the conceptus and the decidua vera. If an ectopic pregnancy is present, the decidua covers the entire endometrial surface (i.e., pseudosac) and there will be no double ring present on the ultrasonogram.

a) Gestational sac

A gestational sac may be seen as early as five weeks' gestation; however, the measurement of the sac's diameter has not proven to be very accurate in dating the pregnancy (i.e., the 95% confidence limits are ± 12 days). **Between 9 and 13 weeks' gestation, the use of the fetal crown-rump length (CRL) in determining gestational age has an accuracy of between ± 2.7 to ± 4.7 days, with a 95% certainty.** In more than 90% of the cases, if the value of 6.5 is added to the crown-rump length, the gestational age in weeks will be predicted within 5–6 days; however, the standard curves are usually available to more accurately assess the value of the crown-rump measurement. Beyond 12 weeks' gestation, the fetal age should be obtained by measuring such parameters as the fetal head biparietal diameter, the femur length, the head circumference, and the abdominal circumference (Table 26-1).

b) Biparietal diameter

The biparietal diameter (BPD) should be obtained on an ultrasonogram as a cross-sectional oval image that is parallel to and slightly above the cantho-meatal line, which includes the falx cerebri, the thalamus, the cavum septum pellucidum, and the medial cerebral artery. In about 5% of patients, the proper plane of measurement cannot be obtained and therefore the BPD cannot be determined. The standard manner of measurement of the biparietal diameter is to measure the distance from the **outer edge** of the skull to the **inner edge** of the opposite wall. There is a 2–3-mm standard error in this measurement. **If the BPD is obtained prior to 26 weeks' gestation, the prediction of the EDC with 95% confidence limits is ± 11 days, and if obtained between 26 and 30 weeks of gestation, it is ± 14 days, whereas beyond 30 weeks' gestation, the accuracy becomes much less (i.e., ± 21 days). The diameter of the fetal skull (i.e., BPD) increases by about 2–3 mm/week up to the last trimester, when it drops to slightly less than 2 mm/week.** Linear array dy-

namic-imaging equipment should be used whenever possible, since most of the reference tables have been constructed from data obtained by either static or linear array dynamic-imaging B-scan equipment. The growth-adjusted sonographic age (GASA) technique, using a second scan, was initially developed to improve the accuracy of the single BPD scan that is taken at 20–24 weeks. Several studies have since shown, however, that two scans apparently provide no improvement in the accuracy over that of a single real-time scan.

A number of ultrasonic formulas have been published on determining the *weight of the fetus*. Those that incorporate the head measurement, the abdominal circumference, and the femur length have the smallest absolute percent errors. One formula that has been derived from low–birth weight infants that seems to have the lowest mean percent error and standard deviation, of 10.9 ± 7.9%, is the following: Log of the predicted birth weight = 1.6961 + 0.02253 (head circumference) + 0.01645 (abdominal circumference) + 0.06439 (femur length).

c) Head circumference

The measurement of the **head circumference (HC)** may be carried out by taking a middle-to-middle measurement of the occipitofrontal diameter (OFD) and the BPD and applying the results to the following formula: HC = [diameter 1 (cm) + diameter 2 (cm)] × 1.57. The resultant value is then plotted on a gestational curve. The head measurement should be taken after 24 weeks' gestation.

The **cephalic index (CI)** may be used to evaluate changes in the shape of the head by the ratio of the BPD:OFD × 100. The CI remains constant throughout pregnancy and is normally 79% ± 8% (± 2 SD). If the ratio is small, then it implies that there is side-to-side flattening of the fetal head. If the ratio is large, then it suggests brachycephaly.

d) Abdominal circumference

The **abdominal circumference (AC)** may be measured with ultrasound at the level of the umbilical vein and perpendicular to the fetal spine. An antero-posterior diameter and a transverse diameter are taken by measuring from "outer to outer." The abdominal circumference is calculated in the same manner as the head circumference, by multiplying diameter 1 plus diameter 2 times 1.57.

TABLE 26-1. Sonographic measurements and gestational age determinations*

Weeks of Gestation	BPD (cm)	Femur Length (cm)	Head Circumference (cm)	Abdominal Circumference (cm)
12		1.0	6.7	5.7
13		1.3	8.2	6.7
14	2.8	1.6	9.6	8.1
15	3.2	1.9	11.0	9.3
16	3.6	2.2	12.4	10.5
17	3.9	2.5	13.7	11.6
18	4.2	2.8	15.0	12.8
19	4.5	3.2	16.2	14.0
20	4.8	3.5	17.4	15.1
21	5.1	3.8	18.6	16.2
22	5.4	4.0	19.8	17.3
23	5.8	4.2	20.9	18.4
24	6.1	4.4	22.0	19.5
25	6.4	4.6	23.0	20.6
26	6.7	4.8	24.0	21.6
27	7.0	5.0	25.0	22.7
28	7.2	5.3	25.9	23.9
29	7.5	5.5	26.8	24.8
30	7.8	5.7	27.7	25.8
31	8.0	6.0	28.6	26.8
32	8.2	6.2	29.4	27.8
33	8.5	6.4	30.1	28.7
34	8.7	6.6	30.9	29.7
35	8.8	6.8	31.5	30.7
36	9.0	7.1	32.2	31.6
37	9.2	7.3	32.8	32.5
38	9.3	7.5	33.4	33.4
39	9.4	7.7	34.0	34.4
40	9.5	8.0	34.5	35.2
41			35.0	36.1
42			35.4	37.0

*All fetal growth measurements correspond to the 50th percentile for that gestational age.

Reprinted with permission from W. F. Rayburn and J. P. Lavin, Jr., *Obstetrics for the House Officer*. Baltimore, Md.: Williams & Wilkins, 1984, p. 3.

The ratio of the head circumference to the abdominal circumference is calculated by the following formula: HC:AC = (BPD + OFD):(anteroposterior diameter of the abdomen + transverse diameter of the abdomen).

The use of the appropriate tables and graphs to determine gestational age from these various measurements will provide for fairly accurate gestational dating.

e) Femur length

The measurement of the fetal **femur length (FL)** by ultrasound has about the same accuracy as the BPD or the head circumference measurements in estimating gestational age. It is interesting that in cases of fetal death, the femur length can be used to estimate the time of death. The femur growth is linear from 12–22 weeks' gestation. If a good measurement can be obtained, the femur length is accurate to within ± 7 days.

It has been suggested that an even greater accuracy may be obtained in dating the pregnancy by combining all of the measurements from the different sonographic procedures (i.e., BPD, head circumference, abdominal circumference, femur length, etc.). This approach has much to recommend it, in that the errors between the individual tests may cancel each other out. As a consequence, there would be less reliance placed upon only one parameter.

f) Fetal sex

In certain situations, such as in X-linked chromosomal disorders, it may be important to determine the fetal sex. While the fetal sex may be determined as early as 14 weeks' gestation, it is generally not until the 18th week that the ultrasonic determination becomes reliable, and not until 24–38 weeks' gestation that the determination becomes easy. Between the 15th and 20th weeks, as many as 70% of fetuses cannot be correctly identified as to sex. If a cross-sectional ultrasonogram can be obtained of the scrotal contents, the testes and the penis may be easily identified in the third trimester. In the female, the labia majora folds may be detected with the labia minora in between them.

c. Fetal growth problems

Intrauterine growth retardation (IUGR) occurs in about 3–7% of pregnancies. **The diagnosis of intrauterine growth retardation may be applied to the infant whose birth weight falls below the 10th percentile for its gestational age.** The perinatal mortality rate in these infants is 10–30 times higher than in the normal fetus.

There are many causes of intrauterine growth retardation. Smoking during pregnancy produces infants who weigh less than normal infants. Alcoholism during pregnancy has been associated with the fetal alcohol syndrome, which consists of congenital abnormalities and intrauterine growth retardation. The use of addictive drugs by the pregnant woman may be associated with IUGR; however, a direct cause-and-

effect relationship has not been established, since these individuals also often have life-styles involving poor nutrition as well as the use of alcohol and cigarettes. In addition, if the maternal weight gain is inadequate, fetal IUGR may occur.

The infant who has severe congenital abnormalities will almost always have an associated IUGR. Abnormalities of the umbilical cord (e.g., velamentous insertion, marginal insertion of the cord) and of the placenta (e.g., infarction, abruption, circumvallate placenta) may be associated with some degree of fetal growth retardation. Multiple pregnancy is almost always associated with fetal growth retardation of one or both infants. Infants who are products of an abdominal pregnancy usually have a greater risk of having congenital anomalies and they are often growth retarded as well.

At times, a particular woman may give birth repeatedly to growth-retarded infants; however, frequently the cause for this type of IUGR is unknown. Intrauterine infections are often associated with IUGR. When the patient has a "flu-like syndrome" or other viral infection during pregnancy, especially during the period of organogenesis, it is important for you to record this information in the patient's record. If an unexplained neurologically damaged infant is subsequently delivered in such a patient, an infectious etiology should be suspected.

Chronic hypertension, especially with superimposed toxemia, may also be associated with fetal growth retardation. Some of these patients will also have an underlying renal disease. In patients with severe cardiac disease, particularly those with cyanotic heart disease, chronic hypoxia may result in an IUGR infant. Individuals who have a severe anemia (i.e., hemoglobin levels of 6 grams or less) will have a smaller oxygen-carrying capacity and may produce growth-retarded infants. The role of maternal hypovolemia, which may be secondary to the failure of the plasma volume to expand appropriately during pregnancy, is unknown; however, growth retardation has been associated with this condition.

1) Diagnosis

The diagnosis of intrauterine growth retardation may be difficult, and it requires a high degree of awareness on the physician's part to detect this problem in patients. Only about one-third of the IUGR cases can be diagnosed antenatally. The failure to diagnose most of these cases is primarily due to inaccuracies in the gestational dating of the pregnancy. **The growth of the infant is reflected in the measurement of the uterine fundal height.** This measurement in centimeters should equal the number of weeks of gestation from about 16 to 34 weeks' gestation. In addition, the superior-inferior uterine fundal measurement on the pelvic examination prior to the 16th week should also equal the number of weeks of gestation. The fetus gains much of its weight during the last trimester; thus, a "plateau effect" of the fundal measurements during weeks 28–34 may be the first indication of IUGR. In patients who have had inadequate weight gain, or in those who have had an intrauterine viral infection early in pregnancy, the fundal measurements may be consistently "behind" the number of weeks of gestation. In many instances, however, this finding may merely reflect an inaccuracy of the gestational dating rather than the presence of IUGR. *If the amniotic fluid volume is also greatly decreased, then IUGR should be strongly considered and delivery should be considered.*

Two types of IUGR have been postulated: (1) symmetrical IUGR, due to congenital abnormalities, intrauterine herpes, cytomegalic inclusion disease, or rubella, and (2) asymmetrical IUGR, secondary to hypertension, renal disease, diabetes with vascular disease, or excessive smoking.

In **symmetrical growth retardation,** both the biparietal diameter of the head and the head circumference, as well as the abdominal circumference, are all less than expected for the gestational age.

In **asymmetrical growth retardation,** the head is spared; thus, the sonographic biparietal diameter and the head circumference (HC) measurements may be normal for the gestational age, although the abdominal circumference (AC) may be reduced (HC:AC ratio above the 95th percentile). The BPD and the femur length may also lag in the later stages of asymmetric growth retardation.

Normally, the head circumference is greater than the abdominal circumference (as measured from the level of the umbilical vein, or ductus venosus) prior to 32 weeks' gestation. After this time the abdominal circumference is about equal to that of the head circumference until about the 36th week, after which the abdominal circumference becomes the larger of the two.

The determination of the fetal weight by sonography can be of benefit in identifying IUGR. When the BPD is utilized, the 95% confidence limits for fetal weight estimations vary from ± 638 grams to ± 980 grams. If the BPD is 9.4 cm or greater, the fetus will weigh 2,500 grams or more in 100% of cases, if hydrocephalus is not present. If the BPD and the cross-sectional views of the thorax are utilized, the fetal weight may be estimated to within ± 660 grams. **The head circumference:abdominal circumference ratio is greater than 1.0 until the third trimester, when the abdominal circumference increases and exceeds the head circumference. In asymmetric growth-retarded infants, the abdomen does not increase in size and the ratio remains at greater than 1.0.**

A recent study has suggested that there is a significant difference between the small-for-gestational-age (SGA) infant and the appropriate-for-gestational-age (AGA) infant in terms of the rate of growth of the fetal abdominal circumference. The mean growth rate of the abdominal circumference for an SGA infant is 6.0 ± 4.9 mm/14 days, as contrasted with that of the AGA infant, who should have 14.7 ± 7.1 mm/14 days. Another study indicated that if the femur length:abdominal circumference ratio was greater than 23.5, then the fetus would have intrauterine growth retardation.

In contrast to an IUGR infant, the infant with **macrosomia** generally weighs more than 4,000 grams. As such, the BPD, head size, and length are all greater than the 90th percentile for the given age. This diagnosis was made antenatally in only about 20% of cases in which the fetus weighed more than 4,500 grams in one study. If the transthoracic diameter of the fetus is more than 1.4 cm greater than the head circumference, then macrosomia may be present. Some authors have suggested that when there is a difference of 1.6 cm in the chest-head circumferences, or when there is a shoulder-head circumference difference of more than 4.8 cm, then infants with these measurements should be highly suspect for possible shoulder dystocia at birth.

The fetal ponderal indices are usually quite low in large fetuses and abnormally high in IUGR infants. These values are relatively constant after 21 weeks' gestation.

1. Femur length: fetal midthigh circumference
   × 100 = 51.8 ± 7.8 (normal range 44–59.6).

2. Tibial length: fetal calf circumference below the knee × 100 = 57.6 ± 9.4 (normal range 48.2–67).
3. Femur length: abdominal circumference × 100 = 22.3 ± 2.4 (normal range 19.9–24.7).
4. Tibial length: abdominal circumference × 100 = 19.3 ± 2.2 (normal range 17.1–21.5).
5. Femur length + tibial length: abdominal circumference × 100 = 41.6 ± 4.2 (normal range 37.4–45.8).

2) Treatment

When IUGR is present, the treatment should be directed toward alleviating the basic causes whenever possible and evaluating the fetal status. Correction of an anemia, the elimination of noxious chemicals and drugs, the improvement of the patient's nutrition, and increased bedrest (in the left lateral decubitus position) may be sufficient to allow the pregnancy to continue for a long enough period of time to gain further fetal maturity. The use of both nonstress and stress tests may help to define the degree of fetal reserve. In many instances, however, the continuation of the pregnancy in these cases is not possible and prompt delivery is necessary. If there is no evidence of fetal distress during labor, the infant may be delivered vaginally. If fetal distress should occur, however, then a cesarean section should be performed. Due to the frequent presence of meconium staining of the amniotic fluid, the mouth and nares of the fetus should be suctioned before the first breath is taken so as to avoid meconium aspiration.

d. Placental/amniotic fluid evaluation

1) Placental grading

The placental site may be visualized by 9–10 weeks after the LMP. **The amniochorionic plate appears as a defined line on the fetal surface of the placenta by 18–20 weeks'** gestation. After the 31st week, maturational changes begin to take place in the placenta (Fig. 26-18). These changes have been divided into grades from 0 to 3. The ultrasonogram for a **grade 0 placenta** shows a homogeneous placenta with an intact amniochorionic plate. A **grade 1** placenta has comma-shaped echogenic areas within the body of the placenta and the amniochorionic plate

may have some undulations. A **grade 2 placenta** is one that has not only the comma-like calcifications within the body of the placenta, but also has basilar calcifications between the placenta and the decidua. At this point, the amniochorionic plate has developed septate indentations that do not reach the basilar plate. In the **grade 3 placenta,** the intercotyledonary septa extend to the basilar plate and calcify. The shadowing effect of these changes cause a Swiss cheese–like effect in the main body of the placenta. If the *placental thickness* exceeds 5–6 cm, then diabetes, Rh isoimmunization, syphilis, or viral infections may be present. Fetal growth retardation or hypertensive disease may be associated with grade 3 placental changes prior to 31 weeks' gestation, whereas patients with diabetes (classes A and B) may have a grade 0 placenta at term.

2) Placental location

The location of the placenta may be identified on an ultrasonogram. **While only 1% of cases of placenta previa are still present at term, ultrasonography has shown that 45% of all placentas are low-lying in the second trimester.** This *placental migration* has only been appreciated in recent years. In cases of abruptio placentae, the presence of a retroplacental sonolucent area representing a blood clot may occasionally be noted in the region of uterine tenderness and pain.

3) Amniotic fluid volume

The amniotic fluid volume should routinely be evaluated during an ultrasonographic examination. The quantity of amniotic fluid is difficult to define; however, it is generally a clinical impression of more or less than normal amounts of fluid about the baby, or the size of the largest pocket of amniotic fluid on ultrasound. If a pocket of amniotic fluid is measured in each of the four quadrants of the abdomen and these amounts are summed, they provide an *amniotic fluid index, which can then be correlated with the gestational age to determine the limits of excess or deficiency (normal term values = amniotic fluid index of 12.9 ± 4.6 cm).* In the presence of *hydramnios,* 20% of the fetuses will have an anomaly, usually involving the gastrointestinal system (i.e., tracheo-esophageal fistula, duodenal atresia), the skeletal system (i.e., chondrodysplasia punctata, achondrogen-

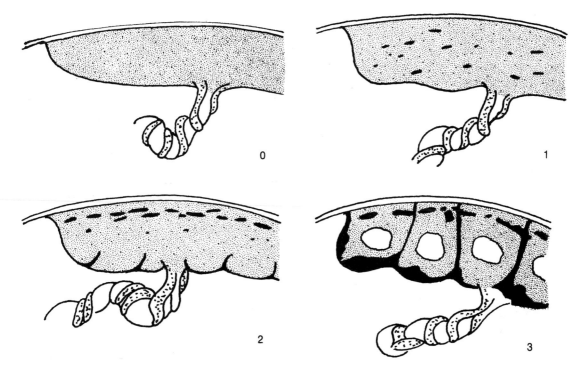

FIGURE 26-18. Ultrasonic classification of placental maturity. Grade 0 has a smooth chorionic plate and clear placental substance. Grade 1 has subtle indentations of the chorionic plate and randomly dispersed echogenic areas in the placental substance. Grade 2 has comma-shaped indentations of the chorionic plate and basally located echogenic densities at the base of the placental substance. Grade 3 has indentations of the chorionic plate that extend to the uterine wall. Echospared or fallout areas are in the placental substance along with irregular densities with acoustic shadowing near the surface. (Adapted from P.A.T. Grannum, R. L. Berkowitz, and J. C. Hobbins, "The Ultrasonic Changes in the Maturing Placenta and Their Relation to Fetal Pulmonic Maturity," *American Journal of Obstetrics and Gynecology* 133 (1979), p. 915.)

esis type I), or of the central nervous system (i.e., anencephaly, hydrocephaly). *Oligohydramnios* may occur in certain fetal congenital anomalies (e.g., renal agenesis) and in a postterm pregnancy.

e. Special fetal evaluations

With the development of sophisticated ultrasound equipment over the past few years, this technique has been used in many new situations with great success. The use of real-time gray-scale ultrasound has allowed physicians to appreciate the subtle shading between body structures. In addition, the use of real-time-directed M-mode echocardiography for the study of the fetal heart has provided a tool for a better under-

standing of fetal cardiac dysfunction and cardiac defects.

Targeted imaging for fetal anomalies (TIFFA) studies have been used for pregnancies in which there is a high risk of birth defects. Such patients may have a history of giving birth previously to a child with a congenital abnormality, or may have elevated alpha-fetoprotein values, IUGR, diabetes mellitus, hydramnios, or exposure to known teratogens. The physician who performs these studies should have the necessary skills as an ultrasonographer to be able to thoroughly examine the fetus to detect the presence of specific congenital defects. Almost every organ system should be visualized individually and evaluated in minute detail. **Due to the need for ex-**

tensive experience and knowledge, these studies should be performed only by specially trained physicians.

In certain cases, surgical procedures other than amniocentesis and intrauterine fetal transfusions have been performed under the direction of ultrasonic imaging. Such problems as obstructive uropathy and obstructive hydrocephalus may be treated in utero by the use of proper shunting procedures. The intramuscular administration of pancuronium bromide to the fetus prior to the performance of intrauterine fetal procedures will eliminate any potentially dangerous fetal movements during these operations.

f. X-ray techniques

The use of X-ray techniques in obstetrics has decreased dramatically since the advent of ultrasound; however, occasionally there is still a need to utilize this modality. Frequently, a roentgenogram of the abdomen is of value in the patient who has a breech presentation and in whom vaginal delivery is contemplated, in order to be certain that there is no evidence of a hyperextended fetal head.

The fetal skeleton may be visualized after 16 weeks and certain skeletal abnormalities may be determined by X-ray examination. Observing the appearance of the ossification centers in the tibia and femur in the third trimester to date the pregnancy, however, has been found to be sufficiently imprecise as to preclude clinical use of this method, since ultrasound has been found to be a much more accurate technique for gestational dating.

The injection of radiopaque water-soluble iodinated media into the amniotic fluid (i.e., an amniogram) to provide contrast between the fetus, the amniotic fluid, and the placenta is another method rarely used now. Placental localization, the fetal configuration, and the ability of the fetus to swallow effectively to produce an in-utero gastrointestinal series, may be appreciated through use of an amniogram X-ray. Monoamniotic twins may also be diagnosed antenatally by an amniogram.

g. Chemical assays

1) Estriol

The measurement of both the urinary and the plasma estriol levels during the third trimester of pregnancy has been used to determine the status of the fetus. The production and excretion of estriol is a cooperative venture that involves the fetus, the placenta, and the mother. The fetus converts dehydroisoandrosterone sulfate (DHAS), from the fetal adrenal gland and from maternal sources, to 16 alpha-hydroxydehydroisoandrosterone sulfate in the fetal liver, and thus provides this precursor to the placenta for its final conversion to estriol. While the fetus plays a role in this metabolic scheme, the placenta also must have the ability to convert this compound to estriol. In some instances, there may be a **congenital lack of the placental sulfatase enzyme that is needed to effect this conversion,** and in this situation, there will be low or absent estriol levels. Finally, the estriol must be transferred to the maternal organism, where it is then excreted in the urine. Certain drugs ingested by the mother, such as phenobarbital, antibiotics, and aspirin, may result in low estriol values. Acute maternal pyelonephritis has also been associated with low estriol urinary excretion values.

There are wide daily fluctuations in the amount of estriol excretion in the urine of pregnant women; however, it has been shown that for any given patient, these values usually only fluctuate by about 20%. Since the plasma estriol levels correlate well with the urinary estriol values, and in addition, are not fraught with the difficulties of obtaining an accurate 24-hour urine collection, the *plasma values* are usually used to assess the estriol level. Due to the variability in the estriol measurements, single values are generally not helpful. Daily values should be obtained and any decreased levels must be verified by demonstrating that they are persistent and significantly different from the mean of the previous values.

PART IV

Abnormal obstetrics

CHAPTER 27

First-trimester bleeding

Case VII. A woman of those who lodged with Pantimides, from a miscarriage, was taken ill of fever. On the first day, tongue dry, thirst, nausea, insomnolency, belly disordered, with thin, copious, undigested dejections. On the second day, had a rigor, acute fever; alvine discharges copious; had no sleep. On the third, pains greater. On the fourth, delirious. On the seventh she died. Belly throughout loose, with copious, thin, undigested evacuations; urine scanty, thin. An ardent fever.

—*Hippocrates (460–370 B.C.)**

· · · · · · · · · · · · · · ·

1. Abortion

a. General considerations

1) Definition

The term "abortion" refers to the delivery of a fetus prior to the time when it can survive. The definition generally accepted for legal purposes is the delivery of a fetus at less than 20 weeks' gestation or with a fetal weight of less than 500 grams. This definition varies somewhat in different states; in Louisiana, for example, the weight value has been decreased to 350 grams. *The incidence of spontaneous abortion is between 10 and 20% of all pregnancies.* Indeed, if the unrecognized fetal losses at the time of the menses were included, it is possible that the abortion rate might approach 50–60%. Infants

---

*Reprinted by permission from Encyclopaedia Britannica, Inc., Great Books of the Western World, vol. 10, "Hippocrates and Galen," Robert Maynard Hutchins, ed. Chicago, Ill.: William Benton, Publisher, 1952, p. 56.

who are delivered early and weigh between 500 and 999 grams have been termed **immature,** whereas those who weigh between 1,000 and 2,499 grams have been called **premature by weight.**

2) Etiology

Spontaneous abortion is most commonly due to chromosomal defects (60%), such as *trisomies, monosomies, and polyploidy.* A "blighted ovum" may also occur, in which case the embryo is markedly degenerated or absent. Hydropic degeneration of the fetal villi will be found on histologic examination in about 60% of the cases of abortion. **In general, the fetus will have been dead for two to four weeks before vaginal bleeding develops and the abortion occurs.** The presence of fetal heart activity detected by ultrasound at 8–12 weeks' gestation is good evidence that the patient may continue to carry the pregnancy (with less than a 3% rate of loss thereafter). The aging of the gametes due to insemination four days before or three days after the time of ovulation may play a role in spontaneous abortion. Any failure of the hormonal mechanisms to prepare the endometrium or to facilitate zygote implantation may also result in an abortion. In addition, the exposure of the embryo to *various viruses, chemicals, or irradiation* during development may also affect the conceptus, by producing either an abortion or a teratogenic effect in those fetuses that are not aborted. Infections by Brucella abortus, Listeria monocytogenes, Toxoplasma gondii, and Mycoplasma hominis have been implicated at various times in human abortion. Space-occupying lesions of the uterus (e.g., leiomyomas, polyps) have been suggested as a cause of abortion.

In cases in which trauma has been implicated

[handwritten margin note: avid that trauma was cause for abort]

as the cause of abortion, it is essential to show that: (1) the conceptus was perfectly normal before the trauma, and (2) the abortion took place within minutes or hours after the trauma, in order for the trauma to be accepted as the cause of the abortion.

b. Threatened abortion

The onset of bleeding and/or lower abdominal cramps in the first 20 weeks of pregnancy, in a patient with intact membranes and a closed cervix, constitutes a threatened abortion. While many patients will successfully carry this type of pregnancy to term, some will not, and it is essential that the patient realize that nothing can be done to prevent an abortion. You can reassure the patient, however, that if she continues to carry the pregnancy, then the fetus will probably have no greater risk of abnormalities than in a normal pregnancy.

The avoidance of heavy physical activity, and especially sexual excitement, perhaps has a valid basis and should be recommended to patients with a threatened abortion, since the latter may cause uterine contractions. The patient should be warned that if her cramps become worse, or if the bleeding becomes heavy, she should notify you. Furthermore, the patient should be instructed to bring in any tissue or clots that she might expel so that they may be examined.

c. Inevitable abortion

An inevitable or imminent abortion is present when the patient presents in the first 20 weeks of pregnancy with bleeding and cramping, a dilated cervix, and/or with associated ruptured membranes, without the passage of tissue. Since there is essentially no chance that the pregnancy can progress any further under these circumstances, the uterus should be emptied immediately.

d. Complete/incomplete abortion

An **incomplete abortion** occurs when part of the tissue is extruded through the cervix, is in the vagina, or is passed. While a complete abortion is one in which all of the products of conception are expelled, this is uncommon in early abortions. Rarely, a blighted ovum may be completely passed as an intact ball of tissue, inside of which there is a sac with clear fluid and no evidence of a fetus. In the majority of early abortions, however, there are still portions of the conceptus remaining inside the uterus. An immediate evacuation of the products of conception by D&C is advisable to prevent excessive bleeding, infection, and undue hospitalization. Rh immunoglobulin should be administered to the Rh negative unsensitized patients.

[handwritten margin note: give Rhogan if necess to prevent sensitization]

e. Missed abortion

A missed abortion is one in which the conceptus has been retained for eight weeks after fetal death; however, the time of fetal death is usually difficult to determine with accuracy. Generally in these cases, the problem is discovered because the uterus is not growing appropriately for the gestational age. Upon ultrasonic evaluation, the pregnancy ring (i.e., the gestational sac) will be indistinct or greatly distorted. In the latter part of the first trimester, no fetal heart activity will be found on ultrasound examination. Since hypofibrinogenemia (i.e., coagulation defects) may occur in a small percentage of patients after about five weeks following fetal death, and since there is a significant emotional burden involved for the woman who is carrying a dead fetus, it is usually recommended that the uterus be evacuated as soon as the diagnosis is made.

f. Habitual abortion

The occurrence of three consecutive abortions prior to 20 weeks' gestation in a patient has been referred to as "habitual abortion." The causes of habitual abortion are difficult to identify, and multiple causes are probably involved in most cases. Certainly, the usual general health considerations, such as nutrition, hormonal activity, and the presence of infective agents should be examined. However, some studies have indicated that when the physician merely establishes a good rapport with the patient and develops a caring approach, the success rate in subsequent pregnancies may dramatically increase. **First-trimester abortions** are due to chromosomal anomalies in more than 50% of the cases. Most commonly, these cases involve trisomy (52%), polyploidy (26%), and monosomy (Turner's syndrome) (15%). A karyotype of the parents may be abnormal in 10% of these patients, and may reveal mosaicism (48%), translocations (44%), or deletions and inversions

[handwritten margin notes: "con'l/forget chromosomal causes 60%" "causes habitual abortion"]

(8%). Hormonal abnormalities have been thought to be implicated in about 25% of patients with habitual abortion. Diabetes mellitus, thyroid dysfunction, and progesterone deficiency (i.e., luteal phase defect) have all been implicated. The infectious agents that have been implicated as possible causes of habitual abortion include Toxoplasma gondii, Mycoplasma (Ureaplasma urealyticum), Brucella abortus, cytomegalovirus, Listeria monocytogenes, Treponema pallidum, and Chlamydia trachomatis. In **mid-trimester abortions,** you should consider the possibility that the patient may have a congenital uterine anomaly (e.g., septum), a uterine malformation (i.e., DES anomaly), cervical incompetence, or a space-occupying lesion of the uterine cavity (e.g., leiomyoma). About 15% of patients with habitual abortion will have such anomalies. Immunologic causes are difficult to evaluate, since the HLA-A and HLA-B antigens, transplantation antigens, transferrin, and the blood types will need to be evaluated in both parents. Seriously ill patients with chronic renal disease, systemic lupus erythematosus, or other conditions may have a history of a poor reproductive performance.

g. Septic abortion

A septic abortion in the past was generally associated with a criminal abortion; however, it may occur in a spontaneous abortion if there has been sufficient bacterial contamination. *The infection is caused by vaginal and intestinal bacterial organisms that ascend into the uterine cavity.* Such organisms include **anaerobic bacteria,** like Peptostreptococcus species, Bacteroides species, and Clostridium perfringens, as well as **aerobic bacteria,** like Escherichia coli, Pseudomonas, enterococcus, and beta-hemolytic streptococcus. With the onset of an infection, endometritis develops, which extends outside of the uterus to produce parametritis, peritonitis, and septicemia. Bacterial endotoxins and exotoxins may produce widespread damage to the patient's microvasculature with **septic shock,** which may lead to a total vascular collapse and death.

The maternal mortality rate from septic abortion varies between 10 and 50%. Whenever uterine tenderness and fever are found in a patient with an abortion, the diagnosis of septic abortion must be strongly entertained. You should rule out infection in other systems to account for the findings (e.g., urinary tract infection). *The urinary output and vital signs should be carefully monitored to detect early evidence of shock.* Appropriate aerobic and anaerobic cultures of the uterus, as well as Gram-stained smears of the uterine secretions, should be obtained. A Gram-stained smear will often provide information as to the most prevalent organism involved in the infection.

The treatment of the patient with a septic abortion consists of the complete evacuation of the uterine contents by a D&C and the intravenous administration of wide-spectrum antibiotics. Usually, penicillin G sodium, 15–20 million units/24 hours; gentamicin sulfate (Garamycin), 3–5 mg/kg/24 hours; and clindamycin phosphate (Cleocin phosphate), 600–1200 mg/day in 2–4 equal doses, will give appropriate coverage for a polymicrobial infection. You should monitor the blood levels of gentamicin (i.e., keep the levels between 8 μg/ml and 10 μg/ml) to avoid undertreatment or toxicity. *Intravenous fluids* (i.e., lactated Ringer's solution) should be utilized to correct for hypovolemic shock. On occasion, a central venous catheter or a Swan-Ganz balloon flotation catheter will provide valuable assistance in the management of the fluid therapy. If severe anemia or hemorrhage is present, then *packed red cells should be given.* The urine flow should be maintained at a rate of at least 30–50 ml per hour. In the past, it was recommended that large doses of corticosteroids should be utilized in the treatment of the septic shock patient; however, some recent studies indicate that the use of methylprednisolone sodium succinate, 30 mg/kg q6h × 4 doses, in septic shock patients may be ineffective. Furthermore, in one study those patients who had elevated creatinine levels or who developed secondary infections after the therapy was begun, there was a higher mortality rate in those treated with methylprednisolone. *Oxygen* should be administered at 6 liters/minute to avoid the adult respiratory distress syndrome (ARDS). Renal failure may occur secondary to the infection or to the hypovolemia, and *dialysis* may become necessary in some patients.

h. Induced, therapeutic, and criminal abortions

1) Definitions

An induced abortion (i.e., voluntary, therapeutic, or criminal) is defined as the deliberate interruption of pregnancy prior to the age of viability. It may be performed at the request of the patient (voluntary or criminal), or upon the recommendation of a physician in cooperation with the patient because of medical reasons (therapeutic) (see Chapter 45). A **therapeutic abortion** is generally done because of the following medical indications: (1) the continuation of the pregnancy would seriously threaten the patient's life or health, (2) the pregnancy was the result of rape or incest, or (3) the fetus would be born with developmental defects that would seriously interfere with the quality of life.

2) Historical aspects

The performance of abortion was illegal in the United States until the decision of the United States Supreme Court in **Roe vs. Wade** in January 1973. In this case, Mrs. Roe of Dallas, Texas, was denied an abortion in 1969 after she had become pregnant as a result of a gang rape. About four years later, the Supreme Court finally ruled that abortion was legal. In 1983, the Supreme Court reaffirmed the legality of abortion. Since that time, considerable controversy has continued to surround the abortion issue in this country.

There are moral, ethical, legal, and societal issues that should be addressed in the consideration of whether abortions should or should not be performed. Some factors that should be considered might include: (1) the national and world population growth, (2) the responsibilities of both the individual and of the society to provide support for a child, (3) the role of the government in regulating such procedures for its citizens, (4) the role of specific moral concerns in the formation of laws for a given individual who may or may not subscribe to such moral tenets, and (5) the role of the government in establishing safety rules in regard to the performance of such medical procedures. These and many more concerns have been voiced concerning the abortion issue, and they will continue to be part of this unsolved dilemma for some years to come.

Criminal abortions used to be more prevalent prior to the Supreme Court's ruling. Since that time, maternal deaths due to criminal abortions have decreased dramatically. On occasion, however, criminal abortions are still seen and may pose a serious threat to the mother's life. Generally, sepsis leading to septic shock has been the main cause of death in these patients. Injuries to adjacent organs (e.g., bladder, rectum) secondary to the perforation of the uterus or of the rectovaginal septum by wooden or metal probes or skewers sets the stage for such pelvic infections. The use of *chemical agents* such as Lysol, which contains a mixture of soap, ortho benzyl-parachlorophenol, ortho phenylphenol, propylene glycol, and alcohol, as a douching agent (or deliberately injected into the uterus) may have profound toxic effects on the mother. The carbolic acid (phenol) and cresol (the three isomers ortho, meta, and para) may initially produce some central nervous system stimulation, followed by depression, coma, cardiorespiratory arrest, and pulmonary edema. These agents are detoxified in the liver and the estrified degradation products are excreted in the urine, which produces a characteristic dark greenish urine due to the positive ferric chloride reaction. The presence of soap in the bloodstream may oxidize the hemoglobin to produce methemoglobin and result in hemolysis and vascular thrombosis. The treatment of these patients consists of the use of broad-spectrum antibiotics, adequate support of the blood volume and cardiovascular needs, and supportive therapy of the renal function (i.e., dialysis). In severe infections, a hysterectomy may become necessary.

2. Ectopic pregnancy

a. Etiology

The incidence of ectopic pregnancy has increased three-fold over the past ten years from about 1:300 to approximately 1:100 deliveries. The risk of death from an ectopic pregnancy from 1970 to 1983 decreased from 35.2 to 5.3 deaths per 10,000 cases. Ectopic pregnancy seems to be more common in nonwhites than in the white population and in the young rather than the old. Significantly, a higher proportion of women with fatal ectopic pregnancies have died at home, rather than in the hospital, illustrating the fact that many nonwhite women and young women do not seek early prenatal care. Histologic studies of the fallopian tubes in patients with a tubal pregnancy have demonstrated evidence of *a previous inflammatory process in as many as 38–42% of cases*, indicating that one of the foremost etiologic factors in the development of an ectopic pregnancy is a previous acute pelvic inflammatory disease (PID). **PID then is the most common cause of ectopic tubal pregnancy. This disease causes the agglutination of the endosalpingeal folds, with the formation of**

blind pockets and a partial occlusion of the tubal lumen.

Other prominent causes of ectopic tubal pregnancy include *transmigration of the ovum (30%), previous ectopic tubal pregnancy (7–25%), and tubal ligation (0.6%).* Patients who have undergone a *tubal anastomosis* have about a 4.4% risk of developing a subsequent ectopic pregnancy. A previous *salpingostomy,* rather than a salpingectomy, for an ectopic pregnancy may also predispose the patient to another ectopic pregnancy. Currently, there is some controversy concerning the role of an *intrauterine contraceptive device* and the occurrence of ectopic pregnancy, but there may be an apparent increased incidence associated with the IUD. One report lists the absolute risk of ectopic pregnancy as being 1.2 : 1,000 woman-years of use in IUD users. Other conditions, which may also produce kinking of the tube and tubal occlusion, include *peritoneal adhesions* secondary to previous surgery, appendicitis, septic abortion, or endometriosis. *Salpingitis isthmica nodosa,* in which the tubal lumen at the isthmical region breaks up into a number of smaller passageways, may also be a cause of ectopic pregnancy.

b. Symptoms

The classic triad of symptoms of ectopic pregnancy include pain (98%), amenorrhea (70–90%), and vaginal bleeding (80%). Typically, the patient will miss her menstrual period by a few days, or by a week or two, and then will begin to have vaginal bleeding in association with lower abdominal cramps, which are often more intense on the side of the ectopic pregnancy. The onset of pain may be gradual, or it may occur dramatically when the patient is *straining* at stool, which then may result in immediate *syncope* and momentary unconsciousness. These symptoms generally occur when the tube ruptures, and they are associated with weakness and *shoulder pain* due to the irritation of the diaphragm by the intraperitoneal bleeding. Upon close questioning, you should be able to elicit *symptoms of pregnancy* (i.e., undue fatigue, breast swelling and tenderness, and nausea and/or vomiting) in about 50% of these cases. The patient may pass a "tissue-like" endometrial cast and initially may be thought to be having an abortion. One might list the **Eight S's** of the findings in an ectopic pregnancy that have been suggested to me by my colleague Dr. Harvey Huddleston,

as (1) **S**kipped period, (2) **S**anguinous vaginal discharge, (3) **S**training at stool with fainting, (4) **S**yncope, (5) **S**houlder pain, (6) **S**hock, (7) **S**anguineous nonclotting blood in the cul-de-sac on culdocentesis, and (8) **S**evere pelvic pain, tenderness, and a mass. The histologic presence of an **Arias-Stella reaction** and **decidua without the presence of chorionic villi,** found in the pathology report of tissue passed from the vagina or tissue obtained in a D&C, should alert you to the possibility of an ectopic pregnancy.

c. Physical findings

Your initial physical examination, and the status of the patient's vital signs, will be important in determining the seriousness of the patient's condition. *Some patients will present with profound shock, tachycardia, a thready pulse, and a distended, rigid abdomen that is filled with blood (15%).* Generally, however, the patient's condition will not be that serious and the pelvic examination may reveal a fullness and *doughy feeling in the cul-de-sac, with an exquisitely tender cervix on motion.* A pelvic mass may be felt in only 50% of patients with ectopic pregnancy. **The pregnancy will be located in the outer third of the tube in 47% of cases, the middle third in 39%, and the inner third in 14%.** The **right tube** is involved in the majority of patients. The mortality rate is about 1 per 1,000 ectopic pregnancies in white women and 3.4 per 1,000 in nonwhite women, with death being due to hemorrhage (85%), infection (5%), or secondary to anesthesia (2%).

The remainder of those patients who have an ectopic pregnancy (85%) will present with minimal to moderate symptoms and, as a consequence, will pose a diagnostic dilemma for the physician. **In the absence of fever, the diagnostic possibilities are: (1) an ectopic pregnancy, (2) a ruptured corpus luteum cyst, (3) a torsion of the tube or ovary, or (4) a threatened or incomplete abortion.** If a significant degree of fever is present (i.e., higher than 38.5° C), then PID, appendicitis, septic abortion, or a tubo-ovarian abscess should be considered.

d. Diagnostic tests
1) hCG

The human chorionic gonadotropin (hCG) molecule is composed of two parts, the alpha and beta subunits.

The beta subunit is specific for the hCG, whereas the alpha subunit is common to all of the glycoprotein hormones (e.g., luteinizing hormone) (see Chapter 19). **The determination of the beta-subunit hCG with a high-sensitivity radioimmunoassay test will allow the identification of a pregnancy within eight days of conception.** It is positive in 96–99% of patients with an ectopic pregnancy. The doubling time of the hCG in normal pregnancy is 1.4–2.2 days (34–53 hrs) during the first 30 days after ovulation, but serial quantitative hCG levels may show lesser values or even decreasing values in an ectopic pregnancy. By 30 days following ovulation, the hCG should be of the order of 1,000 ng/ml (6,000–6,500 mIU/ml) (i.e., 1 ng = 5.6 mIU/ml). In addition, by the time that the hCG has reached this level, the gestational sac should be visible in the uterine cavity on ultrasound.

One study showed that when the hCG level was above 6,500 mIU/ml, then the absence of a gestational sac on the ultrasonogram was indicative of an ectopic pregnancy. The absence of the gestational sac under these conditions had a sensitivity of 100%, a specificity of 96%, a positive predictive value of 86%, a negative predictive value of 100%, and an efficiency of 98%, based upon the 19.4% prevalence of ectopic pregnancies in the group of patients studied.

2) Ultrasonography

Ultrasonography may be used to determine the presence of an intrauterine gestational sac at about five weeks' gestation. A sac that does not have a double-ring effect on one side, owing to the presence of the uterine cavity between the decidua capsularis and the decidua vera, is referred to as a **pseudosac** and is indicative of a possible ectopic pregnancy. If there is a **double echo on one side of the sac,** then an intrauterine pregnancy should be present. If such a sac can be identified as definitely being present, then an ectopic pregnancy is probably not present, since the simultaneous occurrence of an intrauterine pregnancy and an ectopic pregnancy has been said to occur in only 1:30,000 pregnancies. Recent studies seem to indicate, however, that the combination of an intrauterine and an extrauterine pregnancy might be considerably more common than has been previously thought with an incidence of perhaps 1:6,000. The finding of **fetal heart motion** within the uterine cavity also might effectively rule out a diagnosis of ec-

topic pregnancy for the same reason. The abdominal ultrasound technique is accurate in diagnosing ectopic pregnancy in only about 70–90% of the cases. Recently, with the use of a vaginal transducer, the detection of pelvic masses, including ectopic pregnancy, has become much easier.

3) Culdocentesis

Once the diagnosis of an ectopic pregnancy is seriously entertained, and if there is no evidence of shock or compromise in the patient's condition, then a **culdocentesis** should be performed. A culdocentesis should be performed in any patient who presents with symptoms and signs that are highly suggestive of an ectopic pregnancy, in order to determine whether there is unclotted blood in the cul-de-sac (see Chapter 18). **Nonclotting blood may be aspirated in about 85–95% of ruptured ectopic tubal pregnancies, and when found, requires at least a laparoscopy procedure to determine the amount and cause of the bleeding, or in the case of severe bleeding, a definitive laparotomy.** The finding of *serosanguineous fluid* on culdocentesis usually indicates that a corpus luteum cyst has ruptured and that surgical intervention—on the basis of such a minimal amount of intraperitoneal bleeding—is probably not necessary. If there is a strong suspicion that an ectopic pregnancy is present, and if there is doubt concerning the presence of an intrauterine gestational sac, then a laparoscopy should be carried out. In a very early unruptured ectopic pregnancy, however, it may not be possible to visualize any tubal enlargement, even during a laparotomy examination.

4) Treatment

a) Salpingectomy

If an ectopic pregnancy is found to be present, laparotomy is necessary. *The surgical approach may be either radical or conservative.* With a radical approach, a **salpingectomy** is generally performed, especially when the tube has been extensively damaged or when the patient is in shock due to excessive blood loss. A salpingectomy has been utilized in about 75% of cases. **The recurrence rate of ectopic pregnancy in the other tube following salpingectomy is about 12.5%.** A salpingo-oophorectomy has been performed in about 15% of ectopic pregnancy patients when the ovary is involved. Some physicians in the past have utilized the *colpotomy* operative approach to treat an ectopic pregnancy. This procedure is performed by making an incision through the posterior fornix of the vagina into the cul-de-sac where the fallopian tube may be visualized and resected. About 30–40% of ectopic pregnancy patients can be managed in this manner if there is minimal or no intra-abdominal bleeding. A *minilaparotomy* incision can also be used in most patients who do not have serious intra-abdominal hemorrhage. Salpingectomy or salpingostomy can be performed through a *pelviscope (pelvoscopic surgery),* using the coagulation-resection technique, or with electrical or laser procedures, in which an incision may be made into the tube and the products of conception aspirated.

The technique of milking the tube in order to express the products of conception is mentioned only to be condemned, since the recurrence rate of an ectopic pregnancy after this procedure has been shown in at least one study to be doubled (i.e., from 11.6–24.1%). In addition, some patients have required reoperation following this procedure, while an abdominal pregnancy has developed in others, due to the continued growth of the extruded products of conception in the abdominal cavity.

b) Salpingostomy

The conservative approach to the treatment of an ectopic pregnancy consists of a **salpingostomy,** which involves a careful assessment of the unruptured tubal pregnancy. A linear incision is made on the top of the tube over the site of the pregnancy and the products of conception are carefully removed using microsurgical techniques. A needle cautery is used to control the bleeding. Recently, it has been noted that some of these patients may return in six to eight weeks with another episode of intraperitoneal bleeding secondary to a **persistent ectopic pregnancy syndrome.** At the time of the repeat surgery, trophoblastic tissue has often been found at the site of the previous ectopic pregnancy. The persistence of positive quantitative β-hCG values postoperatively may assist in making this diagnosis.

In those patients who have had too much tubal damage to do a salpingostomy, a conservative approach may still be utilized by performing a *segmental resection* of the tube. A microsurgical tubal anasto-

mosis may be performed at this time, or it may be delayed until a later time when a specially trained tubal surgeon can reanastomose the tube. *Rh immunoglobulin should be administered to Rh-negative patients who have ectopic pregnancies and are not sensitized.*

Recently, it has been recommended that patients with ectopic pregnancies may be treated with *methotrexate,* which may be administered over a five-day period and then repeated for a total of three courses to cause the resorption of the conceptus. The safety of this approach, however, has not yet been determined.

e. Other ectopic pregnancies
1) Abdominal pregnancy

An abdominal pregnancy may develop initially in the peritoneal cavity, or it may be secondary to the rupture of the tube or uterus. In the latter case, the products of conception are expelled into the abdominal cavity, where they then develop. This form of ectopic pregnancy occurs in about 1 in 15,000 deliveries (range: 1:780 to 1:50,000). A recent study cited an incidence of 10.9 per 100,000 live births.

The symptoms of an abdominal pregnancy are generally vague and ill defined. **Abdominal pain** that occurs throughout pregnancy, which is usually due to the movements of the fetus against the maternal organs, seems to be the most common symptom. Often, **nausea and vomiting** are present in late pregnancy. Abdominal tenderness is present in 40–100% of patients. **The fetal lie is almost always abnormal (97%), due to the lack of confinement by the uterus.** The fetal parts may be more **prominent to palpation** in 10–30% of cases. An anemia was present in about 70% of the patients included in one study. Moreover, the maternal alpha-fetoprotein values may be abnormally elevated.

The diagnosis of an abdominal pregnancy may be made by demonstrating **fetal parts overlying the maternal spine** on a cross-table lateral roentgenogram. The finding of **maternal bowel gas patterns overlying the fetus** also suggests this diagnosis. The ultrasonogram may demonstrate that the uterus is small and that the placenta is ectopically located. The failure to produce uterine contractions through oxytocin stimulation may assist in defining an abdominal pregnancy in late gestation.

The treatment of an abdominal pregnancy consists of the immediate termination of the

pregnancy by laparotomy. The maternal mortality rate ranges from between 2 and 18%, and the fetal mortality rate is of the order of 50–95%. The incidence of fetal abnormalities in these cases is 20–40%. The possibility of severe hemorrhage at the ectopically placed placental site requires that you have adequate amounts of blood available at the time of surgery. When it is surgically feasible, the placenta should be removed in order to avoid the long-term morbidity of leaving it in situ (i.e., infection, abscess, pain, intestinal obstruction, late hemorrhage, and possible death). If, however, there is a significant risk of a serious hemorrhage if the placenta were to be removed, you should tie off and cut the umbilical cord as close as possible to the placenta and leave the placenta in place. It has been suggested that the patient should be treated postoperatively with methotrexate in order to hasten the absorption of the placenta; however, such chemical necrosis of the placenta may lead to abscess formation and infection. The use of serial ultrasound scans will allow you to follow the course of the placental resolution.

2) Cervical pregnancy

The incidence of an ectopic pregnancy of the cervix is of the order of 1 per 1,000 deliveries (with a range of 1:1,000 to 1:18,000). In order for the cervical pregnancy to be so classified, it must have: (1) the presence of cervical glands opposite the placental attachment, (2) a definite attachment of the placenta to the cervix, (3) a placental attachment below where the uterine vessels enter into the uterus, or below the peritoneal reflection, and (4) no fetal elements inside the corpus uteri. It is obvious that all of these findings can only be determined if a hysterectomy is performed. Clinically, the presence of a dilated, thin-walled, softened cervix that is greatly enlarged over the size of the fundus and a closed internal cervical os strongly suggest a cervical pregnancy. The products of conception will be attached to the endocervix.

Often, a cervical pregnancy may not be diagnosed until a D&C is attempted for a suspected **incomplete abortion** and severe hemorrhage occurs. On the other hand, painless bleeding may initially bring the patient to your attention. Due to the friability of the cervix, a cervical carcinoma should also be considered in your differential diagnosis list. The mortality rate of a cervical pregnancy may be as high as 40–50%; however, prompt control of the bleeding should

prevent such a result. The use of a large catheter (e.g., 28 Fr), with a 75 ml bag inserted into the cervix and a no. 1 chromic pursestring suture placed in the cervix to tamponade the bleeding, may be of benefit in these cases. A *hysterectomy* is frequently necessary in order to control the bleeding.

3) Ovarian pregnancy

An ovarian pregnancy occurs in about 1 per 7,000 deliveries (range 1:2,034 to 1:8,487). This type constitutes about 1% of ectopic pregnancies. Previous pelvic infections may provide a sufficient amount of adhesions to produce an ectopic ovarian pregnancy. Usually, the *Spiegelberg criteria* are utilized to define an ovarian pregnancy. They are: (1) the fallopian tubes must be intact, (2) the pregnancy site must be in the position of the ovary, (3) there must be an ovarian ligament connecting the pregnancy site to the uterus, and (4) there should be ovarian tissue present in the gestational sac wall on histologic examination. The treatment of an ovarian pregnancy requires surgical resection. There may be substantial hemorrhage; however, maternal death is rare in these cases.

4) Cornual and interstitial pregnancies

A **cornual pregnancy** is one that occurs in a rudimentary horn of the uterus, in contradistinction to one that occurs in the interstitial portion of the fallopian tube as it traverses the uterine wall. An ultrasonogram may be able to detect these pregnancies; however, there is little information on this in the literature. The treatment of a cornual pregnancy consists of the excision of the rudimentary horn of the uterus; in addition, an intravenous pyelogram should be performed to detect concomitant renal abnormalities.

In patients who have an **interstitial pregnancy,** a massive hemorrhage may occur due to the restricted area of expansion within the uterine wall and the tendency for the uterine wall to rupture early. A previous cornual resection with a salpingectomy may be the site of the uterine rupture. With rupture, there is often considerable damage to the uterine wall, and a hysterectomy is frequently required to control the bleeding.

5) Intraligamentary pregnancy

The incidence of this very rare form of ectopic pregnancy is between 1:49,000 and 1:184,000. This type of pregnancy develops between the leaves of the broad ligament. Since live-born infants have been delivered in these cases, it has been suggested that conservative management should be followed until about 38 weeks' gestation, with operative delivery at that time. The placenta should be removed if at all possible.

3. Trophoblastic disease

a. Hydatidiform mole

Hydatidiform moles are more common in the Orient than in the Western world. **In the United States and Europe, the incidence is about 1:2,000 pregnancies.** There is an increasing incidence in older women, especially after the age of 45 years. Malnutrition has also been implicated as an etiology. The risk of a second mole in a subsequent pregnancy is 1:60. If the patient has had two moles, then the risk is 1:6.

Traditionally, gestational trophoblastic disease has been classified as: (1) a benign hydatidiform mole, (2) a chorioadenoma destruens (now referred to as an invasive mole), and (3) a choriocarcinoma. In addition, placental-site trophoblastic tumors, which are composed of cytotrophoblastic cells that arise from the placental implantation site, have been identified. The hydatidiform mole may be further classified as: (1) an incomplete mole, or (2) a complete mole.

According to the World Health Organization (WHO) criteria, the diagnosis of gestational trophoblastic disease is based upon the following: (1) high levels of hCG present more than four months after the evacuation of the hydatidiform mole (urinary hCG titer of more than 30,000 IU in 24 hours, or serum titers of more than 20,000 mIU/ml); (2) progressively increasing levels of hCG with a minimum of 3 titers per month; (3) the histologic finding of placental-site trophoblastic tumor or choriocarcinoma at any site; and (4) evidence of metastases to the brain, renal, liver, or gastrointestinal tract, pulmonary metastases of greater than 2 cm in diameter, or more than three metastases present.

The FIGO clinical staging of gestational trophoblastic disease consists of the following: stage I, where the tumor is confined to the uterine corpus; stage II, where the tumor may involve the adnexal structures, but is limited to the genital structures; stage III, where the tumor has metastasized to the lungs, with or without involvement of the genital

structures; and stage IV, where metastatic disease occurs in other sites.

The clinical classification of gestational trophoblastic disease has been based upon whether the tumor is nonmetastatic or metastatic and whether it has a good or a poor prognosis. This classification system divides the patients into those who do not have metastatic disease and those who do have metastases. In the latter category, the patients are divided into low-risk and high-risk patients. **Low-risk patients** have hCG levels of less than 100,000 IU in 24 hours in the urine and of less than 40,000 mIU/ml in the serum; the presence of symptoms for less than four months; no liver or brain metastases; no previous chemotherapy; and antecedent pregnancies that were either moles, ectopic pregnancies, or abortions. **High-risk patients** have hCG titers of more than 100,000 IU in 24 hours in the urine or more than 40,000 mIU/ml in the serum; the presence of symptoms for longer than four months; liver or brain metastases; prior chemotherapeutic failure; and an antecedent term pregnancy. This latter consideration is based upon the fact that gestational trophoblastic tumors that occur after a nonmolar gestation almost always consist of choriocarcinoma, whereas those that arise from a hydatidiform mole are usually an invasive mole.

Another classification scheme for high-risk patients uses a scoring system that takes into account the patient's age (older than 39); incompatible blood-type matings (A × O or O × A) or B or AB blood groups; a tumor size greater than 5 cm; the location of tumor metastases (spleen, kidney, GI tract, liver, or brain); and the number of metastases noted (1–4, 4–8, or more than 8). If there has been a prior chemotherapeutic failure or an antecedent term pregnancy, then the prognosis is poor.

1) Incomplete or partial mole

An incomplete or partial hydatidiform mole is one in which there is a fetus or fetal tissue present in addition to grossly identifiable molar tissue. These moles have a triploid karyotype (69,XXY), (69,XYY) consisting of two paternal and one maternal haploid sets of chromosomes. The extra haploid set of chromosomes is from the father and is due to the fertilization of the ovum by two sperm (i.e., dispermy) or to the failure of sperm meiosis during the first and second reductional divisions (i.e., diandry). Histologically, the hydropic degeneration and trophoblastic proliferation are usually focal in nature. The development of choriocarcinoma in an incomplete mole is thought to be quite rare; however, choriocarcinoma has been reported to occur in a few cases of incomplete moles associated with twins.

2) Complete mole

A complete hydatidiform mole consists of clear, grape-like vesicles only, without a fetus being present. The histologic characteristics of these vesicles are: (1) an enlargement of the villus, with hydropic degeneration and a loss of the blood vessels, (2) varying amounts of syncytial proliferation and atypicality, and (3) an absence of fetal structures or an amnion. The chromosomal complement may vary and may be 46,XX, 45,X, or 46,XY. **In the 46,XX type, both of the X's are of paternal origin, since the fertilized ovum's chromosomes are functionally absent and the paternal haploid sperm (23,X) reduplicates itself after meiosis. The complete mole is thought to be much more prone to produce a local invasion of the uterus (15%) or a choriocarcinoma (4%) than an incomplete mole.**

3) Clinical findings

There are several clinical findings that may lead to the diagnosis of a hydatidiform mole. Spotting, or even massive **hemorrhage,** in the absence of a fetal heart beat, often occurs, and the diagnosis of a threatened abortion may be considered in these cases. In fact, it was shown in one study that partial moles were not diagnosed in 94% of the cases until a D&C had been performed for a suspected incomplete abortion. In rare instances, a patient will pass vesicles per vagina. The **uterus may be enlarged** beyond its appropriate size in about 50% of cases in some series, but in other reports it has been noted to be smaller than the gestational age in as many as 65% of cases. **Hyperemesis gravidarum** occurred in 26% of patients with a complete mole in one study. Symptoms of **toxemia** (i.e., pregnancy-induced hypertension, or PIH), prior to week 24 occurred in 27% of patients who had a mole in this same study. Rarely, an elevation of the plasma thyroxine levels has also been noted with clinical symptoms of **hyperthyroidism** (7%). **Acute respiratory distress,** presumably sec-

ondary to trophoblastic embolization to the pulmonary vasculature, occurred in 2% of the patients in this study.

4) Diagnosis

Confirming a diagnosis of a hydatidiform mole is quite easy once the diagnosis is suspected. **An ultrasonogram will demonstrate the multiple echos (i.e., a vesicular pattern) within the uterine cavity that are characteristic of a hydatidiform mole.** If there is no fetal heart beat and the ultrasonogram demonstrates nonspecific echogenic material in the uterus, then an hCG level of 80,000 mIU/ml or greater will lend support to the diagnosis of a hydatidiform mole. Another diagnostic technique involves the introduction of a radiopaque dye into the uterus by means of amniocentesis. Multiple demilunes of dye-coated hydropic vesicles are also characteristic of a hydatidiform mole and may be seen on an X-ray. The sonogram may also delineate bilateral theca-lutein ovarian cysts. These ovarian tumors will eventually disappear following the complete elimination of the trophoblastic tumor.

5) Treatment

The management of a hydatidiform mole involves two phases: (1) the initial uterine evacuation phase, and (2) the extended follow-up phase that lasts for two years. The patient who desires sterilization may undergo a hysterectomy with conservation of the ovaries. In other patients who desire preservation of their fertility, a D&E using a 12-mm cannula may be carried out. Some authors have suggested that these patients should receive prophylactic chemotherapy at the time of the D&E. After the initial D&E of the molar tissue, the patient should be placed on a low-dose oral contraceptive (i.e., less than 50 micrograms of estrogen) to be sure that a pregnancy does not occur during the time of observation. **About 15–25% of these patients will have persistent trophoblastic disease, so a close follow-up during the first year is essential.** Quantitative human chorionic gonadotropin (β-hCG) titers should be obtained every week until they become negative for at least three weeks, after which time they are followed monthly, if they continue to be normal, for six consecutive months. A *chest roentgenogram* should be obtained initially to serve as a baseline for the future evaluation of the patient regarding possible metastatic disease. Occasionally, a **CT scan of the abdomen or of the brain** may be necessary. An analysis of the **cerebrospinal fluid β-hCG level in relation to the serum levels** may detect very small cerebral metastases if the serum:spinal fluid ratio is less than 60:1. If pelvic adnexal masses are present, then these **theca-lutein cysts** should be observed until they have resorbed; torsion or rupture may occasionally occur. Laparoscopy, with decompression aspiration of these ovarian theca-lutein cysts, may be required in some cases. The *serum chorionic gonadotropin* titers should progressively decrease and become negative if there is no remaining trophoblastic tissue present. If the chorionic gonadotropin levels plateau or increase during the period of observation, then it must be assumed that trophoblastic tissue is still present and that treatment is necessary. Chemotherapeutic treatment consists of the administration of **methotrexate sodium** and **leucovorin calcium** in most low-risk patients. The leucovorin calcium is used to rescue the normal tissues from the folic acid reductase block that is induced by a high dose of methotrexate.

b. Invasive mole

Invasive mole (formerly called chorioadenoma destruens), is quite uncommon. Histologically, **there are villi present;** however, the invasive mole differs from the hydatidiform mole by having an **extensive proliferation of the trophoblastic tissue,** which may invade deep into the uterine muscle. These moles do not usually metastasize to distant organs, but are mainly locally invasive. The treatment of the patient with methotrexate is curative in most cases. The use of the leucovorin calcium (i.e., the citrovorum factor) decreases the toxic effects of methotrexate, which has been referred to as the *folinic acid rescue.* If the tumor is resistant to chemotherapy, a hysterectomy may be necessary to effect a cure.

c. Choriocarcinoma

Choriocarcinoma is rare, and it usually develops from a complete mole. This malignancy is characterized microscopically by the complete absence of chorionic villi. Sheets of syncytiotrophoblastic tissue with marked anaplasia may be seen deep in the tissues in association with necrosis and hemorrhage. *Early metastases to the lungs occurs in 75% of cases, with metastases to the vagina occurring in 30–50% of cases. Metastatic disease to the brain (10%) and liver (10%) carries a poor prognosis. Profuse bleeding may occur in all of the metastatic tumor locations, secondary to the fact that these are highly vascular and friable tumors.*

The diagnosis of choriocarcinoma should be considered when: (1) persistent bleeding occurs after the evacuation of a mole, (2) metastatic lesions are found in the lungs or genital tissues, and (3) the titers of the human chorionic gonadotropin (hCG) plateau or increase during the follow-up observation period.

Methotrexate sodium and dactinomycin (Cosmegen), or combinations of these agents with other drugs have had a significant impact on this disease. About 90% of patients with choriocarcinoma are completely cured today. In the *low-risk* category of patients, the cure rate is essentially 100%. Most of these patients are cured with only one course of methotrexate therapy.

A **high-risk patient** will have one or more of the following findings: (1) a serum hCG level of more than 40,000 mIU/ml, (2) an interval from the pregnancy of greater than four months, (3) hepatic or cerebral metastases, (4) failed prior chemotherapy, (5) a diagnosis of choriocarcinoma on histologic examination, or (6) a placental-site trophoblastic tumor (PSTT). About 74% of patients with only one or two of these factors (excluding PSTT) will respond to primary treatment, whereas only 27% will respond if there are more than three factors present. The placental-site trophoblastic tumor is quite unique and produces low levels of hCG. You should seek expert consultation for the management of these rare PSTT tumors.

The treatment of the high-risk patient may consist of the administration of two different groups of chemotherapeutic drugs, which are administered at intervals of six days (e.g., etoposide, methotrexate sodium, and Actinomycin-D [EMA], in association with cyclophosamide and Oncovin [CO]). This EMA/CO regimen, which was described by K. D. Bagshawe, has been highly successful, with cure rates of 96% being obtained in high-risk patients included in his study since 1980. In patients who become resistant to the EMA/CO regimen, cisplatin (Platinol) may be used, and in patients with brain metastases, intrathecal methotrexate may be administered.

CHAPTER 28

Chemical, infectious, and miscellaneous complications of pregnancy

Modern medicine is a product of the Greek intellect, and had its origin when that wonderful people created positive or rational science.

—Sir William Osler*

1. Drugs, toxins, and irradiation

a. General considerations

While almost any chemical substance may cross the placenta and concentrate in the fetus, some do so more readily than others. **The effects of a chemical or a drug upon the fetal tissues depend upon: (1) when it is administered during the gestational period, (2) the duration of the exposure, (3) the dosage administered, (4) the type of chemical agent, (5) the genetic makeup of both the mother and the fetus, and (6) the coexistence of other chemicals and their interactions with the chemical in question.** Some agents may produce damage to organ systems and cause abnormal development; others may change the growth patterns of a tissue; while still others may cause subtle behavioral or intellectual changes that may only become manifest long after birth. The list of drugs and chemicals that are known to be teratogenic has con-

tinued to increase as new relationships between these agents and fetal abnormalities are further elucidated. It must be kept in mind, however, that a cause-and-effect relationship may not be well established in many instances.

1) Periods of vulnerability

There are several critical periods of vulnerability in which the fetus is at risk. The first critical period is during **the first 13 days of gestation,** when the conceptus demonstrates an "all-or-none" phenomenon (i.e., the conceptus is either killed or it is not affected by the insult). **From about the 13th to the 56th day from conception (or from about day 31 to day 71 after the last menstrual period),** the various organ systems are being formed in the fetus. It is during this time that a chemical insult may produce a congenital abnormality. If an anomaly is produced, then the chemical is referred to as a "teratogen." During **the remainder of the pregnancy,** the fetus is vulnerable to chemical agents, toxins, infections, or drugs, all of which may have subtle influences involving damage to both the intellectual as well as the behavioral capabilities of the fetus, in addition to specific organ systems.

Although the fetus is vulnerable during the **labor and delivery process,** it has been demonstrated that fetal neurological damage often occurs prior to the onset of labor and delivery in many instances. During the **immediate neonatal period,** and then again during **the first few weeks of life,** the fetus is again vulnerable to damage as it attempts to adjust to its extrauterine environment.

---

*Reprinted with permission from Robert Bennett Bean, *Sir William Osler: Aphorisms from His Bedside Teachings and Writings,* William Bennett Bean, ed. Springfield, Ill.: Charles C Thomas, Publisher, 1968, p. 82.

2) Pharmacodynamics

Chemical agents and drugs undergo various interactions in the body before combining with specific tissue receptors to manifest their pharmacologic effect. *This effect may be modified by the extent and rate of absorption, the volume of distribution, the nature and rate of metabolic degradation, and the interactions of the chemical with other compounds.*

a) Oral route

Those physiochemical aspects of the drug that determine the amount and rate of absorption (i.e., its bioavailability), in the case of the oral route, are: (1) the dissolution and solubility of the drug, (2) the gastric and intestinal pH, (3) the gastric emptying time, (4) the intestinal transit time, (5) the presence of other agents that may compete with or block the drug, and (6) the mesenteric blood flow.

b) Parenteral route

In the case of parenteral absorption, the drug's physiochemical characteristics of: (1) water or lipid solubility, (2) degree of ionization, (3) molecular composition, (4) ability to be bound by plasma proteins, and (5) the blood flow at the site of administration (i.e., intramuscular, subcutaneous, epidural), become the determining factors that regulate the absorption of the agent.

c) Other considerations

Since pregnancy imposes striking physiologic changes upon the mother, such as an increased blood volume, a dilutional hypoalbuminemia, and changes in the regional blood flows, and since the fetus is in a compartment that is once-removed from the maternal system, the absorption, distribution, and excretion of any chemical between the maternal and fetal compartments may be quite complex. The fetal circulation is such that the distribution of a drug may vary considerably in different situations. In hypoxic conditions, for example, the peripheral circulation, including the hepatic circulation, may be shut down; thus, the chemicals may bypass the liver entirely and instead attain high concentrations in the fetal brain and heart. Fetal plasma proteins provide for a lesser degree of binding of a drug than the plasma proteins of the adult organism, which allows more free drug to be available to the fetus. Drug distribution is also affected to some extent by the change in the total body water content of the fetus, which decreases from 94% at four months' gestation to 76% at term. Furthermore, in early pregnancy, there is no fat present in the fetus, whereas in the last trimester, fat accounts for about 15% of the body weight at term.

There are four elimination routes for the fetus: (1) the placenta, (2) the fetal kidney, (3) the fetal skin, and (4) the fetal lungs. The placenta is the primary organ for the excretion of fetal waste products. However, the fetal kidneys, lung, and skin offer some intriguing problems with regard to the recirculation of drugs. **The fetus at term has the ability to produce 600–700 ml of hypotonic urine per day. The passage of chemicals via the fetal urine, skin, or lungs may allow them to be recirculated, added to, or preferentially partitioned in the fetus or in the amniotic fluid.**

About 2–3% of infants at birth have congenital abnormalities. At one year of life, this incidence rises to 7.5%, indicating that many anomalies are minor in nature and are not detected until later in life. It is important for you to itemize each medication or chemical that has been used by the patient just prior to and after conception, along with the dosage and frequency of use. The Food and Drug Administration has categorized drugs in an effort to focus attention upon the possible teratogenic effects of these agents (Table 28-1).

b. Identification of chemical abuse

The identification of the pregnant drug addict may be difficult. She may appear to be depressed or nervous during her office visits. She may have bruises on her body, but will deny any marital conflicts. The presence of needle tracts on her arms, or a significant *intolerance to pain,* should suggest that the patient may be an addict. She may complain of a chronic backache, or other pains, that in the past have frequently required narcotics, but which currently are not bothering her. A future "flare-up" of such conditions, however, might seem to be a legitimate reason to her for you to dispense narcotics without a medical workup. She may admit to abuse of alcohol and smoking and may complain of insomnia.

TABLE 28-1. FDA drug categories

The Food and Drug Administration has classified drugs into five categories of teratogenic capabilities as follows:

Category A will apply to drugs for which well-controlled studies in women fail to demonstrate a risk to the fetus. Although such studies can never entirely exclude a risk, a reasonable presumption can be made that when such drugs are used during pregnancy the possibility of fetal harm is remote; however, as with other drugs they should be used during pregnancy only when clearly needed.

Category B indicates either (1) that animal studies have not demonstrated a fetal risk but that there are no adequate studies in women, or (2) that animal studies have uncovered some risk that has not been confirmed in controlled studies in women.

Category C also has two meanings: (1) studies in animals have revealed adverse effects on the fetus and there are no adequate controlled studies in women, or (2) studies in women and animals are not available.

Category D will include drugs that human experience shows to be associated with birth defects, but the potential benefits of the drugs may be acceptable despite their known risks. A category D drug will generally be one indicated for use in a life-threatening situation or serious disease for which safer drugs cannot be used or are ineffective. If a category D drug is given to a pregnant woman, or if the patient becomes pregnant while taking it, the physician should inform her of the potential risk to the fetus.

Category X will include drugs for which fetal abnormalities have been demonstrated in animal or human studies and the potential risks of the drugs clearly outweigh their potential benefits. Such drugs will be contraindicated for use during pregnancy.

FDA recommends that the physician advise the pregnant patient of the potential hazard if she intentionally or inadvertently uses the drug.

Reprinted from FDA *Drug Bulletin* (September, 1979), pp. 23–24.

You should make every attempt to determine which drugs the patient may be using. **The amount of alcohol ingested, the number of cigarettes smoked, and the quantities of other drugs being used should be identified.** An assessment of the patient's emotional status should be made, since many of these people may have severe social and psychological problems. The patient may manifest symptoms that suggest the kind of drug she is using. For example, depression, anxiety, and irritability, may occur in patients who are using amphetamines.

Finding out about the patient's relationship to other members of her family may also be of value in identifying her particular problems. Family members may be able to supply information about the patient's **problems with the law** (e.g., drunk driving, drug arrests) and problems with her neighbors or family. The patient will almost always deny the use of drugs of abuse, and it may be difficult to convince her that you wish to help her even if you do have strong evidence that she is an addict. A display of sensitivity and kindness on your part may be beneficial in developing rapport with the patient. You should bear in mind that the husband may also be a drug abuser, and indeed may supply both himself and his wife with drugs that he obtains from street sources or by forging prescriptions.

1) Alcoholism

The **fetal alcohol syndrome** has been noted in as many as 40% of the infants of mothers who drink **6 alcoholic drinks per day (6 oz)** during the first trimester of pregnancy. This syndrome consists of craniofacial abnormalities, such as a low forehead, a small upturned nose, a sunken nasal bridge, short palpebral fissures, a receding chin, and low-set ears, as well as cardiac defects and multiple joint abnormalities. Intrauterine growth retardation is also present in these infants. The perinatal mortality rate of infants with this syndrome is 17%.

2) Smoking

Smoking cigarettes during pregnancy has been shown to cause about a **200-gram decrease in the infant's birth weight** as compared to infants of women who do not smoke. While the exact number of cigarettes smoked to produce this weight difference is unknown, it does seem to be associated with the use of 10 or more cigarettes per day. In patients who smoke over 15 cigarettes per day, it has been noted that the infant not only weighs less, but also the head circumference and body length are decreased. The time of greatest influence is during the **last four months of pregnancy** and is probably related to the decreased oxygenation of the fetus resulting from the formation of **carboxyhemoglobin** and the decreased uterine blood flow, which is secondary to the **nicotine ef-**

fect. There seems to be a good correlation between the level of **serum cotinine** (i.e., the major metabolite of nicotine) and the reduced fetal birth weight. There is also a slightly increased spontaneous abortion rate and perinatal mortality rate among infants of smoking mothers.

Caffeine consumption of more than 300 mg/day may have an additive effect in patients who smoke more than 15 cigarettes per day. In addition, some concern has been expressed concerning the high cadmium levels present in cigarette smoke in regard to fetal zinc levels and birth weight. Infants with intrauterine growth retardation have been shown to have less leukocyte zinc than normal infants. It has been postulated that the more the woman smokes, the greater the level of cadmium, the greater the placental zinc, and the lower the fetal weight and the fetal red blood cell zinc content, due to the trapping of the zinc in the placenta.

c. Narcotic drug addiction

For a number of years it was thought that heroin addicts were infertile; however, such is not the case. Indeed, the incidence of pregnancy in drug addicts has been on the increase over the past 15 years.

1) Risk factors

The pregnant drug addict of today carries a number of risk factors. These stem from: (1) minimal prenatal care, (2) a history of using more than one drug, (3) poor nutritional status, (4) the use of drugs of variable potency, and (5) the inclusion of a variety of adulterants mixed with the drugs, the results of which are often unknown. Some of the drugs that are commonly used include alcohol, narcotic agents, tranquilizing agents, phencyclidine hydrochloride (PCP, angel dust), cocaine, and tetrahydrocannabinol (THC).

Recently, there has been an increased usage of **cocaine** in all levels of our society. This agent has been further concentrated by certain techniques to produce a highly dangerous form of cocaine called "crack." The early evidence seems to show that the infants of mothers who are addicted to cocaine may undergo withdrawal symptoms in utero, may be small for their gestational age, and may deliver prematurely. In addition, placental abruption has been noted in some cases. Cocaine is vasoconstrictive and affects cat-

echolamine levels, which perhaps accounts for some of these complications.

The pregnant addict and her neonate are subject to a number of medical complications that are related to the addiction and the patient's life-style. *As many as 56% of addicts receive no prenatal care at all. Hepatitis,* and more recently, the *acquired immune deficiency syndrome (AIDS),* occurs more commonly among addicts who share the use of hypodermic needles than in the general population. *The poor nutritional state* of the patient often leads to *anemia* and a *poor weight gain* during pregnancy. Intrauterine growth retardation occurs in 30–50% of heroin users. **Meconium staining of the amniotic fluid occurs in addicted patients.** *Infections,* both at needle sites and in other sites, such as the lungs, heart, and kidneys, may result from a decreased host defense mechanism. Right-sided endocarditis due to infection secondary to intravenous drug abuse has also recently been described in these patients. The life-styles of drug users often includes sexual permissiveness, which may lead to the acquisition of *sexually transmitted diseases,* such as gonorrhea, syphilis, and herpesvirus type 2. Other vaginal infections, such as trichomoniasis, monilial vaginitis, gardnerella vaginalis vaginitis, chlamydial infections, and condyloma acuminatum, are also more common in these patients. A history of a previous premature labor, premature rupture of the membranes, abruptio placentae, and/or a spontaneous abortion may also be more likely in such patients. A maternal urine drug screen may identify illicit drug ingestion.

2) Withdrawal

In the pregnant narcotic addict, it is important that the patient continue to use heroin or methadone, since if she does stop, then the fetus may undergo withdrawal symptoms and die in utero. This is especially important during labor, since fetal withdrawal may be triggered if narcotics are withheld at this time. The **early symptoms of withdrawal** in the pregnant patient may alert you to the fact that you are dealing with an addict, since few patients, if any, will ever admit to their addiction. The presence of twitching and tremulousness may be early signs of withdrawal. The development of such symptoms as sweating, yawning, lacrimation, rhinorrhea, restlessness, dilated pupils, myalgia, muscle twitching, tachycardia, tachypnea, fever, anorexia, nausea, and eventually severe symptoms of extreme restlessness, abdominal pain, vomiting, hypertension, and diarrhea, all indicate that the patient is undergoing withdrawal symptoms.

The patient may first reveal to the physicians and nurses her addiction when she **signs herself out "against medical advice" (AMA)** shortly after delivery; this behavior is due to her drug craving and her inability to obtain illicit drugs in the hospital setting. On occasion, such a patient will appear to be mollified sufficiently to remain in the hospital after you have talked to her, only for you to find out later that the patient's relatives and friends supplied her with the needed drugs while she was still in the hospital.

3) Complications

Withdrawal symptoms can be experienced by the fetus as well as by the mother, and in as many as 33% of pregnant addicts, meconium will be present in the amniotic fluid, presumably due to fetal hypoxia and episodes of withdrawal. *In 18–50% of pregnant addicts, premature rupture of the membranes occurs. There seems to be a five- to six-fold increase in stillbirths among addicts, with one report noting a stillbirth rate of 71:1,000 births.* A low birth weight is very common in the infants of addicts and is probably caused by their prematurity as well as to the poor nutritional status and the life-styles of these mothers. Other pregnancy complications that may occur include toxemia, fetal malpresentation, abruptio placentae, and an increased incidence of puerperal morbidity.

4) Treatment

The physician who treats a **pregnant narcotic addict** must consider the fetus as well as the mother. **Acute detoxification (i.e., withdrawal) should not be performed during pregnancy, due to the potential hazardous effects of such treatment on the fetus.** During withdrawal, it has been demonstrated that there is an increase in the levels of epinephrine and norepinephrine. If the **methadone maintenance program** is utilized in the heroin addict, high doses (i.e., 80 mg+ per day) will effect a blockade and prevent the user from obtaining a euphoric state if she uses heroin illicitly. Conversely, in the low-dose methadone maintenance programs, a lower dose (i.e., 10–40 mg per day) may be administered to merely maintain the patient and prevent withdrawal symptoms from occurring.

Narcotics should be administered to the patient in labor. Meperidine hydrochloride (Demerol) or hydromorphone hydrochloride (Dilaudid) may be used. **Pentazocine lactate (Talwin) should not be used, since it may precipitate withdrawal due to its antagonistic action to narcotics.**

The treatment of the neonate requires a close evaluation of the infant for evidence of a significant weight loss, tremors, general hyperactivity, convulsions, hypertonus, and other signs of withdrawal. This observation should be carried out for at least the first 72 hours, especially if the mother was on methadone, since the onset of the withdrawal symptoms with this drug takes a longer time than with the other narcotics. The long-term effects of narcotic addiction on the neonate are largely unknown. It is thought that it may affect the future personality development and the learning behavior of the infant.

d. Chemical exposure

In the late 1950s and early 1960s, nearly 8,000 cases of phocomelia in newborn infants were found to occur in Europe as the result of the administration of the sedative **thalidomide** to pregnant women. In the past 30 years, it has become evident that the use of **diethylstilbestrol** in pregnant women to prevent abortion was also a mistake, since nearly 500 cases of clear-cell adenocarcinoma of the vagina have occurred in the offspring of these patients, in addition to other genital developmental abnormalities.

In 1953, organic **methyl mercury poisoning** of pregnant women occurred in Minamata Bay in the Kyushu District of Japan as a result of the contamination of the food chain by a plastics factory that discharged its waste material into the bay. The infants of those women who were exposed to methyl mercury had severe brain damage (i.e., cerebral palsy). A similar episode occurred in a family in Alamogordo, New Mexico, in 1970, when the family ate hogs that had been fed seed grain treated with a **methyl mercury–containing fungicide.** In Iraq, thousands of people were exposed to methyl mercury poisoning when they ate bread that had been made from wheat and barley grain that had been treated with a methyl mercury fungicide.

In 1972, an epidemic of **chloracne** occurred among children and adults in Japan who used a particular brand of cooking oil. The contamination of the cooking oil by the leakage of polychlorinated biphenyl (PCB), a heat transfer agent, through corroded pipes was identified as the cause.

Other common pollutants of the atmosphere that have been identified include oxides of nitrogen, oxides of sulfur, carbon monoxide, and hydrocarbons. Food additives and dyes have been used for years to improve the color and taste of food. Moreover, hormones and antibiotics have also been used to improve food products. Household chemicals, adhesives, soaps, and plastics, in addition to numerous aerosols and cosmetic products, add further to the pollution of our environment.

It has only been during the past 30 years or so that the teratogenicity of drugs and chemicals, and the ability of certain drugs to interact with other drugs to cause effects that could be detrimental to both the patient and the fetus, have been appreciated. In earlier years, it was taught that any number of medications could be administered to a patient and that they would not interfere with one another. Similarly, it was thought that environmental chemicals would not cause harm to the fetus. These concepts have since been found to be totally erroneous.

The question might be asked as to why we do not test all drugs and chemicals and find out which ones are dangerous to human beings. Unfortunately, this kind of testing is impossible. In the first place, in order to show a teratogenic increase in the incidence of a given abnormality, such as the incidence of anencephaly, from a background level of 1:1,000 to a level of 2:1,000, which could be attributed to a certain drug or chemical, it has been calculated that it would require the administration of the "suspect" chemical to 23,000 women in the first trimester of pregnancy. In actual practice, however, in order for the change to be recognized clinically, it would require that the background incidence of an anomaly would have to be increased several thousand-fold in order for it to be suspected by the medical practitioner. Thus, literally thousands of women would have to be exposed to a specific teratogen before it would become clinically apparent. Obviously, such experiments on human beings could not ethically be performed, and unfortunately, the effects of drugs and chemicals in the various species of lower animals have not always been the same as in humans. The results of such studies in lower animals must be accepted with a great deal of skepticism in most cases.

e. Irradiation

The use of **diagnostic radiologic procedures** in pregnancy almost never results in a sufficient amount of radiation to cause serious concern for the fetus. It is thought that a radiation dose of less than 5 rads is not teratogenic; however, when the dose exceeds **10 rads,** a therapeutic abortion should be considered. The crude determination of the number of rads involved in different X-ray procedures can be calculated by a radiologist, who can then provide you with an estimate of the dosage involved in a specific X-ray procedure. Radioisotopic studies should not be utilized in pregnancy if at all possible, and this is especially true of radioactive iodine, since the fetal thyroid has a great affinity for iodine.

2. Infections

A number of infectious diseases may involve the fetus and cause congenital anomalies, organ damage, or abortion (Table 28-2). The incidence of viral and parasitic infections during pregnancy has been estimated to be about 5–15%. Damage to the fetus in utero, however, as a consequence of these infections has only been evident in about 1–2% of these pregnancies. Cytomegalovirus, rubella, syphilis, toxoplasmosis, and varicella have all been documented to cause fetal damage.

There are four types of immunizing agents available: (1) immunoglobulin preparations (IG), (2) live vaccines, (3) killed vaccines, and (4) toxoids. Immunoglobulins, killed vaccines, and toxoids may be used in pregnancy; however, *live vaccines* should be avoided in pregnancy.

a. Viral infections

Viral infections in pregnancy are often severe and some carry a risk of fetal involvement. The presence of a maternal viremia may set up inflammatory foci in the placenta with the subsequent transmission of the virus to the fetus (e.g., vaccinia, variola, varicella), or there may be fetal involvement without any discernible placental lesions (e.g., Coxsackie B, mumps, poliomyelitis). It is also possible for viral infections to infect the fetus by the vaginal route (e.g., cytomegalovirus, herpesvirus type 2).

Text continues on p. 410

TABLE 28-2. Documented teratogens

Agent	Effects	Comments
Drugs and Chemicals		
Alcohol	Growth retardation, mental retardation, microcephaly, reduced size of palpebral fissures, various major and minor malformations	Nutritional deficiency states, smoking, and drug use confound data. Risk due to ingestion of one to two drinks per day (1–2 oz) is not well-defined but may cause a small reduction in average birth weight. Fetuses of women who drink six drinks per day (6 oz) are at a 40% risk to show some features of the fetal alcohol syndrome.
Androgens	Pseudohermaphroditism in female offspring, advanced genital development in males	Effects are dose dependent and related to stage of embryonic development. Depending on time of exposure, clitoral enlargement or labioscrotal fusion can be produced. The risk related to incidental brief androgenic exposure is minimal.
Anticoagulants, e.g., warfarin (Coumadin; Panwarfin) and dicumarol	Hypoplastic nose, bony abnormalities, stippling of secondary epiphyses, broad short hands with shortened phalanges, ophthalmologic abnormalities, intrauterine growth retardation, anomalies of neck, central nervous system (CNS) defects	Risk for a seriously affected child is considered to be 25% when anticoagulants that inhibit vitamin K are used in the first trimester. Later drug exposure may be associated with spontaneous abortions, stillbirths, CNS abnormalities, abruptio placentae, and fetal or neonatal hemorrhaging.
Antithyroid drugs, e.g., propylthiouracil, iodide, and methimazole (Tapazole)	Hypothyroidism, fetal goiter	Goiter in fetus may lead to malpresentation with hyperextended head. Effect is in part related to dose and duration of therapy.
Chemotherapeutic drugs, e.g., methotrexate (Mexate) and aminopterin	Increased risk for spontaneous abortions, various anomalies	These drugs are generally contraindicated for the treatment of psoriasis in pregnancy and must be used with extreme caution in the treatment of malignancy. Most authors indicate that cytotoxic drugs are potentially teratogenic. Effects of aminopterin are well documented. Folic acid antagonists used during the first trimester produce up to a 30% malformation rate in fetuses that survive.
Diethylstilbestrol (DES)	Vaginal adenosis, abnormalities of cervix and uterus in females, possible infertility in males and females	Vaginal adenosis is detected in over 50% of women whose mothers took these drugs before the ninth week of pregnancy. Risk for vaginal adenocarcinoma is low. Males exposed in utero may have a 25% incidence of epididymal cysts, hypotrophic testes, abnormal spermatozoa, and induration of the testes.

TABLE 28-2. *(continued)*

Agent	Effects	Comments
Isotretinoin (Accutane)	Increased abortion rate, microtia, nervous system defects, cardiovascular effects, craniofacial dysmorphism, microphthalmos, cleft palate	First-trimester exposure may result in approximately 25% anomaly rate.
Lead	Increased abortion rate and stillbirths	Central nervous system development of the fetus may be adversely affected.
Lithium	Congenital heart disease, in particular, Ebstein's anomaly	Heart malformations due to first-trimester exposure occur in approximately 2%. Exposure in the last month of gestation may produce toxic effects on the thyroid, kidneys, and neuromuscular systems.
Organic mercury	Cerebral atrophy, mental retardation, spasticity, seizures, blindness	Cerebral palsy can occur even when exposure is in the third trimester. Exposed individuals include consumers of contaminated grain and fish. Contamination is usually with methyl mercury.
Phenytoin (Dilantin)	Growth deficiency, mental retardation, microcephaly, dysmorphic features, hypoplastic nails and distal phalanges	Full syndrome is seen in less than 10% of children exposed in utero; up to 30% have some manifestations. Mild to moderate mental retardation is found in two-thirds of children who have severe physical stigmata.
Streptomycin	Hearing loss, VIIIth nerve damage	Animal studies show histologic changes in the inner ear.
Tetracycline	Hypoplasia of tooth enamel, incorporation of tetracycline into bone	Drug has no known effect unless exposure occurs in second or third trimester.
Thalidomide	Bilateral limb deficiencies—days 27–40, anotia and microtia—days 21–27, other anomalies	Of children whose mothers used thalidomide, 20% show the effect.
Trimethadione (Tridione) and paramethadione (Paradione)	Cleft lip or cleft palate, cardiac defects, growth retardation, microcephaly, mental retardation, ophthalmologic abnormalities	Risk for defects or spontaneous abortion is 60–80% with first-trimester exposure. A syndrome including V-shaped eyebrows, low-set ears, high arched palate, and irregular dentition has been identified.
Valproic acid (Depakene)	Neural tube defects	Exposure must be prior to normal closure of neural tube during first trimester to get open defect. Neural tube defects can be diagnosed by alpha-fetoprotein or ultrasound. Incidence of neural tube defects in exposed fetuses is 1–2%.
Infections		
Cytomegalovirus (CMV)	Microcephaly, retardation of somatic growth, brain damage, and hearing loss	Although 0.5–1.5% of newborns may have CMV colonization, the frequency of severe defects due to CMV at birth is approximately 0.1/1000 newborns.

(continued)

TABLE 28-2. *(continued)*

Agent	Effects	Comments
Rubella	Cataracts, deafness, heart lesions, plus expanded syndrome including effects on all organs	Malformation rate is 50% if mother is infected during first trimester. Rate of permanent organ damage decreases to 6% by midpregnancy. Immunization of children and nonpregnant adults is necessary for prevention. Immunization is not recommended during pregnancy, but vaccine virus has not been shown to cause the malformations of congenital rubella syndrome.
Syphilis*	If severe infection, fetal demise with hydrops; if mild, detectable abnormalities of skin, teeth, and bones	Penicillin treatment is effective for Treponema pallidum eradication to prevent progression of damage. Severity of fetal damage depends on duration of infection of fetus during gestation.
Toxoplasmosis*	Possible effects on all organs; severity of manifestations dependent on duration of disease	The initial maternal infection must occur during pregnancy to place fetus at risk. Toxoplasma gondii is transmitted to humans by raw meat or exposure to infected cat feces. Incidence of fetal infection is as low as 15% in the first trimester increasing to approximately 75% in the third trimester; however, the severity of congenital infection is greater in the first trimester than at the end of gestation. Treat with pyrimethamine and sulfadiazine (2,3).
Varicella*	Possible effects on all organs including skin scarring and muscle atrophy	Frequency of congenital varicella is low. Zoster immune globulin is available for newborns exposed in utero during last few days of gestation.
Radiation		
X-ray therapy	Microcephaly, mental retardation	Medical diagnostic radiation (less than 10 rads) has little or no teratogenic risk.

*Syphilis, toxoplasmosis, and varicella may be classified as "fetal pathogens" since they produce damage to fully or partially formed tissues by direct infection—they are not limited to inducing abnormal development during organogenesis.

Reproduced with permission from American College of Obstetricians and Gynecologists, "Teratology," *ACOG Technical Bulletin* 84 (1985), pp. 2–4.

The amount of damage that the fetus sustains with a transmitted viral infection is dependent upon the time of gestation that the infection takes place, the ability of the virus to destroy fetal cells, the amount of the initial inoculum, and the ability of the virus to replicate in the fetal tissues. Infections during the period of organogenesis (i.e., 13–56 days' gestation) may cause developmental defects in the fetus, whereas later fetal infections may produce organ damage secondary to the ravages of the infection itself.

1) Rubella

Only about 15% of patients are susceptible to rubella. The occurrence of rubella in pregnancy, especially during the first trimester, however, is cause for considerable concern that the fetus may develop the rubella syndrome. The incubation period is about 14–21 days.

The infection in the mother may present as a mild febrile illness with a rash, and occasionally with myalgia and joint pains. The rash is often prominent on the face and is accompanied by an enlargement of the posterior cervical and postauricular lymph nodes. Rarely, encephalitis may occur. *The viremia precedes the clinical symptoms by 5–7 days, and the patient is the most contagious about 1–2 days before the development of the rash. Infection during the first trimester carries an overall risk of 20% for fetal anomalies, with the risk being possibly as high as 50% in the first month, 22–25% in the second month, and 7–10% during the third month.* The incidence of spontaneous abortion is increased, and the virus may be recovered from the abortion material in 50–90% of these cases. Infection in the second and third trimesters may result in infectious sequelae in the fetus. *The most frequent anomalies that are seen in the rubella syndrome are cataracts, cardiac lesions (patent ductus arteriosus), hearing impairment, mental retardation, and low birth weight, although lesions may be seen in almost any organ system.* The congenitally involved infant may shed the virus for months or years afterwards.

The management of the pregnant patient who has been exposed to rubella consists of first determining the patient's baseline **immune status.** If a hemagglutinating inhibition (HI) antibody test that is drawn either prior to the exposure or within a few days of the exposure is positive (i.e., a titer of 1:16 or greater), then the patient should be considered to be immune to rubella and should not be at risk. If, on the other hand, the titer is of the order of 1:8, then a repeat titer should be obtained in seven days and should be run in conjunction with the initial titer. If the results are the same, then the patient may be considered to be immune. Any titer less than 1:8 is considered to represent susceptibility, and a baseline specimen and one obtained 3–4 weeks later should be run simultaneously to determine any rise in the titer that would be due to an infection by the rubella virus. A positive rubella culture of the pharynx obtained after exposure to rubella will also provide positive evidence of infection. The use of gamma globulin in patients who have been exposed to rubella is a controversial topic, but it probably should be given, since it may mollify the infection. Should a confirmed rubella infection occur within the first trimester, then a therapeutic or voluntary abortion should be considered.

Women who are not pregnant but who are susceptible to the rubella virus should be vaccinated. It is recommended that the patient be placed on an adequate birth control program one month prior to the vaccination and that these birth control measures be continued for another three months afterwards to prevent conception during this time. In patients who were pregnant at the time of vaccination with HPV 77, the rubella virus was recovered from 21% of 28 abortions. Those who carried their infants to term had babies that appeared normal; however, rubella-specific IgM protein was present in 10% of these infants, indicating that an intrauterine infection had occurred. It would appear that the risk of fetal involvement from vaccination is small, perhaps less than the 20–25% risk of a naturally acquired infection. The vaccination of children in a household in which the mother is pregnant apparently does not present a risk, even though the virus may be shed from the pharynx for 7–28 days following vaccination.

2) Herpesvirus group

The members of the herpesvirus group are herpes simplex virus, Epstein-Barr viruses, varicella-zoster virus (VZ), and the cytomegalovirus (CMV).

a) Herpes simplex virus

There are two types of the herpes simplex virus (HSV). HSV type 1 is an infection of nongenital tissues ("fever blisters"), whereas HSV type 2 is usually a sexually transmitted disease. It is possible to find either virus involved at both sites in individuals who practice orogenital intercourse (see Chapter 11).

About 1–2% of all pregnancies are complicated by infections with the herpesvirus. In a **primary infection,** the clinical symptoms of headache, myalgia, fever, atypical lymphocytosis, and generalized lymphadenopathy are associated with vesicular lesions that are filled with a clear liquid and are quite painful.

The presence of multinucleated giant cells with intranuclear inclusion bodies on exfoliated cells in a Papanicolaou smear is suggestive of a herpesvirus infection. If these cytopathic effects are found in a viral tissue culture, the diagnosis is confirmed. Occasionally, a Papanicolaou smear will uncover the herpesvirus as the etiology of a cervical erosion or cervicitis.

Apparently, the herpesvirus may infect the fetus transplacentally; however, it more commonly infects the fetus during its passage through the birth canal at the time of delivery, causing a disseminated infection 7–21 days after delivery. An ascending infection may occur after the rupture of the membranes, and perhaps even when the membranes are intact. Fetal involvement may occur in the form of a vesicular rash, microcephaly, chorioretinitis, or central nervous system calcifications.

If there is evidence during pregnancy of a herpetic infection (HSV type 2) after 20 weeks' gestation, then the chance of an intrauterine infection may be increased. If other evidence is available sonographically to indicate fetal intrauterine growth retardation, then it has been suggested that an amniocentesis should be performed and cultures carried out to determine whether the virus is indeed present. *Patients who have genital herpetic lesions at the time of labor should be delivered by cesarean section to prevent the fetus from being exposed to the virus during the delivery process. The previous concern about the length of time that the membranes have been ruptured is no longer considered in making this decision.*

b) Epstein-Barr virus

Chronic Epstein-Barr virus (CEBV) disease resembles mononucleosis with its symptoms of unexplained fatigue and illness. The patients are usually white females between the ages of 13 and 52 who may experience myalgia, arthralgia, fever, sore throat, and headaches. Little is known about this disease and its effects on pregnancy.

c) Varicella-zoster virus

Both shingles (zoster) and chickenpox (varicella) are caused by the varicella-zoster virus (VZV), a DNA herpesvirus. **Chickenpox** is rare in pregnancy, but when it occurs, it may be severe and may include varicella pneumonia, which is often fatal. The incidence of varicella-zoster infections in pregnancy has been estimated to be about 1–5:10,000 pregnancies. While about 80–95% of all adults are immune to varicella, those who are susceptible to infection will manifest fever, malaise, and a pruritic rash between 10 and 20 days after exposure. These symptoms will then last for 7–10 days. Although a viremia is usually present, only about 24% of the fetuses of patients with chickenpox in one study were infected. Another report stated that there was only about a 2% chance of fetal damage from an in-utero exposure. Infants affected may have widespread disseminated organ disease, which is associated with a high neonatal mortality rate, or they may have only a few skin lesions and a mild infection. When the infection is contracted within the first trimester, as many as 10% of these infants may develop a congenital syndrome consisting of limb hypoplasia, chorioretinitis, cutaneous scars, cataracts, cortical atrophy, and microcephaly. **If the mother contracts chickenpox immediately prior to or shortly after delivery, then the infant should be treated with varicella-zoster immune globulin (VZIG) (1.25 ml), a high-potency pooled immune serum derived from patients who are recovering from zoster infections.** Isolation of both the mother and the infant should be carried out after delivery. The complement fixation test (CF), the immune adherence hemagglutination test (IAHA), the fluorescent antibody membrane antigen test (FAMA), and the enzyme-linked immunosorbent assay (ELISA) for chickenpox can be carried out to detect antibodies to VZV.

The development of shingles **(zoster)** in pregnancy is quite rare. It does not increase the risk for the mother, and the fetus is seldom involved. The disease represents a reactivation of the VZV in the dorsal root ganglia with the development of vesicular lesions along a dermatome distribution.

d) Cytomegalovirus infection

The cytomegalovirus causes a congenital infection in 0.5–2.0% of all newborns, but only about 10% of these will manifest evidence of the disease. The virus is widespread in nature and is common in the bodily secretions (i.e., milk, semen, vaginal secretions) of people who live in crowded and unsanitary conditions. *Once infected, the organism remains in the tissues, with periodic reactivation and viral shedding thereafter.* The cervix is frequently involved in these infections. The virus can be isolated in about 3% of pregnant patients in the first trimester, 5% in the second trimester, and 8% in the third trimester. The urinary tract (5%), breast milk (15%), and pharynx (2%) also harbor the virus. The recovery of cells from the urine containing intranuclear inclusion bodies serves to establish the diagnosis, and the fluorescent antibody test (FA), and the complement fixation test (CF) are also helpful in making the diagnosis. The indirect hemagglutination and ELISA tests are specific for CMV and may be utilized to test for antibodies.

In cases where *a primary CMV infection occurs during pregnancy, central nervous system abnormalities occur in about 1.2% of the fetuses.* In these infants, hepatosplenomegaly, jaundice, petechiae, and low birth weight are prominent findings. As many as 15% of these infants may later be found to have defects in the auditory or ocular systems. Many infants may be infected during their passage through the birth canal but may not manifest symptoms until later. If the infants are infected, 90% eventually develop blindness, epilepsy, mental retardation, spastic diplegia, hearing loss, and optic atrophy. Viral transmission also occurs in up to 58% of nursing infants who have infected mothers. There is no known method of prevention of these infections, nor is there any known treatment.

3) Mumps

Mumps is caused by a paramyxovirus, which is an RNA virus. *The occurrence of mumps in pregnancy is uncommon.* Clinically, mumps involves a viremia, which, after 2–3 weeks, is followed by parotid gland inflammation. In addition to the parotitis, there may be pancreatitis, oophoritis, or meningoencephalitis; however, in most cases the disease is rather mild. If the infection occurs in the first trimester, the incidence of spontaneous abortion is doubled. Vertical transmission to the fetus can be demonstrated by the presence of the mumps virus in the fetus or by immunologic findings. Nonpregnant females at risk should be given a live attenuated mumps virus vaccine to produce active immunization. This vaccine apparently induces a long-lasting immunity in 95% of the recipients. **It is contraindicated in pregnancy, however, since it is a live vaccine.** The administration of pooled immunoglobulin after exposure is not protective and thus not indicated.

4) Enterovirus infections

The enteroviruses include the poliovirus, the echovirus, and the Coxsackie viruses. Immunization policies have nearly eliminated polioviruses in the United States, although outbreaks of polio still periodically occur. **Polio in pregnancy has a higher maternal mortality rate than in nonpregnant women, and there is an increased fetal wastage.** While Coxsackie B virus infections also have a high stillbirth and prematurity rate, the other Cox-

sackie viruses and echoviruses do not seem to be as detrimental to pregnancy. There is no specific method of preventing infections with the echovirus or of the Coxsackie viruses. An inactivated poliovirus vaccine may be given to a pregnant woman if she is planning to be in an area where polio is highly endemic.

5) Influenza

The antigenic characteristics of the virus that produces influenza change frequently. Indeed, annual changes in the virus have been noted, which makes the prevention of this disease difficult. The viral strains A, B, and C are prominent in the myxovirus group. These viruses are about 100 nm in size, and they are RNA viruses. They contain nucleocapsids within a lipid envelope, which has glycoprotein spikes containing **hemagglutinin** and **neuraminidase.** While neuraminidase-derived antibodies may limit the spread of the disease, the hemagglutinin-derived antibodies will prevent the infection. **Changes in these two antigens (i.e., neuraminidase and hemagglutinin) are responsible for the changing antigenic patterns of the influenza viruses from year to year.**

The act of coughing or sneezing disseminates viral particles in an effective manner. These particles invade the nasopharynx and the lower bronchial tree and cause the clinical infection known as influenza. If immunoglobulin A (IgA) is present, the infection is stopped; if absent, then a replication of the virus occurs and an infection ensues. The severity of the infection is related to the cellular immunity and to the presence of immunoglobulin G (IgG) antibodies. Pregnant women have a moderate impairment of cell-mediated immunity in the second and third trimesters, which makes them more susceptible to this infection. **The clinical illness occurs after an incubation period of 1–3 days and lasts for about 3–4 days. The fever is typically higher than 101° F and is accompanied by chills, headache, myalgia, malaise, and a dry, unproductive cough.** The leukocyte count is normal or low, and the chest film is negative. Patients with underlying cardiopulmonary disease are also more susceptible to influenza and are more prone to succumb to the illness. Secondary bacterial pneumonia may also occur in these patients.

While the amniotic fluid may harbor viral particles, congenital abnormalities resulting from influenza have not been detected in humans.

The diagnosis of influenza may be made when hemagglutinin and complement fixation antibodies show a four-fold increase in the serum titer. **Vaccination may be carried out in pregnant women in the second and third trimesters if they are in a high-risk category (e.g., cardiovascular disease, chronic pulmonary disease, diabetes mellitus, Addison's disease).** Since these are totally inactivated vaccines, there should be no concern about teratogenicity; however, the Centers for Disease Control (CDC) has suggested that they should not be used in the first trimester. The CDC has also suggested that **amantadine hydrochloride** should not be used for prophylaxis in pregnant women.

b. Bacterial infections

1) Group B streptococci

During the past 10–15 years, an increasing number of neonatal infections have been found to be due to the *group B streptococci*. This bacterial organism is common in the upper respiratory tract, the gastrointestinal tract, and the genital tract. *Vaginal colonization occurs in 5–30% of pregnant women and may result from contamination from the rectum or by sexual transmission.* Culture evidence in one study demonstrated that group B streptococci were present in 26% of their population and in 31% of those patients with chorioamnionitis. An infant may be colonized during passage through the birth canal, but only about 1–2% of these infants will develop an active group B streptococcal infection. **Postpartum endometritis, with fever that occurs within the first 24 hours, should alert you to the possibility that a group B streptococcus infection may be present.** A cervical Gram stain has been found to have a 93% sensitivity, a 69% specificity, a 33% positive predictive value, and a 98% negative predictive value.

Two forms of group B streptococcus infection have been described in the infant: the early-onset type and the late-onset type. The **early-onset type** of infection usually occurs within the first 24 hours after delivery. It consists of symptoms of a rapidly developing septicemia, meningitis, or pneumonitis and is associated with shock and death in 40–60% of cases. All five strains of the bacterium may be involved. The **late-onset form** of disease generally occurs one or more weeks after delivery and may involve a more insidious onset of symptoms. Meningitis seems to be more common in the late-onset form of the disease, and *the serotype III strain is almost always involved in the late-onset form.* A culture of group B streptococci will generally show a mucoid colony surrounded by a zone of hemolysis on a blood agar plate. The bacteria can be separated into immunologic serotypes on the basis of their type-specific capsular polysaccharide antigens (i.e., type I_a, I_b, I_c, II, and III).

The colonization of the mother with group B streptococci may occur at any time throughout the pregnancy. The treatment of the patient has been of little value in eradicating the organism, as rapid recolonization occurs in most of the patients. The identification of the organism in the vagina of patients who are at high risk *(i.e., patients with prolonged rupture of the membranes, premature delivery, and low–birth weight infants)* has prompted the suggestion that such infants should be treated with 50,000 units of penicillin immediately after delivery. This procedure has been effective in decreasing fetal colonization and may be beneficial in eliminating serious sequelae.

2) Enterococci

The enterococci are represented most commonly by **Streptococcus faecalis,** a gram-positive coccus that is included in the Landsfield group D streptococci classification. These organisms are found in the genital tracts of about 10% of asymptomatic women, and in 25% of women with a postoperative endometritis following cesarean section. The antibiotics of choice for the treatment of this organism are a combination of penicillin and an aminoglycoside, such as gentamicin. Vancomycin hydrochloride may be used if the patient is allergic to penicillin. Ampicillin may be used in mild infections.

3) Escherichia coli

The most common aerobic gram-negative organism in the female genital tract is E. coli. It has been thought to be pathogenic in only 10–20% of pelvic infections; however, it is frequently seen in the bloodstreams of patients who have septic shock. While E. coli is susceptible to β-lactam antibiotics, including several of the new penicillins and cephalosporins, the drugs of choice are the aminoglycosides.

4) Staphylococcus aureus

This organism is found in the genital tracts of about 10% of asymptomatic women. It is also present in essentially 100% of patients who have toxic shock syndrome. Moreover, this organism is found to be present in 15–20% of women who have postoperative pelvic infections. About 85–95% of these organisms produce β-lactamase, which makes them resistant to penicillin, ampicillin, and the newer penicillins. Staphylococci are usually susceptible to the β-lactamase-resistant penicillins of the methicillin-nafcillin group, and to clindamycin and the cephalosporins.

5) Peptostreptococci

These organisms are very common in female genital tract infections and are present in 20–60% of pelvic infections. Peptostreptococci are susceptible to cephalosporins, penicillins, clindamycin, and metronidazole.

6) Bacteroides

Bacteroides bivius is the most common anaerobic organism in pelvic infections and is representative of the anaerobic gram-negative organisms. It has been found in 20% of patients with postpartum endometritis or chorioamnionitis and in as many as 40% of patients with pelvic infections. B. bivius is susceptible to clindamycin, metronidazole, the newer penicillins, and the newer cephalosporins.

Bacteroides disiens has been found to be present in 2–15% of women with genital infections. This organism is susceptible to the same antibiotics as B. bivius.

Bacteroides fragilis is less commonly found. It is susceptible to clindamycin, chloramphenicol, cefoxitin, and metronidazole.

7) Mycoplasmas

The **Mycoplasma hominis** organism is found in 30–50% of sexually active women and seems to be involved in intrapartum and postpartum infections. A more common mycoplasma organism is **Ureaplasma urealyticum,** which is present in 60–80% of sexually active patients. The antibiotics of choice in the treatment of mycoplasma infections are tetracycline and erythromycin.

8) Listeriosis

Listeriosis is caused by **Listeria monocytogenes,** a motile gram-positive bacillus that may exist in aerobic or microaerophilic conditions. It is a common inhabitant of the human intestinal tract and is also widely found in animals and in the soil. Recently, it was implicated in a large outbreak of perinatal listeriosis that was traced to Mexican-style cheeses and a contaminated dairy herd. **It is generally nonpathogenic, except in individuals who have some impairment of their host defense mechanisms (i.e., due to diabetes mellitus, alcoholism, or in immunosuppressed patients).** The infection may take the form of meningoencephalitis or disseminated sepsis, or it may involve specific organ systems, such as in arthritis or endocarditis.

When listeriosis occurs in the pregnant patient, it is most commonly seen in the last trimester. The patient may present with nonspecific flu-like symptoms of fever, chills, general malaise, myalgia, headache, and back pain. The blood cultures in these patients may be positive, and *premature labor or spontaneous abortion may occur.* The treatment consists of the administration of penicillin or ampicillin in high doses for 2–3 weeks. Neonatal infections may involve skin rashes, pneumonia, or meningitis.

9) Chlamydia trachomatis

Chlamydia trachomatis has been increasingly implicated in neonatal conjunctivitis and pneumonia (see Chapter 12). The conjunctivitis occurs about 5–14 days after birth and affects about 25–50% of the neonates who are exposed to maternal chlamydial cervicitis. Neonatal ocular prophylaxis with silver nitrate does not prevent the infection; however, it is thought that erythromycin ointment may be effective. Late pneumonia occurs in 10–20% of these infants. The treatment of choice in a chlamydial infection consists of the administration of erythromycin, tetracycline, or sulfonamides. Amoxicillin or ampicillin may also be used.

c. Protozoans

1) Toxoplasmosis

The protozoan **Toxoplasma gondii** produces a multisystem disease. It is usually contracted from cats who are allowed to hunt rodents, as human contact with the cat feces may infect the patient. In addition, the eating of rare meat from animals that have grazed in contaminated fields might also convey the disease. Cooking contaminated meat with a temperature of over 60° C will kill the infectious cysts. Almost 25% of all women in the United States have positive evidence of having had an infection with T. gondii. Acute toxoplasmosis has been estimated to occur in 0.5% of all pregnancies. The parasitemia that results from an infestation may cross the placenta and infect the fetus. The transmission to the fetus may also occur in chronic carrier states, when the trophozoites enter the maternal circulation. Maternal disease will involve the fetus in the first trimester in 15% of cases, in the second trimester in 25% of cases, and in the third trimester in 65% of cases. The disease in the fetus is similar to that of cytomegalic inclusion disease, in that severe intrauterine growth retardation, hydrocephalus or microcephalus, central nervous system (CNS) calcifications, chorioretinitis, microphthalmia, thrombocytopenia, jaundice, and fever may be noted.

The indirect immunofluorescent test and the Sabin-Feldman dye tests are thought to be diagnostic for toxoplasmosis. These tests will become positive about 2–3 weeks after an active infection begins. A significant increase in serial titers distinguishes a recent infection from a chronic one. An ELISA test may also be used.

The treatment of a Toxoplasma gondii infection is with pyrimethamine and folinic acid; however, due to the teratogenicity of pyrimethamine, it should not be used in the first trimester. Sulfonamides (e.g., sulfadiazine) have also been used effectively to treat this disease. The maternal disease is self-limited with a good prognosis.

3. Central nervous system disease

a. Epilepsy

1) Incidence

The incidence of epilepsy in pregnant women is approximately 0.15–0.44%. If a patient who is not eclamptic has her first seizure during pregnancy, a seizure workup should be carried out, including an electroencephalogram, skull films, a CT scan, a lumbar puncture, a complete blood count (CBC), a serum sodium, a serum calcium, a serum glucose, and a drug screen. An effort should be made to determine whether the seizures are *generalized or focal* and to determine how often they occur. In patients who have an established diagnosis of epilepsy, *about 50% will notice no change in the frequency of their seizures during preg-*

nancy, whereas slightly more than one-third will experience an increased frequency, and less than 15% will have a decreased frequency. The fatigue and sleeplessness of early pregnancy, as well as the lack of medication compliance that occurs with hyperemesis, may also cause an increase in the seizures. Serum levels of anticonvulsive medications decrease during pregnancy due to the increased blood volume and to the uncertain intestinal absorption of the drug in the presence of hyperemesis or hypomotility of the bowel. Since all of the anticonvulsive medications cause thrombocytopenia and a decrease in coagulation Factors II, VII, IX, and X, and because of the vitamin K deficiency, bleeding may be increased during pregnancy in epileptics who are treated with these medications.

2) Treatment

The treatment of pregnant epileptic patients should consist of a single anticonvulsive medication, whenever possible, and it should be administered in the lowest effective dose. Usually, however, phenytoin sodium (Dilantin) and phenobarbital are prescribed, although carbamazepine (Tegretol) or primidone (Mysoline) may also be utilized. Ethosuximide (Zarontin) and clonazepam (Klonopin) have been used for petit mal epilepsy; however, there may be a risk of birth defects. Trimethadione (Tridione) and valproic acid should be avoided in pregnancy due to the possibility of developing a **trimethadione embryopathy,** or, in the case of valproic acid, a fetal spina bifida. **The fetal hydantoin syndrome may occur in patients who take phenytoin during pregnancy. This syndrome consists of craniofacial abnormalities, mental retardation, growth retardation, and other anomalies;** however, there is some controversy as to whether it is entirely due to the drug or whether epilepsy and the abnormalities are linked regardless of treatment. Midline fusion defects (i.e., cleft lip or palate) are ten times more frequent and septal heart defects are four times more common in these patients. Diazepam, phenytoin, phenobarbital, or pentobarbital may be given intravenously in patients who are in status epilepticus. Carbamazepine (Tegretol) may be used in pregnancy (Pregnancy Category C), but since the milk contains about 60% of the maternal blood levels, nursing should probably be proscribed.

Supplemental medications for epileptic patients

during pregnancy include folic acid (1 mg) and iron and vitamins, including vitamin K supplementation during the last few weeks.

b. Paraplegia

The occurrence of pregnancy in paraplegic patients poses some special problems. Spinal cord injury does not interfere with fertility. During pregnancy, **urinary tract infections are common,** due to the relative stasis of the urine, or secondary to repeated catheterizations. Acute pyelonephritis, urinary calculi, and cystitis are common in paraplegic patients, and long-term antibiosis should be instituted with methenamine mandelate (Mandelamine) or nitrofurantoin. If an **anemia** develops during pregnancy, tissue resistance is reduced in these patients and "bed sores" **(i.e., decubitus ulcers)** may become a problem. The hemoglobin should be maintained above 10 grams/dl and the hematocrit above 30%. While oral iron is of benefit, it also may cause constipation in the paraplegic patient, so stool softeners should be prescribed in these patients in conjunction with the iron supplements.

These patients can be classified into three groups as follows: (1) those with a lesion below T11, T12, or L1 (sensory afferents from the uterus), (2) those with a lesion from T5 or T6 to T10, which results in a painless labor, and (3) those with a lesion above T5 or T6 (above the splanchnic outflow), which results in autonomic hyperreflexia.

Autonomic hyperreflexia (autonomic stress syndrome or mass reflex) may occur with the distention of any hollow viscus, such as the bladder or intestine, in patients who have a spinal cord lesion above the T5 or T6 vertebra. This response consists of paroxysmal hypertension, bradycardia or tachycardia, headache, flushing, diaphoresis, nasal stuffiness, cardiac irregularities, convulsions, and coma. **These paroxysms may be severe enough to result in cerebral hemorrhage and death.** It has been suggested that this response is secondary to the release of catecholamines.

Labor contractions are usually painless in paraplegic women. The uterus will contract even after the severance of its nerve supply, and labor will be painless if the spinal cord transection is above the 10th thoracic vertebra. In order to prevent **autonomic hyperreflexia,** it is necessary to insert a Foley catheter at the onset of labor to avoid bladder distention. Fetal heart rate monitoring should be instituted. The administration of diphenhydramine hydrochloride (Benadryl), promethazine hydrochloride (Phenergan), or diazepam (Valium) for the autonomic hyperreflexia, and hydralazine hydrochloride (Apresoline HCL) or phentolamine mesylate (Regitine), trimethaphan camsylate (Arfonad) or sodium nitroprusside (Nipride) to treat the hypertension, should be utilized as necessary. The outcome for the fetus should be good if any complications involving the mother are promptly corrected.

4. Reproductive tract disease

a. Adnexal torsion

Adnexal torsion during pregnancy is rare; however, the tortuosity of the veins along the fallopian tube may produce a twisting effect to the tube to cause torsion (see Chapter 15).

b. Incarceration of the uterus

In rare instances, the pregnant uterus may remain in a retroflexed position during the first 3–4 months of pregnancy and may fail to rise out of the pelvis, **resulting in an incarceration of the uterus in the true pelvis.** The patient may present with lower abdominal pain and cramps, and even with spotting. Urinary and fecal obstruction may also occur. The abdominal examination will reveal an absence of the fundus. On pelvic examination, the cul-de-sac will be found to be filled with the tender, retroflexed uterus, and the cervix will be displaced upwards behind the symphysis pubis. Gentle pressure on the uterus with the patient in the knee-chest position will often elevate the uterus out of the pelvis and resolve the problem, but the patient must be watched closely over the succeeding few weeks to prevent a recurrence. The use of a Hodge's pessary may temporarily help to keep the uterus more anterior and out of the true pelvis. After about 4–5 months, the uterus will be too large to incarcerate again in the pelvis. Occasionally, the uterus may have to be replaced back into the abdominal cavity under general anesthesia.

c. Sacculation of the uterus

On rare occasions, a diverticulum or a sacculation of the uterus occurs. Frequently, this very thin-walled sac may contain the placenta. The **etiology of this condition is unknown,** but it has been observed that the sacculation does not necessarily occur in subsequent pregnancies.

d. Uterine torsion

There is normally a dextrorotation of the uterus in pregnancy due to the effect of the solid fecal contents present in the descending and rectosigmoid colon (in contrast to the fluid contents in the right ascending colon), which tends to force the uterus to rotate into the right paracolic gutter. On extremely rare occasions, such dextrorotation of the uterus may become excessive and may embarrass the uterine circulation.

5. Neoplastic disease

a. Carcinoma of the cervix

Cervical dysplasia and carcinoma-in-situ do not need to be treated during pregnancy; treatment can usually be safely deferred until the pregnancy is completed, if the patient's lesion is monitored closely. A colposcopic evaluation of the cervix, with directed biopsies, should be performed initially in an effort to rule out invasion.

The extent of an invasive cancer of the cervix during pregnancy cannot be adequately staged and is frequently underestimated. In the past, it was thought that the delivery of an infant through a carcinomatous cervix would jeopardize the patient and that her prognosis would be much worse. Although the cervix may fail to dilate, or more probably will lacerate and produce severe hemorrhage, it would appear that the patient's prognosis is not affected by vaginal delivery. Nonetheless, the prevailing mode of delivery for the patient with an invasive cervical carcinoma is by cesarean section. In stage I cervical disease, a radical hysterectomy and a bilateral pelvic lymphadenectomy following the cesarean section has been shown to be effective. In more extensive disease, radiation therapy should also be utilized.

In early pregnancy, patients with invasive cervical cancer should receive external irradiation to effect an abortion. A D&C should then be performed to remove the products of conception, and then appropriate intracavitary radiation applicators can be placed in the cervix and uterus for definitive treatment. In mid-pregnancy, patients with invasive disease may undergo a hysterotomy with the removal of the products of conception prior to the administration of radiation therapy. In the late second trimester, it is sometimes possible to delay the therapy for a few weeks in an effort to allow the fetus an additional amount of time to attain enough maturity to survive a premature delivery by cesarean section, after which the appropriate treatment of the cancer can then be instituted. It is unknown whether such a delay in treatment jeopardizes the patient's ultimate prognosis, but it does at least allow the patient the option of obtaining a viable infant.

b. Breast carcinoma

The occurrence of carcinoma of the breast in pregnancy should be managed in the same manner as in the nonpregnant patient (see Chapter 16). If the patient is at less than 20 weeks' gestation, then the incidence of spontaneous abortion is minimal. If the pregnancy has advanced to the third trimester, then a premature delivery is not very common and definitive therapy, such as a mastectomy or tumor resection, should be accomplished. The tumor tissue should be evaluated for the presence of estrogen and progesterone receptors; however, these receptors are often absent in these patients. Adjuvant chemotherapy should be administered in patients with positive nodes and in those with evidence of metastatic disease. Subsequent pregnancies may be considered after one to two years if there is no further evidence of persistent tumor.

6. Miscellaneous diseases

a. Collagen disease

1) Systemic lupus erythematosus

The presence of systemic lupus erythematosus (SLE) is not uncommon in pregnancy. This disease is more prevalent in blacks, American Indians, and oriental women. **The laboratory findings may consist of a positive antinuclear factor, positive LE preparations, and a false positive serological test for syphilis in a patient who presents with the clinical findings of a butterfly malar rash (70–80%), arthritis (90%), convulsions, and renal disease. Other clinical findings include**

weight loss, fever, fatigue, pleuritis, pericarditis, photosensitivity, and psychosis.

In about 65% of patients, SLE does not affect the pregnancy. **In established cases of SLE, the patient will do well during pregnancy if there is clinical evidence of a remission during the six months preceding conception.** In the 30–35% of patients who have an exacerbation of their disease during pregnancy only 10% will experience significant morbidity. **Patients who present with pregnancy-induced hypertension (PIH), especially with convulsions, may be indistinguishable from those who have lupus nephropathy with neurologic sequelae.** The presence of lupus-induced hemolytic findings of leukopenia, hemolysis, and thrombocytopenia may further lend false support to the diagnosis of pregnancy-induced hypertension (PIH) with the HELLP syndrome (i.e., **H**emolysis, **E**levated **L**iver enzymes, and **L**ow **P**latelet count) instead of SLE.

Recently, a **lupus anticoagulant** has been identified in patients who have systemic lupus erythematosus as well as in some patients who do not have evidence of lupus. It is an IgG immunoglobulin that inhibits coagulation. The diagnosis should be strongly suspected by demonstrating a **prolonged activated partial thromboplastin time using platelet-poor plasma.** About 50–90% of lupus patients who have the lupus anticoagulant will also have a false-positive test for syphilis. Interestingly, although bleeding problems do not seem to occur in the clinical situation, an opposite effect of **arterial and venous thrombosis** seems to be more prevalent, occurring in 25–70% of individuals who have the lupus anticoagulant. The effect of the lupus anticoagulant on the fetus includes spontaneous abortion and fetal death. If lupus erythematosus (with the lupus anticoagulant) is not appropriately treated during pregnancy, then the fetal wastage may be as high as 98%. When low-dose aspirin, 75 mg/day (i.e., one baby aspirin) and high-dose corticosteroids (e.g., 40–60 mg of prednisone per day) are administered to these patients, the salvage rate is reversed, with nearly a 100% fetal survival.

Anticardiolipin (ACL) antibody, an antiphospholipid antibody, either alone or in conjunction with the lupus anticoagulant antibody, is associated with recurrent pregnancy losses and IUGR. Steroids also seem to improve the outcome in these patients. Those patients who have either lupus anticoagulant antibodies or anticardiolipin antibodies, or both, should

be maintained on immunosuppressive therapy for 4–8 weeks' postpartum to prevent postpartum thrombosis.

Nephropathy, along with hypertension and proteinuria, may develop in SLE and may lead to severe renal insufficiency or to the nephrotic syndrome. It is uncommon for pregnancy to occur in a woman who has a BUN of greater than 30 mg/dl, or a serum creatinine value of 3 mg/dl or more. Pregnancy-induced hypertension is often superimposed upon the hypertension that already exists in such patients. The treatment of SLE may involve the use of glucocorticoids or cytotoxic agents in doses that will suppress the clinical activity of the disease, and neither of these agents has been found to cause any developmental defects in the infants of these patients. Oral contraceptives should not be used in these patients in between pregnancies.

On rare occasions, the newborns of mothers who have systemic lupus erythematosus will develop a neonatal lupus erythematosus syndrome. **Congenital heart block** and endomyocardial fibrosis have also been described in these neonates.

2) Rheumatoid arthritis

Rheumatoid arthritis is a chronic inflammation of the joints characterized by a proliferative reaction of the synovial membranes. About three-fourths of the affected individuals are women, and the symptoms usually begin to appear between the ages of thirty and seventy. An insidious onset of fatigue, joint stiffness, weakness, and arthralgia is followed by joint swelling. The course of the illness is one of exacerbations and remissions. Other manifestations include vasculitis, the Sjögren's syndrome, pleurisy, pericarditis, neuropathy, lymphadenopathy, pulmonary nodules, and rheumatoid nodules.

Rheumatoid arthritis does not have an effect on pregnancy; however, pregnancy does have an effect upon the arthritis, with nearly three-fourths of the patients experiencing some relief of their symptoms. About 90% of these patients will have an exacerbation of their disease within two months' postpartum. Therapy with salicylates and corticoids has been effective.

b. Skin lesions

Most skin lesions have no appreciable effect on pregnancy, and neither does the pregnancy have any effect on the lesion. There are some dermatoses, however, which are peculiar to pregnancy.

A pregnancy-induced **pruritic eruption** of purplish or reddish-brown papules may occur during pregnancy. Treatment with corticoids has been recommended, since the perinatal mortality rate may be increased in the untreated patient.

Finally, **herpes gestationis** is a disease that occurs in pregnancy consisting of large papules or bullae and involving the skin of the abdomen and the extremities. Treatment with corticoids has also been beneficial in this condition.

c. Carpal tunnel syndrome

The median nerve of the hand passes under the transverse carpal ligament at the wrist. Occasionally, the edema of pregnancy may cause swelling of the median nerve with the resulting symptoms of tingling and cramping of the fingers **(i.e., the carpal tunnel syndrome).** The patient will generally complain of tingling and numbness of the hand (i.e., her hand has "gone to sleep") upon arising in the morning. Percussion of the wrist may elicit pain and tingling (Tinel's sign). A flexion splint worn during sleep may provide relief. Occasionally, cortisone injections may be necessary. A similar, although less common condition involving entrapment of the **posterior tibial nerve** below the medial malleolus may also occur in pregnancy.

d. Bell's palsy

Idiopathic facial nerve paralysis occurs in about 0.05% of pregnant women. The treatment consists of a 10-day course of prednisone, 40–60 mg per day.

CHAPTER 29

Cardiac disease

What can one hear with one's fingers? Vocal fremitus and a sharp second sound.

—*Sir William Osler**

1. Cardiac arrhythmia

Perhaps the most common types of arrhythmia seen in pregnancy are the various kinds of tachyarrhythmia (i.e., paroxysmal supraventricular tachycardia, atrial flutter, and atrial fibrillation). They may occur in association with certain medications (e.g., antiasthmatic preparations, decongestants), or they may be caused by the ingestion of caffeine-containing beverages such as colas, coffee, or tea. The elimination of such dietary factors may obviate the need for specific treatment. In addition, fatigue and the occurrence of anxiety-producing situations should be avoided. If medical treatment for these conditions becomes necessary during pregnancy, the usual drugs may be utilized (e.g., cardiac glycosides, quinidine, lidocaine, procainamide, disopyramide, beta-adrenergic blocking agents, and verapamil), and if necessary, electrical cardioversion may also be used without danger to the fetus.

Permanent bradycardia is usually due to an atrioventricular block. Pregnancy in these patients is well

tolerated if there are no other cardiac problems involved.

2. Cardiomyopathy

Peripartum cardiomyopathy has been defined as a cardiac disease that: (1) occurs during the peripartum period, (2) occurs in a patient who has had no previous history of cardiac problems, and (3) is attributable to no known etiology. While a number of known etiologies have been proposed, such as hypertensive disease, viral myocarditis, idiopathic myocardial degeneration, beriberi heart disease, autoimmune myocarditis, or familial causes, none of these conditions have been accepted as the etiologic cause of peripartum cardiomyopathy.

The incidence of peripartum cardiomyopathy has been estimated to be of the order of 1:1,300 to 1:4,000 pregnancies. It occurs in whites and orientals, but appears to be more common in blacks in the United States. It is often *more common in multiparous black women,* and the incidence of twins in cases associated with cardiomyopathy is of the order of 7–10%. **The maternal mortality rate is 30–60%, while the fetal death rate is about 10%.**

The patient with cardiomyopathy usually experiences symptoms of dyspnea, cough, edema, and tachyarrhythmia that develop from about the seventh month of pregnancy up to five months' postpartum. **The autopsy findings include dilatation and enlargement of all four chambers of the heart, which is pale and flabby.** If the patient survives, the subsequent prognosis is poor if the heart size does not return to normal within six months, or if congestive heart failure again develops during a subsequent pregnancy.

---

*Reprinted with permission from Robert Bennett Bean, *Sir William Osler: Aphorisms from His Bedside Teachings and Writings,* William Bennett Bean, ed. Springfield, Ill.: Charles C Thomas, Publisher, 1968, p. 38.

3. Acquired heart disease

a. Mitral stenosis

Mitral stenosis is caused by rheumatic fever and is the most common type of acquired heart lesion. Due to the obstruction of the blood flow between the left atrium and the left ventricle, any demands for an increased cardiac output, such as occurs in pregnancy, may cause an increased atrial pressure. This pressure is then transmitted to the pulmonary system, producing transudation of fluid into the pulmonary alveolar walls (i.e., pulmonary edema). A pulmonary capillary wedge pressure (PCWP) of greater than 28 mm Hg is associated with pulmonary edema (i.e., via a Swan-Ganz balloon flotation catheter). These pressure changes in the left atrium may also lead to atrial fibrillation and the development of an atrial mural thrombus and possible embolization. The treatment of this valvular lesion may require mitral commissurotomy or the placement of an artificial heart valve. Anticoagulation should be utilized if atrial fibrillation occurs. The usual cardiac treatment regimens, such as digitalis, low-sodium diet, and bedrest are recommended as necessary. Rheumatic fever prophylaxis should be given during pregnancy, and subacute bacterial endocarditis (SBE) prophylaxis should be administered during delivery. **Epidural block is the anesthetic of choice for delivery in patients with mitral stenosis.**

b. Mitral insufficiency

This type of lesion is generally well tolerated during pregnancy; however, it is occasionally necessary to replace the valve during pregnancy. Rheumatic fever and SBE prophylaxis should be administered to these patients. Epidural anesthesia is effective in the management of these patients during delivery.

c. Aortic stenosis

Although this type of lesion is rarely seen in pregnancy, when it does occur, it produces an obstruction of the aortic outflow stream from the left ventricle. **As a consequence, any pregnancy demands for an increased cardiac output may not be met, which could lead to an episode of sudden dyspnea, chest pain, syncope, and death. The maternal mortality rate has been reported to be 17% in these cases, whereas the perinatal mortality rate**

is 31%. Since these patients may not be able to compensate for the decreases in the venous return and in the systemic vascular resistance that occurs with epidural anesthesia, other types of anesthesia should be used for delivery.

d. Aortic insufficiency

This type of cardiac lesion is rarely associated with congestive heart failure, but when it is, conventional medical therapy is usually successful in pregnant patients. If endocarditis occurs, or if medical therapy is ineffective, the aortic valve should be replaced with an artificial valve. Epidural anesthesia may be used for delivery.

e. Tricuspid and pulmonary valve lesions

Usually these types of lesions are associated with severe involvement of the mitral and aortic valves. A newly defined entity of **right-sided endocarditis** has been reported in relation to drug addiction, due to the use of intravenous drugs of abuse.

4. Congenital heart disease

Congenital heart disease is much more common today in pregnancy because of the newer advances in both the diagnosis and the treatment of many of these cardiac lesions. **The risk of a mother having a child with a congenital heart defect that is similar to her own is about 2–4%.**

a. Septal defects

Left-to-right shunting occurs with septal defects due to the pressure gradient between the arterial and venous sides of the vascular system. If the septal defect is large and there is a considerable amount of shunting, then pulmonary hypertension and right ventricular failure will ultimately occur. Spontaneous closure occurs in perhaps 50% of patients who have small septal defects. Larger defects generally have to be closed surgically.

b. Coarctation of the aorta

A complicated coarctation of the aorta is associated with an increased maternal mortality rate. A bicuspid aortic valve, a weakening of the aortic wall, or an atrial septal defect may be present as the complicating lesion. Due to the risk of aortic rupture with the increased cardiac output of pregnancy, strict rest and minimal physical activity should be prescribed. SBE prophylaxis is indicated at the time of delivery, and epidural anesthesia should not be used.

c. Tetralogy of Fallot

This anomaly consists of the presence of: (1) pulmonary stenosis, (2) an intraventricular septal defect, (3) an overriding aorta, and (4) right ventricular hypertrophy. The degree of pulmonary stenosis present is the main factor in determining the direction of the shunting (i.e., left-to-right, balanced, or right-to-left), the amount of cyanosis, and the amount of blood flow to the lungs.

With the decreased peripheral resistance that occurs with pregnancy, there is an increase in the right-to-left shunting, and also an increase in the cyanosis, due to the decreased pulmonary flow. If the mother's hematocrit exceeds 60% and/or there is a decreased oxygen saturation of the arterial blood to below 80%, then the prognosis is poor. The number of live-born infants and their birth weights is indirectly proportional to the amount of cyanosis that is present. A decrease in the systemic vascular resistance would increase the right-to-left shunt, so epidural anesthesia is contraindicated.

d. Eisenmenger's syndrome

This entity consists of pulmonary hypertension associated with either a reversed or a bidirectional shunt in: (1) the aorticopulmonary area, (2) the atrial septal region, or (3) the ventricular septal area. Left-to-right shunting through the septal defect initially causes an increase in the pulmonary vascular resistance and eventually causes pulmonary hypertension. *When the pulmonary pressure becomes sufficiently elevated, the shunt then reverses; the blood is then shunted away from the lungs and cyanosis develops.* **When this condition occurs in pregnancy, the maternal mortality rate is 60% (ventricular septal defect); 44% (atrial septal defect); and 41% (patent ductus arteriosus). The perinatal mortality rate has been reported to be 28%.** The incidence of intrauterine growth retarda-

tion, which is probably secondary to the cyanosis and the lack of oxygen transport to the fetus, is 30%. It is obvious that Eisenmenger's syndrome is a serious problem in the pregnant patient and requires the sophisticated management of a team approach. Epidural anesthesia should not be utilized for delivery in these patients.

e. Primary pulmonary hypertension

As with the secondary form of pulmonary hypertension (i.e., Eisenmenger's syndrome), primary pulmonary hypertension during pregnancy also carries a grave prognosis for both the mother and the child.

f. Mitral valve prolapse

The incidence of this condition in pregnancy has been reported to be about 5–10%; however, a mid to late systolic click or systolic murmur has been noted in as high as 17%. It may be associated with Marfan's syndrome, atrial septal defect secundum, von Willebrand's disease, autoimmune connective tissue disease, hyperthyroidism, or coronary artery disease. Cardiac arrhythmia has been noted to be present in these patients by many investigators. Chest pain, dyspnea, dizziness, fatigue, palpitations, and anxiety are also commonly seen, as are transient ischemic attacks (TIA). Although sudden death has been described in 60 of these patients, this outcome is a rare one. Beta-blockers have been recommended for those patients who have arrhythmia. Anticoagulants have been recommended for patients who have recurrent ischemic attacks in spite of antiplatelet therapy (i.e., aspirin, dipyridamole). SBE prophylaxis is indicated at delivery.

g. Idiopathic hypertrophic subaortic stenosis

This lesion is due to an autosomal dominant gene. Due to the aortic outflow obstruction, a history of dyspnea, chest pain, and syncope may be elicited. These patients generally do well in pregnancy; however, some may experience an increase in their symptoms. Beta-adrenergic blocking agents have been used with success in these patients. SBE prophylaxis is indicated at delivery.

h. Marfan's syndrome

This syndrome is an autosomal dominant disorder that is characterized by a number of mesodermal tissue defects (i.e., aneurysm of the aorta, subluxation of the optic lens, arachnodactyly, and cystic lung disease). Marfan's syndrome accounts for most of the dissecting aneurysms that occur in pregnant women under 40 years of age. **Pregnancy interruption should be considered because of the seriousness of this type of lesion.**

5. Cardiac surgery (valvotomy and commissurotomy)

In many instances, cardiac patients may be managed effectively during pregnancy by medical treatment alone. In others, however, surgical treatment becomes necessary. The most ideal patients for cardiac surgery are those who have symptoms *only on activity*. Patients who have symptoms *at rest* have a poor prognosis. Closed valvotomy has an overall mortality rate of about 3% whether it is performed in the pregnant or in the nonpregnant state.

Cardiac valve replacement is performed as a cardiopulmonary bypass procedure and involves the use of either a mechanical or a bioprosthetic valve. **There are a number of mechanical prostheses available, such as the caged-ball (Starr-Edwards), caged-disk (Beall-Surgitool), and the tilting-disk (Bjork-Shiley) types of valves. The bioprostheses consist of the homograft and the heterograft (i.e., a glutaraldehyde-treated porcine valve, which is also called a xenograft).**

While the mechanical valves are more durable, they carry a greater risk with regard to embolism (3–6%), and thus require the long-term administration of anticoagulants to the patient, which during pregnancy can cause serious problems. The tissue grafts do not require anticoagulation therapy; however, they are more prone to develop valvular calcification and may require earlier replacement.

6. Myocardial infarction and ventricular aneurysms

Coronary artery disease leading to myocardial infarction occurs in about 1:10,000 live births and carries a mortality rate of 28–32%. The mortality rate is highest in late pregnancy and in the early puerperium, with death occurring most commonly in patients who deliver within two weeks of the infarction. While coronary occlusive disease may be present in many of these patients, there are also reports of infarction occurring in patients who have had normal coronary arteries on follow-up angiographic studies. In these instances, spasm of the coronary arteries or embolization with subsequent recanalization has been suspected. In the presence of a dissecting aneurysm of the coronary artery, death usually occurs; however, one instance of survival has been reported. When patients who have a ventricular aneurysm fail to respond to medical management, surgery may be lifesaving.

7. Invasive cardiac monitoring

The use of a special pulmonary catheter (i.e., the Swan-Ganz balloon flotation pulmonary artery catheter) to monitor central vascular events provides the clinician with a tool of inestimable value in the management of patients with cardiovascular problems. The pulmonary artery catheter is usually inserted into the internal or external jugular vein or the subclavian vein and is then advanced and positioned to record: (1) the continuous pulmonary artery pressure (PA) when the balloon is collapsed, and (2) the pulmonary capillary wedge pressure (PCWP) when it is inflated. The proximal port may be used to administer fluids, draw blood samples, or to measure the central venous pressure (CVP). The distal port may also be used to collect blood samples from the pulmonary artery. The measurement of **cardiac output (CO)** can be carried out by using the thermodilution technique.

The **stroke volume (SV)** is the amount of blood that is pumped per contraction. The *cardiac index and the stroke index* may be calculated from the cardiac output and the stroke volume by dividing these values by the body surface area. Information concerning the preload may be obtained from the ventricular filling pressures and the cardiac output. By plotting the **CVP** or the **PCWP** against the **CO**, a Starling curve of ventricular function may be developed. It has been assumed in this instance that the CVP or PCWP represents the cardiac muscle fiber length, whereas the CO represents the cardiac muscle fiber shortening. A failing heart must function at a higher preload, or filling pressure (i.e., CVP or PCWP), in order to produce the same cardiac output as the normal heart. The **preload** on the heart may be increased by the administration of intravenous fluids or blood; it may be decreased by the administration of diuretics, vasodilators, or phlebotomy. The **afterload** on the heart consists of the ventricular wall tension during systole, which is dependent upon the pulmonary and systemic vascular resistances. An increase in the afterload causes a worsening of cardiac failure due to the fact that both the stroke volume and the cardiac output decrease. Alpha-adrenergic agents, such as phenylephrine, cause an increase in the afterload. The afterload or systemic vascular resistance may be decreased by hydralazine hydrochloride or sodium nitroprusside. The **contractile, or inotropic, state of the heart** may be defined as the force and velocity of the ventricular contractions when the preload and afterload are held constant. If there is cardiac failure present with a low cardiac output, the preload and afterload may be manipulated to obtain the best situation. If this approach fails, the cardiac output may be increased with beta-sympathomimetics, such as dopamine hydrochloride or isoproterenol hydrochloride (Isuprel), which will increase the cardiac output immediately.

The **heart rate** may also affect the cardiac output. Bradycardia or heart block is unusual in pregnant patients; however, if it is present, it may interfere with the cardiac output. Atropine will increase the heart rate and improve the cardiac output in these cases. In patients with sustained tachycardia, the diastolic filling and shortened systolic ejection time may also compromise the cardiac output and lead to cardiac failure and myocardial ischemia; thus, the cause of the tachycardia should be determined and corrected. In other patients without a defined reason for the tachycardia, propranolol, hydrochloride (Inderal), digoxin, or verapamil may be indicated in an effort to limit the heart rate.

The usual pregnant values for some of these parameters in the third trimester are: (1) cardiac output = 5.0–6.0 l/min, (2) central venous pressure = 5–12 mm Hg, (3) pulmonary capillary wedge pressure (PCWP) = 5–12 mm Hg, (4) heart rate = 84 bpm, (5) mean arterial pressure = 86 mm Hg, (6) stroke volume = 76 ml/beat, and (7) systemic vascular resistance = 800–1,400 dynes $\times$ sec $\times$ cm^{-5} (see Chapter 37).

8. Cardiac arrest in pregnancy

Pregnant patients who are perfectly healthy may suffer cardiac arrest from pulmonary embolism, anesthesia problems, hemorrhagic shock, drug overdosage, or with seizures secondary to pregnancy-induced hypertension (PIH). In general, however, young pregnant patients are healthier than the older cardiac patients, who may have long-standing medical conditions, and are thus able to withstand cardiac arrest much better, as long as the resuscitation efforts are successful.

a. Cardiopulmonary resuscitation (CPR)

When cardiac arrest occurs in pregnancy, the physician or other health-care professional who sees the patient first should determine the patient's status and briefly attempt to arouse her. If this is unsuccessful, then a precordial thump should be administered (i.e., a sharp blow from a height of 20 cm to the midsternum). (The principles of resuscitation as taught by the American Heart Association should be thoroughly understood.) The patient should be placed quickly on a firm surface or on the floor, the head tilted back, and the neck lifted forward to **straighten out the airway.** The health-care professional should then follow these procedures: Begin **mouth-to-mouth resuscitation,** using four breaths in rapid succession, while the nose is pinched shut. Check the carotid pulse, and if it is absent, then begin **external chest compression.** You should position your hands, one over the other, over the lower half of the sternum above the xiphoid process, and then, using a 1:1 compression-release ratio, begin with depression of the sternum to about 4–5 cm with each compression. If you are alone during the resuscitation procedure, you should do 15 sets of compressions at a rate of 80 per minute, interrupting each set with a set of two breaths (i.e., **2:15**). If there is someone to help you, then you should give one breath for every 5 compressions (i.e., **1:5**), which should be given by your partner at a rate of 60 per minute. This rate should be maintained until you are relieved, or until the patient begins to breathe on her own. Do not interrupt the resuscitation for more than 30 seconds to check for the pulse or to intubate the patient. Tilt the pregnant patient to the left side slightly with a pillow under the right hip to get the pregnant uterus off of the inferior vena cava. A bag-and-mask ventilation may be used if available, or an endotracheal intubation may be performed, with the administration of 100% oxygen. **Suction equipment** should be immediately available. Once the tube has been placed, you should check to be certain that it is not below the bifurcation of the trachea by listening for breath sounds and making sure that they are equal bilaterally.

Once the cardiopulmonary resuscitation (CPR) is in progress, then other specific problems will need to be addressed. The most experienced CPR team member should appoint one person to record the time and the events as they subsquently transpire. Cardiac monitoring leads should be placed on the chest and an **electrocardiogram (ECG)** should be obtained. If the ECG shows a regular heartbeat in the absence of a pulse and respiration (electromechanical dissociation), the diagnoses of tension pneumothorax, cardiac tamponade, or hypovolemia must be considered. The discovery of ventricular fibrillation, ventricular tachycardia, complete asystole, or electromechanical dissociation may be considered to be potentially lethal findings.

Ventricular fibrillation consists of either low-amplitude, or more commonly, high-amplitude spikes on the ECG and requires defibrillation treatment using energy levels of 200–300 J of direct current. This treatment should not affect the fetus. A conductive paste is applied to the paddles, and then one paddle should be placed to the right of the sternum beneath the clavicle while the other is placed to the left of the left nipple at the cardiac apex. After the energy setting has been made, you should instruct the team to stand clear, and discharge. The discharge lasts for between 4 and 12 msec. If the fibrillation still persists after the first shock, it may be repeated at the same setting. CPR should be continued on the patient while the paddles are charging. For subsequent attempts, use the maximal setting of 360 J and give the countershocks in sets of two.

In the past, it was recommended that sodium bicarbonate, 1 mEq/kg (75–100 mg), be given initially, with half this dose being repeated every 10 minutes; however, this agent is no longer recommended because of the buildup of sodium and the need to correct the respiratory acidosis by the blowing off of the carbon dioxide. Intubation should also be carried out.

If the initial set of defibrillation attempts are unsuccessful, *bretylium tosylate* (Bretylol), 5 mg/kg I.V. (350–500 mg) may be given initially, followed by 10 mg/kg I.V. (750–1000 mg) after the next set of defibrillation attempts. After the use of bretylium, or as an alternative to it, *lidocaine* (Xylocaine), 1 mg/kg, may be administered as an initial bolus, followed by 0.5 mg/kg 10 minutes later. This dosage may be repeated every 10 minutes until a total of 225 mg has been administered, after which an I.V. infusion of 2–4 mg per minute may be given.

Another alternative to bretylium or lidocaine therapy is the administration of 100 mg of *procainamide hydrochloride* (Pronestyl) over a period of five minutes. While administering this drug, you should watch for the appearance of hypotension or a 50% increase in the QRS complex. After a total dose of 1 gram has been reached, the maintenance dosage is 1–4 mg per minute.

Asystole may respond to 0.5–1.0 mg I.V. of *epinephrine*. Atropine, 1.0 mg I.V., may be administered. *Isoproterenol hydrochloride* (Isuprel) may be administered in an infusion of 2–20 μg per minute. A pacemaker should be placed as soon as possible.

Electromechanical dissociation may be managed by intubation with 100% oxygen and the administration of *epinephrine,* 0.5–1.0 mg I.V. initially. The epinephrine may be repeated every five minutes. An *isoproterenol* infusion at 2–20 μg per minute may be administered. You should attempt to identify the presence of a cardiac tamponade, a tension pneumothorax, or hypovolemia, and treat it appropriately.

CHAPTER 30

Vascular disease

Medicine is the science of uncertainty and an art of probability.

—*Sir William Osler**

1. General considerations

Venous problems occur in 5–30% of pregnant women. Varicose veins and hemorrhoids are therefore quite common in pregnancy. In view of the fact that the enlarging gravid uterus compresses the inferior vena cava, as well as the iliac veins and the abdominal aorta, it becomes obvious that an increased vascular pressure in the lower extremities must be transmitted to the venous system to cause the subsequent development of varicosities, venous stasis, and edema.

There is a two- to three-fold linear increase in the venous pressure in the femoral veins during pregnancy, which results in venous pressure values of the order of 20 cm of H_2O or more. Another result of obstruction to the blood flow in the lower extremities is the decrease in the *blood flow velocity,* which in the third trimester falls to nearly half of the normal values, except when the patient assumes the lateral decubitus position.

With the increasing levels of progesterone in pregnancy, there is a gradual decrease in the peripheral vascular resistance, which results in **an increased venous distensibility and an effective doubling of the venous volume.**

a. Supine hypotensive syndrome

A compression of the inferior vena cava and the iliac veins by the gravid uterus occurs in almost all pregnant women when they assume the supine position. When this occurs, the venous return to the right heart from the lower extremities may be severely restricted, causing a decreased cardiac output, hypotension, pallor, sweating, and tachycardia. **This reaction occurs in about 2% of pregnant patients and has been termed the "supine hypotensive syndrome."** In those patients who manifest this syndrome, the treatment consists of placing the patient on her left side so as to shift the uterus off the inferior vena cava. *Fortunately, most patients have an adequate collateral circulation, by which the blood flow is shunted around the obstruction through the ascending lumbar and azygos veins, and thus they do not have any symptoms.*

b. Varicose veins

1) Etiology

Varicose veins initially appear during pregnancy in 10–20% of women. While pregnancy per se does not cause the development of varicose veins, it does aggravate the condition once it appears. *In 60% of patients who develop varicose veins, a positive history of varicose veins in other family members exists. Presumably, this type of inheritance is polygenic.*

Three different theories have been suggested to explain the development of varicose veins. The *first theory* proposes that there is a hereditary

*Reprinted with permission from Robert Bennett Bean, *Sir William Osler: Aphorisms from His Bedside Teachings and Writings,* William Bennett Bean, ed. Springfield, Ill.: Charles C Thomas, Publisher, 1968, p. 129.

component in the walls of the veins that makes them more distensible.

The *second theory,* which is perhaps the most widely accepted hypothesis, suggests that the varicose veins are the result of **incompetent venous valves.** There are no valves in the inferior vena cava or in the common iliac veins; however, **there is one valve in either the external iliac vein or in the common femoral vein.** If this valve is incompetent, as it is in some patients who have a family history of varicose veins, then a retrograde flow may occur whenever there is an increase in the femoral venous pressure, such as can occur in pregnancy. **As a consequence, when the iliofemoral valve becomes incompetent, an increased head of hydrostatic pressure below this point causes the saphenous vein to dilate, thus forcing the valves in this system to also become incompetent. When this happens, superficial varicosities result.**

The *third theory* postulates that the varicose veins develop as a result of **incompetent perforating veins connecting the deep and the superficial venous systems.** With exercise, the muscular pump drives the blood from the deep venous system out to the superficial venous system. The distention that is caused by this shunting will ultimately cause the superficial venous system valves to fail and become incompetent, resulting in varicosities.

During pregnancy, the increased venous distensibility, secondary to the increased levels of progesterone, combined with either a congenitally absent venous valve or the development of an incompetent valve in the iliofemoral region, may result in the development of varicose veins. The increase in the venous pressure due to the obstruction of the inferior vena cava by the gravid uterus aggravates this incompetency of the valves even further.

2) Symptoms

The primary symptoms associated with superficial saphenous varicose veins of the legs include aching soreness, fatigue, and a feeling of heaviness in the legs. Usually, these symptoms are not very prominent initially, and the patient will complain more of the unsightly appearance of the varicosities rather than the symptoms.

Deep vein involvement causes edema and a brownish discoloration of the skin, which may be associated with induration and ulceration. These findings are not seen in superficial venous disease.

3) Prognosis and treatment

Nearly all varicosities (i.e., 90%) will regress to some degree following the end of pregnancy. Surgical vein stripping is generally performed at 6–12 weeks following delivery if there are still significant varicosities present. During pregnancy, *support hose* are beneficial, since they decrease the amount of blood flow in the legs and may compress the veins sufficiently to allow the venous valve cusps to regain their competence. *Bedrest in the left lateral decubitus position* allows for a more normal blood flow velocity in the lower extremities and relieves the inferior vena cava obstruction that occurs in the supine position. Elevating the legs will add to the above factors, allowing for a more normal circulation to occur in the legs and preventing excessive edema. *The woman should be cautioned about prolonged standing or sitting, as well as about crossing her legs when sitting.* Trauma to the legs by the use of inappropriate padding of the delivery stirrups (or by the absence of padding) should be avoided.

c. Hemorrhoids

Hemorrhoids develop during pregnancy as a result of the increased venous distension and the obstruction of the rectal venous system. Due to the fact that there is an increased level of progesterone during pregnancy, which decreases the intestinal peristalsis, there is an increased transit time of the feces in the gut. This process results in additional absorption of fluid by the large intestine, which causes *constipation.* **The pregnant patient will often strain harder at stool, adding even more pressure to the rectal venous system, which results in an increased pressure in the hemorrhoidal veins to produce hemorrhoids.** The patient should be encouraged to drink large amounts of water during her pregnancy (i.e., 6–8 eight oz glasses per day) and to develop the daily habit of attempting to have a bowel movement at about the same time each day when she can go to the bathroom without interruption. Mild stool softeners may be used, but harsh laxatives should be avoided. Following a bowel movement, any prolapsed hemorrhoids should be replaced into the anus. If thrombosis of a hemorrhoid should occur, surgical removal may become necessary, since these may be quite painful. Soothing anesthetic or antibacterial ointments may also provide satisfactory relief of the minor symptoms of pain and swelling.

2. Venous thrombosis

a. Incidence

The clinical incidence of deep vein thrombosis is of the order of 1:2,000 in antepartum patients and about 1:700 in the postpartum period. In one study of gynecologic postoperative patients, the incidence of abnormal ^{125}I fibrinogen leg scans was 19%. **After major abdominal surgery, the incidence of positive evidence of thrombosis varies between 14 and 33%.** Most of these patients, however, never manifest clinical signs of thrombosis in spite of having positive leg scans; **the incidence of clinical thrombosis is about 2% in these patients.** *The incidence of puerperal thromboembolism in women who receive estrogens in the postpartum period for the suppression of lactation is increased tenfold over the normal rate.* By way of comparison, the risk of thromboembolism in women who take birth control pills is increased on the order of about seven-fold over the normal rate.

The usual sites for deep vein thrombosis in the lower extremities are in the left iliofemoral venous segment, in the pockets of the valve cusps, and in the veins of the soleus muscle. Calf vein thrombosis is more common than thrombosis of the thigh veins.

b. Etiology and mechanism of coagulation

The classic Virchow triad of: (1) blood flow stasis, (2) vascular endothelial trauma, and (3) alterations in the coagulability mechanisms of the blood, remain as valid today as an explanation for the causation of thrombosis as they were in R. Virchow's time nearly 100 years ago.

There are two pathways by which the process of coagulation may be activated, and they are: (1) the **intrinsic pathway** and (2) the **extrinsic pathway.** In the **intrinsic pathway,** the process is activated when the blood contacts a nonendothelial surface, such as when an injury occurs to a blood vessel with the exposure of the underlying collagen. Platelets adhere to the collagen and aggregate under the influence of adenosine diphosphate (ADP) and platelet factor 3 (PF3). The cascade of events then includes the activation of Factor XII, Factor XI, and Factor IX. In the presence of platelet phospholipid, calcium, and Factor VIII, Factor X becomes activated. This, in turn, causes the activation of Factor V, which converts prothrombin to thrombin, and the thrombin then converts fibrinogen to fibrin. These soluble fibrin monomers are then converted to fibrin polymers, which are insoluble and precipitate from solution (Fig. 30-1).

The **extrinsic pathway** is much simpler and is triggered by the exposure of the blood to a "tissue thromboplastin." This substance combines with Factor VII and activates Factor X, which then proceeds along a common pathway with that of the intrinsic mechanism to form deposits of fibrin.

During pregnancy, the plasma fibrinogen increases by 50%. Factors VIII and XII are also elevated. Factor XI is often decreased, as is antithrombin III and the heparin cofactor. There have been reports of pulmonary embolism in patients who have a hereditary deficiency of antithrombin III.

Factors II (prothrombin), VII (proconvertin, a stable factor), IX (the Christmas factor), and X (the Stuart-Prower factor) are all **vitamin K dependent.** The various coagulation factors are: I (fibrinogen), II (prothrombin), III (the tissue factor, or thromboplastin), IV (calcium), V (proaccelerin, or the labile factor), VII (proconvertin, a stable factor), VIII (antihemophilic factor, antihemophilic globulin), IX (the Christmas factor), X (the Stuart-Prower factor), XI (plasma thromboplastin antecedent), XII (the Hageman factor), and XIII (fibrin stabilizing factor).

c. Diagnosis

When edema (i.e., increased leg circumference), a palpable superficial cord, and calf tenderness are noted in the leg, the diagnosis of superficial vein thrombosis can usually be made without difficulty. The treatment consists of elevating the leg, applying local heat, bedrest, and the administration of analgesics. If the patient fails to respond to these measures, a deep vein thrombosis should be suspected. Furthermore, if deep calf tenderness is present along with a positive Homans' sign (i.e., calf pain on dorsiflexion of the foot), fever, and tachycardia, then the possibility of a **deep vein thrombosis** should again be strongly considered.

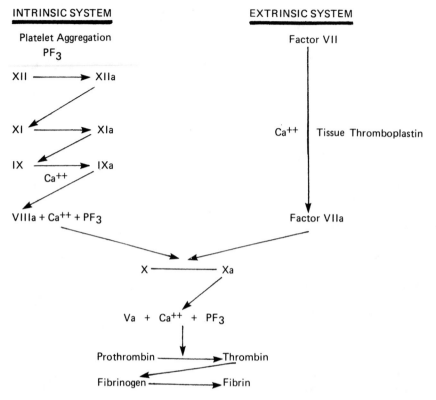

FIGURE 30-1. The activation of the blood coagulation factors that lead to the production of fibrin. (PF3 = platelet factor 3)

The ^{125}I fibrinogen scan is contraindicated in pregnancy. The Doppler ultrasonographic technique, while considered to be of value in some centers, seems to have a sensitivity of only 55% in patients with calf vein thrombosis. Plethysmographic techniques using a strain gauge, an air cuff, or impedance have been quite sensitive in diagnosing major venous thromboses, except for in the calf veins. All of these techniques have been found to be much less sensitive in the diagnosis of calf vein thrombosis than in diagnosing other types of thrombosis. **Venography** is apparently the most effective imaging technique for demonstrating lower extremity thrombi in pregnancy, although there is a minimal risk of radiation exposure (about 1 rad), even with pelvic shielding.

d. Therapy

The primary therapy for deep vein thrombosis is anticoagulation with intravenous heparin so-

dium, which should be administered in sufficient dosage so as to keep the partial thromboplastin time at approximately 1.5–2.0 times its normal value. Usually, an initial dose of 10,000 units of heparin followed by a continuous infusion of about 1,000 units per hour is administered for seven days. Subcutaneous heparin may then be used for the remainder of the treatment period. While there is some evidence that heparin may cause an increased risk of perinatal loss, the evidence has not been considered to be conclusive. In one study, it was reported that heparin was associated with an incidence of prematurity as high as 14% and an incidence of stillbirths of 13%.

The use of *warfarin is contraindicated* during the first three months of pregnancy, and relatively contraindicated throughout the remainder of pregnancy, due to the fact that it may cross the placenta and cause a **warfarin embryopathy** early in pregnancy, or **fetal bleeding** later in pregnancy. Warfarin can be given during nursing, however, since it is highly bound to protein and does not enter the breast milk in appreciable amounts.

About 5% of patients with deep vein thrombosis will require ligation of the inferior vena cava for recurrent pulmonary emboli. The use of such agents as streptokinase and urokinase to lyze the clots is contraindicated in pregnancy and during the first five days postpartum.

e. Prophylaxis

The use of **low-dose heparin therapy** (i.e., 10,000–15,000 units/day) prior to **elective gynecologic surgery** has been advocated in an effort to prevent postoperative venous thrombosis. Although the incidence of intraoperative bleeding does not seem to be increased with this therapy, about 1–2% of these patients will develop wound hematomas.

3. Postpartum ovarian vein thrombosis

a. Incidence

Since the first case report of postpartum ovarian vein thrombosis (POVT) was published in 1956, there have been more than 70 cases reported in the literature. It has been estimated by some authors that the incidence of POVT is 1:600 deliveries. Thus, it is obvious that most of these cases must go unreported or are just not clinically recognized.

b. Pathophysiology

During pregnancy, the ovarian veins undergo tremendous dilatation, with their capacity being increased as much as 60 times over the normal amount. In addition, there is evidence of a *decreased velocity of the blood flow* in the peripheral veins during the third trimester of pregnancy, which probably also includes the ovarian vessels. This *relative stasis* of the venous blood flow in the patient is further compounded in the postpartum period by bedrest and inactivity. Venous stasis allows platelet aggregation and the adhesion of the platelets to the vessel walls.

Several well-known *biochemical alterations* take place in the clotting mechanism during pregnancy. The increased levels of Factors VII and VIII, the increased platelet aggregation, the increased prothrombin, and the hyperfibrinogenemia have all been im-

plicated as reasons for the increased coagulability during pregnancy.

Vascular endothelial injury causes the release of adenosine diphosphate (ADP) and platelet factor 3 (PF3), which instigates the clotting cascade and the eventual formation of a thrombus. The pelvic and genital tract trauma that occurs during labor and delivery, as well as the bacterial contamination of these structures, may also provide conditions suitable for the initiation of the clotting mechanism. **Endometritis has been suspected or proven in nearly one-third of patients with POVT—an incidence that is considerably higher than the rate of occurrence in the general population.** It is possible that bacterial invasion of the pelvic veins may occur by a direct extension from a pelvic cellulitis, which results in a perivascular inflammation with subsequent endothelial injury. Such an injury could then become a nidus for the development of a thrombus.

c. Clinical findings

The POVT syndrome usually occurs in the immediate postpartum state; however, in some cases, it may be delayed for several weeks. The symptoms consist of fever and abdominal or lower quadrant pain. Nausea and vomiting, ileus, and rebound tenderness of the abdomen may also be present. On physical examination, a large, **sausage-shaped mass** may be palpated in the paracolic gutter. This mass almost always occurs on the **right side** but occasionally it may occur bilaterally. Rarely does POVT occur only on the left side. The patient's temperature is usually elevated to slightly more than 100°F, and a mild leukocytosis (i.e., at 10,000 WBC/mm^3) is usually present. The mass may be difficult to define, due to tenderness and guarding. It may measure up to 10 cm in diameter and will usually extend from the pelvic area cephalad toward the lower pole of the kidney.

d. Diagnosis

When doubt exists as to the diagnosis of POVT, and the literature indicates that this is frequently the case, then a variety of tests can be utilized. *The detection of a sausage-shaped paracolic mass, either on clinical examination or on examination under anesthesia, is strong evidence of POVT.* Computer-assisted tomography (CT) scanning is often helpful in defining the mass of dilated vessels in the paracolic mass. Ultrasonography may also be helpful in identifying the dilated vascular channels in the mass.

e. Treatment

The treatment of choice in POVT consists of the intravenous administration of broad-spectrum antibiotics and heparin anticoagulation. When such a regimen is instituted, the fever should defervesce within 48–72 hours and the patient should begin to improve symptomatically. Should this regimen fail to cause a defervescence of the fever and improvement in the patient's condition within this time period, then another diagnosis should be strongly considered.

If the initial diagnosis was not POVT and an exploratory laparotomy was carried out only to find a sausage-shaped paracolic mass, then two courses of action are open to you: (1) close the patient while maintaining meticulous hemostasis and begin heparin anticoagulation, or (2) very carefully and gently completely excise the mass in a retrograde fashion from the inferior vena cava inferiorly toward the uterus, using minimal manipulation so as to not cause systemic embolization. Postoperatively, following complete excision of the mass, the antibiotics should be continued. There is some controversy concerning the use of anticoagulants in the postresection patient. The risk of *wound hematomas* is increased if anticoagulants are used, but on the other hand, there still may be a risk of pulmonary embolism and death, which might be prevented by the use of anticoagulants. This decision requires careful judgment on the part of the physician.

4. Pulmonary embolism

Perhaps as many as 100,000 people die from pulmonary embolism as the direct cause of death in the United States each year. The mortality rate for all cases that are diagnosed clinically and treated is about 8%. The incidence of pulmonary embolism in pregnancy has been estimated to be about 1:2,500.

a. Clinical findings

The traditional signs of pulmonary embolism in order of frequency, according to one study, are: (1) tachy-

pnea (92%), (2) pleuritic pain or chest pain (88%), (3) dyspnea (84%), (4) apprehension (59%), (5) cough (53%), (6) tachycardia, of greater than 100 bpm (44%), (7) fever of more than 37.8°C (43%), (8) hemoptysis (30%), (9) diaphoresis (36%), and (10) syncope (13%). *Clinically, the presence of tachycardia, dyspnea, pleuritic pain, and apprehension, with an arterial pO$_2$ of 80 torr or less, should strongly suggest the diagnosis of pulmonary embolism.*

b. Diagnosis

The diagnosis may often be difficult to confirm. The presence of an infiltrate on the chest X-ray film may confuse the diagnosis, although a pleural effusion may be noted in 60% of patients with a pulmonary embolism. A **ventilation/perfusion lung scan** utilizing xenon[133] may increase the accuracy of the diagnosis considerably. The most effective diagnostic technique in cases of pulmonary embolism is **pulmonary angiography;** however, the morbidity of this procedure is 1%, and the mortality has been estimated to be of the order of 0.5%, although this may be much lower in skilled hands. Pulmonary angiography should not be performed on patients who have a right ventricular end-diastolic pressure of 20 mm Hg or greater, since a number of deaths from this procedure have occurred in such individuals.

c. Treatment

The primary therapy for pulmonary embolism is intravenous heparin therapy. In those patients who have had a massive pulmonary embolism, and who survive long enough, an *embolectomy* may be performed, either by a direct surgical approach or by the use of the intravenous catheter. In these individuals, the systolic blood pressure falls to less than 90 mm Hg during the first hour after embolization, the PaO$_2$ is less than 60 torr, and the urine output is less than 20 ml/hr. An embolectomy procedure in these patients may be lifesaving.

5. Intracranial hemorrhage and stroke

a. Intracranial hemorrhage

Intracranial hemorrhage usually occurs in patients who have either a berry aneurysm or an

intracranial vascular malformation. The sudden onset of a severe headache, dizziness, nausea, vomiting, and sweating, in the presence of hypertension and a stiff neck, should alert you to the possibility of an intracranial hemorrhage. The cerebral spinal fluid will be bloody initially, but as time passes, it will become xanthochromic.

Since exertion or Valsalva's maneuvers are responsible for one-third of all subarachnoid hemorrhages, the bearing-down maneuvers that are associated with labor and delivery are particularly hazardous for the patient. In severe intracranial hemorrhages, the patient may become comatose, with dilated pupils, and subsequently develop focal neurologic signs. The prognosis is guarded in such patients.

Cerebral angiography or a CT scan can be used to define the location of the hemorrhage. The fetus should be delivered vaginally, since a cesarean section offers no special advantages.

b. Stroke

The incidence of cerebral infarction in pregnant women is about 1:26,000 live births. **In pregnant patients, arterial occlusions, rather than venous occlusions, are the most common cause of strokes.** About 35% of such occlusions involve the middle cerebral artery, and 20% are found in the internal carotid artery. *Although vertebrobasilar strokes are more common in oral contraceptive users than in the general population, such involvement in pregnancy is rare.*

Emboli in pregnancy usually originate in the heart. Atrial fibrillation carries a 10–23% risk of embolism in pregnancy. As a consequence, patients who have chronic atrial fibrillation are candidates for long-term anticoagulation therapy. Since patients who have a mechanical heart valve implant have a 3–6% risk of embolism, these patients are also candidates for long-term anticoagulation. Some authors have recommended that tissue cardiac valve should be used in women of childbearing age, since the risk of embolism with this approach is less than 2% and anticoagulation is not considered to be necessary (see Chapter 29).

c. Ischemic infarction

Ischemic infarction of the brain can occur in patients who have prolonged episodes of sustained hypoten-sion, which results in the development of diffuse cerebral edema, decreased blood flow to focal areas of the brain, and then localized areas of necrosis. The classic Sheehan's syndrome is an example of a focal necrosis of the pituitary gland secondary to a prolonged episode of hypotension with decreased blood flow in the distribution of the inferior hypophyseal artery.

d. Prolapsed mitral valve

The prolapsed mitral valve syndrome occurs in about 10% of young adults (see Chapter 29). In the past few years, this syndrome has been increasingly associated with pregnancy-related strokes.

e. Subacute bacterial endocarditis

In patients who have subacute bacterial endocarditis (SBE), a sudden focal neurological deficit may develop as a vegetative embolization occurs. **In pregnancy, the most common bacterium involved in SBE is Streptococcus viridans.** In about 8% of the cases, enterococci are the infective agents, especially after an abortion, after a term delivery, after the insertion of an intrauterine device (IUD), or after a dilatation and curettage (D&C) of the uterus. Transient ischemic attacks (TIA) or strokes have been reported in patients more than a year after an initial episode of treated SBE, apparently as the result of the embolization from the sterile valvular vegetations.

f. Hemoglobinopathy

Pregnant patients with sickle cell anemia (SS) or sickle cell hemoglobin C disease (SC) are at risk for developing occlusion of major cerebral arteries. Strokes that occur in sickle cell anemia patients are due to the *sickling effects of the red blood cells,* whereas in patients with SC disease, it appears that stroke is more commonly due to *fat embolism.* In SC disease, the embolic event usually follows shortly after a long-bone fracture or following an infarction of the bone marrow.

g. Other causes of stroke

Due to the possible development of *mural thrombi* in the dilated chambers of the heart in patients with peripartum cardiomyopathy, it has been recommended that anticoagulant therapy be utilized to prevent the possibility of embolization. In those patients who have a patent foramen ovale, an increase in the right atrial pressure (e.g., secondary to pulmonary hypertension, as a result of a pulmonary embolus) might allow an embolus from the lower extremities to cross over into the arterial circulation. Such an event would produce an arterial embolization to the brain and result in a stroke. Thrombocytopenic purpura may result in transient ischemic attacks and strokes, and metastatic choriocarcinoma to the brain may result in either stroke or cerebral hemorrhage.

CHAPTER 31

Pulmonary disease

The four points of a medical student's compass are: Inspection, Palpation, Percussion, and Auscultation.
—*Sir William Osler**

1. Asthma

Asthma is a condition in which there is a stimulation of the airways in such a manner as to produce bronchial smooth muscle contraction, mucosal edema, and a hypersecretion of mucus, which results in an acute obstructive lung disease that can be reversed by therapy. A number of **triggering stimuli** have been identified, such as upper respiratory tract infections, smoke, fog, cold air, exercise, emotional stress, and various air pollutants, including specific allergens (e.g., ragweed, pollen, molds).

a. Incidence

Asthma occurs in only 0.4–1.3% of pregnant patients, in contrast to an incidence of 2.6–3.1% in the general population. During pregnancy, the incidence of the attacks and their severity become worse in 25% of patients who have asthma, remains the same in 35%, and improves in 40%. In one study, 5.7% of the patients were severely involved, and it was in this group of patients that two-thirds of the maternal deaths occurred, 35% of the low–birth weight infants were found, and 28% of the perinatal deaths were

noted. Most patients with asthma, however, tolerate pregnancy quite well.

b. Symptoms

Asthmatic attacks occur at irregular intervals with the patient being entirely normal in the interim. **The initial symptoms** include tightness in the chest and a sensation of not being able to breathe associated with sneezing or coughing. Dyspnea ensues, with wheezing and difficulty in expelling air. Confusion, cyanosis, and weakness may occur in severe cases.

c. Treatment

The treatment of asthma consists of oral methylxanthines (i.e., theophylline, aminophylline) and predominantly beta-2 sympathomimetics (i.e., metaproterenol sulfate, terbutaline sulfate). Theophylline inhibits the enzyme phosphodiesterase, which causes the degradation of cyclic AMP (cAMP). As a result, intracellular cAMP increases, resulting in bronchodilatation due to smooth muscle relaxation. Theophylline or aminophylline, 6 mg/kg, should be infused intravenously over 20 minutes in an acute attack, and then if the response is favorable, oral medication may be used. If continued I.V. therapy is essential, then the patient may be maintained on 0.9 mg/kg/hr by means of a constant infusion pump. Blood levels should be checked periodically to ensure that an overdose does not occur.

Epinephrine (1:1,000 solution), 0.3–0.5 ml, can be given subcutaneously every 20 minutes in an acute situation; however, its short duration of action precludes its use as long-term therapy. It also should be used cautiously in patients with tachycardia or cardiac disease.

---

*Reprinted with permission from Robert Bennett Bean, *Sir William Osler: Aphorisms from His Bedside Teachings and Writings,* William Bennett Bean, ed. Springfield, Ill.: Charles C Thomas, Publisher, 1968, p. 103.

Cortisone may be utilized in patients who are hospitalized with severe symptoms. The peak effect of the corticosteroids may not occur for as long as 3–9 hours, so their use must be anticipated. Hydrocortisone, 4 mg/kg q4h initially followed by 3 mg/kg q6h, should be administered to patients who have needed corticosteroids in previous episodes, whereas in those who have never had corticosteroids before, 4 mg/kg in one dose is usually adequate. In patients who require continued cortisone administration, oral prednisone, 60 mg, may be substituted after 2–3 days and the dose may then be gradually decreased by 5–10 mg every 2–3 days. While there has been some controversy concerning the possible adverse effects of cortisone on fetal development, there is no conclusive evidence that there are any deleterious effects on the fetus.

Oxygen should be administered if the arterial pO_2 is less than 70 mm Hg. The replacement of fluids is also essential in the treatment of the asthmatic patient who is pregnant. If the patient has an elevated temperature and shows evidence of an infection, then you should administer intravenous broad-spectrum antibiotics after appropriate cultures have been obtained.

The management of labor and delivery in the asthmatic patient is no different from that of the normal patient. The delivery should usually be by the vaginal route and cesarean section should be reserved for obstetric indications only. Prostaglandin $F_{2\alpha}$ is a bronchoconstrictor, and if used in the asthmatic patient to control a postpartum hemorrhage, it may precipitate an acute attack. If general anesthesia is used, halothane anesthesia is preferred over cyclopropane.

2. Tuberculosis

a. Incidence

The occurrence of a pulmonary infection with *Mycobacterium tuberculosis* has decreased dramatically since the turn of the century due to the development of wide-ranging public health measures to improve sanitation and the discovery of effective treatment regimens. **The mortality rate has decreased from 200:100,000 to 10:100,000 over the past 80 years. About 1–3% of all pregnancies will be associated with tuberculosis in this country, especially in high-risk areas in the southeastern United States, where the disease is indigenous.** The recent increased incidence of this disease has been due to the immigration of women from Mexico and Southeast Asia.

b. Symptoms

The patient may present with a low-grade fever, night sweats, weight loss, anorexia, and respiratory symptoms, such as a cough that is productive of sputum or blood.

c. Diagnosis

Tuberculosis may be suspected in the presence of the typical symptoms; however, in many instances, a positive tuberculin skin test may be the first thing that is noted during pregnancy in a patient who previously had a negative skin test. Such tuberculin skin test **converters,** and patients who present with symptoms suggestive of tuberculosis, should have a chest roentgenogram performed. The purified protein derivative (PPD) tuberculin skin test (first strength) becomes positive 4–12 weeks after exposure. It rarely gives a false positive result, and the incidence of false negative tests is stated to be less than 2%. This test remains positive for life in 96–97% of patients. *A positive sputum acid-fast smear and a tuberculosis culture demonstrating the Mycobacterium tuberculosis bacillus will provide confirmatory evidence of the diagnosis of an active tuberculosis infection.* The sputum smear is positive 75% of the time in patients with active tuberculosis, while a culture is essentially 100% positive in such patients. *Routine chest roentgenograms are no longer recommended in the pregnant population* unless there are clinical or laboratory findings suggestive of pulmonary pathology, including tuberculosis.

d. Treatment

The usual indications for therapy are: (1) inactive disease that has not been treated previously, (2) active untreated disease, and (3) patients who have recently converted to a positive PPD test within the past year. Patients with a recently converted positive PPD test who do not exhibit clinical symptoms or findings do not need to be treated in pregnancy.

The treatment of active tuberculosis during pregnancy usually requires more than one drug. The treatment should be carried out over a prolonged period of time, although some investigators have recently recommended short courses of therapy. **The use of** isoniazid (INH) and ethambutol hydrochloride for a period of 18–24 months may be used in established cases of tuberculosis in pregnancy; however, supplemental pyridoxine should be given (i.e., 50 mg/day) to prevent INH-induced peripheral neuropathy. Streptomycin should not be used in pregnancy, due to its fetal ototoxicity. Isoniazid and rifampin appear to be safe in pregnancy and provide another therapeutic combination often used in short courses of therapy (i.e., 9–12 months).

Since tuberculosis does not affect the course of pregnancy, therapeutic abortion is never indicated on the basis of this disease alone. **A reactivation of tuberculosis occurs in 5–10% of patients during pregnancy.**

e. Congenital and neonatal tuberculosis

Congenital tuberculosis occurs only rarely. **The infant is most susceptible to contracting the disease at the time of delivery and should be isolated immediately from an untreated mother with active tuberculosis, and in addition should probably receive INH therapy or BCG (bacillus of Calmette-Guérin) vaccination.** The BCG vaccine is given to infants of mothers with active tuberculosis who have not been adequately treated. It is also administered to individuals who are PPD negative and in high-risk situations.

3. Pneumonia

Pneumonia is one of the leading causes of nonobstetric deaths. The incidence of pneumonia in pregnancy is about 0.1–0.8%. This disease may be caused by bacterial, mycoplasmal, viral, or fungal organisms. **Bacterial pneumonia** *(e.g., Streptococcus pneumoniae)* generally has a more abrupt onset than mycoplasmal pneumonia and is usually accompanied by severe symptoms, such as fever, chills, a productive cough, and pleuritic chest pains. These patients may go into premature labor if the fever is persistent. The treatment of choice in a bacterial pneumonia usually consists of high doses of intravenous penicillin administered until the patient is afebrile for 24–48 hours. In addition, supportive measures consisting of oxygen, fluid replacement, and temperature control should be instituted.

In **mycoplasmal pneumonia,** a nonproductive cough, sore throat, and fever may develop over the course of several days. *This clinical syndrome is associated with patchy infiltrates in the lung fields on a chest roentgenogram. The laboratory studies will reveal the presence of cold agglutinins and complement fixation antibodies to mycoplasma.* The treatment consists of a course of *erythromycin* therapy.

A viral pneumonia involving varicella (chickenpox) is a rare disease entity in pregnancy, but when it occurs in pregnant women it carries a maternal mortality rate of 45%. It may be associated with an infectious vesicular eruption of the skin, pleuritic pain, cough, and dyspnea that gradually resolve over the course of about two weeks if the patient survives (see Chapter 28).

The occurrence of an **influenzal pneumonia** usually develops after an initial flu-like syndrome and frequently involves not only the influenza virus but other secondary bacterial invaders as well (see Chapter 28).

A **fungal pneumonia** involving **coccidioidomycosis** has been reported in from 1:500 to 1:1,000 pregnancies and is seen primarily in the southwestern United States. This disease tends to become disseminated in 0.2% of cases. In the undisseminated form, there is little risk to the mother or the fetus. In the untreated disseminated form, the maternal mortality rate may be as high as 90%. *Amphotericin B* is the treatment of choice for the disseminated form of the disease.

4. Cystic fibrosis

Cystic fibrosis is a hereditary disease that is transmitted as an autosomal recessive. It occurs in about *1:2,000 births* and appears to be much less common in the black population. Previously, the survival of a patient with this disease beyond the age of 10 years was quite uncommon; however, with the new advances in the diagnosis and treatment of cystic fibrosis, nearly 20% of these individuals have survived into their teenage years and some of them are now entering the reproductive age groups.

These individuals have decreased or absent pancreatic enzyme function, which produces a malabsorption syndrome. An excessive amount of sodium and chloride are excreted in the sweat. The plugging of the small bronchioles by the *abnormal mucus production,* which impairs the respiratory efforts and ventilation, may be a prominent finding. Secondary pulmonary infection often occurs in these patients, due to the poor physiologic pulmonary toilet. The diagnosis can be made by sweat tests and by nail clipping tests to determine the amount of sodium and potassium present.

The pregnancy outcome in patients with cystic fibrosis is quite poor with a *maternal mortality rate of about 10%*. Moreover, intrauterine fetal growth retardation may occur secondary to the fact that the mother has such poor gastrointestinal absorption and nutrition during pregnancy.

5. Alpha₁-antitrypsin deficiency

A deficiency of alpha₁-antitrypsin is a hereditary trait characterized by an early onset of a gradually progressive obstructive lung disease with the development of a cough and dyspnea. Aggressive pulmonary toilet, including the avoidance of alcohol, sedatives, infections, fatigue, and the elimination of smoking, will assist in retarding the deterioration of the pulmonary functions. As long as the pulmonary function is not too compromised, there is apparently no effect on the pregnancy.

6. Sarcoidosis

This granulomatous disease is of unknown etiology. Sarcoidosis is a multisystem disease in which there may be involvement of the pulmonary system, the skin (i.e., erythema nodosum), the liver, the spleen, the ophthalmologic system, and the central nervous system. The pulmonary lesions occur in three stages: (1) adenopathy of the hilar and peritracheal areas, (2) reticular and/or nodular infiltrates of the lung with hilar adenopathy, and (3) adenopathy with pulmonary fibrosis.

The treatment of sarcoidosis usually involves the use of *corticosteroids*. Some patients may improve during pregnancy, and the disease has no effect on the pregnancy per se as long as there is no respiratory embarrassment. Relapses may occur in the puerperium.

7. Aspiration pneumonia (Mendelson's syndrome)

In 1946, C. L. Mendelson drew attention to the pulmonary syndrome that occurs when there has been an aspiration of the gastric contents. While this may occur especially at the time of the induction or the recovery from general anesthesia, it may also develop at any time that the patient's swallowing or consciousness is impaired. The low pH of the gastric contents causes bronchospasm, severe hypoxemia, cyanosis, apnea, and tachycardia, and if particulate matter is present, a plugging of the smaller bronchioles will occur.

The treatment of aspiration pneumonia consists of the support of the vital signs, positive end-expiratory pressure (PEEP) ventilation with adequate ventilatory volume control, and large doses of corticosteroids. A Swan-Ganz catheter is sometimes effective in monitoring the fluid replacement. While the use of corticoids is controversial, the administration of methylprednisolone sodium succinate (Solu-Medrol) I.V. in high doses has been recommended by some authors. The development of a fever, increased sputum production, and roentgenographic changes indicate the presence of an infection and the need for broad-spectrum antibiotic therapy. The usual aerobic and anaerobic mouth flora will often be present.

8. Adult respiratory distress syndrome (ARDS)

The occurrence of an adult respiratory distress syndrome (ARDS) has been attributed to the development of an acute diffuse epithelial and endothelial injury to the lung that results in fluid accumulation, secondary to surfactant damage and the increased hydrostatic forces. ARDS may occur as the result of a variety of causes, such as sepsis (39%), pulmonary aspiration (30%), hypertransfusion (24%), and pulmonary contusion (17%); the first two causes are more commonly seen in the obstetric patient. Other causes include cardiopulmonary bypass (1.7%), pneumonia (12%), burns (2.3%), fractures (5.3%), and disseminated intravascular coagulopathy (DIC) (12.5%).

The patient will initially become tachypneic as the oxygen requirements increase. Hypoxemia, decreased lung compliance, and leukopenia then develop. The administration of 100% oxygen is usually required and an endotracheal tube may become necessary, with the application of positive end-expiratory pressure (PEEP) at a level of between 8 and 12 cm of water (range 5–15 cm). The patient may later be weaned from this mechanical ventilation when the improvement in the resting minute ventilation becomes less than 10 l, the respiratory rate decreases to less than 20, and the forced vital capacity (spirometry) increases to at least 1 l. The use of high levels of pressure while using PEEP may result in a lung leak. Furthermore, PEEP may be detrimental in some cases because it may decrease the venous return and the cardiac output. If there is evidence of anemia or hypovolemia, then these conditions should be appropriately corrected with the administration of blood and crystalloids. Diuretics may be used to reduce the cardiac preload and the hydrostatic forces. If hypotension is present, it may be necessary to administer dopamine to maintain an adequate cardiac output and blood pressure. Broad-spectrum antibiotics should be administered to these patients to combat any underlying infection that may be present. The use of corticoids has been recommended, and the administration of low-dose heparin sodium may be effective in preventing pulmonary embolism. The combination of a low pH, a low bicarbonate level, a peripheral blood smear with less than 10% band forms, and a rising blood urea nitrogen (BUN) level are poor prognostic factors in these patients.

CHAPTER 32

Gastrointestinal disease

A physician who treats himself has a fool for a patient.
—*Sir William Osler**

1. Duodenal ulcer

A duodenal ulcer (i.e., peptic ulcer) is *an erosion into the mucosa and the underlying muscularis mucosa of the duodenum.* The patient generally has a history of epigastric pain or reports a burning sensation that occurs prior to meals and is relieved by food. The patient may relate to you that the use of antacids (e.g., Tums or Rolaids) has also provided relief of the pain and "heartburn."

During pregnancy, almost all patients with a duodenal ulcer get better and become asymptomatic. *The diagnosis can be made by using a flexible endoscope to visualize the lesion.* Diagnostic roentgenographic studies (i.e., upper GI series) are usually deferred until after the pregnancy is over because of the possible radiation hazards to the fetus.

The treatment of a duodenal ulcer is based upon the use of *antacids and diet.* Some of the newer medications, such as cimetidine and H_2 blockers, should be avoided until further information is available concerning their effects in pregnancy.

---

*Reprinted with permission from Robert Bennett Bean, *Sir William Osler: Aphorisms from His Bedside Teachings and Writings,* William Bennett Bean, ed. Springfield, Ill.: Charles C Thomas, Publisher, 1968, p. 53.

2. Inflammatory bowel disease

The effect of inflammatory bowel disease (i.e., Crohn's disease or regional enteritis, and ulcerative colitis) on the pregnant patient was considered with some pessimism in the past. Although it was previously thought that patients with inflammatory bowel disease did poorly in pregnancy, this has not been found to be the case, *except perhaps in the case of ulcerative colitis.* In Crohn's disease, there is no greater risk of having a premature delivery, a stillbirth, or a congenital abnormality; however, the abortion rate may be slightly higher (10–25%). As a consequence, when inflammatory bowel disease is under good control, there is little reason to be overly pessimistic about the course of the pregnancy in such patients. About 50% of these patients will experience a flare-up of their disease in pregnancy, and the same number will experience a relapse of their disease in the postpartum period. The complications of inflammatory bowel disease are no more frequent in pregnant women than they are in those who are not pregnant; however, they may be more difficult to detect because of the relative contraindication to using certain diagnostic techniques (e.g., radiologic procedures).

The treatment of inflammatory bowel disease is essentially the same for both Crohn's disease and ulcerative colitis. In the patient who has active disease, an initial dose of *prednisone,* 20–40 mg, may be given each morning with a gradual reduction in the dosage as the patient improves.

Sulfasalazine, another drug that has been used in nonpregnant patients, should not be used in pregnancy unless it is absolutely necessary, since its effect on the fetus is unknown. Other agents typically used for symptomatic relief of inflammatory bowel disease, such as codeine, Metamucil, Amphojel, Pepto-Bismol, or Lomotil, may be used as necessary.

3. Cholestatic jaundice and cholecystitis

a. Cholestatic jaundice

This syndrome was originally described in Swedish women in late pregnancy who complained of *pruritus and jaundice*. As many as 18–44% of affected women have relatives who have had a similar episode of pruritus and jaundice during pregnancy. Cholestatic jaundice occurs in about 1:1,500 pregnancies in the United States and is second only to viral hepatitis as a cause of jaundice. Since it also occurs in women who take oral contraceptives, it has been postulated that a relationship may exist between cholestatic jaundice and the estrogens and progesterone present in pregnancy.

Usually, the **pruritus,** which can be quite severe, develops in the third trimester and is followed in 1–2 weeks by the occurrence of jaundice, with dark urine and light stools. Fever, nausea and vomiting, and abdominal right upper quadrant pain are absent in these patients. The differential diagnosis should include viral hepatitis, drug-induced hepatic injury, cholecystitis, sepsis/pyelonephritis, acute fatty liver of pregnancy, toxemia (pregnancy-induced hypertension), hemolytic anemia, and megaloblastic anemia of pregnancy.

The laboratory studies will reveal an elevated alkaline phosphatase and an elevated bilirubin, particularly the direct-reacting fraction, which will be slightly elevated to about 5 mg%. The serum transaminase levels (i.e., serum glutamic-oxaloacetic transaminase, or SGOT, and serum glutamic-pyruvic transaminase, or SGPT) are generally less than 250 sigma units. *The values of the serum bile acids (i.e., cholic, chenodeoxycholic, and deoxycholic acid) may increase* up to 100-fold. The deposition of the bile acids in the skin causes pruritus.

The therapy is symptomatic in nature. An attempt is made to lower the serum and skin levels of bile acids by treating the patient with cholestyramine resin (Questran), 4 grams t.i.d. in a liquid suspension. There are no other effects of this condition on the mother, except for perhaps a slightly increased risk of premature labor and of fetal loss.

b. Cholecystitis

Acute cholecystitis is rare in pregnancy and has been reported to occur in about 1:16,000 pregnancies. **Biliary colic occurs as a pain in the right upper quadrant of the abdomen and is secondary to the obstruction of the cystic duct. Acute cholecystitis occurs when this obstruction leads to inflammation of the gall bladder. If the common bile duct becomes obstructed, severe nausea and vomiting, fever, and jaundice may occur.** Moreover, if the ampulla is temporarily obstructed, pancreatitis may develop.

Gallstones are usually formed from cholesterol, although on rare occasions, they may be made of calcium bilirubinate. *Whenever the bile becomes supersaturated with cholesterol, crystallization of the cholesterol takes place.* In the presence of large amounts of chenodeoxycholic acid, the cholesterol secretion is decreased and supersaturation does not occur. Estrogens and progesterone increase the risk of stone formation by increasing the biliary cholesterol saturation.

The diagnosis of gallstones can be made by the use of ultrasonography or with intravenous cholangiography (IC). The use of a *HIDA technetium scan* (i.e., **H**–technetium radical diisopropyl, **IDA**—imino diacetic acid), however, has proven to be as accurate as the IC and has the added advantage of not exposing the fetus to as much radiation or to the risk of allergic reactions.

When acute cholecystitis occurs in pregnancy, treatment is primarily symptomatic in nature and consists of fluid and electrolyte replacement, nasogastric suction, and antibiotics. Surgery is rarely necessary during pregnancy, but it should be performed in the interconceptional period in patients who have had one or more attacks of cholecystitis during pregnancy.

4. Infectious hepatitis

Since the discovery of the hepatitis B antigen in 1963, it has been shown that there are at least three primary forms of hepatitis: (1) hepatitis A, (2) hepatitis B, and (3) non-A, non-B hepatitis.

Recently, a fourth type, delta-hepatitis, has been noted as a coinfective agent with acute hepatitis B.

a. Hepatitis A

Viral hepatitis A (infectious hepatitis) is caused by the hepatitis A virus (HAV), which is a 27-nm single strand ribonucleic acid (RNA) surrounded by a nucleocapsid. It is classified as an enterovirus which is a type of picornavirus. This disease occurs in patients who are in the lower socioeconomic groups. The transmission of the HAV occurs under conditions of poor hygiene, including poor sanitation, and through contaminated food (e.g., shellfish) and water. It may also be transmitted by sexual contact. About 38% of the cases of acute hepatitis in the United States are due to the hepatitis A virus.

The greatest period of infectivity is during the two weeks preceding the onset of jaundice. The incubation period is 15–50 days. The patient usually presents with an abrupt onset of a *flu-like syndrome,* which may be severe, with abdominal pain, fever, malaise, anorexia, nausea and vomiting, jaundice, and pruritus. It is often more severe in adults than in children, with a mortality rate of about 0.6%. **Rarely, vertical transmission to the fetus may occur.**

The laboratory values generally show a marked elevation of the SGOT and SGPT levels, as well as an elevation of the alkaline phosphatase, serum cholesterol, and bilirubin values. Acute and convalescent sera will detect IgM class anti-HAV and total anti-HAV antibodies. Anti-HAV IgG antibodies develop during the clinical illness and are then detectable for life (i.e., life-long immunity). Approximately 30–50% of all adults will show serologic evidence of a previous infection with HAV.

The treatment of hepatitis consists of rest and good nutrition. Close contacts should receive immune serum globulin (0.02 ml/kg I.M.) within 14 days of exposure. If administered early in the incubation period, its prophylactic success is of the order of 80–90%.

b. Hepatitis B

The hepatitis B virus (serum hepatitis) (HBV) is the most common cause of acute and chronic hepatitis and occurs as a result of exposure to the saliva, semen, and blood or blood products of infected individuals.

There are about 200,000 cases in the United States each year, and about 250 of these people will die. Health-care workers, homosexuals, drug abusers, and patients who require frequent blood products are at an increased risk for contracting this disease.

The hepatitis B virus has a 42-nm double-stranded circular DNA genome with a nucleocapsid core surrounded by an outer lipoprotein envelope. It is a member of the Hepadnaviridae family. The intact virus is known as a "Dane" particle. The Australia antigen, hepatitis-associated antigen, or, as it is now called, the HB_sAg, is a surface antigen (outer lipid envelope) and is also found on the 22-nm spherical and tubular forms. The subtypes of the HB_sAg surface antigen are "adw," "adr," "ayw," and "ayr." The determinant "a" is common to all HB_sAg antigens. **HB_sAg may be identified in the serum as early as 7–14 days following exposure to the hepatitis B virus, and it occurs about 7–10 days before the onset of the clinical symptoms.** The presence of HB_sAg does not distinguish between a chronic or an acute infection. The concomitant presence of the HB_sAb antibody is indicative of a noninfectious state, whereas without the antibody, then it is indicative of a chronic carrier state. An antibody to the core antigen HB_cAg (the nucleocapsid core), anti-HB_c (IgM), develops during the infection and persists for many years. HB_eAg, a third antigen, is reflective of the infectivity of the virus. It is usually present early in the disease and disappears after about 6–8 weeks if the hepatitis does not become chronic. HB_eAg, HBV-associated DNA polymerase enzyme activity, and HBV DNA have all been found in the serum at the onset of the illness. These markers have been associated with the replication of HBV and correlate with the infectivity of the blood. By the time the HBV replication has ended, antibodies HB_eAg appear and the patient's infectivity is markedly diminished.

In the United States, about 0.1–0.5% of the population are carriers of HBV. Following exposure to the HBV, adults should receive 0.06 ml/kg I.M. (or 5 ml) of HBIG within 24 hours, in conjunction with 1.0 ml (20 μg) I.M. of vaccine within seven days, and then again at one month and at six months following exposure.

The greatest period of infectivity is during the two weeks preceding the onset of jaundice. The incubation period is long (average 60–120 days). The onset of hepatitis B is more insidious than that of hepatitis A and consists of symptoms of anorexia, malaise, nausea and vomiting, abdominal pain, skin rash, jaundice, and arthralgia. **Vertical transmission to the fetus is common (65%), especially during the third trimester, in both the chronic carrier and in the patient with active disease.** Prematurity is increased, according to some studies. Transmission of the disease to the fetus may take place either transplacentally or during the passage of the fetus through the birth canal; in cases where transmission to the fetus occurs, either a chronic carrier state (up to 90%) or a fulminant hepatic disease with fetal death may result. The incidence of the development of the carrier state is inversely proportional to the age at which the infection is contracted, with only about 6–10% of young adults who contract the disease becoming chronic carriers.

Hyperimmune serum (HBIG) (0.5 ml, or 10 µg I.M.) should be administered to the fetus within 12 hours of birth. The hepatitis B vaccine should also be given within 12 hours of birth, again at 1 month, and then again at 6 months of age (0.5 ml, or 10 µg I.M.), for a total of 3 doses. The use of the combined HBIG and hepatitis vaccine soon after birth has been shown to be about 85–95% effective in preventing the development of the HBV carrier state. Routine testing of all prenatal patients, as well as the subsequent treatment of the infants, is cost-effective. The treatment of the mother consists of good nutrition and rest.

c. Non-A, non-B hepatitis

Non-A, non-B hepatitis seems to occur mostly in patients who have a **posttransfusion hepatitis,** which accounts for 90% of these cases in the United States. The exact virus or viruses involved in non-A, non-B hepatitis, are unknown; however, the virus may be transmitted by the fecal-oral route in some instances. The incubation period is 30–160 days. Chronic hepatitis may occur in 20–70% of the patients who contract non-A, non-B hepatitis, while only about 8% of those who contract the disease will become carriers. The treatment is the same as in the other forms of hepatitis, except that immune globulin treatment of the infant is not recommended. If it is administered, it has been suggested that it be given in the same dosage as has been described for hepatitis B.

d. Delta hepatitis (HDV)

This 35–37 nm virus consists of defective RNA genetic material and a protein delta antigen coated with

$HB_s Ag$ surface antigen (lipid envelope). The infection occurs in conjunction with a hepatitis B viral infection, either as a coinfection or as a superinfection. Those individuals who are at risk for HBV, such as parenteral drug addicts, homosexuals, and hemophilia patients, are also at risk for the delta virus infection. The delta antigen can be detected in the serum early in the course of the infection. This agent appears to be associated with chronic hepatitis in as many as 50% of the cases.

5. Acute fatty liver in pregnancy

Acute fatty liver in pregnancy (AFLP), also called acute obstetric yellow atrophy, or acute fatty metamorphosis of the liver, has been thought in the past to be quite rare, with an estimated incidence of the order of 1:1,000,000. However, recent evidence indicates that this entity might be much more prevalent than was formerly thought, with an incidence of about **1:13,000.** In addition, the maternal mortality rate in these cases was reported to be as high as 75% in the past, with a fetal mortality rate of 74%. More recent reports indicate that the maternal mortality rate may be close to zero and the fetal mortality rate may be of the order of between 10 and 22%.

a. Clinical findings

AFLP appears to be limited to the **third trimester** and is more commonly associated with **primigravidas** who have **multiple gestations** than with multiparous women. **Preeclampsia and eclampsia has been noted in 46% of these patients.** The patient may initially present with nausea and vomiting associated with malaise and fatigue. Various degrees of upper quadrant distress or abdominal pain may also be present. Jaundice (90%) without pruritus will usually occur within one week of the onset of symptoms and may be associated with an altered sensorium or coma. Premature labor or vaginal bleeding may occur. Toxemia with hypertension, edema, and proteinuria is often present, and the patient may manifest tachycardia without fever.

b. Diagnosis

In patients with AFLP, there may be severe hypoglycemia and an elevation of the uric acid, blood urea nitrogen, and creatinine levels. In addition, hyper-bilirubinemia may be present, with an elevation of both the direct and the indirect fractions and elevated amylase levels. A moderate elevation of the SGOT over the SGPT may occur. These changes are different from those of the patient with acute hepatitis, where the SGOT may be greatly elevated to over 1,000 U/l. Hyponatremia may also occur.

Anemia, leukocytosis (more than 15,000/mm³), and thrombocytopenia (i.e., less than 50,000/mm³) may develop secondary to hemorrhage and intravascular hemolysis (i.e., DIC). The peripheral blood smear will usually show target cells, normoblasts, basophilic stippling, toxic granulations, and giant platelets. There may be a prolongation of the partial thromboplastin time (PTT) and the prothrombin time. Factor V and other clotting factors, such as antithrombin III, may be decreased.

Ultrasound has not been helpful in these cases; however, the use of computerized tomography (CT), and magnetic resonance imaging (MRI) of the liver have been of assistance. While a liver biopsy will make a definitive diagnosis, the presence of DIC will often make this diagnostic technique too dangerous. If a *specimen of liver* is obtained, the use of a special solution of oil-red O stain on the **fresh tissue** will confirm the diagnosis.

The differential diagnosis should include: (1) hepatic dysfunction of pregnancy and toxemia (HELLP syndrome), (2) drug abuse, (3) chemical/alcohol exposure, (4) viral hepatitis (hepatitis A, hepatitis B, or hepatitis non-A, non-B), (5) cholestasis of pregnancy, (6) hemolytic uremic syndrome, (7) cholecystitis, and (8) systemic lupus erythematosus.

c. Treatment

The treatment of AFLP is immediate delivery and the use of intensive supportive therapy of the patient. The early diagnosis of AFLP and the prompt termination of the pregnancy have been largely responsible for the recent improvement in both the maternal and fetal survival rates. Following the delivery of the infant by the most expeditious method, the patient's condition will frequently deteriorate rapidly. The DIC, the anemia, and the hypoglycemia should be corrected by the administration of fresh frozen plasma (or cryoprecipitate), packed red blood cells, and glucose solutions. The fluid management may require a central venous pressure catheter.

The administration of cimetidine (Tagamet) may prevent serious bleeding from the gastrointestinal tract, and broad-spectrum antibiotics should be utilized to prevent the development of a serious infection.

6. Acute pancreatitis

It has been estimated that 65% of all cases of pancreatitis in pregnancy are due to gallstones. Pancreatic involvement should be considered in pregnant patients who have severe epigastric pain associated with persistent nausea and vomiting and jaundice. The detection of elevated levels of *serum lipase and amylase may be helpful in making the diagnosis.*

The treatment for acute pancreatitis is essentially the same type of symptomatic therapy that is utilized in acute cholecystitis. It consists of fluid and electrolyte replacement, nasogastric suction, and antibiotics. If there is biliary tract involvement, the clinical course of the pancreatitis usually begins to resolve within two days. If the symptoms persist beyond this time, you should suspect that the pancreatitis may be due to alcoholism, or, in rare cases, to other lesions, such as a stenosis of the sphincter of Oddi or a carcinoma of the head of the pancreas.

7. Hyperemesis gravidarum

The diagnosis of hyperemesis gravidarum is usually reserved for severe cases of nausea and vomiting that require hospitalization. The vomiting reflex originates in the central nervous system, which coordinates the closure of the epiglottis, the contraction of the pyloric region of the stomach, the relaxation of the fundal region of the stomach, and the increase in abdominal pressure, which pushes the gastric contents up into the esophagus to be expelled. **"Morning sickness" occurs in about one-third of all pregnant women during the first 2–3 months of pregnancy.** In most of these patients, the symptoms are mild and only occur upon awakening. The symptoms in another one-third of patients may persist throughout the day in a more severe form. If the nausea or vomiting becomes excessive, the patient should be hospitalized for the restoration of her fluid and electrolyte balance. **When the husband develops nausea and vomiting instead of the pregnant woman, it has been termed the "couvade" syndrome.**

a. Incidence

In some reports, the incidence of severe hyperemesis is about 1:250–1:350 pregnancies. In others, it has been reported to occur in 1.6% of white patients and 0.71% of black patients. Hyperemesis has been thought to be more common in patients who smoke, who weigh more than 77 kg, and who are primigravidas and adolescents. In many of these patients, emotional and psychological factors either instigate or aggravate hyperemesis. One author has characterized such women as being of moderate intelligence with histrionic personalities, who have strong maternal attachments and have demonstrated immature behavior. These patients commonly are under stress and have a low level of social support. The cause of hyperemesis is unknown, but high chorionic gonadotropin values have been implicated, since the highest values occur during the early part of the pregnancy when the nausea and vomiting are most prevalent. The high incidence of severe hyperemesis in patients with a hydatidiform mole, which also is associated with high levels of chorionic gonadotropins, seems to be supportive of this theory.

b. Diagnosis

The finding of a decreased skin turgor and dry mucous membranes, associated with a high specific gravity of the urine and the presence of ketones in the urine, will provide you with a crude estimate of the severity of the emesis and the degree of dehydration. The diagnoses that should be considered in patients with hyperemesis are: (1) appendicitis, (2) liver disease, such as cholecystitis or hepatitis, (3) hiatal hernia, (4) intestinal obstruction, and (5) hydatidiform mole. Appropriate tests should be obtained, depending upon the severity of the patient's symptoms and the clinical picture.

c. Treatment

The treatment of hyperemesis requires a sympathetic physician who can reassure the patient that the condition is self-limited. *Frequent small feedings of bland liquids and solids, such as toast or crackers, alternating with broth or tea, are often helpful. Greasy and spicy foods should be avoided. Full meals, as well as adverse cooking odors, should also be avoided.* Carbonated beverages are often tolerated better than milk or other fluids. The patient should use **hard Christmas candy** upon awakening, letting it dissolve slowly in her mouth, since this will usually alleviate the initial morning nausea.

Various tranquilizers and antiemetics have been used with success in some patients. Drugs that have been used to treat hyperemesis include meclizine hydrochloride (Bonine) and promethazine hydrochloride (Phenergan).

If acidosis, dehydration, and weight loss occur, the patient should be hospitalized and her electrolytes and fluids replaced by intravenous infusion. In the rare instance in which the I.V. fluids and a bland diet do not prove to be adequate in the management of the patient, you may be forced to resort to gastric feedings or parenteral nutrition.

8. Pica

The term "pica" refers to the craving for strange foods or for bizarre materials by the pregnant patient. While the desire for odd combinations of foods, such as dill pickles and ice cream, elicits smiles and knowing nods from the patient's family and friends, the craving for clay, baking powder, baking soda, ice, or starch is quite a different thing. Ice, snow, and frost craving have been considered to be a sign that the patient may have an iron deficiency anemia. Starch and clay ingestion are often found in patients who are economically disadvantaged. Indeed, clay from certain areas of the country may be avidly sought after by the patient as being of better quality than clay in other areas.

While these materials do not usually cause problems when ingested in small quantities, the absorption of iron and other nutrients may be impaired when large amounts are eaten. There is one report of pica in a nonpregnant patient in which the ingested clay was shown to be a potassium binder. The patient presented with muscle weakness and hypokalemia.

9. Ptyalism

Ptyalism is the name that is applied to excessive salivation. In these cases, the various substances that stimulate the glands should be identified and eliminated from the diet.

CHAPTER 33

Urinary tract disease

The art of the practice of medicine is to be learned only by experience; 'tis not an inheritance; it cannot be revealed. Learn to see, learn to hear, learn to feel, learn to smell, and know that by practice alone can you become expert.

—*Sir William Osler**

Women who have severe chronic renal disease, as evidenced by a blood urea nitrogen (BUN) of greater than 30 mg/dl and a creatinine concentration above 2.0 mg/dl, will have difficulty in pregnancy. Hypertension, with superimposed preeclampsia, may occur in more than 40% of these cases. The perinatal morbidity and mortality rate is increased in patients with chronic hypertension, and further increased if superimposed preeclampsia occurs. Intrauterine growth retardation and fetal distress is common in hypertensive patients.

1. Asymptomatic bacteriuria

Asymptomatic bacteriuria (ASB) occurs in 2–12% of pregnant patients. If the bacteriuria is not treated, then about 25–30% of these patients will later develop acute pyelonephritis during the pregnancy, as opposed to only 2–3% of those patients who have been treated.

A culture of a clean-catch specimen of urine should be obtained on all pregnant patients. **A colony count of 100,000 per milliliter of urine, on two consecutive cultures, in the absence of clinical symptoms of urinary tract disease, confirms asymptomatic bacteriuria.**

Patients with sickle cell trait, toxemia, or diabetes mellitus, are thought to have an increased risk of having asymptomatic bacteriuria. As many as 40% of patients with ASB show evidence of an upper urinary tract disease, such as a silent or asymptomatic pyelonephritis. Another cause of urinary tract infection is faulty hygiene, and the patient should be cautioned to wipe backward rather than frontward after a bowel movement to avoid labial and urethral contamination. Coitus may also cause trauma and contamination of the urethral area.

Specific receptors for the fimbria of the Escherichia coli organisms have been demonstrated on the surface of the uroepithelial cells of the urologic tract. Whether there are quantitative differences in the number of receptor sites in patients who are more susceptible to urinary tract infections is unknown. The frequency of urinary tract infections may be related to the ability of the bacteria to adhere to mucosal or squamous cells. **A substance called "uromucoid" has been isolated. It is a polysaccharide, which is very hydrophilic, and it interposes water between the bacteria and the surface membrane.** This uromucoid is decreased in some individuals, and is markedly decreased in the absence of estrogen (e.g., during menopause). A lack of uromucoid might cause some women to be more susceptible to urinary tract infections. This explanation might also account for the marked decrease in urinary infections in older women after instituting therapy with vaginal estrogen cream.

Certain virulence factors have also been described that enhance the ability of the organism to set up an

*Reprinted with permission from Robert Bennett Bean, *Sir William Osler: Aphorisms from His Bedside Teachings and Writings*, William Bennett Bean, ed. Springfield, Ill.: Charles C Thomas, Publisher, 1968, p. 129.

infection. K antigens, a capsular substance that allows E. coli to evade the phagocytes, have been described. Coliform bacteria have been found to have a mannoside-receptor type of pili that apparently allows the bacterium to attach itself easily to the uroepithelium. Some studies have shown that patients who have a blood substance known as "P" are more susceptible to urinary tract infections and that this substance is associated with a particular galactosugar. It has been suggested that perhaps certain sugars that are ingested may coat the pili receptor sites and act to prevent the adherence of bacteria on the pili receptors. Moreover, a naturally produced protein, the Tamm-Horsfall (TH) protein, has been shown to occlude receptor sites and prevent the adherence of bacteria so that it can then be flushed out of the urinary tract with normal urination.

A patient with ASB should be treated with an appropriate antibiotic and should have at least one follow-up negative culture after the therapy is completed. Treatment failure may occur in as many as 20–30% of patients, secondary to preexisting renal disease, resistant bacterial organisms, or patient noncompliance.

2. Acute pyelonephritis

Urinary tract infections are one of the most common causes of hospitalization in pregnancy. The infection not only poses problems in terms of sepsis to the mother, but it also places the fetus at risk for damage secondary to maternal fever, antibiotic therapy, and possibly premature labor. **The diagnosis of acute pyelonephritis should be considered whenever a patient presents with symptoms of frequency of urination, dysuria, suprapubic pain, costovertebral angle tenderness, fever, and chills.**

The diagnosis of pyelonephritis is assured when a urine culture indicates that there are more than 10^5 bacteria per milliliter of urine and a urinalysis shows the presence of pyuria. The most common bacterial isolates are those of the Enterobacteriaceae species, the most common organism being Escherichia coli, with its five serotypes K1, 2, 3, 12, and 13. Other gram-negative organisms include the Klebsiella and Proteus species. In addition, the Pseudomonas and Staphylococcus species may also be present.

Although it has been suggested that it would be beneficial to be able to distinguish between infections of the bladder (i.e., lower tract disease) and those involving the kidney (i.e., upper tract disease), there are currently no reliable simple techniques to make this determination. Fluorescent-antibody-coated bacteria can usually be seen in patients who have upper tract infection, but they also may be found in as many as one-third of the patients who have a lower tract infection. The definitive test for upper tract involvement is a renal biopsy; however, this approach is rarely indicated. Furthermore, such a distinction would perhaps offer little in the management of the patient, since the organisms in both places should be susceptible to the usual antibiotics that are utilized. If the infection is in the upper tract, then a longer course of therapy should be administered or the patient should receive such antibiotics as kanamycin, gentamicin, or tobramycin, which should sterilize the urinary tract.

A variety of drugs have been used to treat acute pyelonephritis, such as sulfonamides, ampicillin, and cephalosporins. The treatment of acute pyelonephritis commonly consists of the administration of intravenous antibiotics, such as ampicillin, 1.0 gram every 4–6 hours, until the patient is afebrile for 24–48 hours. Some authors recommend oral ampicillin for an additional 10–14 days. Since the conditions in the renal system during pregnancy are quite favorable for the development of urinary tract infections (i.e., ureteral dilatation, decreased peristalsis, relative stasis of the urine, increased pH, decreased osmolality conducive to the growth of E. coli, and increased estrogen levels, which may impair leukocytic function), follow-up cultures are necessary to be certain that the infection has been cured by the course of antibiotic therapy. Patients who have a recurrence of their infection should be considered as candidates for long-term antibiotic therapy for the duration of the pregnancy. An agent such as nitrofurantoin (Macrodantin) may be used for long-term therapy. It should be noted, however, that recent evidence indicates that short-term therapy may be as effective as long-term therapy.

3. Acute and chronic glomerulonephritis

The occurrence of **acute glomerulonephritis** in pregnancy is quite rare and has been estimated to occur in about 1 in 40,000 pregnancies. The treatment of this condition in pregnancy is no different than in the nonpregnant patient. The control of the hypertension, and of the electrolyte and fluid balance, is essential to avoid complications. *Superimposed toxemia should be guarded against, since it may increase the perinatal morbidity.* With adequate medical therapy to control the blood pressure, including salt restriction, the pregnancy should progress uneventfully to a satisfactory conclusion.

In **chronic glomerulonephritis,** the outcome of the pregnancy is usually dependent upon whether severe renal disease and hypertension are present. If hypertension is present, one investigator found a fetal survival rate of only 55%, whereas in its absence, the survival rate was 93%. Proteinuria is commonly present; the amount of protein in the urine may progress to the amount that is usually seen in patients with the nephrotic syndrome.

4. Nephrotic syndrome

While the most common cause of the nephrotic syndrome is thought to be membranous or membranoproliferative glomerulonephritis, other conditions, such as chronic glomerulonephritis or lipoid nephrosis, have also been reported to be involved. *The presence of edema, severe proteinuria (more than 5 grams in 24 hours), and hypoproteinemia (i.e., the nephrotic syndrome) does not appear to influence the outcome of pregnancy appreciably, unless hypertension or azotemia is also present.* The risk of thromboembolism (e.g., renal vein thrombosis) due to hyperlipidemia, edema, and other changes in the coagulation system in pregnancy is thought to be increased in patients with nephrotic syndrome. A high-protein diet is essential in these patients in order to replace the amount that is lost in the urine. In addition, these patients are more susceptible to infections and should be followed closely with frequent urine cultures.

5. Urinary calculus

A renal calculus may occur in about 1:1,000 pregnancies. During pregnancy, the dilatation of the renal pelvis and ureters is associated with a decreased peristalsis, which is secondary to the increased progesterone secretion and perhaps also to some degree to the mechanical obstruction of the ureters by the enlarging uterus. *These changes cause a relative stasis of the urine flow and lead to an increased risk of infection.* Chronic infections may predispose the individual to the formation of kidney stones. Since most of the stones in pregnancy are made of calcium, hyperparathyroidism should be ruled out. A serum urate determination should also be obtained. *Recurrent urinary tract infections should be treated with antibiotics and followed closely with posttherapy cultures throughout the pregnancy.*

When acute pyelonephritis does not respond to the administration of appropriate antibiotics, the astute physician should suspect that a renal calculus may be present. A "single-shot" intravenous pyelogram (IVP) will often demonstrate the stone. The presence of urease-containing bacterial organisms in the urine may be significant, since they may cause alkalinization of the urine and the resultant precipitation of calcium phosphate. *Cystinuria is an uncommon cause of renal calculi, but if present, it may be treated with D-penicillamine.* You should also be aware of the milk-alkali syndrome, in which an excessive ingestion of antacids, alkali, and sodium bicarbonate by the patient causes the formation of renal calculi.

The management of a renal calculus is dependent upon: (1) when it occurs in pregnancy, and (2) whether there is complete or incomplete obstruction of the ureter. **If there is complete obstruction of the ureter, the blockage must be immediately relieved.** There are two approaches that have been utilized in the management of stones: (1) dilatation and exploration of the ureter, with the hope that the stone will be passed or removed, and (2) abdominal surgical exploration with the removal of the stone. During the first two trimesters, the surgical removal of the stone can usually be easily accomplished; however, in the third trimester, the bulk of the uterus may prevent an adequate exposure of a stone in the lower ureter. In such a situation, if the obstruction of the ureter is complete, then it may be advisable to perform a nephrostomy and reserve definitive treatment until after the pregnancy is over.

6. Diabetic glomerulosclerosis (Kimmelstiel-Wilson's syndrome)

Over the course of about 15 years, most diabetics develop a nephropathy that has been described as a nodular or diffuse glomerulosclerosis. The usual vascular changes involve the arteries of the kidney and consist of intimal and medial hyalinization, atheromatous changes in the large vessels, and mesangial proliferation in the glomeruli, with a thickening of the basement membrane. *This basement membrane thickening is referred to as a Kimmelstiel-Wilson's nodule.* **Since there are widespread vascular changes throughout the body in diabetes, the involvement of the retinal vessels, with aneurysms and arteriosclerotic changes, tends to parallel those that are seen in the kidney.**

The clinical features of diabetic nephropathy consist of hypertension, proteinuria, and azotemia. Asymptomatic bacteriuria may also be more common in pregnant diabetics (i.e., about 15–18%). The presence of asymptomatic bacteriuria should be identified and treated to prevent the progression of the infection to an acute pyelonephritis and the possibility of developing diabetic ketoacidosis.

7. Severe renal disease and renal transplantation

Patients who have chronic renal failure and who are undergoing dialysis may become pregnant (about 1:200), although only a few will produce full-term infants. A number of such patients have now been reported, and of about 15 patients in one series, 2 had stillbirths, and 11 had infants that were premature by weight (i.e., under 2,000 grams). The occurrence of hypotension and vaginal bleeding appears to be the only maternal complications noted with the dialysis procedure itself. Recently, nine cases were reported in which the course was complicated by diabetes mellitus. There was one maternal death and two fetal losses reported in this series.

The incidence of pregnancy in women who have had a renal transplant is about 1 in 50. **Pregnancy should be deferred until 18–24 months after a renal transplantation and until there is no evidence of graft rejection present.** *Only 45–65% of living donor kidneys and 30–35% of cadaver kidneys are functional after five years.* Should the renal function deteriorate in such patients during pregnancy, then consideration should be given to terminating the pregnancy.

About 26–30% of transplant patients will develop pregnancy-induced hypertension. **In addition, urinary tract infections (17%), premature rupture of the membranes, premature labor, premature delivery (33–52%), and intrauterine growth retardation (IUGR) (8–45%), are also more common.** No fetal congenital malformations have been noted in patients with a renal transplant, in spite of the fact that all of the reported patients have been treated with cortisone supplementation during pregnancy and at the time of delivery. The rejection rate of the kidney is the same as in the nonpregnant patient (9%).

The management of the pregnancy following renal transplantation should include, in addition to the normal studies, the following: (1) biweekly visits until 28 weeks' gestation, then weekly visits, (2) early ultrasound dating of the pregnancy, (3) periodic laboratory studies, including antibody titers for the cytomegalovirus (CMV) and the herpes simplex virus (HSV), plus cervical smears and cultures for HSV, (4) a glucose tolerance test as indicated, and at 26–28 weeks' gestation, (5) multiple sonographic studies in the third trimester to detect intrauterine growth retardation (IUGR), (6) nonstress and stress tests in the third trimester, and (7) a serum HB_sAg test prior to delivery to determine the need for the administration of hepatitis B immune globulin (HBIG) to the infant. The renal function tests should be monitored at periodic intervals throughout the pregnancy. The serum creatinine should be less than 2 mg/dl, and there should be minimal proteinuria and hypertension. Although 60–70% of patients who have had renal transplants do well in pregnancy, about 20–50% will require cesarean section for obstetric reasons.

Postpartum contraception should not include oral contraceptives (due to the higher risk of thromboembolism and hypertension) or an intrauterine device (due to the risk of infection) in an immunosuppressed patient.

CHAPTER 34

Endocrine/metabolic diseases

Acquire the art of detachment, the virtue of method, and the quality of thoroughness, but above all the grace of humility.

—*Sir William Osler**

1. Diabetes mellitus

In the days before insulin became available, diabetes mellitus in pregnancy resulted in a 30% maternal mortality rate and a 65% perinatal mortality rate. With modern treatment, the fetal mortality rate has decreased to about 3–5%. *Diabetes mellitus is a metabolic disorder that occurs whenever there is an absolute or relative lack of insulin available to the individual.* In the initial stages, when the body is unable to appropriately handle the glucose load from a meal, then postprandial hyperglycemia results (i.e., an abnormal glucose tolerance test). If the insulin lack becomes more severe, then fasting hyperglycemia develops (i.e., overt diabetes mellitus).

One classification system lists **type I diabetes,** an insulin-dependent form of diabetes (previously called juvenile diabetes), and **type II diabetes,** an insulin-independent form of diabetes (previously known as a maturity-onset diabetes). The American College of Obstetricians and Gynecologists' classification system has proven to be more useful in the management of the pregnant diabetic patient (Table 34-1). *The levels*

*Reprinted with permission from Robert Bennett Bean, *Sir William Osler: Aphorisms from His Bedside Teachings and Writings,* William Bennett Bean, ed. Springfield, Ill.: Charles C Thomas, Publisher, 1968, p. 72.

of the circulating glucose, either while fasting or after a 100-gram glucose load in a three-hour glucose tolerance test, will differ depending on whether the glucose is measured in the whole blood or in the plasma. The plasma glucose levels are slightly higher than those in whole blood.

a. Incidence

The incidence of gestational diabetes is approximately 3–12% in pregnancy, whereas the incidence of insulin-dependent diabetes mellitus in pregnancy is only about 0.1–0.5%. About 60,000–90,000 American women develop gestational diabetes each year. Ideally, **preconceptional counseling** should be carried out on all diabetic patients prior to the onset of pregnancy. Those patients who are known diabetics should be regulated and their condition optimized prior to conception for the best pregnancy results. In one report, when diabetes was under good control prior to conception, the incidence of fetal anomalies was 1.1%, whereas in those patients who were not controlled prior to eight weeks' gestation, the incidence of anomalies was 6.6%. Patient education, by means of media campaigns and posters, and by the physician's emphasis on the importance of optimal care during pregnancy for the diabetic, would go a long way toward diminishing the damaging fetal effects of this disease. The infants of diabetic mothers are at risk for congenital anomalies (6–8%) (e.g., brain, kidney, limbs, and heart), macrosomia, prematurity, the respiratory distress syndrome, and death, in addition to the metabolic derangements in the neonatal period of hypoglycemia, hypocalcemia, and hyperbilirubinemia. In addition, polycythemia and renal vein thrombosis may occur in the neonate. If the maternal glucose level is closely controlled during preg-

TABLE 34-1. Classification of diabetes in pregnancy

Pregestational diabetes

Class	Age of onset (year)	Duration (year)	Vascular disease	Therapy
A	Any	Any	0	A–1, diet only A–2, insulin
B	>20	<10	0	Insulin
C	10–19 or	10–19	0	Insulin
D	10 or 20		Benign retinopathy	Insulin
F	Any	Any	Nephropathy	Insulin
R	Any	Any	Proliferative retinopathy	Insulin
H	Any	Any	Heart disease	Insulin

Gestational diabetes

Class	Fasting glucose level		Postprandial glucose level
A–1	< 105 mg/dl	and	< 120 mg/dl
A–2	≥ 105 mg/dl	and/or	≥ 120 mg/dl

Reprinted with permission from American College of Obstetricians and Gynecologists, "Management of Diabetes Mellitus in Pregnancy," *ACOG Technical Bulletin* 92 (1986), p. 1.

nancy, it is thought that the risk of these complications may be decreased considerably.

b. Diagnosis

The presence of diabetes should be suspected in obstetric patients who have: (1) diabetes in a parent or sibling, (2) a history of delivering a previous infant weighing 9 lbs or more (more than 4,000 grams), (3) glucosuria, (4) a previous unexplained stillbirth or neonatal death, (5) a previous congenital abnormality, or (6) obesity (i.e., body weight of more than 200 lbs). Additional reasons for evaluating a patient for possible glucose intolerance are: (1) hydramnios, (2) excessive thirst, (3) recurrent urinary tract infections, and (4) persistent monilial vulvovaginitis.

A **glucose screening test** (i.e., 50 grams of glucose orally) should be administered routinely to all pregnant patients at 26–28 weeks' gestation. The plasma fasting blood sugar (FBS) level should be less than 105 mg/dl, and the plasma glucose level taken one hour after an oral glucose load should be less than 140 mg/dl to be considered normal. Values in excess of these levels should be investigated with a full three-hour glucose tolerance test to be certain that

the diagnosis of diabetes mellitus is not missed. **The plasma glucose concentrations for the oral glucose tolerance test, after a 100-gram glucose load, should be less than 105 mg/dl (FBS), 190 mg/dl (one hour), 165 mg/dl (two hours), and 145 mg/dl (three hours).** If any two of the three hourly values are elevated, then the test is considered positive and the diagnosis of gestational diabetes or Class A diabetes is assured. If the FBS is also abnormal, then the diagnosis is overt diabetes, Class B diabetes, or greater (i.e., Class B, C, D, etc.) if the patient was diabetic prior to pregnancy.

Once the patient has been diagnosed as having diabetes, she should be followed at two-week intervals until 20 weeks' gestation, and then weekly thereafter throughout the rest of the pregnancy, with fasting blood sugars (FBS) and two-hour postprandial blood sugars (two-hour PP) to evaluate the degree of glucose control that has been achieved by the treatment protocol of an American Diabetic Association (ADA) diet and/or insulin regimen. **If the plasma FBS exceeds 105 mg/dl or if the two-hour PP plasma sugar is more than 120 mg/dl, then insulin should be instituted, or increased if the patient is already on it, to achieve proper control (i.e., an average glucose level of 80–84 mg/dl).** From

15–19 weeks' gestation, an alpha-fetoprotein test should be obtained to screen for neural tube defects. Between the 16th and 20th weeks, the gestational dating should be verified clinically (i.e., quickening, fetal heart tones, fundal measurements) and an ultrasonic evaluation should be considered to evaluate the gestational dating. A detailed ultrasonic evaluation of the fetus should be performed to detect fetal abnormalities. Beginning at about 30–32 weeks' gestation, nonstress (NST) FHR testing may be performed every 3–4 days to evaluate the status of the fetus. Contraction stress tests (CST) should then be utilized whenever there is a nonreactive NST. The patient may be instructed in the technique of monitoring her baby's activity at home. The recording of 10 fetal movements in a 12-hour period has been considered to be normal. Fetal growth evaluations using the ultrasonogram should be carried out every 2–4 weeks in the third trimester. The fundal measurements will also assist you in detecting fetal macrosomia.

c. Treatment

1) Diet

In initiating either an ADA diet and/or insulin treatment of the obstetric patient, you should admit the patient to the hospital where her blood sugars can be monitored daily and the treatment protocol can be adjusted appropriately. *The basic management of diabetes relies upon the proper intake of carbohydrates, proteins, and fats in the form of an ADA diet.* A total maternal weight gain of 22–27 lbs is recommended. The total calories should not fall below 2,000 calories per day. The daily caloric intake should be about 17 calories per pound of ideal body weight plus 300 calories. Usually, at least 2,100–2,400 calories are given to avoid any weight loss, since it is not advisable for a patient to lose weight during pregnancy.

About 50–60% of the calories of an ADA diet are made up of carbohydrates, 18–22% of protein, and 25% of fat. These values may vary somewhat depending upon the degree of control and the investigator's management protocol. Usually the distribution of the calories is spread out over four meals per day in the following manner: 2/7, 2/7, 2/7, and 1/7; however some authors have used a distribution of 10% (breakfast), 7.5% (mid-morning snack), 30% (lunch), 7.5% (mid-afternoon snack), 30% (dinner), 7.5% (evening snack), and 7.5% (bedtime snack).

2) Insulin

Insulin treatment should generally include a mixture of an intermediate-acting insulin preparation (e.g., NPH insulin) and a short-acting insulin preparation (e.g., regular insulin). **A ratio of 2:1 (NPH:regular insulin) in the morning and a 1:1 ratio prior to the evening meal is usually effective.** As a consequence, two-thirds of the NPH dose will be given in the morning and one-third at night. With regard to regular insulin, one-half is given in the morning and the other half at night. **The usual blood sugar "panels" are drawn at 7:00 A.M., 11:00 A.M., 4:00 P.M., and 10:00 P.M., which occur just prior to breakfast, lunch, dinner, and the evening snack.** Since NPH insulin has a relatively long effect (i.e., about 12 hours), the 7:00 A.M. and 4:00 P.M. blood sugar values reflect the adequacy of the dosage of the evening and morning NPH dosage, respectively. Since the regular insulin has a shorter action (i.e., about 4 hours), the 11:00 A.M. and 10:00 P.M. blood sugar values reflect the morning and evening regular insulin dosage, respectively. Usually, the fasting blood sugar values should be between 70 and 80 mg/dl, and the two-hour postprandial blood sugar values at between 100 and 120 mg/dl.

The initial number of insulin units that should be administered may be calculated as a factor of the patient's body weight in kilograms, according to some authors; however, the values used in this calculation vary according to the time of gestation and the severity of the diabetes. The suggested multiplying factor in one scheme is 0.6 (first trimester), 0.7 (second trimester), and 0.8 (third trimester). Another method of approximating insulin requirements is to calculate the 24-hour dosage as 0.7 unit/kilogram body weight (from 6–18 weeks' gestation), 0.8 unit/kilogram body weight (18–26), 0.9 unit/kilogram body weight (26–36), and 1.0 unit/kilogram of body weight (36–40). You should be certain that the patient is complying with her diet and that her activity levels have not changed appreciably while in the hospital before you change to a different dosage regimen. The use of pump-insulin therapy is of benefit in achieving optimal euglycemia; however, if the patient can administer three or more daily injections of insulin, this method also will result in optimal blood sugar levels. In many cases, especially in indigent or poorly compliant patients, such a degree of control cannot be achieved.

The goal of therapy is to achieve normoglycemia and to maintain the patient as close to a euglycemic state as possible. Ketoacidosis should be avoided, since there is evidence that it may be associated with a decrease in the intellectual ability of the infant. **The degree of metabolic control that has been achieved over the preceding 4–6 weeks may be evaluated by measuring the percentage of hemoglobin that has been glycosylated (i.e., hemoglobin A$_{1c}$).** Tight metabolic control may be important in preventing an intrauterine fetal death, macrosomia, or fetal malformations.

3) Delivery

The management of the pregnant diabetic requires mature judgment with regard to *the timing of the delivery.* It was recognized many years ago that early delivery (i.e., prior to the beginning of the 37th week) in diabetic patients resulted in prematurity and fetal death secondary to the respiratory distress syndrome (RDS). On the other hand, a delay in the delivery beyond the 37th week often resulted in an intrauterine fetal demise due to the diabetes. Thus the delivery was scheduled for the 37th week. This approach has since been found to be too crude and inexact to be useful in the management of the diabetic patient.

In recent years, with the development of new techniques to monitor the fetal status, the delivery of the diabetic patient can be tailored to each individual patient's needs so as to obtain the maximum degree of fetal maturity consistent with a maximum of fetal safety. Nonstress tests (NST), contraction stress tests (CST), estriol determinations, and ultrasonic monitoring for fetal growth and congenital defects should be performed periodically from about 32 weeks' gestation until delivery in diabetic patients. In addition, the detection of fetal lung maturity by means of the amniotic fluid lecithin/sphingomyelin ratio (L/S ratio), and especially the determination of the presence of phosphatidylglycerol (PG), has been helpful in determining the timing of delivery. The presence of PG in the amniotic fluid gives considerable assurance that RDS will not occur if delivery takes place. In addition, the use of the biophysical profile tests (i.e., fetal activity, tone, cardiac reactivity, breathing motions, and the amniotic fluid volume) may add even more information to your assessment of the fetal status.

During labor, the patient should be maintained in a

euglycemic state by the administration of 5% dextrose in water with added regular insulin, so as to provide 0.5–2 units per hour (e.g., 10 U regular insulin in 1,000 ml of 5% dextrose in water, infused at 100 ml/h). You should strive to keep the plasma glucose at a level between 80 and 100 mg/dl. The plasma glucose values should be obtained every two hours throughout labor. Prolonged serial inductions should probably not be utilized if the membranes are ruptured, since the diabetic patient is at an increased risk for the development of amnionitis. Electronic fetal monitoring should be carried out during labor on these patients.

Following delivery, the insulin requirements of the patient may decrease dramatically. In many instances, insulin may not be required during the first 24–48 hours; however, blood glucose levels should be obtained every six hours and a lower dosage of insulin gradually reinstated as necessary.

4) Complications

Pregnant patients with diabetes are susceptible to the development of pregnancy-induced hypertension (PIH) and chronic hypertension. **The development of hydramnios has been noted in up to 31% of pregnant diabetics, and this finding seems to be an ominous sign. Pyelonephritis occurs in 1.5–12% of pregnant diabetic patients. The neonatal mortality rate is of the order of 1–5%; 30–50% of these perinatal losses will be due to congenital anomalies, most commonly involving abnormalities of the heart, the nervous system, and the skeleton.**

In Class A through Class C diabetes, there is an increased incidence of fetal macrosomia. You should measure the fundal height of the diabetic patient to determine if there is excessive fetal growth (e.g., a fundal measurement more than 38 cm at term), and observe the patient closely in labor for any delay in the descent of the fetus that might indicate *cephalopelvic disproportion.* You should be alert to the possibility of *shoulder dystocia* in those patients with fetal macrosomia who deliver vaginally (see Chapter 38).

The infant of a diabetic mother is susceptible to hypoglycemia, hypocalcemia, and hyperbilirubinemia in the early neonatal period. **There is a 5–6-fold increase in the incidence of RDS in infants of diabetic mothers.** The L/S ratio may not be reliable in diabetics, but the presence of PG is indicative of maturity. You should be careful in your follow-up care of the Class A diabetic patient following delivery, and should encourage her to reduce her weight and maintain it at the appropriate level, since a high proportion of patients with gestational diabetes eventually develop overt diabetes mellitus (i.e., 60% of the obese patients versus 20% of the nonobese patients). All diabetic patients should probably be delivered either at, or prior to, 40 weeks' gestation.

2. Diabetes insipidus

a. Incidence

Diabetes insipidus is uncommon in pregnancy, with only approximately 100 cases having been reported, and it has no effect upon the onset and course of labor. About 50% of patients with diabetes insipidus worsen in pregnancy, 15% do not change, and the rest improve. Diabetes insipidus may be secondary to a decrease in the secretion of antidiuretic hormone (central diabetes insipidus), or secondary to peripheral resistance to this hormone (nephrogenic diabetes insipidus).

b. Symptoms

The symptoms of diabetes insipidus consist of polyuria, polydipsia, and a urinary output of from 4–15 liters/day. The water deprivation test may be helpful in diagnosing the disease. Urine osmolality and specific gravity should be measured with each voided specimen until no further increases occur in these values, or until the patient has lost as much as 3% of her body weight. To determine whether the cause of the diabetes insipidus is central or peripheral, five units of aqueous vasopressin are administered subcutaneously at the end of the test; only the patients with central diabetes insipidus will decrease their urinary output and increase the urine osmolality.

c. Treatment

The treatment of diabetes insipidus consists of: (1) the parenteral administration of aqueous Pitressin (5–10 units q4-6h), or (2) the use of a long-acting vasopressin tannate in oil (1.5–5.0 pressor units q24-48h p.r.n.). All of the infants that have been born of mothers with diabetes insipidus have apparently been normal.

3. Adrenal disorders

a. Addison's disease

1) Etiology

While Addison's disease is rare in pregnancy, it does occur, and it may be difficult to diagnose. *The cause of Addison's disease in 70% of the cases is autoimmune disease.* In rare cases, an acute adrenal insufficiency may occur in association with severe systemic meningococcal infections (Waterhouse-Friderichsen syndrome). **One of the most common causes of relative adrenal insufficiency today is the chronic suppression of the adrenal gland by exogenously administered corticosteroids. Any patient who has had corticosteroids within eight months of a stressful event, such as a delivery or a cesarean section, should probably receive corticosteroid support during these stress periods.**

2) Symptoms

Chronic fatigue, weakness, weight loss, anorexia, nervousness, hypoglycemia, and increased skin pigmentation may initially be confused with the symptoms of pregnancy and the diagnosis of Addison's disease may be overlooked; however, the continued weight loss and the nausea and vomiting should alert you to this diagnosis. An adrenal crisis is heralded by severe nausea and vomiting, diarrhea, and dehydration and is associated with an elevated temperature.

While electrolyte disturbances may be present, including hyponatremia, hypercalcemia, and hyperkalemia, in association with increased creatinine and blood urea nitrogen levels in patients with severe symptoms, in mild cases there may be no changes at all. In **primary adrenal insufficiency,** the adrenocorticotropic hormone (ACTH) levels are elevated (i.e., greater than 250 pg/ml). Also, the plasma cortisol values will be less than 10 μg/dl. **The diagnosis may be confirmed by either the short or the long ACTH test.** The short test consists of the administration of 0.25 mg of synthetic ACTH (Cortrosyn) as a bolus I.V., after obtaining a baseline cortisol level. Repeat cortisol values are then obtained in 30 and 60 minutes. If the cortisol level increases 10 μg/dl over the baseline values, then Addison's disease is not present. In the long test, synthetic ACTH, 0.25 mg in 500 ml of 5% dextrose in normal saline, is administered q12h I.V. for 48 hours. A baseline cortisol and one every 12 hours is obtained. A rise in the plasma cortisol of more than 30 μg/dl accurately rules out Addison's disease.

3) Treatment

Therapy for Addison's disease includes the administration of prednisone or cortisone acetate, along with 9-fluoro-hydrocortisone each day. While some physicians will give two-thirds of the dose of cortisone in the morning and one-third of the dose at night, the dosage will sometimes have to be adjusted according to the individual patient's needs.

If an acute *Addisonian crisis* occurs, the patient will develop hypotension, fever, and vomiting. The treatment consists of an emergency intravenous administration of adequate fluids (5% dextrose in normal saline) and cortisone hemisuccinate (Solu-Cortef) 200 mg in a bolus, and then 100 mg per each liter of 5% dextrose in isotonic saline solution.

In patients who have received adrenal suppression within the preceding eight months and who are undergoing surgery, 100 mg of cortisone should be administered in 5% dextrose and normal saline q8h × 24 hours, after which time the dosage may be reduced by 50 mg/day until the patient can return to oral medication (i.e., about 4–5 days).

The infants of mothers who have Addison's disease have been normal and, in most cases, have not shown evidence of adrenal suppression.

b. Cushing's syndrome

1) Etiology

Cases involving an excessive secretion of ACTH by the pituitary gland (Cushing's disease) should be differentiated from those involving an excessive secretion of cortisone secondary to an adrenal tumor (Cushing's syndrome), although both conditions will result in an excessive secretion of glucocorticoids. Usually, patients who have Cushing's disease have an **ACTH-secreting adenoma** of the pituitary gland. Cushing's syndrome, on the other hand, is due to **adrenal hyperplasia** in 70% of cases and adrenal tumors in 20%, with the remainder of the cases being due to the ectopic ACTH syndrome.

2) Symptoms

Cushing's syndrome (or disease) is a chronic, insidious disease that is manifested by truncal obesity, weakness, easy bruisability, plethora, hypertension, abdominal striae, buffalo hump, emotional disturbances, osteoporosis, hirsutism, and amenorrhea (66%) or oligomenorrhea (20%). Probably less than 50 cases of Cushing's syndrome (or disease) in pregnancy have been reported, which is due to the fact that most patients with Cushing's syndrome are anovulatory.

The dexamethasone-suppression screening test may be used to diagnose this syndrome. In this test, 1 mg of dexamethasone is given at 11:00 P.M., and then an 8:00 A.M. plasma cortisol is obtained. A value of greater than 5–6 μg/dl indicates Cushing's syndrome (or disease). This test is not helpful in pregnancy, however, due to the elevated levels of transcortin and corticosteroid-binding globulin (CBG), which elevates the plasma cortisol levels. Since the diurnal variation is lost in Cushing's syndrome, a comparison of the morning plasma cortisol values (7:00–9:00 A.M.) with those in the evening (9:00–10:00 P.M.), may be useful.

The dexamethasone-suppression test is performed by administering 0.5 mg of dexamethasone q6h × 48 hours **(low-dose test),** or by the administration of 2.0 mg of dexamethasone in the same manner **(high-dose test).** Normal patients will suppress their cortisol secretion with the low-dose test, whereas the patient with Cushing's syndrome will require the higher dose to suppress the cortisol level. If an adrenal tumor or an ACTH-secreting tumor is present, the high-dose test generally will not suppress the plasma cortisol. The use of a CT scan in these patients may assist in confirming the diagnosis of an adrenal tumor. Very high values of plasma cortisol are found in the ectopic ACTH syndrome (i.e., ACTH in excess of 400 pg/ml).

There appears to be an increased fetal wastage in patients who conceive with Cushing's syndrome. Abortion and stillbirth are greatly increased, and only a few normal infants have been reported. Premature labor occurs frequently.

3) Treatment

Pituitary adenomas may be resected via a transsphenoidal approach. The use of cyproheptadine, a serotonin antagonist, will suppress ACTH in many, but not all, patients. In primary adrenal disease during pregnancy, adrenalectomy may result in the delivery of a normal infant. When adrenalectomy is performed in cases of Cushing's syndrome, some patients may develop a pituitary tumor with elevated ACTH levels and hyperpigmentation *(Nelson's syndrome)*. With proper corticosteroid and mineralocorticoid replacement therapy, these patients also can have a successful pregnancy.

c. Congenital adrenal hyperplasia

1) Etiology

Congenital adrenal hyperplasia (CAH) is a hereditary disorder due to an autosomal recessive trait that involves one or more enzymatic defects in the biosynthesis of corticosteroid compounds. The most common defect (in 90% of affected patients) is in the *21-hydroxylase enzyme,* which converts 17-hydroxyprogesterone to 11-desoxycortisol, the immediate precursor to cortisol. Due to the reduced production of cortisol, an increase in ACTH secretion occurs, which results in a secondary hyperplasia of the adrenal gland in an attempt to maintain the normal secretion of cortisol. **Other enzymatic defects** involve 18-hydroxylase and 18-hydroxydehydrogenase **(aldosterone deficiency),** 11β-hydroxylase and 21-hydroxylase **(corticoids and aldosterone deficiency),** 17α-hydroxylase **(deficiency of androgens, estrogens, cortisol, and aldosterone),** and the 3-beta-ol-dehydrogenase enzymes **(deficiency of all steroid hormones).**

2) Symptoms

Almost all patients who have CAH will develop **virilization,** which is due to the ACTH drive on the adrenal gland (producing an increased secretion of androgens) in an effort to obtain a normal output of cortisol. As a consequence, many of these patients are infertile, due to amenorrhea or oligomenorrhea. Often, the disease appears at birth in infants whose mothers or fathers show no stigmata of the disease, because the gene expresses itself only in the homozygous condition (i.e., autosomal recessive). These infants may also show some ambiguity in their external genitalia at delivery. The antenatal diagnosis may be accomplished by analyzing the amniotic fluid for increased levels of delta-[5] and delta-[4] compounds as well as 17-hydroxyprogesterone.

3) Treatment

The treatment of adrenal hyperplasia consists of supplying enough cortisone or prednisone to return all of the metabolic parameters to normal. Patients under treatment have essentially normal pregnancy outcomes, except for perhaps a slightly increased spontaneous abortion rate (20%). *If a patient has CAH, the risk of producing an affected child is between 1:100 and 1:200. If a previous child has the disease, then there is a 25% risk that a subsequent child will be affected.*

d. Primary aldosteronism

Primary aldosteronism is a rare condition that is characterized by hypertension and hypokalemia secondary to the excessive secretion of aldosterone. The diagnosis may be suspected by low renin levels and a failure of the renin to increase after the administration of furosemide. (Renin levels are increased throughout normal pregnancy.) In addition, increased serum or urine aldosterone levels and high levels of urinary potassium are present in this condition. *In 70% of these cases, there will be a unilateral adrenal adenoma.* A CT scan or the performance of a percutaneous catheterization of the adrenal veins to measure the amount of serum aldosterone and renin secretion may be helpful. The treatment consists of the surgical resection of the adrenal tumor.

e. Pheochromocytoma

Only 0.5% of the cases initially diagnosed as hypertension are due to a pheochromocytoma. This type of tumor also occurs in about 5% of patients who have neurofibromatosis. Hypertension (82%) associated with weakness and palpitations (36%), flushing, tremor, sweating (33%), and headaches (66%) may occur as periodic attacks in these patients. *This diagnosis may be confirmed by finding elevated levels of the catecholamines (epinephrine and norepinephrine) and their metabolites* (vanillylmandelic acid, or VMA, and metanephrine). The localization of the adrenal tumor may be accomplished by means of a CT scan, venography, and by vena cava catheterization to obtain venous samples for catecholamine determinations. The primary treatment is the surgical resection of the tumor. The use of blocking agents, such as phenoxybenzamine hydrochloride or phentolamine, should be administered prior to surgery in order to block the effect of the norepinephrine. The administration of propranolol hydrochloride (Inderal), 20–40 mg/day, may be useful in controlling the tachycardia.

In the undiagnosed patients reported in one series, the maternal mortality rate was 48%. When death occurred, it happened most commonly within 72 hours of delivery and was caused by arrhythmia, cerebrovascular accidents, shock, and acute pulmonary edema. *The fetal mortality rate in these cases was 54%. As many as 30% of patients with a pheochromocytoma will be diagnosed for the first time during pregnancy.* There is some evidence that the use of alpha-blocking agents will reduce both the fetal and maternal mortality rates. The use of a combined cesarean section with the simultaneous resection of the tumor may also have merit. Toxemia occurs in 43% of these patients, and intrauterine growth retardation, stillbirth, and spontaneous abortion are more common in these patients than in the general population.

4. Thyroid disorders

a. Hyperthyroidism

1) Incidence

Hyperthyroidism occurs in about 1:500 pregnancies (0.2–0.3%) and is associated with the delivery of smaller than normal infants and a slightly increased neonatal mortality rate. While this condition may occur in association with trophoblastic disease, it is more commonly associated with a diffuse toxic goiter (Graves' disease), a toxic nodular goiter (Plummer's disease), a chronic autoimmune thyroiditis, or a subacute thyroiditis.

2) Symptoms

Symptoms of hyperthyroidism include tachycardia, heat intolerance, insomnia, diarrhea, palpitations, nervousness, tremor, weakness, fatigability, increased appetite, and weight loss. **The pulse is usually over 100 bpm and will fail to slow with Valsalva's maneuver.** A bruit may be present over the thyroid gland. The development of pretibial edema (5%) is pathognomonic of Graves' disease.

3) Diagnosis

When hyperthyroidism occurs during pregnancy, the thyroxine (T_4) levels are generally elevated above 15 μg/100 ml and the resin triiodothyronine uptake (RT_3U) is in the normal range. The diagnosis may be confirmed by finding an elevated free thyroxine index (FT_4I).

4) Treatment

There are two approaches to the treatment of hyperthyroidism in pregnancy: medical and surgical. Since ^{131}I thyroid ablation cannot be used in pregnancy, medical therapy involving the use of antithyroid drugs, such as methimazole (Tapazole) or propylthiouracil (PTU), is required. PTU blocks the conversion of T_4 to T_3 and inhibits thyroid hormone synthesis. Since *aplasia cutis congenita* (i.e., scalp lesions) occurs in the infants of those patients who have received methimazole, **PTU is the preferred drug for treatment.**

PTU, 100–150 mg t.i.d., p.o., is administered initially to obtain control of the hyperthyroidism, and then the dosage is reduced to the *lowest dose necessary to maintain the patient in a euthyroid condition.* A T_4 level can be obtained after 2–3 weeks, and at one-month intervals thereafter, to determine the effectiveness of therapy. The reduction of the tachycardia and an increase in the patient's weight are also good indicators of progress.

Maternal hypothyroidism must be guarded against, since about 1–5% of the fetuses of mothers receiving PTU will develop hypothyroidism and a goiter. Since the antithyroid drugs cross the placenta, the dosage of the drug may be important. The presence of normal amounts of maternal thyroxine, which may cross the placenta to some small extent, seems to prevent the development of hypothyroidism or goiter in the fetus; however, the addition of thyroxine to the therapeutic regimen does not seem to be effective in preventing fetal goiter and hypothyroidism. *Testing monthly for T_4 values is of benefit in following these patients. If the T_4 level falls too low, then the PTU should be decreased. If the T_4 level increases, then the PTU should be increased.* In about 2–7% of these patients, side effects such as skin rashes, pruritus, nausea, arthralgia, or drug fever occur. Rarely, acute agranulocytosis may occur after months of therapy. A sore throat and fever often heralds the onset of this complication.

There may be an increased neonatal mortality rate and an increase in low–birth weight infants in patients with hyperthyroidism. Moreover, neonatal thyrotoxicosis may occur if there is a transfer of thyroid-stimulating immunoglobulins to the fetus. In mothers who ingest or are injected with iodine during pregnancy (e.g., cough medicines, radiopaque dyes in medical procedures), fetal hypothyroidism occurs at a rate of 1:10,000 births. Usually, fetal hypothyroidism and goiters are transient in nature, but mental retardation may occur (i.e., cretinism).

5) Preparation for surgery

Propranolol hydrochloride (Inderal) should be utilized in the control of hyperthyroidism in patients who are being prepared for surgical therapy (i.e., subtotal thyroidectomy) and for those who have a thyroid storm. Usually, propranolol hydrochloride (Inderal), 40 mg q6h, with Lugol's iodine, 5 drops b.i.d., is administered for 2–7 days to control the disease and the vascularity of the thyroid gland prior to surgery. Such a surgical procedure should be performed in the second trimester if at all possible. Currently, however, medical therapy is considered the treatment of choice for hyperthyroidism in pregnancy.

6) Thyroid storm

A *thyroid storm* may occur in association with surgery or in other stressful situations, such as infection or delivery. The symptoms consist of tachycardia, nausea and vomiting, severe dehydration, high fever (above 103° F), and cardiovascular collapse, which may lead to death in as many as 20–25% of cases. The treatment involves the administration of propylthiouracil (300 mg q4h), sodium iodide (1 gram I.V. 1 hour after the propylthiouracil × 24 hours), lithium (300 mg t.i.d.), propranolol hydrochloride (Inderal) (40 mg p.o. q6h), and dexamethasone (8 mg/day), in addition to other supportive measures, such as antipyrexia therapy and adequate fluid replacement.

b. Hypothyroidism

1) Etiology

Hypothyroidism is not very common in pregnancy, since many women with this disease are also anovulatory. If pregnancy does occur, there seems to be an increased incidence of spontaneous abortion and congenital anomalies. The etiology of hypothyroidism is usually previous treatment of hyperthyroidism with either surgery or radioactive iodine; however, a few cases may be secondary to Hashimoto's autoimmune thyroiditis.

2) Symptoms

Symptoms of hypothyroidism include dry skin, cold intolerance, constipation, coarse hair, sluggish mentation, and irritability. *The diagnosis of hypothyroidism may be detected by finding T_4 and T_3 levels, and the resin triiodothyronine uptake (RT_3U) value, at below normal levels, in association with a greatly elevated thyroid-stimulating hormone (TSH) level.*

3) Treatment

The treatment of hypothyroidism consists of the administration of levothyroxine, 50 μg/day for 2–3 weeks, after which the thyroid function tests should be repeated, especially the TSH test, which is a sensitive indicator of primary hypothyroidism. The usual dosage will be about 100–200 μg/day, but it should be tailored to the patient's response. The TSH level should decrease to below 6 μU/ml, and the T_4 level should return to the normal range for pregnancy.

CHAPTER 35

Hematologic disease

Educate your nerve centres so that not the slightest dilator or contractor influence shall pass to the vessels of your face under any professional trial.

—*Sir William Osler**

1. Iron deficiency anemia

a. Incidence

The incidence of iron deficiency anemia in pregnancy varies from one socioeconomic group to the next and may occur in as many as 55% of all patients. Since 75% of all anemias in pregnancy are due to iron deficiency, it should be the primary diagnostic consideration in the anemic pregnant patient.

b. Diagnosis

The definition of iron deficiency anemia is somewhat arbitrary, but the average hemoglobin (Hb) values in women who have had a sufficient amount of iron therapy during pregnancy can provide a baseline for comparison. In several studies, it has been shown that the normal pregnant woman who has received iron supplementation throughout pregnancy will have a hemoglobin level above 12.0 g/dl. In contrast, women

*Reprinted with permission from Robert Bennett Bean, Sir William Osler: Aphorisms from His Bedside Teachings and Writings, William Bennett Bean, ed. Springfield, Ill.: Charles C Thomas, Publisher, 1968, p. 90.

who were not treated with iron had levels below this value. *Thus, the average normal hemoglobin values in pregnancy range between 11.5 and 12.5 g/dl.* Since the hemoglobin values normally decrease in early pregnancy, secondary to the expansion of the plasma volume occurring at a different rate than that of the red cell mass (i.e., physiologic anemia of pregnancy), *the usual definition of anemia has been stated to be a hemoglobin value of less than 10 g/dl, or a hematocrit (HCT) or packed cell volume (PCV) of less than 30%.*

Most women who do not receive supplemental iron during pregnancy will become anemic, since the iron requirement of pregnancy is about 1,200 mg. The usual diet is generally insufficient to provide enough iron to fulfill this need (i.e., the normal diet contains 5–6 mg iron per 1,000 calories).

The consequences of anemia (i.e., usually in severe anemia of less than 6 g/dl) in pregnancy may include postpartum hemorrhage, infection, and a failure of the patient to recuperate rapidly from childbirth, which may result in a prolonged hospitalization. It also has implications for the fetus, in that there is a decreased oxygen-carrying capacity of the blood when the patient is anemic, which might play a role in prematurity, low–birth weight infants, fetal distress, and death.

The laboratory diagnosis of iron deficiency anemia involves the identification of a microcytic, hypochromic anemia (i.e., Hb of less than 10 g/dl, or HCT of less than 30%) with a mean corpuscular hemoglobin concentration (MCHC) of less than 30 g/dl, a serum iron level of less than 30 μg/dl, a serum iron binding capacity of more than 400 μg/dl, and a transferrin saturation of less than 15%.

459

c. Treatment

Oral iron supplementation is the preferred mode of therapy for iron deficiency anemia. Ferrous sulfate is effective and inexpensive; the other iron preparations on the market (i.e., ferrous fumarate, ferrous gluconate) are more expensive and are no more effective than ferrous sulfate. *About 20% of the iron complex administered is released as elemental iron, of which about 180–240 mg (given in divided doses, usually after meals) are needed daily.* A resolution of the anemia should occur in most cases after about six weeks of therapy; however, iron therapy should be continued for an additional period of time to replenish the iron stores.

Parenteral iron (i.e., administered intramuscularly or intravenously) may be given as a dextran or sorbitol complex (e.g., Imferon) in noncompliant patients who need correction of their anemia. Mild complications occur in 8–10% of patients who receive parenteral iron and include skin staining, pyrexia, headache, palpitations, and a metallic taste. Major problems, such as phlebitis, serum sickness, and anaphylaxis, occur in 0.5% of patients.

The use of *blood transfusions* should be reserved for patients who have an HCT of less than 20–25%, unless infection is present or operative delivery is considered, in which case they should be transfused to an HCT of greater than 30% and an Hb of more than 10 g/dl to avoid unnecessary complications.

2. Megaloblastic anemia

Megaloblastic anemia is relatively uncommon in pregnancy and is secondary to a folic acid deficiency in almost all cases (99%), with a deficiency of vitamin B_{12} (i.e., pernicious anemia) being a rare disorder (i.e., 1:8,000 pregnancies). Some very rare diseases that produce megaloblastic anemia and are unresponsive to folic acid therapy are the Lesch-Nyhan syndrome, DiGuglielmo syndrome, and pyridoxine-responsive anemia. Folate deficiency secondary to gastrointestinal absorption problems may also occur in certain malabsorptive syndromes (i.e., tropical sprue, postgastrectomy complications, diabetes mellitus). **In addition, the use of anticonvulsant medications, such as the hydantoin derivatives, may result in a folate deficiency.**

a. Diagnosis

Patients who have megaloblastic anemia usually complain of weakness, dizziness, malaise, dyspnea, and in very severe cases, they may manifest cardiac failure. A laboratory evaluation will reveal a *macrocytic, normochromic anemia,* with the mean corpuscular hemoglobin concentration (MCHC) and the mean corpuscular hemoglobin (MCH) being normal; however, the *mean corpuscular volume (MCV) will be greatly elevated* to levels of the order of 150 cu μ/cell (normal values are 70–90 cu μ/cell). **Hypersegmented neutrophils,** stippling, Howell-Jolly bodies, and Cabot's ring bodies on the peripheral blood smear provide further assistance in confirming the diagnosis of megaloblastic anemia. Nucleated red blood cells (RBC) may also be seen on the smear in the more severe cases. The serum iron saturation and the uric acid levels will be elevated, whereas the unsaturated iron binding capacity (UIBC) will be decreased. The normal RBC life span is reduced from 120 days to 60 days. Leukopenia and thrombocytopenia may be present in severe cases.

b. Treatment

The minimum daily requirement of folic acid in pregnancy is 100 μg/day; however, due to absorption and storage problems, 0.5–1.0 mg/day has been recommended. *Thus, the treatment of megaloblastic anemia in pregnancy is 1 mg of folic acid per day, notwithstanding the small risk of masking pernicious anemia.* Patients with pernicious anemia are frequently infertile, and in addition, are generally much older than women in the reproductive age group. Within one week of therapy, the white blood cell count and the platelet count should return to normal and the reticulocyte count should increase. Since many of these patients are also iron deficient, *iron should be administered as well as folic acid.* While not all authorities would agree that folic acid should be given routinely in pregnancy, it probably should be given in patients who are at risk for folate deficiency, such as in multiple pregnancies or in patients who are on hydantoin medication for epilepsy.

3. Sickle cell disease

The sickle cell hemoglobinopathies consist primarily of sickle cell anemia (SS disease),

sickle cell–hemoglobin C disease (SC), and sickle cell–thalassemia disease (STh).

a. Sickle cell anemia

Sickle cell disease, when inherited in the heterozygous form, is called **sickle cell trait (AS),** and it occurs in 1:10 black Americans. **Women with sickle cell trait do not have difficulties with their pregnancies** because HbA is also present, but they do exhibit an increased incidence of **asymptomatic bacteriuria.**

Hemoglobin S probably originated as a genetic structural mutation that protects against malaria. *It involves a substitution of valine for glutamic acid in the sixth position from the N-terminal in both of the beta chains of hemoglobin, which allows for the sickling of the cell in hypoxic situations.* While there are 150 different structural variants of hemoglobin, most of them are very rare, except for the SS, SC, and STh conditions.

Sickle cell anemia (SS) is the homozygous condition and occurs in 1:1,800 black Americans. The spontaneous abortion rate is slightly increased and the incidence of severe *sickle cell crises* is greatly increased in pregnant women with this anemia. The maternal mortality rate is 0–25%, with a perinatal mortality rate of 20–35%. Maternal morbidity may involve severe anemia, megaloblastic crises, acute sequestration of sickled erythrocytes, pneumonia, pulmonary embolism, antepartum hemorrhage, pyelonephritis, toxemia, and crises involving the bones, the abdomen, or the cerebrum.

1) Pathophysiology

The sickling of the RBCs is dependent upon many factors, such as the pH, the temperature, the state of oxygenation, the concentration of both HbF and HbS, and the condition of the cell membrane and the extracellular osmotic pressure environment. *Sickling may be triggered especially by infections and conditions that produce hypoxia. The initiation of the sickling process in the microcirculation, with the continued sequestration of the RBCs in the microvasculature, leads to further hypoxia and a further promulgation of the process in various organs.* This process results in pain crises, which may involve many different organ systems, including the skeleton, the brain, and the skin.

2) Diagnosis

The presence of hemoglobin S can be demonstrated by **hemoglobin electrophoresis.** Sickle cell anemia (SS) is usually normochromic and normocytic, unless a concomitant iron deficiency anemia is present. There is often an increase in the reticulocytes and thrombocytes during crises, as well as an elevation of the liver enzymes. A urine culture should be carefully checked in patients who have sickle cell anemia or sickle cell trait, since asymptomatic bacteriuria is more prevalent in these patients than in the general population.

3) Treatment

Patients with sickle cell anemia should be followed closely in pregnancy in order to try to prevent trauma or infection and to quickly diagnose an incipient sickling crisis. The occurrence of pain, fever, or infection requires immediate hospitalization. An evaluation of the HCT and Hb should be carried out frequently to identify the progression of the anemia. Both iron and folic acid, in normal dosages, should be administered throughout the pregnancy. Other symptomatic therapy that has been recommended includes the use of analgesics, oxygen, bed rest, transfusions, and hydration.

While the previous therapy for sickle cell patients has generally been only symptomatic, recent evidence has suggested that a new approach in the treatment of these patients may be beneficial. This treatment consists of the use of *partial exchange transfusions.* Beginning at about 24–28 weeks' gestation, or even earlier if necessary, buffy-coat-poor-washed-red-cell (BCPWRC) transfusions are administered to increase the HbA level and the HCT to preselected levels. It has been stated that the HbS should be kept below 50% of the total hemoglobin in order to prevent a crisis. This procedure may have to be repeated about every six weeks, or whenever the HbS increases above a preselected level (50%), the HCT falls below a preselected level (25%), a crisis occurs, or labor develops.

4) Pregnancy outcome

The maternal mortality rate in patients with sickle cell anemia is of the order of less than 1% in most of the recent series. Painful crises occur in almost all reported series. The other major complications include pyelonephritis (2–12%), pneumonia (3–15%), endometritis (2–10%), pulmonary embolism (1–9%), and cardiac failure (1–5%). The incidence of spontaneous abortion in patients with sickle cell anemia is between 20 and 35%. The incidences of intrauterine growth retardation and premature labor are also increased. Stillbirths occur in 5–13% of these patients and are usually associated with severe crises.

b. Sickle cell–hemoglobin C disease

Sickle cell–hemoglobin C disease (SC) is a mild disease in the nonpregnant woman. It occurs in about 1:1,200 black Americans. The structural defect in the hemoglobin molecule is similar to that of sickle cell anemia, except that the amino acid lysine is substituted for glutamic acid in an identical position on both of the beta-chains.

1) Symptoms

The morbidity of this disease is increased appreciably during pregnancy, with attacks of *bone pain and pulmonary embolism occurring periodically*. While patients with SC disease seem to have fewer crises than SS disease patients, the complications that do occur, such as aseptic bone necrosis, acute pulmonary emboli, marrow emboli, renal papillary necrosis, and ocular lesions, are usually more severe. *The emboli consist of necrotic bone marrow fat and cellular material.* There is also an increased incidence of postpartum hemorrhage. There is a 12% reported incidence of spontaneous abortion, stillbirth, and neonatal death. **The maternal mortality rate has been reported to be 2–10%, and the perinatal mortality rate is 10–60%.**

2) Treatment

The treatment of SC disease consists of supportive measures similar to those used in SS disease patients. In addition, the prophylactic use of partial exchange transfusions, beginning at about 24–28 weeks' gestation, has proved to considerably reduce the maternal morbidity in these patients. An attempt is made with the transfusions to lower the percentage of HbS to a safer level and to maintain the HCT above 30–35%. While there may be some significant complications associated with the transfusions, the benefits probably outweigh the disadvantages.

c. Sickle cell–thalassemia disease

Sickle cell–thalassemia disease (STh) is relatively uncommon (1:3,300) and has the same morbidity rate as sickle cell anemia and sickle cell–hemoglobin C disease. This disease occurs when an HbS gene is inherited along with a beta-thalassemia gene. The maternal mortality rate has been noted to be 0–5%, with a perinatal mortality rate of 9–15%. Folic acid, 1.0 mg per day, should be administered to these patients in pregnancy. The use of partial exchange transfusions, beginning at 24–28 weeks' gestation, are as effective in this disease as they are in SS disease. In general, these patients should be treated similarly to those who have SS and SC disease.

4. Hemolytic anemia

a. Autoimmune hemolytic anemia

Autoimmune hemolytic anemia may occur in pregnancy and may be associated with positive antiglobulin tests (i.e., indirect and direct Coombs test). Either IgM or IgG antierythrocyte antibodies may be present. The IgM antibodies do not cross the placenta, in contrast to the IgG antibodies, which do cross the placenta. This anemia is usually a normocytic, normochromic anemia. There is destruction of the erythrocytes with an elevation of the serum bilirubin levels and the development of jaundice. Treating these patients with prednisone seems to be effective in decreasing the rate of hemolysis.

b. Pregnancy-induced hemolytic disease

A hemolytic disease that is related to pregnancy has been described in very rare instances, but *no etiologic agent* has been identified in these cases. It occurs during pregnancy and resolves after the pregnancy is over. Treatment with corticosteroids appears to be effective in this condition.

c. Glucose-6-phosphate dehydrogenase deficiency

In about 2% of black women, a specific enzymatic defect present in the erythrocyte—a *glucose-6-phosphate dehydrogenase deficiency (G6PD)*—allows the erythrocyte to hemolyze in the presence of certain oxidant drugs.

5. Aplastic anemia

Aplastic anemia is often associated not only with a decrease in the red blood cells but also with thrombocytopenia and leukopenia (i.e., pancytopenia). The bone marrow is hypocellular in these patients. This disease can pose a grave problem in pregnancy. While transfusions may be used, they may be detrimental to the retention of a future bone marrow graft. A bone marrow transplantation may be used; however, immunosuppressive therapy will be necessary for several months after the procedure to avoid a graft-versus-host disease and graft rejection. Antithymocyte globulin has also been suggested as a treatment in patients who cannot find a suitable histocompatible donor.

6. Thrombocytopenia

a. Immune (or idiopathic) thrombocytopenic purpura (ITP)

In this disease, antibodies are formed against the platelets, which are then destroyed by the macrophages of the spleen, liver, and bone marrow (i.e., the reticuloendothelial system). The reason for the production of antibodies is unknown. The antibody is of the IgG type and is specific for a platelet-associated antigen. The affected platelets have a reduced survival time; instead of lasting the normal 9–12 days, they may last anywhere from only a few minutes to perhaps 3 days. The normal platelet count in pregnancy is 150,000 to 350,000/mm^3. Platelet values of less than 100,000/mm^3 are diagnostic of thrombocytopenia. These antibodies are capable of crossing the placenta and affecting the fetus. If the fetus becomes severely thrombocytopenic, it is at great risk for intracranial hemorrhage during delivery.

The maternal mortality rate of patients with ITP is probably essentially zero today, due to the use of corticosteroids; however, in earlier times, it was about 4%. The main risk to the mother is hemorrhage, which occurs in 5–25% of patients who have an episiotomy or lacerations. Spontaneous bleeding may occur with platelet counts of less than 20,000/mm^3. **In the face of a cesarean section in cases of thrombocytopenia, it is recommended that platelet transfusions be given prior to the procedure in order to avoid severe hemorrhage.** During pregnancy, corticosteroids should be administered, ini-

tially at a dose of 1–1.5 mg/kg of nonpregnant weight per day for two weeks, and then at a reduced dosage, in order to maintain the platelet count at levels greater than 50,000–100,000/mm^3.

The perinatal mortality rate of ITP is of the order of 15–25%. Fetal death in these cases has been attributed mainly to intracerebral hemorrhage and prematurity. **Neonatal thrombocytopenia has been reported in as many as 50–70% of the neonates born to women with this disease, but it appears to be self-limited and usually resolves after 1–2 months.** Since labor may cause intracerebral hemorrhage in the fetus in these cases, it has been recommended that all of these infants should be delivered by cesarean section. The status of the fetus can be determined by fetal scalp blood platelet counts. In one series, if the scalp blood platelet count was less than 50,000/mm^3, a cesarean section was performed. Unfortunately, however, cesarean section may not always prevent the hemorrhagic phenomena in the neonate.

In one report, a patient who had refractory ITP and an autoimmune IgG erythrocyte panagglutinin was treated with high doses of intravenous gamma globulin (I.V. IgG) during pregnancy. Although the patient had severe thrombocytopenia and also had the erythrocyte panagglutinin in her serum at the time of delivery, the infant was noted to have a normal platelet count and a negative direct antiglobulin test. It was postulated by the authors that the treatment may have prevented the passage of the maternal antibodies across the placenta.

b. Drug-induced thrombocytopenia

A decrease in the platelet count may occur secondary to the administration of certain drugs. Medications such as quinidine, quinine, sulfonamides, methyldopa, and digitoxin have been implicated in this type of thrombocytopenia. The platelet count will return to normal after the discontinuation of the drug.

c. Thrombotic thrombocytopenic purpura (TTP)

Thrombotic thrombocytopenic purpura (TTP) is an uncommon condition consisting of a clinical pentad: (1) microangiopathic hemolytic anemia (hemoglobin of less than 10 mg/dl, reticulocytes greater than 5%), (2) thrombocytopenia (usually less than 75,000/mm^3),

(3) fever (higher than 38.3° C or 101° F), (4) renal abnormalities (BUN of less than 40 mg/dl, creatinine of less than 3 mg/dl), and (5) neurologic symptoms. **Of these five, the neurologic complaints, the thrombocytopenia, and the hemolytic anemia are the major criteria needed to make the diagnosis.** In addition, the presence of at least two of the symptoms of fever, renal abnormalities, microthrombi on tissue biopsy, or the absence of intravascular coagulopathy should be present to make the diagnosis of TTP. There have been probably no more than 70 cases of this condition reported at the present time. **In contrast to ITP, TTP is confined to the maternal compartment and does not involve the fetus, except through the severity of the maternal illness.**

The patient may complain of fever, headache, nausea and vomiting, abdominal pain, jaundice, and/or musculoskeletal pains. In addition, she may note weakness and generalized malaise. Bruises may be evident on the skin secondary to the low platelet count. **TTP has been associated with toxemia of pregnancy in nearly half of the reported cases.**

The small arterioles throughout the body in these cases are periodically occluded with hyalinized platelet-fibrin thrombi. The peripheral blood smear usually shows red cell fragmentation, a few nucleated red cells, and thrombocytopenia. While prostacyclin and thromboxane have been implicated, the exact mechanism of their action is unknown. **Thromboxane is released from the platelets and causes platelet cohesion and the constriction of the smaller arterioles. Prostacyclin has just the opposite effect.** A balance between these two prostaglandins is the normal state of affairs. Pregnancy and the use of birth control pills may sometimes trigger functional damage to the endothelial cells, which in turn induces a series of events involving interactions between the platelets and the endothelial cells. In the absence of a *platelet-aggregating factor inhibitor* (a normal plasma component), the *platelet-aggregating factor* present in the plasma of patients with TTP causes multiple platelet aggregates and the local occlusion of the microcirculation. When this occurs, thromboxane is released as well as beta-thromboglobulin, which attaches to the endothelial cells to prevent the production of prostacyclin. As a consequence, the delicate balance between thromboxane and prostacyclin is tilted in favor of thromboxane, which then may produce the clinical manifestations of TTP.

The treatment of TTP consists of *exchange transfusions, plasmapheresis, and normal plasma transfusions.* It is thought that the transfused plasma contains the missing *platelet-aggregation factor inhibitor,* which would account for the success of the treatment. Platelet transfusions should be avoided, since they may aggravate the condition. Antiplatelet agents such as aspirin, dipyridamole, or dextran 70 have been noted to be effective. **The maternal mortality rate ranges between 10–60%, with death being secondary to renal failure or brain hemorrhage. The fetal mortality rate is also high.**

d. Postpartum hemolytic-uremic syndrome

The postpartum hemolytic-uremic syndrome (HUS) was first reported in 1968 and consists of vomiting, diarrhea, and an influenza-like illness that begins about two months' postpartum. Recently, seven nonpregnant patients have been reported with HUS in association with gastroenteritis with an E. coli serotype 0157:H7. Many patients with this syndrome will also have severe microangiopathic hemolytic anemia, thrombocytopenia, and evidence of renal disease. Some patients will be found to have disseminated intravascular coagulation (DIC). Furthermore, oliguria, proteinuria, and hematuria may be noted. **The mortality rate in patients who have HUS is about 60%; when death occurs, it is often secondary to the severe renal disease and the hypertension.** Since there are vascular occlusions present in the medium-sized vessels of the kidney in this disease, it has been postulated that a local renal intravascular coagulation may be the initiating factor. There is no specific treatment for the postpartum hemolytic uremic syndrome. The combination of dipyridamole (Persantine) and aspirin may decrease the systemic embolization and the consumption of platelets.

7. von Willebrand's disease

This **autosomal dominant** inherited bleeding disorder is characterized by a prolonged bleeding time and a deficiency of plasma Factor VIII von Willebrand's factor. About 27% of patients with von Willebrand's disease have been reported to have excessive bleeding with abortion, delivery, or in the puerperium. **The deficiency of the Factor VIII–related antigen**

(VIII R:Ag) or the von Willebrand's factor antigen (VWF:Ag), results in a bleeding diathesis. The most common form of the disease is **type I**, which is generally mild and is characterized by a prolonged bleeding time and low plasma levels of the Factor VIII von Willebrand's factor antigen, and of the ristocetin cofactor (RiCof). A dysfunctional von Willebrand's factor characterizes the other forms of the disease that have been classified as **type II**, which include subtypes IIA (most common), IIB, IIC, and IID. The administration of estrogens (or the presence of pregnancy) and the infusion of **desmopressin** (a derivative of the natural antidiuretic hormone) may be of benefit in patients with the type I disease. Type I patients may be delivered vaginally and their bleeding should be closely monitored. Patients who have type IIA disease should be treated with **cryoprecipitate** and **desmopressin**. Desmopressin should not be administered, however, to patients with type IIB disease, since it may cause thrombocytopenia. The **type III** disease is a rare condition in which there is a quantitative homozygous abnormality of Factor VIII. In these patients, the bleeding is severe and there are no measurable amounts of RiCof or VWF:Ag present. In patients with type IIA or type III disease, the fetus may be involved with the bleeding diathesis. It has been recommended that in these patients a **cesarean section should be performed** to avoid bleeding complications in the newborn infant. The administration of cryoprecipitate will assist in controlling the bleeding during cesarean section. An anticoagulated sample of cord blood should be obtained at delivery for analysis of the clotting factors. The cells should be centrifuged off and the plasma kept on ice until it can be tested.

8. Leukemia

It has been estimated that acute and chronic leukemias occur in 1:75,000 pregnancies. **Acute myelocytic leukemia is three times more common than acute lymphatic leukemia.** Chronic myelocytic leukemia is the chronic form of leukemia that is found in pregnancy. You should strongly suspect leukemia in any patient who has anemia, granulocytopenia, thrombocytopenia, immature white blood cells present in the peripheral blood smear, lymphadenopathy, and hepatosplenomegaly.

Although the disease apparently is not adversely affected by pregnancy, the pregnancy may be influenced greatly by the presence of leukemia. The need for chemotherapeutic agents may bring up the possibility of performing an abortion; however, there is little evidence that the administration of chemotherapeutic agents will cause adverse fetal effects if given during the second and third trimester. **In fact, the incidence of fetal abnormalities is less than 10% even when chemotherapy is utilized in the first trimester.** Intrauterine growth retardation, however, has been noted in infants whose mothers received chemotherapeutic drugs.

Acute leukemia can be rapidly fatal for pregnant women, and part of the risk to the fetuses is due to the poor survival rate of the mothers. In one report, all of the mothers died by the 7th month of pregnancy. The use of combination chemotherapy may produce remissions in as many as 50–80% of the mothers, and in view of the consequences of providing no therapy at all, chemotherapy should probably be used in these patients in the second and third trimesters. The removal of the abnormal peripherally circulating leukemic cells by leukophoresis has also been of benefit in some cases. Labor and delivery in the leukemia patient should be no different than in a normal patient, and cesarean section should be reserved for obstetric reasons.

9. Hodgkin's disease

Hodgkin's disease occurs in 1:1,000 to 1:6,000 pregnancies and is the most common type of lymphoma that complicates pregnancy. These patients usually experience symptoms of weight loss, night sweats, and fever and are found to have an enlargement of one or more lymph nodes. The disease is not affected by the pregnancy, and the pregnancy is unaffected by the disease, except for the effects of irradiation and chemotherapy, which are the main modalities of treatment.

If megavoltage irradiation therapy is utilized, then the pelvic contents should be shielded whenever possible. If the fetus receives a significant dose of radiation early in pregnancy, then a therapeutic abortion should be considered. The use of chemotherapy in the second and third trimesters does not seem to affect the fetus adversely. Vinblastine sulfate has been used effectively, and has not been reported to cause fetal abnormalities.

CHAPTER 36

Surgical problems in pregnancy

Advice is sought to confirm a position already taken.
—*Sir William Osler**

1. Incompetent cervix

An incompetent cervix may be defined as one that fails to retain a pregnancy because of painless effacement and dilatation between 14 and 28 weeks' gestation. It occurs in 1:500 to 1:2,000 pregnancies. This entity was first described in 1950 by A. F. Lash and S. R. Lash, who suggested that it could be prevented by performing a corrective surgical procedure on the cervix in the interval between pregnancies. Since this time, other procedures have been developed that have essentially replaced the Lash procedure. These procedures consist of the McDonald, the Wurm, and the Shirodkar cervical cerclage techniques (see Chapter 26).

This silent effacement and dilatation of the cervix usually begins to develop at about 14–16 weeks' gestation, when the uterine cavity is completely filled by the conceptus. The uterine enlargement up to this point has been accomplished by hormonal effects; however, from this time onward, the conceptus will exert pressure on the uterus to expand it even further. This pressure is transmitted to the uterine walls and to the cervix, and if the cervix is incompetent, then a premature delivery may occur.

---

*Reprinted with permission from Robert Bennett Bean, *Sir William Osler: Aphorisms from His Bedside Teachings and Writings,* William Bennett Bean, ed. Springfield, Ill.: Charles C Thomas, Publisher, 1968, p. 91.

a. Etiology

There are three etiologic factors that may be involved in the development of an incompetent cervix: (1) congenital, (2) traumatic, and (3) functional.

In patients who have a **congenitally malformed uterus,** such as a bicornuate uterus or a septate uterus, other anomalies may also be present, such as a congenitally shortened cervix. An incompetent cervix may be present in as many as one-third of these cases.

Approximately one-third of patients with incompetent cervices will have a history of **cervical trauma.** The most common causes are a D&C, a D&E, cervical lacerations, conization of the cervix, a mid-forceps delivery, or a breech extraction, all of which may result in excessive stretching or laceration of the collagenous fibers of the cervix.

A few patients may have a degree of **functional impairment of the cervix,** which may allow for the silent dilatation of the cervix in the presence of such conditions as multiple gestation or hydramnios, where the uterus has been over-distended. It has been suggested that an increased amount of smooth muscle tissue in the cervix will lead to incompetence. In some instances, these patients may have had repeated episodes of premature births.

b. Diagnosis

The diagnosis of an incompetent cervix may be made in between pregnancies by the easy passage of a no. 9 Hegar's dilator through the internal os of the cervix, or by the use of a hysterosalpingogram to demonstrate an abnormally widened internal cervical os. The ultrasonic detection of abnormal isthmic diameters may assist in confirming this diagnosis. **Clinically, the diagnosis is frequently based upon the pre-**

vious obstetric history of a painless, progressive effacement and dilatation of the cervix leading to the delivery of a premature infant.

c. Treatment

The primary treatment of an incompetent cervix is a cerclage operation (see Chapter 26). This operation may be performed as early as 12 and 14 weeks' gestation, if on ultrasonic evaluation there is a viable pregnancy with good fetal cardiac motion. The diagnosis may become evident between the 16th and the 28th week of gestation (i.e., because of silent cervical effacement and/or dilatation), or it may have been made in the interval between pregnancies with special testing to determine the condition of the internal cervical os. The fetal salvage following a cerclage procedure is of the order of about 80%, whereas without surgery it may be only about 20–40%. The adherence to specific criteria and the initiation of early surgical intervention produces the best results. This surgical procedure should be accomplished before the cervix becomes dilated beyond 3 cm. At the onset of labor at term, the cerclage suture can be severed to allow for a vaginal delivery. The contraindications to the placement of a cervical cerclage suture include such conditions as uterine bleeding, ruptured membranes, uterine contractions, and chorioamnionitis.

2. Acute appendicitis

Acute appendicitis occurs in about 1:2,000 pregnancies and appears to occur with almost equal frequency throughout each of the trimesters. If the patient presents with nausea and vomiting associated with a fever and abdominal pain, the diagnosis of acute appendicitis should be strongly considered. Due to the upward displacement of the appendix secondary to the enlarged gravid uterus, the site of the pain and tenderness of an acute appendicitis may be shifted considerably above the usual place at McBurney's point. **Since there may be some difficulty in the walling off of the infection due to this displacement, widespread peritonitis resulting from the rupture of an acutely inflamed appendix is more common in pregnant women with appendicitis than in nonpregnant individuals.** When this occurs, abortion, premature labor, or a fetal loss of about 10–15% may result. It is therefore essential

that surgery be performed without delay when this diagnosis is considered. **It is perfectly permissible to have as high as a 20% diagnostic error rate in this condition (i.e., a normal appendix instead of a pathologic appendix), since the risk of generalized peritonitis that would occur with the rupture of a true appendicitis, especially in the last trimester, could be catastrophic for both the mother and the fetus.**

As with all surgery during pregnancy, hypotension and hypoxia should be carefully avoided. The tissues should be handled gently and the hemostasis should be meticulous. The administration of intravenous broad-spectrum antibiotics should be carried out, and the appendix should be removed prior to its rupture. If this is accomplished, then the patient will usually do quite well.

3. Bowel obstruction

A bowel obstruction in pregnancy should not be difficult in most instances to diagnose. The obstruction is usually due to adhesions; however, in some cases it may be due to a volvulus. Nausea, vomiting, and colicky abdominal pain, associated with abdominal distention and loud high-pitched peristaltic rushes, should suggest this diagnosis. An upright X-ray film demonstrating air-fluid levels may be used to confirm the diagnosis.

After 6–8 hours, if the obstruction is not relieved surgically, oliguria may develop as increasing amounts of fluid and electrolytes pour into the distended bowel. A nasogastric tube should be inserted, and the patient should receive adequate amounts of fluid and electrolytes. A dilute solution of barium may be administered to determine the exact location of the obstruction prior to surgery. The definitive therapy of intestinal obstruction requires surgery.

4. Dental surgery

Frequently, you will be asked by your patient's dentist as to whether the patient may undergo dental surgery during pregnancy. Generally, if the dental condition can be managed medically, then the surgery should be postponed until the pregnancy is over. On occasion, however, medical treatment may not be effective and surgery may have to be performed. Whenever possible, it is best for the surgery to be performed during the second trimester, so that if a spontaneous first-trimester abortion should occur, it will not be erroneously attributed by the patient to the dental procedure.

5. Traumatic injuries

a. Acute accidents

1) Introduction

About 6.9% of women are injured during pregnancy; however, the actual incidence of injuries may be even higher than this, since many such accidents go unreported. The awkwardness of the pregnant woman, due to the change in her center of gravity and her inability to see obstructions, predisposes her to more injuries than usual. The frequency of minor trauma increases with each trimester, from about 8.8% in the first trimester, to 40% in the second, and to 52% in the third trimester. The main cause of injury in pregnant women is accidental falls, vehicular accidents, and piercing instruments. Women are now involved in 177 automobile accidents for every 100 million miles driven, as compared to 204 accidents for every 100 million miles driven by men.

2) Automobile accidents

Most of the injuries that result in death in pregnant women are due to automobile accidents. During head-on automobile crashes, the driver's chest usually strikes the steering wheel. The front-seat passenger does not have this restriction and is generally driven by inertia through the windshield. The rear-seat passengers are usually somewhat protected by the back of the front seats. If there are any lateral impacts on the automobile, it will mainly affect the occupants on the side of the impact. If the passengers are ejected from the automobile, the risk of serious injury or death will be increased by the secondary impact of the individual on the ground, brush, trees, or highway. In recent times, there has been some concern expressed over the use of seat belts by pregnant women, and the risk to the fetus that such abdominal compression might engender during an accident. **Studies have shown that accidents cause fewer deaths in pregnant women who have worn seat belts (3.6%), since they were not thrown out of the car, as compared with those women who did not use seat belts and who were killed by being ejected from the automobile (7.8%). The most common cause of fetal death in these instances has been shown to be the death of the mother.**

The use of the lap belt alone, which allows the mother to jackknife over the belt upon impact, may result in significant uterine injuries, such as a rupture of the uterus or *abruptio placentae*. The addition of the **shoulder harness,** however, partially eliminates this problem and decreases the amount of deceleration force that is transmitted to the hips and the uterus by distributing it more evenly to the upper body. The fetus may be squeezed considerably by a seat belt as the uterus flattens and deforms secondary to the continuing inertia as the crash occurs. While fetal skull fractures or other crushing injuries of the fetus have been reported in cases where the mother was flexed over the lap belt buckle during an accident, these injuries are unusual, and other severe maternal injuries were usually also present, such as fractures of the pelvic bone. Severe internal maternal injuries, such as a liver or splenic rupture, may also cause fetal death.

a) Management

Some of the immediate maternal life-threatening injuries that occur in vehicular trauma include tension pneumothorax, cardiac tamponade, rupture of the spleen, laceration of the liver, rupture of the uterus, subdural hematoma, and epidural hematoma. A **thorough physical examination** should be carried out as soon as the patient's vital signs have been stabilized, since as many as 25% of serious, life-threatening injuries are not recognized prior to death. The initial management of seat belt injuries consists in the preservation of the vital functions involving the airway and the control of the blood pressure in the mother. **The ABCs of the initial emergency management include: A—airway management; B—breathing and adequate ventilation of the patient; and C—circulation management and the maintenance of the blood pressure at adequate levels to perfuse the vital organs.** These goals may be accomplished by the administration of *oxygen,* by placing the patient on her left side to *eliminate the supine hypotensive syndrome,* by the replacement of adequate amounts of *blood and fluids,* and by the *electronic monitoring of the fetal heart rate.* This latter evaluation might prove to be a more sensitive indicator of the mother's condition, since impending maternal shock should affect the uterine blood vessels early and result in fetal distress, even though the mother may still be able to maintain her blood pressure and pulse within normal limits. A real-time ultrasonogram may detect the immediate physical status of the fetus.

The detection of an increase in the uterine tonus may suggest the diagnosis of a possible abruptio placentae (see Chapter 37). This is the most common type of injury, since traumatic compression of the uterus may dislodge the placenta. In 5% of patients in late pregnancy who have been in severe automobile collisions, the violent harmonic motions that are set up in the amniotic fluid result in the separation of the placenta. Since abruptio placentae has been known to develop slowly, it is advisable to observe the patient in the hospital for at least 24 hours in order to detect this possible development. The finding of fetal red blood cells in the maternal bloodstream (i.e., Kleihauer-Betke test) during this period of observation might be of assistance in making this diagnosis, and the use of an ultrasonogram to detect a retroplacental clot may also be of benefit.

The problem of spontaneous abortion or abruptio placentae following an automobile accident has medicolegal implications. You may be asked in a court of law whether the fetus died as the result of the accident. The answer lies in the following considerations: (1) the **pregnancy should have been entirely normal** up until the time of the accident (i.e., there should be no history of previous bleeding or cramps, or the passage of a blighted ovum, which was not causally related to the accident), (2) there should be **a close relationship in time** (i.e., minutes or hours) between the accident and the premature rupture of membranes, spontaneous abortion, or fetal death, (3) the pathology report of the **conceptus should be entirely normal,** and (4) there should be **no other possible etiology** for the final event. For example, if abruptio placentae occurs a week after an automobile accident in a patient who has chronic hypertension, the accidental etiology should be subject to considerable doubt since hypertension and abruptio placentae are often seen together in nonaccident patients.

3) Gunshot wounds

The presence of a bullet wound in the abdomen of a pregnant woman presents a great danger to both the mother and the fetus. The vital organs that might be affected by the trauma, both fetal and maternal, usually can only be surmised by considering the trajectory of the bullet. The larger the uterus, the greater the chance that the uterus and the fetus will sustain an injury. Only 19% of the gunshot wounds to the uterus will have associated intestinal injuries. **Fetal injuries have been noted in between 59 and 89% of uterine gunshot wounds, with a perinatal mortality rate of between 41 and 71%. Generally, more than 90% of gunshot wounds to the abdomen will require operative management of the intra-abdominal injuries.**

The presence of peritoneal irritation, with guarding and tenderness, are the best signs to indicate that an exploratory operation should be performed. The close monitoring of both the mother and the fetus may provide additional definitive information. A roentgenogram might show the location of the bullet or its fragments; however, an exploratory laparotomy will often be necessary to define the situation. In cases of severe uterine involvement with bleeding and extensive damage, a hysterectomy may become necessary. In situations in which the fetus has been damaged by a bullet fragment, a cesarean section may be necessary. A cesarean section should not be performed, however, just because an exploratory laparotomy has been performed, if there are no injuries to the fetus or to the uterus. Indeed, if the fetus has minimal injuries, healing may take place in utero and the fetus may be delivered vaginally at a later time. Unfortunately, it is often difficult to determine the extent of the fetal injuries without doing a cesarean section. This is especially true if there is damage to the uterus. An **amniocentesis** might detect the presence of severe fetal bleeding, whereas an **amniogram** (i.e., the addition of radiopaque dye into the amniotic fluid) might detect the location of the bullet fragments in relation to the fetal body (i.e., superficial or deep). A real-time ultrasonogram may also be of help. A pediatric surgeon should be present at the delivery in order to remove any bullet fragments from the infant.

4) Stab wounds

Stab wounds are less common during pregnancy than bullet wounds. These wounds should be divided into upper and lower abdominal wounds. Those that occur in the upper abdomen more frequently miss the gravid uterus and injure the small bowel, the liver, or the spleen, whereas in the lower abdominal wounds, the uterus and the fetus are more commonly involved. **About 30% of all stab wounds do not penetrate the abdomen completely.** Posterior stab wounds in the flank or back are difficult to assess, due to the fact that the retroperitoneal space may be involved. In such wounds, injuries to the large bowel, a major blood vessel, or other viscera may occur. The patient should be hospitalized and evaluated by a **computerized tomography (CT) scan** to determine if there is a retroperitoneal hematoma. If the kidneys or ureters are in the area of injury, **intravenous pyelography (IVP)** may be necessary as well, especially if hematuria is present. An exploratory laparotomy and a surgical evaluation of the extent of the injury is utilized more often in the posterior stab wounds.

a) Management

To avoid an unnecessary exploratory laparotomy, it is sometimes possible to clean the wound, pass a no. 16 or no. 18 French catheter into it, and instill radiopaque dye into the cavity **(sinography)** to determine the degree of penetration. If the dye does not appear in the peritoneal cavity on a roentgenogram, then conservative wound therapy may be elected. If the peritoneal cavity has been penetrated, then it may be possible to determine the degree of intraperitoneal bleeding by utilizing a **peritoneal lavage technique, using 1,000 ml of saline.** In the nonpregnant individual, the amount of red blood cells (RBCs) (more than $100,000/mm^3$ for stab wounds, or more than $5,000/mm^3$ for gunshot wounds) and white blood cells (more than $500/mm^3$) present in the lavage fluid is often used to determine the need for an exploratory laparotomy. This amount of blood in a urinary catheter, a peritoneal lavage tube, or a chest tube will prevent you from reading a newspaper through the tubing, as a crude assessment of the bleeding. If the peritoneal lavage fluid is returned through a Foley catheter or through a chest tube, then an exploratory laparotomy will be necessary. The presence of bile, bacteria, vegetable fibers, or elevated enzyme values, such as amylase or alkaline phosphatase (i.e., enzymes released by the injured bowel), may further help define the presence of a significant intra-abdominal injury. A **retrograde cystogram** can be used to detect a bladder penetration. **Continuous electronic fetal monitoring** will assist in detecting fetal distress due to maternal injury or blood loss. The

presence of fetal distress might prompt you to perform a cesarean section.

In about 1:330 cases, an upper abdominal stab wound lacerates the diaphragm and may later lead to bowel obstruction and possible strangulation, which may be lethal to the mother. If surgery is undertaken to repair a diaphragmatic laceration, then it has been recommended that a cesarean section should also be peformed if at all possible in order to avoid the straining (i.e., Valsalva's maneuver) that might occur at the time of vaginal delivery.

6. Hemorrhagic shock

Hemorrhagic shock occurs when the patient loses enough blood to become hypotensive (i.e., more than 25–30% of the blood volume). The loss of about **15% of the blood volume** results in postural hypotension. With a **30% blood loss,** the *skin becomes cold and clammy* and the patient becomes *hypotensive, tachycardic, and tachypneic, with oliguria and metabolic acidosis.* With a loss of **45%** of the blood volume, the same findings as above will be present along with *cardiac failure and coma.*

When a large blood loss occurs, the patient's physiologic mechanisms will attempt to shift the blood flow from the nonvital organs to support the vital organs, such as the heart, brain, and kidneys. *This process results in peripheral vasoconstriction and causes the skin to become cool, pale, and moist.* The *heart rate increases* in an effort to maintain the cardiac output in spite of the diminished blood volume. As the oxygen supply to the organs becomes increasingly depressed, mental confusion and oliguria develop. The tissues of the body shift to an anaerobic metabolism in the absence of sufficient amounts of oxygen, then pyruvic and lactic acids accumulate, which leads to the development of *acidosis.* As this metabolic acidosis increases, it eventually leads to cellular death and autolysis, irreversible shock, and then finally to the death of the individual.

The initial signs of shock consist of air hunger, tachycardia, anxiety, apprehension, diaphoresis, hypotension, and a thready pulse. In such a situation, you should make every effort to stabilize the patient's condition and provide cardiopulmonary support. **Oxygen** should be administered to the patient by mask or by nasal catheter at a rate of 8–10 l/min, if the patient is conscious and the airway is open. **If the patient is unconscious and is not ventilating effectively, then an endotracheal intubation should be accomplished and positive pressure ventilation carried out.** The blood pressure should be maintained by the administration of dopamine hydrochloride or other beta-adrenergic stimulators, such as metaraminol bitartrate or ephedrine. **Dopamine hydrochloride,** 200 mg, should be mixed in 500 ml of sodium chloride solution and administered at 2–5 μg/kg/min with an infusion pump and the blood pressure titrated. *The use of Military Anti-Shock Trousers* (**MAST**) may be indicated in a massive hemorrhage when the blood pressure cannot be maintained by other means. The leg portions of the MAST will not interfere with uterine blood flow, in contrast to the abdominal portion.

Several large-bore needles (14-gauge) should be placed *intravenously, or a venous cutdown instituted, in order for you to maintain an open vascular channel for fluid and blood administration.* A central venous pressure (CVP) catheter or a Swan-Ganz catheter may become necessary in severe shock in order to monitor the CVP or PCWP in cases of significant volume depletion. *The arterial blood gases and the pH should be monitored at periodic intervals.* Several units of blood should be typed and cross-matched as soon as possible; however, you should infuse 5% dextrose in normal saline (or lactated Ringer's solution)

until the packed cells and plasma are ready. If absolutely necessary, type O Rh-negative blood with a low titer of anti-A and anti-B may be used. In order to correct for the occurrence of a transfusion-associated coagulopathy, you should consider the administration of 1 unit of fresh frozen plasma for every 4–5 units of packed cells given to the patient. The use of fresh frozen plasma for this purpose, however, should be based upon a demonstrated coagulation problem. The administration of 10 units of platelets for every 8 units of packed red blood cells has also been advocated.

If the patient is bleeding from a traumatic wound, or postoperatively following abdominal surgery, it is axiomatic that the **bleeding must be controlled.** This may require the exploration of the abdomen to determine the extent and the source of the bleeding. If dopamine hydrochloride is being administered, avoid the use of cyclopropane or halogenated hydrocarbon anesthetics because of the risk of serious arrhythmia.

The fluid and electrolyte balance must also be monitored carefully. The **urine output** should be maintained at more than 30–50 ml/hour. Volume loading with 500–1,000 ml of sodium chloride solution may improve the urine output. The CVP or PCWP readings are of value in assessing the fluid requirements of the patient.

CHAPTER 37

Obstetric problems of pregnancy

In ancient Egypt, two great physicians were known. Thoth, the physician to the gods, and Imhotep, a historic physician (ca. 2600 B.C.), who by the sixth century B.C. had displaced Thoth as the chief healing god of Egypt. Clearly, Imhotep was the first real physician in the Western world to stand out in ancient times. Later, the Greek god of healing, Asclepios, was combined with Imhotep, the Egyptian god of healing, as Asclepios-Imhoutes. Both were replaced by Hippocrates (460–370 B.C.), whose teachings and tenets have persisted into modern times in the form of the Hippocratic oath and the Corpus Hippocraticum.

—D. R. Dunnihoo

1. Abruptio placentae

a. General considerations

Hemorrhage has been listed as one of the classic causes of maternal death. Due to the advances that have occurred in obstetrics residency training, anesthesia, antibiotics, and in the availability of blood banking facilities, the high maternal mortality rate that was noted in 1935 (582:100,000) decreased to 107.2:100,000 in 1945, 47:100,000 in 1955, 12.8:100,000 in 1975, 8.9:100,000 in 1982, and finally 7.8:100,000 in 1985. **The three main causes of maternal death today are pulmonary embolism, pregnancy-induced hypertension (PIH), and hemorrhage.** The availability of whole blood and blood components is one of the essential factors in preventing serious consequences, or even death, from obstetric hemorrhage.

Whenever there is a separation of a normally implanted placenta prior to the delivery of an infant,

abruptio placentae is said to be present. Usually, the bleeding engendered by this separation dissects beneath the membranes and is discharged through the cervix to produce *external vaginal bleeding.* On occasion, however, the blood may accumulate beneath the placental detachment site *(i.e., concealed hemorrhage),* which not only remains concealed from view, but may add further pressure to the detachment site and cause additional abruption of the placenta as the blood dissects beneath it. Also, the bleeding may erupt into the amniotic fluid. In a small number of cases, the bleeding may cease, and if the abruption involves less than 50% of the placental area, then the pregnancy may continue. A fetal-to-maternal hemorrhage is uncommon, but it can occur and may be diagnosed by obtaining a maternal peripheral blood smear in order to conduct a Kleihauer-Betke test.

b. Incidence

Abruptio placentae occurs in about 1% of all deliveries (range 0.3–1.6%). It seems to be more common in patients who are over the age of 35, and in women of high parity. The perinatal mortality rate is about 36.5% overall (range 19–87%) and is almost entirely dependent upon the amount of abruption present. The recurrence of abruptio placentae in subsequent pregnancies has been stated to be about 5.6–17.3%.

c. Etiology

While the **etiology of abruptio placentae** is unknown, several causes have been advanced: (1) *trauma,* such as a kick to the abdomen (which may shear the placenta off of the uterine wall by the sharpness of the blow), rebound from a seat belt decompression in a car accident, or decompression of the uterus after a sudden release of amniotic fluid by the rupture of the membranes in a patient with hydramnios, (2) *a short umbilical cord*, (3) *PIH or chronic hypertension*, (4) *an inferior vena cava obstruction* (although the ligation of the inferior vena cava for the treatment of thromboembolism does not seem to cause any problem), and (5) *a folic acid deficiency* (however, this etiology has not held up in more recent studies). Recently, the presence of prolonged preterm premature rupture of the membranes was reported to be associated with abruptio placentae in nine patients. Presumably, the natural mechanisms that lead to normal placental separation at delivery were thought to be responsible for the abruptio placentae in these patients.

d. Clinical findings

The classic clinical findings in severe abruptio placentae include vaginal bleeding, a tense uterus, absent fetal heart tones, and shock. In a moderate placental abruption, the diagnosis may not be so obvious, and only mild to moderate vaginal bleeding with an increased uterine tone may be present. Some increased uterine irritability and lower abdominal discomfort will usually be noted, and there may be a mild degree of fetal distress. Clinically, the findings in patients who have a mild form of abruptio placentae may resemble the normal release of the mucus plug (i.e., "bloody show") with the associated contractions of early labor. **The presence of uterine tenderness and an increased uterine resting tone, however, should lead you to suspect the diagnosis of abruptio placentae.**

e. Management

The management of the patient with abruptio placentae is dependent upon the condition of the mother and the fetus. An immediate assessment of the *maternal blood loss* and the monitoring of her vital signs is essential as you begin to replace the blood loss with the intravenous administration of blood and balanced salt solutions. **Electronic fetal monitoring** should also be instituted immediately to detect any evidence of *fetal distress*. An ultrasonic evaluation of the placental location should be carried out, and the presence of a retroplacental blood clot should be identified. *If fetal late decelerations or*

bradycardia occurs, or if the mother's blood loss cannot be reasonably managed by repeated transfusions, then a cesarean section should be performed. You should be aware of the fact that, **in the presence of a dead fetus, the maternal heart rate may be reflected in the fetal ECG electrode, which may falsely lead you to think that the fetus is still alive and is experiencing bradycardia.** Thus, it is essential to check the observed "electronic fetal heart rate record" against the pulse rate of the mother prior to performing an emergency cesarean section for "fetal distress."

In the past, the presence of bleeding into the uterine muscle in cases of abruptio placentae (i.e., a *Couvelaire uterus*) was thought to prevent the uterine muscle from contracting after delivery leading to postpartum hemorrhage. As a consequence, the presence of this condition was considered to be an indication for a hysterectomy; however, *such a finding at the time of cesarean section is no longer considered to be an indication for a hysterectomy.*

If fetal distress is not present and the mother's condition has been stabilized, then the membranes should be ruptured and an internal fetal monitor applied. Labor should be induced with oxytocin in these patients, and delivery should be anticipated within a reasonable time, as long as the condition of the mother and fetus remains stable. In the past, delivery was usually expected within about six hours; however, this time restriction is no longer utilized, and the condition of the mother and fetus is now considered in making the decision about delivery.

In cases of abruptio placentae that are severe enough to kill the fetus, about 30% develop **consumptive coagulopathy or disseminated intravascular coagulation (DIC).** In this condition, the fibrinogen levels decrease considerably and the blood fails to clot. Clinically, a tube of the patient's blood should be obtained at periodic intervals so that the onset of clotting can be observed. This approach will allow you to make a crude assessment of the level of the blood fibrinogen present (i.e., delayed clotting indicates a blood fibrinogen level between 100 and 150 mg/dl; no clotting indicates a blood fibrinogen level of less than 100 mg/dl).

The use of packed red blood cells to replace the blood loss and cryoprecipitate and fresh frozen plasma to correct coagulation problems is recommended in DIC. Cryoprecipitate contains Factors I, V, VIII, and XIII. It has been recommended in von Wil-

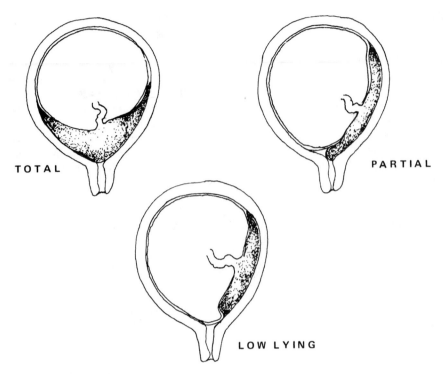

FIGURE 37-1. Types of placenta previa.

lebrand's disease and hemophilia A, in addition to its use in DIC. If packed red blood cells are administered, it has been recommended that one unit of fresh frozen plasma should be given for every four units of packed red blood cells, since it will provide a sufficient amount of clotting factors to support coagulation.

2. Placenta previa

a. Types of placenta previa

The incidence of placenta previa is about 1:200 deliveries, and it seems to be more common in multiparas than in primigravidas. Early ultrasonic studies have noted that up to 45% of all pregnancies have been shown to have a low-lying placenta in the second trimester. The placenta apparently "migrates" away from the internal cervical os as the pregnancy progresses, since less than 1% of all pregnancies still show a placenta previa at term. **Placenta previa has been classified as follows:** (1) **low-lying pla-**

centa, in which the placenta is implanted in the lower uterine segment, (2) **marginal placenta previa,** in which the placenta is implanted at the margin of the internal cervical os, (3) **partial placenta previa,** in which the placenta is implanted in such a manner as to partially cover the internal cervical os, and (4) **complete placenta previa,** in which the placenta covers the entire internal cervical os (Figure 37-1). Another condition that may be confused with placenta previa, called **vasa praevia,** involves a velamentous insertion of the cord with the umbilical vessels overlying the cervical os, which may produce vaginal bleeding.

b. Etiology

The **etiology of placenta previa** may be related to: (1) defective vascularization of the decidua of the uterus (e.g., resulting from multiparity or previous cesarean section), (2) implantation of the placenta on other areas of the uterus in which there is defective decidua (e.g., lower uterine segment), or (3) it may be due to an overly large placenta, as may be seen in Rh isoimmunization erythroblastosis or in a multiple gestation. Occasionally, placenta accreta, increta, or percreta may be associated with placenta previa. In contrast to an abruptio placentae, placenta previa usually presents with painless bleeding, which is frequently recurrent, but not severe. The diagnosis may often be established by an *ultrasonic localization of the placenta*. The possibility of a *vasa praevia* (i.e., a presentation of the fetal vessels inserting into the membranes) as the cause of the bleeding should be considered and efforts should be directed toward detecting the presence of fetal red blood cells in the bloody vaginal discharge (i.e., Kleihauer-Betke test, Apt test, Ogita test).

The **Apt test** consists of mixing 2–3 ml of bloody fluid with an equal volume of water, which is then centrifuged for two minutes at 2,000 rev/min. One part of 1% NaOH solution is mixed with five parts of the clear supernatant liquid and the color change is observed after two minutes. Maternal blood changes from pink to yellow-brown, while fetal blood remains pink. Another test **(Ogita test)** only requires two test tubes containing 10 ml of 0.1 N potassium hydroxide. A few drops of vaginal blood is added to one tube and the same number of drops of maternal blood is added to the other tube. If the tubes turn yellowish-brown within 20 seconds, then there is no fetal blood present. If the vaginal blood tube remains pink, then fetal blood is present. While the presence of fetal blood can be detected by these tests, or even by a simple Wright's stain for nucleated fetal red cells, this condition is so rare that such testing is not done in many hospitals in the United States. Unfortunately, most of the infants who have a vasa praevia do not survive, since even a small amount of fetal blood loss may be lethal to the fetus.

You should also *examine the vagina with a sterile speculum* to rule out extrauterine causes of bleeding. This examination should be accomplished carefully, and should include a careful palpation of the vaginal fornices in an effort to define the presence of a placenta previa. As long as you do not put your finger in the cervical os and disrupt the placenta, severe bleeding should not occur with these examinations.

c. Treatment

In a patient who has a placenta previa, who has only minimal to moderate bleeding, and who is at less than 37 weeks' gestation, the treatment of choice is to transfuse the patient as necessary and to maintain the patient in the hospital or at home under close observation. **If the gestational age is beyond 37–38 weeks, then a pelvic and cervical examination under a "double setup" (i.e., the patient in the operating room, prepped, draped, and ready for an immediate cesarean section) may be performed.** If a total placenta previa is established, either prior to such an examination (e.g., by ultrasonogram) or during the examination, then an immediate cesarean section should be performed, since a further prolongation of the pregnancy beyond 37 weeks will be of no further benefit to the fetus. If, on the other hand, the double setup examination determines that there is only a low-lying or partial placenta previa present (the amount of partial coverage of the cervical os is dependent upon the dilatation of the cervix), then a vaginal delivery may be possible. *In this instance, if the cervical os is dilated, then the membranes should be ruptured, a fetal electrode applied to the fetal scalp, and labor induced with intravenous oxytocin.* Should severe hemorrhage or fetal distress occur, then delivery should be accomplished by cesarean section. Due to the accuracy of the ultrasonic evaluation, most cases of placenta previa are now diagnosed before an examination under a double setup becomes necessary, and the patient may then undergo an elective cesarean section. The major cause of perinatal death in patients who have a placenta previa is prematurity.

3. Hypertensive disease of pregnancy

a. Pregnancy-induced hypertension (PIH)

For many years, the term **toxemia of pregnancy** has been used to define a group of disorders that variably includes hypertension, proteinuria, edema, and convulsions. The Committee on Terminology of the American College of Obstetricians and Gynecologists have suggested that **hypertension** should be defined as a rise of 15 mm Hg diastolic and a rise of 30 mm Hg systolic blood pressure, or a systolic blood pressure value of 140 mm Hg over a diastolic blood pressure of 90 mm Hg, with the blood pressure values being obtained on two occasions at least six hours apart.

The diagnosis of **preeclampsia** is defined as *hypertension,* with one or both of the findings of *edema* *and proteinuria,* after 20 weeks of pregnancy, with the single exception being that of a molar pregnancy, in which the diagnosis of preeclampsia may be made prior to 20 weeks' gestation. The diagnosis of **eclampsia** may be made whenever there are *convulsions* in a patient who has preeclampsia. In patients who have a sustained elevated blood pressure prior to 20 weeks' gestation, the diagnosis of **chronic hypertension** may be applied. If the findings of preeclampsia or eclampsia are found in the latter part of pregnancy in conjunction with chronic hypertension, then the term **superimposed toxemia** (i.e., hypertension with superimposed preeclampsia or eclampsia) should be used. The finding of hypertension alone during the last half of pregnancy and during the first 24 hours' postpartum has caused confusion and has been termed *gestational hypertension.* Similarly, the finding of greater than a 1+ pitting edema after a 12-hour bedrest, or a weight gain of more than 5 lbs per week, has been categorized as *gestational edema.* The isolated occurrence of proteinuria without the appearance of edema, hypertension, or other renal or vascular disease has been termed *gestational proteinuria.*

b. Classification of toxemia

Recently, attempts have been made to devise a new classification system of toxemia in order to incorporate these different definitions into one coherent concept. **In doing so, the term "toxemia" has been changed to "pregnancy-induced hypertension" (PIH), which has been classified by some authorities into the following categories: (1) hypertension (a) without proteinuria or edema, (b) with proteinuria and/or edema (preeclampsia), either mild or severe, or (c) with proteinuria and/or edema and convulsions (eclampsia), (2) chronic hypertension alone, and finally, (3) chronic hypertension with or without superimposed preeclampsia or eclampsia.**

1) Preeclampsia, eclampsia, and chronic hypertension

The diagnosis of **preeclampsia** has been classically described as the presence of hypertension (as defined above) in association with either edema, and/or proteinuria, after 20 weeks' gestation, except for cases involving a hydatidiform mole. The edema may be generalized, but frequently involves the face and hands, and is especially noticeable upon arising in the morning. The proteinuria may consist of a variable amount of protein excretion throughout the day; the presence of more than 300 mg in a 24-hour specimen is considered to be significant.

Preeclampsia may be considered to be severe when: (1) the blood pressure values are at least 160 mm Hg systolic and 110 diastolic, with the patient at bedrest, on two occasions at least six hours apart, (2) the proteinuria is at a level of at least 5 grams per 24 hours, or more than 3+ or 4+ on a semiquantitative evaluation, (3) there is oliguria with less than 400 ml per 24 hours, (4) there are cerebral and visual disturbances, (5) there is pulmonary edema or cyanosis, (6) there is right upper quadrant pain (epigastric pain), (7) there are elevated liver function tests, and/or (8) thrombocytopenia is present. The presence of this latter group of findings—**H**emolysis (i.e., microangiopathic hemolytic anemia), **E**levated **L**iver function tests, and **L**ow **P**latelet counts, have been termed the **HELLP syndrome** and have been considered to provide evidence of severe PIH. **Disseminated intravascular coagulation (DIC)** may also occur in severe cases. This acquired coagulopathy is characterized by decreased fibrinogen levels and bleeding, and it may occur in a number of gynecologic conditions, such as toxemia, fetal death, abruptio placentae, amniotic fluid embolism, sepsis, carcinomatosis, and in transfusion complications. The bleeding is secondary to the consumption of platelets, fibrinogen, and factors V and VIII. The delivery of the fetus and the emptying of the uterus will promptly correct this bleeding diathesis.

Studies have shown that there is an increase in the rate of perinatal loss if hypertension alone is present, and that this loss is further augmented if proteinuria is also present. Proteinuria alone, however, does not seem to have an influence on the perinatal mortality rate. **In one recent report, asymptomatic bacteriuria was noted to be increased in preeclamptic patients (19%).** These patients had lower than normal levels of total serum protein and albumin, and were also noted to have a higher incidence of anemia than non-preeclamptic patients.

Chronic hypertension may predispose a patient to the development of a superimposed toxemia (25–30%) later in pregnancy. A blood pressure in the hypertensive range prior to 20 weeks' gestation, or a systolic blood pressure in excess of 180 mm Hg in the third trimester, should alert you to the possibility that toxemia may be superimposed upon an underlying chronic hypertensive disease. Usually, the systolic blood pressure will not exceed 180–190 mm Hg in cases of toxemia unless chronic hypertension is also present. Other conditions that may produce hypertension include renal disease, lupus erythematosus, chronic glomerulonephritis, diabetic nephropathy, and pheochromocytoma. Due to the decreased uterine blood flow, and consequently, a decrease in the intervillus space blood flow in these hypertensive patients, intrauterine fetal growth retardation and fetal death are more prone to occur. In addition, abruptio placentae occurs in 5–10% of patients who have chronic hypertension.

a) Pathophysiology

The basic underlying disease process in toxemia is **vasospasm.** This observation was first noted as early as 1918, and it would seem to explain essentially all of the manifestations of toxemia. The vasospasm increases the peripheral vascular resistance, which then in turn increases the blood pressure. The localized vasospasm in the various organs may result in hypoxia, necrosis, and hemorrhage.

Studies have shown that normal pregnant women develop a resistance to the administration of angiotensin II, whereas patients who are destined to develop toxemia seem to have an increased sensitivity to angiotensin. The **angiotensin sensitivity test** involves the intravenous administration of **angiotensin.** Those patients who undergo an increase in their diastolic blood pressure of 20 mm Hg over the baseline at about 30 weeks' gestation with less than normal amounts of angiotensin per kilogram of body weight will frequently develop PIH later in pregnancy. In one study, the administration of calcium supplementation in such patients during pregnancy seemed to result in a reduced "vascular sensitivity" and a decreased incidence of PIH (4.5% vs. 21.2%). This vascular hypersensitivity may be further demonstrated by the **rollover test,** performed at 28–32 weeks' gestation, in which the patient's diastolic blood pressure is measured when her position is changed from the side to the back. The majority of patients whose diastolic blood pressure increases by 20 mm Hg during this test will develop pregnancy-induced hypertensive disease at a later date in pregnancy.

Recently, there has been some evidence that prostacyclin and thromboxane A_2 may be involved in the vascular changes in pregnancy and perhaps in the development of toxemia. **Prostacyclin is a prostaglandin and is a potent vasodilator and an inhibitor of platelet aggregation. In contrast, thromboxane A_2 has exactly the reverse capabilities, in that it is a vasoconstrictor and will induce platelet aggregation.** During pregnancy, the maternal and fetal circulations are widely dilated and have a low vascular resistance. Since the decidua, chorion, amnion, trophoblast, umbilical cord, uterine blood vessels, and the endometrium may all produce prostacyclin, it is possible that the regulation of the umbilical blood flow and of the maternal vasculature may be due to the release of prostacyclin.

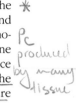

PC vs TxA₂

*

PC produced by many tissue

In contrast, **thromboxane A_2** may also be produced in many tissues associated with pregnancy, such as the placenta, decidua, amnion, chorion, and the myometrium, in order of decreasing production. The maternal platelets also produce increasing amounts of thromboxane A_2 during pregnancy. **Thromboxane A_2 may be involved in the production of the platelet aggregation and vascular vasospasm changes that occur in preeclampsia.** Either a deficiency of prostacyclin, or an excess of thromboxane A_2, might therefore be involved in the development of toxemia. Interestingly, magnesium sulfate, which is the current treatment of choice for PIH, acts as a stimulant for the production of prostacyclin. In addition, it has been demonstrated that there is an increased production of placental progesterone in patients with mild preeclampsia. Since progesterone inhibits the production of placental prostacyclin, the relatively higher levels of thromboxane in relation to prostacyclin may be secondary to this inhibition. Future studies may elucidate the effects of these prostaglandins more completely.

It was demonstrated many years ago that pregnant toxemic patients usually have a lower blood volume (i.e., hypovolemia) than normally occurs in pregnancy. Thus, instead of having a 30–50% increase in the blood volume, the patient's blood volume might be similar to that of the nonpregnant woman. As a consequence, the vasospasm that occurs in toxemia maintains the decreased volume of the vascular bed, which would then account for the filling of the vascular bed in spite of the absence of the usual pregnancy-induced volume expansion. One study demonstrated that the cardiac output and the stroke volume of PIH patients with small-for-gestational-age infants were significantly lower than in normal pregnancy. *There is a 20% decrease (from normal pregnancy values) in the renal plasma flow, and a 32% decrease in the glomerular filtration rate, in patients with PIH. The uterine blood flow is lower by about 50–70%, which accounts for the intra-uterine growth retardation and the increased incidence of fetal distress seen in patients with PIH.*

The low glomerular filtration rate in the presence of PIH results in a decrease in the clearance of uric acid and an increase in the uric acid plasma values. Microscopically, the renal glomeruli are enlarged about 20% and contain dilated loops of capillaries that show swollen endothelial cells **(i.e., glomerular capillary endotheliosis).** A subendothelial deposit of homogeneous protein material, probably a derivative of fibrinogen, has been thought to be characteristic, but perhaps not pathognomonic, for preeclampsia. Hemorrhagic necrosis of the peripheral portion of the liver lobule (i.e., *periportal necrosis*) used to be considered pathognomonic of eclampsia; however, there is now doubt concerning this concept as well. Hemorrhage beneath the liver capsule may occur in rare cases and may lead to the rupture of the capsule with massive intra-abdominal bleeding. Focal hemorrhagic lesions, varying from small petechiae to gross bleeding and edema, have been noted in the brains of patients who have died from eclampsia.

The increased vasospasm associated with PIH is undoubtedly reflected also in the perfusion of the intervillus space. Studies have indicated that the normal blood flow to the placenta at term is about 500–700 ml per minute, but that only one-third of this amount may be present in preeclamptic patients. Studies that have compared the diameter of the myometrial spiral arteries in both normal and toxemic women have shown a decrease in the arterial diameter of up to 40% in toxemia patients. The histologic evaluation of the uteroplacental arteries has also shown endothelial damage and other changes in the walls of the vessels.

b) Clinical aspects

Although PIH generally occurs in about 5–7% of private practice patients, it is often seen in a higher percentage of patients attending clinics that serve an indigent, low socioeconomic population. The disease is more commonly seen in the young primigravida patient, but older patients with chronic hypertension also may be seen with superimposed toxemia. The incidence of eclampsia is of the order of 1:1,000–1:1,500 deliveries. According to some reports, there does seem to be a familial tendency for the development of PIH in certain families, perhaps due to a recessive gene. It is possible that toxemia may be due to an inherited enzme deficiency for the production of certain prostaglandins.

The occurrence of excessive weight gain in a pregnant patient may herald the onset of **preeclampsia.** A gain of more than 2 lbs/week, or 6 lbs/month in the third trimester, should alert you to the possibility of impending preeclampsia. The discovery of *edema* of the fingers or face is even more suggestive of the diagnosis. An increase in the blood pressure to hypertensive levels and the appearance of proteinuria and/or edema completes the clinical picture of PIH.

c) Treatment

Once the diagnosis of PIH has been made, the patient should be hospitalized and placed at bedrest in the left lateral decubitus position. As close observation is essential, these patients should not be managed in an outpatient setting unless the diagnosis is very questionable. **The ultimate treatment of PIH requires delivery of the fetus and the placenta.**

If the patient is near term (i.e., past 37 weeks), the delivery may be easily accomplished, by the elective induction of labor, without undue problems for either the mother or the fetus. However, when the patient requires an earlier delivery, then the risk of fetal prematurity, RDS, or fetal death becomes increasingly higher as the gestational age decreases. Occasionally, strict bedrest may gain some time in mild cases of toxemia before delivery becomes necessary. Twice a week nonstress tests, weekly contraction stress tests, and weekly biophysical profiles should usually be accomplished on these patients if the delivery is delayed. In addition, the patient's creatinine clearance should be monitored at weekly intervals. If the patient's blood pressure cannot be controlled with bedrest, and if the level of proteinuria increases, then consideration should be given to the delivery of the fetus.

Once delivery has been decided upon, which usually occurs because the patient's condition has worsened, then you should stabilize the patient by the administration of magnesium sulfate, either by intramuscular injection or by continuous intravenous infusion, in an attempt to prevent or control convulsions. If the blood pressure is excessively elevated, the judicious administration of hydralazine (Apresoline) to lower the blood pressure may decrease the risk of a cerebral vascular accident.

Magnesium sulfate is the drug of choice for the treatment of PIH. It may be administered in one of the following regimens: (1) an initial loading dose of 4 grams I.V., followed by 1 gram per hour; (2) a 4-gram IV, followed by a maintenance dose of 3 grams per hour; (3) a loading dose of 10 grams I.M., followed by 5 grams I.M. q6h; (4) in severe preeclampsia—a loading dose of 4 grams I.V. and 10 grams I.M. initially, followed by 5 grams I.M. q4h; in mild preeclampsia—a loading dose of 10 grams I.M., followed by 5 grams q4h I.M.; (5) a loading dose of 4 grams I.V., followed by 1–2 grams per hour I.V.; and (6) a loading dose of 6 grams in 100 ml of 5% dextrose in water administered over 15 minutes, followed by a 2-gram maintenance dose per hour. The recommended range of the serum magnesium level is 4.3–8.4 mg/dl. **The patient should be evaluated periodically (i.e., hourly during I.V. dosage, and prior to each dose in those patients who are receiving I.M. dosage) for the presence of patellar reflexes, urine output of more than 25–30 ml/h, and a respiratory rate of more than 12 breaths per minute.** The patellar reflexes will disappear at a magnesium serum level of 10–12 mg/dl, at which point the patient may complain of a feeling of warmth, flushing, muscle weakness, and slurred speech. Respiratory arrest will occur at magnesium serum levels of 15–17 mg/dl, and cardiac arrest will occur at 30–35 mg/dl. **Calcium gluconate** is the antidote for magnesium poisoning and should always be available at the patient's bedside during magnesium sulfate therapy.

Usually, a 4- to 6-gram I.V. dose of magnesium sulfate will produce a serum level of 5–9 mg/dl within 60 minutes, and with the subsequent administration of a 2-gram/hour maintenance dose, a serum level of 4–8 mg/dl will be produced. The I.M. dosage regimen for mild PIH listed as no. 4 above will result in serum levels of between 3 and 6 mg/dl. Magnesium sulfate is not an antihypertensive agent. Its main effect apparently is its ability to prevent convulsions. The amount of depression in the neonate may be related to the dosage of magnesium sulfate administered to the mother just prior to delivery, so the lower dosage levels are preferred if the PIH can be controlled.

In severe cases, the cardiac status should be carefully monitored by means of a Swan-Ganz balloon flotation catheter. The normal values that may be found are as follows: (1) cardiac output (CO) = 5–6 l/min; (2) central venous pressure (CVP) = 5–12 mm Hg; (3) pulmonary artery pressure (PAP) = < 30/15; (4) pulmonary capillary wedge pressure (PCWP) = 5–12 mm Hg; (5) stroke volume index (SVI) = CO divided by the heart rate times the body surface area = 35–45 ml/beat/m^2; (6) mean arterial pressure (MAP) = systolic blood pressure plus 2 times diastolic blood pressure divided by 3 = 85–95 mm Hg; (7) systemic vascular resistance (SVR) = MAP minus CVP times 79.9 divided by the CO = 800–1,400 dyne-sec/cm^{-5}; (8) pulmonary vascular resistance (PVR) = mean pulmonary arterial pressure minus PCWP times 79.9 divided by the CO = 150–250 dyne-sec/cm^{-5}; and (9) left ventricular stroke work index (LVSWI) = SVI times (MAP − PCWP) times (0.0136) = 51–61 g-min/m^2.

The *pulmonary capillary wedge pressure* (PCWP) reflects the pressure of the left atrium. It also correlates with the left ventricular end-diastolic pressure (LVEDP). *The LVEDP, in turn, reflects the preload on the left ventricle.* **Starling's curve of cardiac function** represents the relationship of the cardiac preload and the force of contraction. The greater the preload, the greater the force of contraction, up to the point where the curve levels off. The value of PCWP may increase to levels as high as 33 mm Hg in pulmonary edema. The CVP value may not truly reflect the status of the vascular volume in the preeclamptic patient, whereas the PCWP has been shown to be more accurate. The LVSWI value reflects the left ventricular function more accurately than does the cardiac output. *The SVR represents the afterload against which the heart must function.* Due to the vasospasm that is present in toxemia, the SVR is always high in these patients. The SVR and CO have an inverse relationship (i.e., CO decreases as SVR increases). There are no important changes in the PVR in toxemia; however, this parameter is of significance in the management of some other cardiac problems. **About 1% of these patients will have complications secondary to the use of a Swan-Ganz catheter.** These problems include cardiac arrhythmia, pneumothorax, hemothorax, pulmonary infarction, thromboembolism, and sepsis.

The delivery of the fetus of a patient with PIH generally should be carried out under local or pudendal anesthesia for a vaginal delivery, or under general anesthesia if by cesarean section. In patients with PIH, epidural or spinal anesthesia should probably be avoided because of the toxemia-induced hypovolemia and the risk of developing severe hypotension with subsequent splanchnic blockade. In general, however, the method of anesthesia should be individualized according to the severity of the PIH. The administration of a loading dose of intravenous fluids to patients prior to the use of regional anesthesia may prevent a hypotensive reaction.

The fetus should be closely monitored throughout labor with an electronic fetal heart rate monitor. Variable and late decelerations of the fetal heart rate have been noted to occur in a significant number of patients with severe pregnancy-induced hypertension.

4. Isoimmunization

a. Rh disease

1) Incidence

About 13% of all marriages are potentially incompatible for the Rh factor; however, the incidence of Rh isoimmunization is considerably less than 0.5%. **The $Rh_o(D)$ antigen varies widely between the races; it is present in 85% of white Americans, in 99% of black Americans, in 93% of orientals, and in 66% of the members of the Basque population in France and Spain.**

2) Historical aspects

Prior to the advent of amniocentesis and amniotic fluid bilirubin studies by **D.C.A. Bevis** in the early 1950s, when only the maternal history of having previously had an infant affected by hemolytic disease and the indirect Coombs test values could be used to determine the severity of the erythroblastotic process, the estimated fetal loss rate with Rh isoimmunization was of the order of 30%. With the advent of amniocentesis and the selective delivery of the fetus using the **Liley** amniotic fluid bilirubin graph, the fetal mortality rate fell to about 10%. With the use of the intrauterine fetal transfusion procedure, which was first performed by **A. W. Liley,** in 1963, about 70% of the severely involved fetuses beyond 28 weeks' gestation have been salvaged; however, since this procedure is

only necessary in about $1:2,000$ $Rh_o(D)$-sensitized pregnancies, it has not contributed appreciably to the lowering of the fetal mortality rate.

Patients may become sensitized to a number of different blood group antigens other than the Rh factor. **ABO incompatibility** occurs when the **mother has group O blood** with anti-A and anti-B in her serum and **the fetus has group A, B, or AB blood.** The infant will become jaundiced within the first 24 hours following delivery, with a variable amount of anemia and hyperbilirubinemia. While the jaundice is usually mild in the fetus, it may be more severe on occasion. Other **irregular blood groups** may also involve the fetus in an isoimmunization problem. The blood groups Kell, Duffy, and Kidd are the ones most commonly involved in sensitization (Table 37-1).

3) Sensitization

If the $Rh_o(D)$-negative mother is exposed to the $Rh_o(D)$ antigen, she may become sensitized to the antigen and begin to produce antibodies against it. Sensitization may occur secondary to a mismatched blood transfusion, or more commonly, it may occur as the result of the transplacental passage of fetal erythrocytes into her bloodstream, either during the course of the pregnancy or at the time of the delivery. Once sensitization has occurred, further exposure to the $Rh_o(D)$ antigen in subsequent pregnancies will again stimulate the production of $Rh_o(D)$ antibodies. These antibodies, once produced, will transfer back across the placenta into the fetal circulation and cause hemolysis of the fetal erythrocytes. As more and more erythrocytes are destroyed, the fetus first becomes anemic, and then later, as the anemia becomes severe, will develop cardiac failure and will finally die. This syndrome of anemia, erythroid hyperplasia of the bone marrow, extramedullary hematopoiesis, subcutaneous edema, ascites, hydrothorax, hepatosplenomegaly, and cardiac failure has been termed **erythroblastosis fetalis.** The edema of the fetal body and the collection of serous fluid in the body cavities has been called **hydrops fetalis.**

4) Periodic evaluation

A $Rh_o(D)$-negative maternity patient should have an initial indirect Coombs test performed on her first visit and then should have repeat tests done at 20, 24, and 28 weeks' gestation, in an effort to detect the first

TABLE 37-1. Antibodies causing hemolytic disease

Blood group system	Antigens related to hemolytic disease	Severity of hemolytic disease	Proposed management
Rh	D	Mild to severe	Amniotic fluid studies
	C	Mild to moderate	Amniotic fluid studies
	c	Mild to severe	Amniotic fluid studies
	E	Mild to severe	Amniotic fluid studies
	e	Mild to moderate	Amniotic fluid studies
Lewis		Not a proved cause of hemolytic disease of the newborn	
I		Not a proved cause of hemolytic disease of the newborn	
Kell	K	Mild to severe with hydrops fetalis	Amniotic fluid studies
	k	Mild to severe	Amniotic fluid studies
Duffy	Fy^a	Mild to severe with hydrops fetalis	Amniotic fluid studies
	Fy^b	Not a cause of hemolytic disease of the newborn	
Kidd	Jk^a	Mild to severe	Amniotic fluid studies
	Jk^b	Mild to severe	Amniotic fluid studies
MNSs	M	Mild to severe	Amniotic fluid studies when IgG titer is high
	N	Mild	Expectant
	S	Mild to severe	Amniotic fluid studies
	s	Mild to severe	Amniotic fluid studies
Lutheran	Lu^a	Mild	Expectant
	Lu^b	Mild	Expectant
Diego	Di^a	Mild to severe	Amniotic fluid studies
	Di^b	Mild to severe	Amniotic fluid studies
Xg	Xg^a	Mild	Expectant
P	PP$_1$P^k (Tj^a)	Mild to severe	Amniotic fluid studies
Public antigens	Yt^a	Moderate to severe	Amniotic fluid bilirubin studies
	Yt^b	Mild	Expectant
	Lan	Mild	Expectant
	En^a	Moderate	Amniotic fluid bilirubin studies
	Ge	Mild	Expectant
	Jr^a	Mild	Expectant
	Co^a	Severe	Amniotic fluid bilirubin studies
Private antigens	Co^{a-b}	Mild	Expectant
	Batty	Mild	Expectant
	Becker	Mild	Expectant
	Berrens	Mild	Expectant
	Biles	Moderate	Amniotic fluid bilirubin studies
	Evans	Mild	Expectant
	Gonzales	Mild	Expectant
	Good	Severe	Amniotic fluid bilirubin studies
	Heibel	Moderate	Amniotic fluid bilirubin studies
	Hunt	Mild	Expectant
	Jobbins	Mild	Expectant
	Radin	Moderate	Amniotic fluid bilirubin studies
	Rm	Mild	Expectant
	Ven	Mild	Expectant
	Wright^a	Severe	Amniotic fluid bilirubin studies
	Wright^b	Mild	Expectant
	Zd	Moderate	Amniotic fluid bilirubin studies

Modified from L. Weinstein, "Irregular Antibodies Causing Hemolytic Disease of the Newborn: A Continuing Problem," *Clinical Obstetrics and Gynecology* 25, no. 2 (1982), pp. 331–332.

Reprinted with permission from The American College of Obstetricians and Gynecologists, "Management of Isoimmunization in Pregnancy," *ACOG Technical Bulletin* 90 (1984), p. 2.

sign of sensitization (i.e., the presence of antibodies). When an antibody titer of about 1:16 or greater is detected, it becomes necessary for you to follow the patient throughout the rest of her pregnancy by *utilizing amniocentesis for the determination of the bilirubin content of the amniotic fluid.* The level of antibody titer at which amniocentesis should first be instituted, however, should be determined in your own particular laboratory. In my experience, a titer as low as 1:32 may be associated with severe erythroblastosis and fetal death. The severity of the erythroblastotic process, and the condition of the infant, is reflected in the amount of bilirubin present in the amniotic fluid, since bilirubin is the product resulting from the breakdown of the fetal red blood cell hemoglobin. If there is no evidence of sensitization at 28 weeks' gestation, then $Rh_o(D)$ immune globulin may be given to protect the mother from sensitization until the time of delivery.

5) Amniocentesis

Since it is technically difficult to perform an intrauterine transfusion on the fetus prior to about 22–24 weeks' gestation, the first diagnostic amniocentesis is generally delayed until this point in time. Repeat amniocenteses are then carried out as necessary thereafter, according to the degree of severity of the erythroblastosis fetalis. **Approximately 10 ml of amniotic fluid should be obtained by amniocentesis and placed in a brown bottle to shield it from light. It should then be analyzed by means of a scanning spectrophotometer from 350–700 mμ. in order to detect a bilirubin peak at the 450-mμ. wave length.** The values obtained are then plotted on a three-phase semilogarithmic paper, with the baseline drawn between 375 and 525 mμ. While some investigators prefer to draw the baseline between 368 and 525 mμ, the important consideration is that it should be kept consistent from one tracing to the next. The difference between the peak and this baseline at the 450-mμ wave length represents the delta optical density (ΔO.D.) value for bilirubin (Fig. 37-2).

There are several additional aspects of the spectrophotometric scan that should be considered. If there is a single peak at 410–420 mμ, in addition to the 450-mμ wave length peak, then there is *meconium contamination* of the amniotic fluid present. If

there is a peak at the 410–420 mμ wave length in addition to the 450-mμ peak, and also additional small peaks at 540 mμ and at 575 mμ (i.e., the Soret band), then this represents *blood contamination.* If there is a peak at 410 mμ, in addition to the 450-mμ peak, and also another small peak at 620–623 mμ, then this is indicative of the presence of *methemalbumin.* Methemalbumin is often present in the severely involved fetus. Finally, if you plot the slope of the baseline between 375 and 525 mμ in successive graphs, you will note that the slope becomes steeper when the fetal condition worsens and becomes less steep when the ΔO.D. values decrease. It should be remembered that there will be an increased level of bilirubin present in the amniotic fluid even in the Rh(D)-positive patient. This level is usually in the moderate involvement zone of Liley's gestational graph from about 20 weeks until late in pregnancy, when it gradually drops into the zone indicating minimal to no involvement.

The ΔO.D. is plotted on a Liley gestational graph according to the number of weeks of gestation (Fig. 37-3). **This graph provides information as to the severity of the erythroblastosis in relationship to the week of gestation and is divided into three zones: (1) the minimal-to-no-involvement zone, (2) the moderate involvement zone, and (3) the severe involvement zone.** If two or more of these plotted values fall within the upper two zones, then further follow-up amniocenteses will be required in order to determine the optimal time for the delivery of the fetus. If the values are in the severe zone, and the infant is at less than 31–32 weeks' gestation, then an intrauterine transfusion should be considered. Beyond 32 weeks, the infant will almost always do better in the nursery and should be delivered. The knowledge of the fetal salvage rate in your nursery at the various gestational ages and fetal weight levels should help you in making this decision.

A recent technique that has been used in the management of Rh-sensitized patients in some centers is the **percutaneous umbilical blood sampling (PUBS) technique.** The risk of fetal loss with this procedure is about 1%; however, the ability to define the hematocrit level of the fetus more precisely with this method provides the physician with a much more accurate approach to the management of these patients than was provided by previous methods.

6) Prophylaxis

In patients who have not yet been sensitized to the $Rh_o(D)$ antigen, it is important to try to prevent such sensitization from occurring. It has been found that as little as 0.5 ml or less of $Rh_o(D)$ blood may cause sensitization. As a consequence, **possible sensitization may occur as the result of an amniocentesis, an abortion, or an ectopic pregnancy, as well as during pregnancy and delivery.** In order to prevent this from occurring, it has been recommended that $Rh_o(D)$ immune globulin should be administered in these patients. Throughout pregnancy, there is a small leakage of fetal red cells across the placenta into the mother's bloodstream, and this is especially true at the time of delivery. Because of this, it has been recommended that $Rh_o(D)$ immune globulin be given to the unsensitized patient at 28 weeks' gestation and then again within 72 hours after the delivery (the latter is given only if the infant is Rh(D) positive). **Although a 1.6% failure rate occurs when only the postdelivery dose of $Rh_o(D)$ immune globulin is given, this can be reduced to about a 0.1% failure rate when the 28th-week dose is added to the regimen.** If there is a massive bleeding from the fetus to the mother at the time of delivery, then an additional amount of immune globulin should be administered to protect the patient. It has been estimated that 300 µg of immune globulin will counteract 30 ml of whole blood or 15 ml of fetal red blood cells.

7) Erythroblastosis

If the fetus is delivered with erythroblastosis fetalis, the fetal plasma bilirubin level will increase rapidly and the infant will become jaundiced. If the infant cannot degrade the bilirubin quickly enough, perhaps due to the immaturity of its liver enzymes, then the plasma bilirubin may rise to levels exceeding 20 milligrams per 100 ml (mg%). When this occurs, there is a risk that the bilirubin may affect the basal ganglia and hippocampal areas of the fetal brain, causing mental retardation and spasticity **(i.e., kernicterus).** In order to prevent this increase in the bilirubin, the judicious use of *exchange transfusions and phototherapy* have been found to be beneficial. If the fetus is very anemic at delivery as a result of erythroblastosis, associated with obvious edema of the entire body (i.e., hydrops fetalis), then cardiac failure is present. An immediate exchange transfusion will be required in such cases, which requires the presence at the delivery of expert pediatric assistance to care for the infant.

8) Nonimmune hydrops

Due to the decrease in hydrops secondary to Rh isoimmunization, nonimmune hydrops has become the more common form of hydrops fetalis that is seen in clinical practice today. Nonimmune hydrops occurs in about 1:3,700 pregnancies. This entity may occur as the result of: (1) **hematologic problems** (i.e., fetomaternal or twin-to-twin transfusion, α-thalassemia, G6PD deficiency), (2) **congenital heart disease** (i.e., Tetralogy of Fallot, septal defects, subaortic stenosis, arrhythmia), (3) **pulmonary abnormalities** (i.e., pulmonary hypoplasia, cystic adenomatoid formation), (4) **renal anomalies** (i.e., polycystic kidneys, renal venous thrombosis, hydronephrosis), (5) **intrauterine infections** (i.e., cytomegalovirus, toxoplasmosis, syphilis), (6) **chromosomal abnormalities** (i.e., Turner's syndrome, trisomy 18, 21, and XX/XY mosaicism, tuberous sclerosis), (7) **diabetes mellitus,** and (8) **umbilical cord problems** (i.e., thrombosis of the umbilical vein, hemangioma of the cord).

The collection of serous fluid in the body cavities is probably caused by a number of mechanisms, some of which are due to cardiac failure, others of which are unknown. The treatment involves the delivery of the fetus, if it is of a viable gestational age. Since **pulmonary hypoplasia** will occur in more than 42% of these infants, significant problems in the neonatal period should be anticipated.

5. Postdatism

A term pregnancy has been defined as one that lasts between 38 and 42 weeks of gestation (i.e., 266–294 days). About 80% of all pregnancies are carried to term. The term **premature** has been used to define the cessation of pregnancy prior to the 38th week of gestation, while the terms **postterm pregnancy** and **postdatism** refer to pregnancies that continue beyond 42 completed weeks. About 7–10% of all pregnancies are premature, and about 2–11% are postterm; however, the determination of the true

Text continues on p. 486

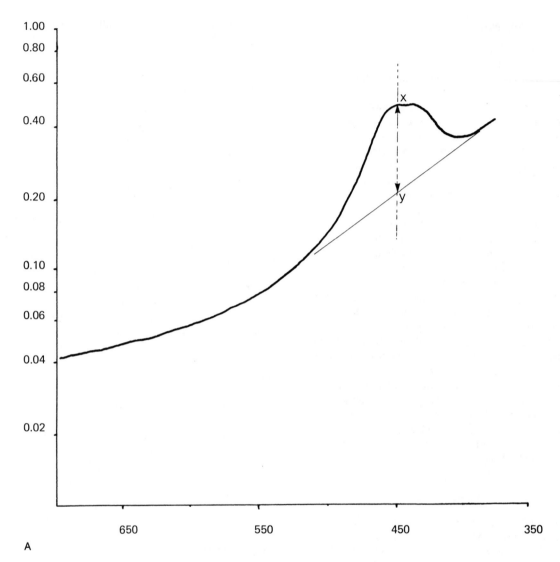

A

FIGURE 37-2. (A) Diagrammatic representation of a spectrophotometric scan of amniotic fluid containing bilirubin. The line of the base is drawn from 368–375 to 525 mμ to illustrate the baseline curve had there been no bilirubin present. The absorption peak of bilirubin is at 450 mμ. The difference between the peak at 450 mμ and the baseline constitutes the delta O.D. (Δ optical density) value. (B) (1) Normal bilirubin curve. If there is a single peak at 410–420 mμ, in addition to the 450-mμ wave length peak, then there is *meconium contamination* of the amniotic fluid present. (2) If there is a peak at 410 mμ, in addition to the 450-mμ peak, and also another small peak at 620–623 mμ, then this is indicative of the presence of *methemalbumin*. Methemalbumin is often present in the severely involved fetus. (3) If there is a peak at the 410–420-mμ wave length, in addition to the 450-mμ peak, and also additional small peaks at 540 mμ and at 575 mμ (i.e., the Soret band), then this represents *blood contamination*. Finally, if the slope of the baseline is plotted between 375 mμ and 525 mμ in successive graphs, the slope will become steeper when the fetal condition worsens and will become less steep in those cases in which the Δ O.D. values decrease.

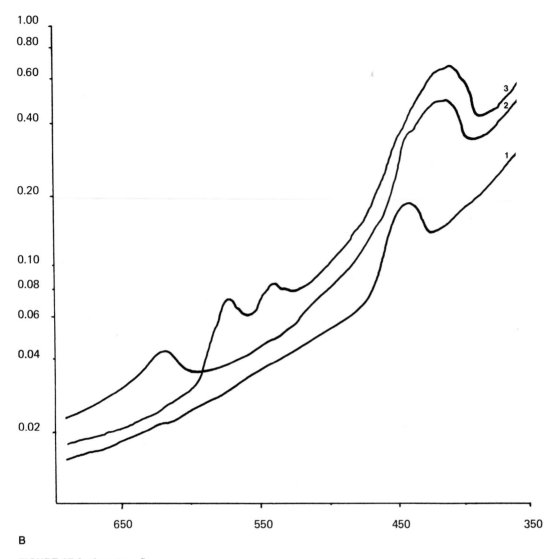

B

FIGURE 37-2. *(continued)*

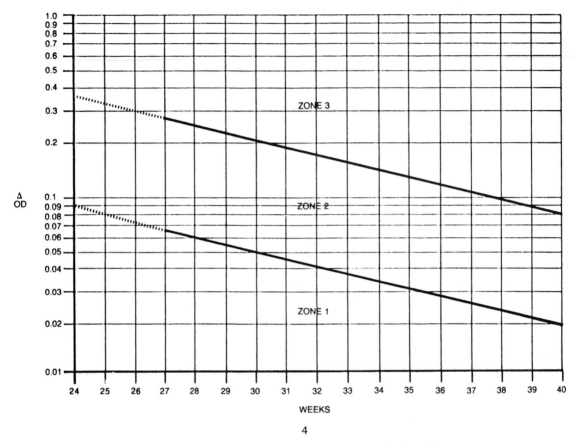

FIGURE 37-3. Modified Liley graph used to predict degrees of sensitization. The dotted line represents a linear extrapolation from the original Liley data (solid line). Zone 1 represents the area that indicates minimal-to-no involvement of the fetus. Zone 2 is moderate involvement. Zone 3 is severe involvement. (Reprinted with permission from American College of Obstetricians and Gynecologists, "Management of Isoimmunization in Pregnancy," *ACOG Technical Bulletin* 90, 1986, p. 4.)

gestational age is often quite inaccurate. Poor gestational dating constituted one of the most pressing problems in obstetrics in the past and it still complicates the management of many obstetric problems. The new ultrasonic techniques have made great advances in resolving this problem. Prolonged pregnancies are more common in primigravida patients.

a. Fetal weight variations

The gestational age should not be confused with the weight of the fetus. The two may at times correlate, in which case we might say that the *fetus is appropriate for gestational age* (AGA) (i.e., the fetal weight falls between the 10th and the 90th percentiles). On other occasions, however, the fetus may be *small for gestational age* (SGA) (i.e., the weight falls below the 10th percentile), or it may have intrauterine growth retardation. In infants who are larger than normal, the designation of *large for gestational age* (LGA) (i.e., the weight falls above the 90th percentile) or *macrosomia* may be applied (Fig. 37-4).

Infants who show evidence of weight loss and who have been subjected to chronic distress should be considered to be **dysmature** instead of postmature. Various studies have shown that the mean fetal birth weight at term is about 3,335 grams, with a range from 3,280–3,400 grams. The fetal weight is influenced by the sex of the fetus (males weigh more than females), the race (white infants weigh more than black infants),

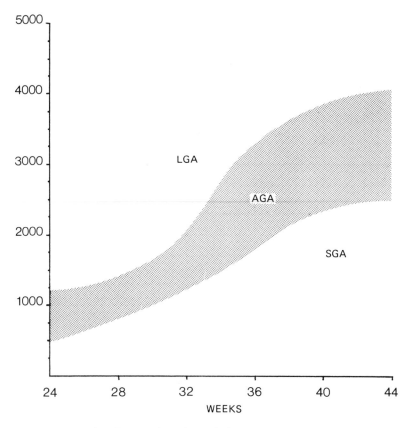

FIGURE 37-4. Classification of newborns by birth weight and gestational age: (LGA) Large for gestational age; (AGA) Appropriate for gestational age; (SGA) Small for gestational age.

parity (babies of multiparous women weigh more than those of primigravidas), and the maternal height and weight (greater maternal height and weight may be related to larger infants).

b. Etiology

Although the exact cause of labor has not been fully defined, it has been shown that certain conditions seem to be associated with **prolonged gestation.** *They are: (1) fetal adrenal hypoplasia, (2) placental sulfatase deficiency, (3) fetal anencephaly, (4) absent fetal pituitary or adrenal gland, and (5) extrauterine pregnancy.* Since the installation of cortisol into the amniotic fluid has been shown to induce labor in a prolonged pregnancy, it is possible that a deficiency in fetal cortisol may be responsible for delaying the onset of labor. It is thought that the fetus triggers the onset of labor by excreting a substance into the am-

niotic fluid, which results in the release of phospholipase A_2 to produce arachidonic acid, which in turn produces prostaglandin PGE_2 and PGF_{2_α} in the uterine decidua. The prostaglandins then stimulate the uterine muscle to cause contractions (i.e., labor) (see Chapter 24). All of the conditions that are known to prolong pregnancy are associated with a lower than normal estrogen level. In normal pregnancy, estrogens are involved in the production and storage of glycerophospholipids in the fetal membranes. The glycerophospholipids are the precursors of the arachidonate compound.

c. Fetal outcomes in postdatism

There are two possible outcomes in the post-term fetus. The fetus may continue to grow and become larger (LGA) (60–80%), or it may cease to grow, lose weight, and become a dysmature

infant (20–40%). In the *first instance,* the fetal size becomes the problem as the gestation advances beyond term, and the incidences of *cephalopelvic disproportion and/or shoulder dystocia* become increasingly more common, due to the large size of the infant. In the *second instance,* the amniotic fluid gradually decreases (oligohydramnios), the fetus loses weight, and it subsequently experiences **cord compression problems** with **fetal distress** and the release of meconium into the amniotic fluid. As the placenta ages and becomes less efficient in transferring oxygen and nutrients, there is a loss of the subcutaneous tissue and a desquamation of the skin of the fetus, who, when born, looks like a "little old man" with an apprehensive facies **(the postmaturity or dysmaturity syndrome).** In some cases of postterm pregnancy, the placental insufficiency may be very severe and fetal death may ocur in utero. Death presumably results from extreme fetal distress secondary to placental insufficiency and/or cord compression.

d. Diagnosis

To make a clear diagnosis of a postterm pregnancy requires that the pregnancy be accurately dated. An ultrasonic evaluation of the fetal crown-rump length at 7–14 weeks' gestation has an accuracy of ±4.7 days; the femur length between weeks 12 and 22 has an accuracy of ±6.7 days; and the measurement of the biparietal diameter between weeks 17 and 26 has an accuracy of ±11 days. These ultrasonic parameters may provide an additional check upon the clinical gestational dating observations (i.e., the last menstrual period, the quickening date, the first date that the fetal heart tones were first heard, and the uterine fundal measurements between weeks 16 and 34). Ultrasonic biparietal diameter measurements should generally not be used beyond the 26th week for pregnancy dating, since their accuracy decreases at that point to ± 14–21 days.

e. Management

Any patient who goes beyond term should be kept under close surveillance after 41 weeks' gestation, unless there is earlier evidence of such factors as decreased amniotic fluid, decreased fundal measurements, or decreased fetal activity, which might prompt an earlier institution of techniques to assess the fetus. **When the gestational dating in a patient is** **thought to be accurate, the patient's cervix is favorable for the induction of labor, and there has been no evidence of fetal compromise, labor should probably be induced at the completion of the 42nd week of gestation.** Those patients who do not have accurate gestational dating should be tested with **nonstress tests (NST) every 3–4 days,** and/or with **contraction stress tests (CST) once a week.** In addition, an **ultrasonic evaluation should be performed each week** to assist in detecting whether there is any decrease in the amniotic fluid (i.e., oligohydramnios). Variable decelerations (cord compression) may sometimes be seen on the fetal heart rate monitor if oligohydramnios is present. The **biophysical profile,** using the NST, fetal body movements, amniotic fluid volume, fetal tone, and fetal breathing movements, may be employed in assessing the fetal status (see Chapter 26).

In the management of the postterm delivery, it is necessary to use continuous electronic monitoring of the fetal heart tones and the uterine contractions throughout labor in order to detect any evidence of fetal distress. Many postterm pregnancies have meconium in the amniotic fluid, and great care should be taken at the time of the delivery to suction the infant carefully prior to the first breath in order to try to prevent the *meconium aspiration syndrome,* which can result in severe pulmonary hypertension that may end in fetal death. In many instances, however, since the fetus may have already aspirated meconium in utero, it may not always be possible to prevent this syndrome. You should plan to have pediatric support in the delivery room to provide immediate care for these high-risk infants.

If the postterm infant is macrosomic, with a fundal measurement of greater than 40 cm, then you should be alert to the possibility that *cephalopelvic disproportion or shoulder dystocia may occur. In such instances, it is well to be prepared to perform a cesarean section.* An estimated fetal weight of 4,500 grams or more has been suggested by some authors as being an indication for an elective cesarean section.

6. Fetal distress

a. Onset

Fetal distress occurs whenever the fetus is deprived of either nutrients (chronic metabolic deficiency) or oxygen (acute and chronic re-

spiratory placental insufficiency). Intrauterine growth retardation, for example, is the result of chronic fetal distress. Acute fetal distress is most commonly noted during parturition, when the fetus is under close scrutiny during labor. In recent years, however, with the use of antepartum nonstress and stress testing, there is a greater appreciation of the fact that fetal distress can occur at any time in pregnancy and that it does not occur just during the labor process. **Furthermore, it has become evident in recent studies that as many as 50% of the cases of cerebral palsy are associated with a perfectly normal course of labor and delivery, implying that the fetal damage had to have occurred "silently" (i.e., unrecorded) at an earlier time in the pregnancy.** While our litigious society has placed the blame for these damaged infants upon the physician, it is entirely possible that the physician's contribution to these tragedies may be far less than previously supposed.

b. Fetal monitoring

The pioneering development of the electronic fetal monitor by Dr. Edward Hon in the 1960s, and its general acceptance by practicing physicians in the 1970s, has been a major advance in obstetrics in this century in detecting fetal distress. The monitoring of the fetal heart rate (FHR) may be accomplished by using either an *external* or an *internal* FHR electrode and a uterine pressure sensor.

The **external FHR monitoring** method involves the use of an electronic abdominal receiver, which may consist of a **phonocardiographic,** an **ultrasonographic,** or an **electrocardiographic** transducer to record the FHR. Because these external appliances could not provide a good FHR signal and variability interpretation, a computerized computation of the signal, called **autocorrelation,** was recently introduced. The uterine contractions are qualitatively evaluated by an abdominal **tocodynometer,** which senses the uterine contractions by monitoring the displacement of a pin in the transducer that is against the maternal abdomen (Fig. 37-5).

The **internal method of FHR monitoring** consists of the application of a spiral electrode to the scalp of the fetus in order to record the FHR in beats per minute (bpm) on a moving strip chart. The external tocodynometer may be used in conjunction with the internal electrode, or if more accuracy is desired, then an **intrauterine plastic catheter** may be placed in the amniotic sac to **quantitatively** record the intrauterine pressure in mm of Hg, which is then graphically recorded on the bottom of the FHR strip chart. This moving strip chart is separated into two sections: (1) a 4-cm vertical scale (25 mm Hg/cm for a total of 100 mm Hg) for the recording of the uterine contraction pressures in mm of Hg, and (2) a 6-cm vertical scale (30 bpm/cm for a total of 30–210 bpm) for the recording of the FHR in bpm. The strip chart speed that is usually utilized is 3 cm/minute.

c. Terminology

The terminology that has been accepted in fetal heart rate (FHR) monitoring involves the following terms. The **baseline FHR** is the fetal heart rate recorded over about a five-minute period in between the uterine contractions. The **periodic FHR** is the heart rate change that occurs in association with a uterine contraction (Table 37-2).

There are two main periodic FHR patterns: accelerations and decelerations. A fetus that is in good condition may exhibit no periodic changes, or **accelerations** of the fetal heart rate may occur with the movements of the fetus or with the uterine contractions. These accelerations are thought to be representative of a fetus who is in good physiologic condition.

The **decelerations** that occur on a periodic basis

TABLE 37-2. Fetal heart rate terminology

Baseline FHR changes:	
Normal	120–160 bpm
Moderate tachycardia	161–180 bpm
Marked tachycardia	> 181 bpm
Moderate bradycardia	100–119 bpm
Marked bradycardia	< 100
Periodic FHR changes:	
Accelerations	> 15 bpm
Decelerations	
Early	decreased 10–40 bpm
Late	decreased 5–60 bpm
Variable	decreased 10–60 bpm
Variability:	
Average 4–9% of baseline	
Minimal < 3% of baseline	
Marked >15% of baseline	

NB. beware of over dx due to sophisticated monitoring

incr rate of c-sections w fetal monitoring

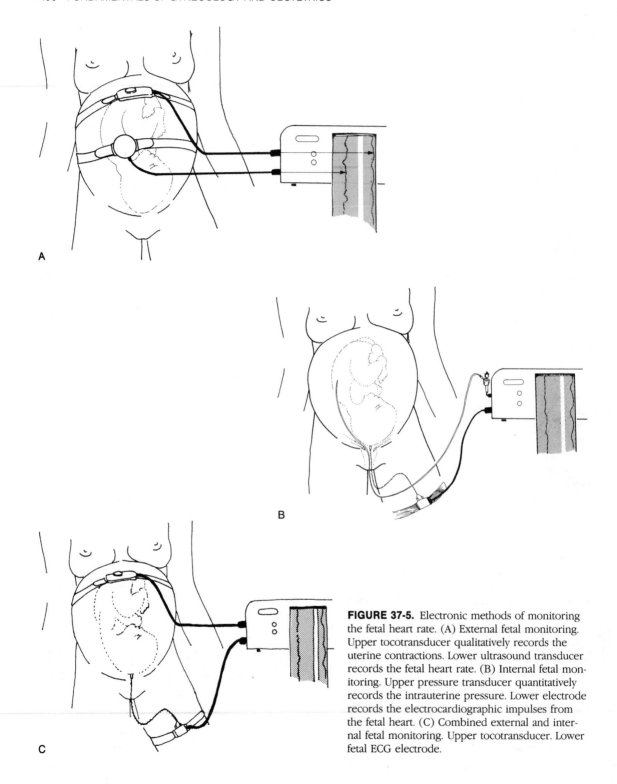

FIGURE 37-5. Electronic methods of monitoring the fetal heart rate. (A) External fetal monitoring. Upper tocotransducer qualitatively records the uterine contractions. Lower ultrasound transducer records the fetal heart rate. (B) Internal fetal monitoring. Upper pressure transducer quantitatively records the intrauterine pressure. Lower electrode records the electrocardiographic impulses from the fetal heart. (C) Combined external and internal fetal monitoring. Upper tocotransducer. Lower fetal ECG electrode.

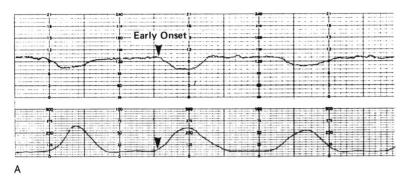

A

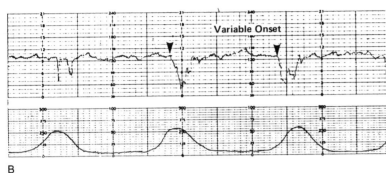

B

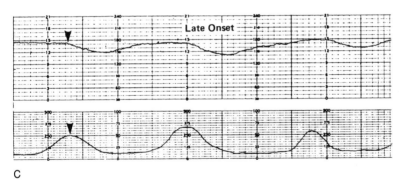

C

FIGURE 37-6. Basic periodic fetal heart rate patterns. Note the onset of the deceleration in relationship to the onset of the uterine contraction in each panel. (A) An early deceleration due to head compression. (B) A variable deceleration due to umbilical cord compression. (C) A late deceleration due to uteroplacental insufficiency.

in association with uterine contractions may be benign or may be representative of fetal distress (Fig. 37-6). **The early deceleration, or head compression pattern,** is a smooth deceleration that begins and ends at the same time as the contraction (i.e., an upside-down mirror image of the contraction). This pattern has no clinical significance and does not indicate that fetal distress is present. **A late deceleration, or the uteroplacental insufficiency pattern,** is also a smooth deceleration; however, it starts *after* the uterine contraction begins and persists *beyond* where the contraction has finished. This is the most *ominous FHR pattern,* and even when the decrease in beats per

minute is quite small, severe fetal distress should be considered to be present. **The variable deceleration, or cord compression pattern,** may have either a V-shaped, W-shaped, or squared-off U-shaped appearance (Fig. 37-7). The onset may occur at any time in relation to the uterine contraction (i.e., variable onset), but it is **always abrupt in onset and abrupt in its return to the baseline.** This is the *most common* type of deceleration pattern and it has been shown to be due to compression of the umbilical cord. If this pattern is persistent and severe, the fetus may be severely compromised. The replacement of the amniotic fluid (i.e., amnioinfusion) with 400–

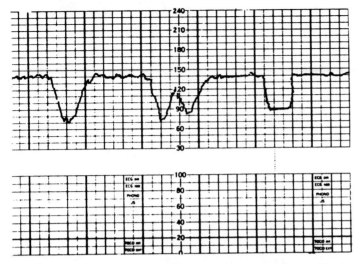

FIGURE 37-7. The tracing shows three different forms of a variable deceleration. From left to right: A V-shaped form that is often seen in premature infants; a W-shaped form; and a square-wave form. The latter two wave forms are most commonly seen.

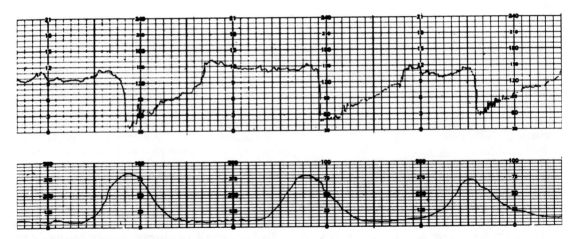

FIGURE 37-8. Variable decelerations with late recovery.

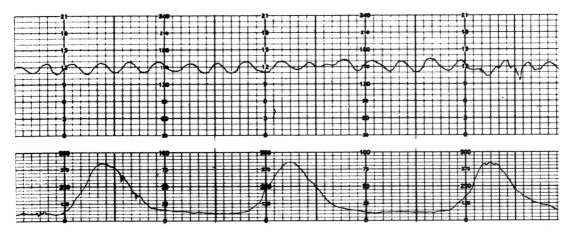

FIGURE 37-9. Sinusoidal fetal heart rate pattern.

800 ml of saline may eliminate this pattern in some patients who have oligohydramnios; however, the amount of infusion should be monitored carefully. **The presence of a nuchal cord may be identified antepartum or during early labor by the manual compression of the fetal neck area while monitoring the fetal heart rate.** (Note: either an acceleration or variable deceleration may occur if a nuchal cord is present.) A nuchal cord may also be identified on an ultrasonogram. Umbilical cord compression may be present in as many as 25–30% of laboring patients. **A combined pattern (i.e., a combined variable deceleration with a late deceleration; variable with late recovery; or late variables)** usually begins with an abrupt onset as with the variable deceleration, but instead of returning to the baseline abruptly, it returns very slowly and extends beyond the time of the uterine contraction like that of a late deceleration. This pattern is indicative of increased fetal distress, and it usually begins to replace the variable deceleration pattern after the latter has persisted for a long period of time (Fig. 37-8). The **sinusoidal pattern** is a rolling, somewhat smooth, undulating baseline that has been described in severely anemic fetuses (e.g., due to Rh disease, abruptio placentae, or fetomaternal transfusion) (Fig. 37-9). In addition, fetal hypoxia, acidosis, and chorioamnionitis have been associated with this pattern. **The criteria** that have been suggested to define a sinusoidal pattern are as follows: (1) the baseline should be stable at 120–160 bpm with regular oscillations at 2–5 cycles per minute and of a 5–15 bpm

amplitude, and (2) there should be no areas of normal baseline variability present. When these criteria are present, the fetus is usually in serious difficulty. In some cases, however, the administration of alphaprodine hydrochloride (Nisentil), or even meperidine hydrochloride (Demerol), has been associated with this pattern without any ill effects being noted in the fetus. Butorphanol tartrate (Stadol) administration has also been associated with a benign sinusoidal rhythm pattern.

The baseline variability, consisting of a rolling slow wave (3–5 per minute) with a superimposed fast wave (140 per minute), has been attributed to the interaction of the sympathetic and parasympathetic autonomic nervous systems in controlling the normal fetal heart rate. A loss of this control, with a flattening and smoothing of the FHR baseline, has been considered to be indicative of possible fetal compromise (Fig. 37-10). **There are several factors, however, that will cause a decrease in the baseline variability: (1) prematurity, (2) a fetus who is asleep, (3) the administration of sedative medications, such as meperidine hydrochloride, barbiturates, and phenothiazines, and (4) severe hypoxic fetal distress.**

On occasion, **fetal rhythm disturbances may occur in utero.** The presence of maternal fever may result in fetal tachycardia. Rarely, a fetal supraventricular tachycardia may be noted. Fetal bradycardia may occur as the result of a fetal heart block, which may be due to a viral infection, a congenital heart defect, or may be secondary to maternal lupus erythematosus.

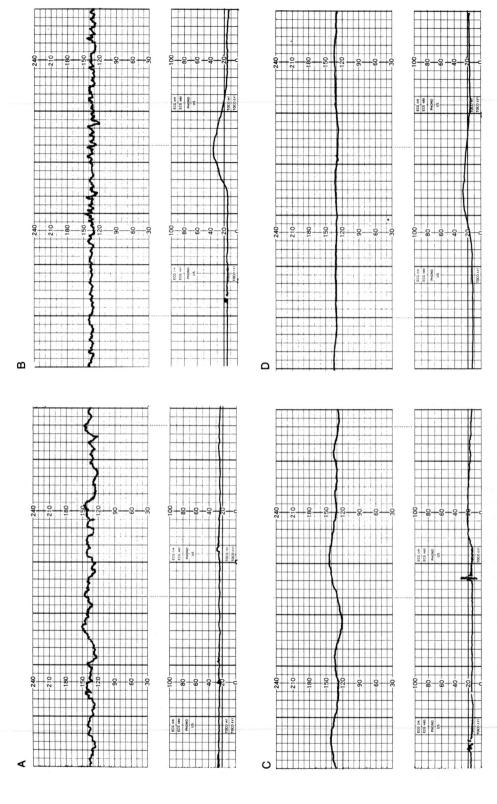

FIGURE 37-10. Baseline variability. (A) Normal baseline variability. (B) Decreased long-term variability. (C) Decreased short-term variability. (D) Absent variability.

494

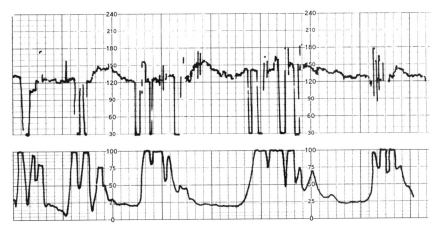

FIGURE 37-11. Fetal cardiac arrest episodes. Note the abrupt drop of the FHR to the baseline and the immediate return (i.e., cardiac arrest episodes).

While fetal cardiac arrhythmia is generally benign, close pediatric observation during the first few days of life should be carried out. *Sinus arrest episodes* in the fetus during labor may have significance for the immediate neonatal period, and the infant should be closely monitored in an effort to try to prevent a crib death. **Episodes of fetal cardiac asystole** may occur in association with the descending limb of a variable deceleration (type 1), or in association with a preceding severe late or variable deceleration, and are usually associated with an absent baseline variability (type 2). In my experience, these cardiac arrest episodes have also been seen in patients with mild variable decelerations, and they do not always seem to be associated with the downward limb of a variable deceleration. In one infant who had had a number of brief sinus arrest episodes prior to delivery, the newborn decompensated in the nursery about 32 hours after delivery and later showed evidence of severe brain damage (Fig. 37-11). In another case, an infant who had occasional sinus arrest episodes during labor suddenly died in the nursery on the third day postpartum. The Apgar scores of both of these infants at delivery were normal. It has been suggested that the type 1 sinus arrest episodes are due to an **over-reactive vagal response,** whereas the type 2 episodes are probably due to **asphyxial damage to the cardiac control centers.** In both of the above-mentioned cases, the mechanism involved was probably an over-reactive vagal response.

Complications that have been attributed to the use of electronic monitoring of the FHR are trauma to the fetal scalp (secondary to the electrode), perforation of the uterus by the intrauterine catheter, and an increased incidence of intrauterine infection; however, these problems have been relatively uncommon, and when they do appear, they are usually not severe.

d. Fetal scalp blood sampling

In some clinical situations, it is of value to assess the pH of the fetal scalp blood. This is particularly true in the patient who develops a cord compression pattern (i.e., variable decelerations) late in labor. Since this pattern may at times be tolerated for quite a while without unduly endangering the fetus, it is important to determine the level of the fetal blood pH in such a patient. A pH value above 7.25 is normal, whereas a pH of between 7.25 and 7.20 is borderline. When the pH value falls below 7.20, then it is considered to be abnormal and represents acidosis. The fetal pO_2, pCO_2, and the base excess can also be determined. The pO_2 value of the fetal scalp blood is about 28–33 mm Hg. In one study, there was a 98% correlation between the scalp blood pH and the base excess, and the health and status of the fetus.

The technique of fetal scalp blood sampling consists of first visualizing the fetal scalp through an amnioscope (Fig. 37-12). The scalp is wiped clean of mucus and a silicon-soaked swab is then applied to the fetal scalp to assist in the formation of the bead of blood. A special lancet with a 2-mm blade is then

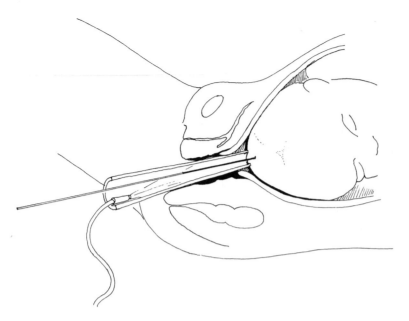

FIGURE 37-12. Fetal scalp blood sampling.

used to stab an incision in the scalp. The bead of blood is then drawn up into a heparinized glass capillary tube. An iron flea may be added to the capillary tube for mixing purposes, the tube sealed at each end, and the specimen immediately analyzed on a blood-gas-acid-base machine. The scalp blood sampling technique may be used in other clinical situations, such as idiopathic thrombocytopenic purpura (ITP), where a blood smear and a platelet count may be of value.

The main complication that has been attributed to fetal scalp blood sampling procedure has been fetal hemorrhage. A dry cotton swab should be applied to the sampling site throughout the period of one contraction in order to prevent undue bleeding; however, on occasion a bleeding diathesis in the fetus has resulted in a severe hemorrhage.

e. Management

Whenever periodic FHR decelerations occur, they should be identified as to their type and severity. **The immediate treatment of periodic FHR decelerations (other than early decelerations, which are benign) consists of: (1) the administration of oxygen at 6 l/min, (2) the movement of the patient to one side or another (in order to move the uterus off of the inferior vena cava or the fetus off of the umbilical cord), and (3) the discontinuance of an oxytocin drip.** The maternal blood pressure should be checked immediately. If there are variable decelerations and the membranes have just ruptured, then an immediate sterile vaginal examination should be performed to detect a possible prolapsed umbilical cord. The continued observation of an ominous FHR pattern, such as late decelerations, should not exceed about 30 minutes, and if they cannot be corrected with the above maneuvers within this time, then a cesarean section should probably be performed in most cases.

If the fetal scalp blood pH is less than 7.20, the procedure should be immediately repeated. If the second specimen reveals a similar value, and the mother's blood pH is normal, then delivery should be carried out immediately. If, on the other hand, the pH values on repeated sampling remain above 7.20, then continued observation of the course of labor may be safely carried out.

Any infant who has manifested evidence of fetal distress, either on the electronic fetal monitor or on fetal scalp sampling during labor, should have a cord blood pH and blood gases obtained at the time of delivery to validate the fetal status. The **normal umbilical artery values** should be as follows: pH = >7.25; base deficit = 0–10; pO_2 = 18 torr; and pCO_2 = 40–48 torr. The **normal umbilical vein**

values are: pH = 7.35; base deficit = 0–5; pO_2 = 28–30 torr; and pCO_2 = 38 torr.

The range of values in **severe respiratory acidosis for the umbilical artery** are: pH = 6.8–7.0; base deficit = 15–25; pCO_2 = 60–120 torr. The range of values in **severe respiratory acidosis for the umbilical vein** are: pH = 6.8–7.15; base deficit = 10–25; and pCO_2 = 40–50 torr.

The range of values in **severe metabolic acidosis for the umbilical artery** are: pH = 6.8–7.0; base deficit = 15–25; and pCO_2 = 45–55 torr. The range of values in **severe metabolic acidosis for the umbilical vein** are: pH = 6.8–7.0; base deficit = 15–25; and pCO_2 = 40–50 torr.

7. Multiple gestation

a. Incidence

The incidence of twinning is 1:79 in the black race, 1:100 in the caucasian race in the United States, and 1:155 in Japan. The occurrence of twinning is due most commonly to the fertilization of two separate ova (i.e., dizygotic, or fraternal twins), with only about one-third of twinning (i.e., 1:250 births) being due to the fertilization of only one egg (i.e., monozygotic, or identical twins). The occurrence of triplets or quadruplets occurs in a similar manner. While the incidence of dizygotic twinning increases with maternal age and parity, monozygotic twinning remains relatively constant. *As the number of fetuses increase in a pregnancy, the sex ratio changes and begins to favor the female.* In the United States, the percentage of females in all singleton fetuses is 48.41%, in twins it is 49.15%, in triplets 50.46%, and in quadruplets 53.52%.

b. Types of twinning

Dizygotic twinning is the fertilization of two separate ova during an ovulatory cycle, whereas monozygotic twinning is the fertilization of one ova and then a later division of that zygote into two or more separate individuals. In monozygotic twinning, if the division occurs during the *first three days,* then two embryos, two amnions, and two chorions will develop **(i.e., diamniotic, dichorionic)** (Fig. 37-13). If the division does not occur until the fourth through the eighth day, then only one chorion will be present **(i.e., diamniotic, monochorionic).**

Shortly after eight days, only one amniotic sac will be present, and the monozygotic twins will be contained in a **monoamniotic monochorionic sac.** Should the division of the zygote occur even later, then the fetuses will be connected as *conjoined twins* **(i.e., Siamese twins). The determination of the number of layers of the amnion and of the chorion between the fetuses at birth will detect the type of zygosity in more than half of the cases of multiple gestation.** The correlation of the major blood groups will usually confirm monozygosity; however, in difficult cases, tissue antigen typing may be necessary.

At times, there may be vascular anastomosis between the monozygotic fetuses. If the arteriovenous connections are extensive, one fetus may receive more blood than the other **(twin-twin transfusion syndrome),** which may result in hypervolemia, polycythemia, cardiac failure, and increased urine output (i.e., hydramnios). Rarely, one fetus may be reduced to a malformed monster or "homunculus."

Superfetation is the occurrence of two fertilizations in two separate ovulatory cycles. This phenomenon has not been demonstrated in humans, but has been seen in the mare. **Superfecundation,** on the other hand, is the occurrence of two separate fertilizations within one ovulatory cycle, but at two different coital episodes. This has been demonstrated in humans—in one case, a black man and a white man supposedly fathered a set of twins, of which one was white and the other a mulatto.

Twinning seems to have a hereditary component, with the maternal genotype being more important in this determination than the father's genotype. With advancing age and parity, twinning seems to increase up to the age of 40, and up to a parity of seven. The use of the ovulation inducing agent clomiphene citrate in infertility patients has been associated with an increased incidence of twinning. Human menopausal gonadotropin therapy in infertility patients also increases the incidence of multiple pregnancies (three or more fetuses) up to 20–40%. The increased numbers of fetuses in patients who undergo in-vitro fertilization and embryo transplant are due to the deposition of more than one blastocyst into the uterine cavity in an effort to improve the conception success rate. In cases where infertility patients conceive an excessive number of fetuses (e.g., 5 or more), selective fetal destruction has recently been advocated in order to provide a better

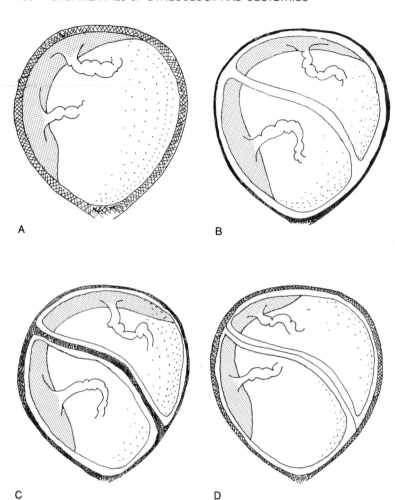

FIGURE 37-13. The placenta and membranes in twin pregnancies. (A) Monochorionic, monoamniotic, and one placenta occurs when the cleavage of the zygote occurs after the 8th day. (B) If the cleavage of the zygote occurs between the 4th and 8th days, after the chorionic cells have been defined, the two amniotic sacs will be covered by a single chorion; monochorionic, diamniotic. (C) If the division of the zygote occurs within 72 hours, then both amnions and chorions will develop; dichorionic, diamniotic. (D) If the membranes of two twins, who are dizygotic, fuse, then they may appear to be identical twins at birth.

environment and salvage rate for the remaining fetuses.

c. Diagnosis

The diagnosis of multiple gestation should be suspected when the fundal measurements do not match the number of weeks of gestation in early pregnancy. The differential diagnoses that should be entertained in such cases, when the uterus is obviously larger than the dates would suggest, are: (1) incorrect dates, (2) hydatidiform mole, (3) multiple gestation, (4) myomatous uterus, (5) a large adnexal mass, and (6) hydramnios.

Leopold's maneuvers should always be carried out in the more advanced pregnancies in an attempt to identify the fetal lie. In the case of multiple fetuses, it is frequently difficult to separate two or more fetuses in the second trimester; however, during the third trimester, this becomes increasingly easier to do, unless the patient is quite obese. The detection of two or more fetal heart rates by either a Doppler ultrasonic unit or by a fetoscope may be possible beyond 18 weeks' gestation, but the physician should be sure that the rates are clearly different. *Ultrasonography will easily identify two fetuses, but when more fetuses than that are present, then this determination becomes more difficult, due to the confusion of the fetal parts.* If more than four fetuses are suspected to be present, it may be necessary to obtain an abdominal X-ray. This approach should be delayed until well beyond the 18th to the 20th week of gestation, since the fetal skeletons may not be sufficiently opaque prior to this time. An amniogram will define the presence of monoamniotic twinning, since the placement of radiopaque dye into one twin's amniotic sac will show whether both of the fetuses lie within a common sac. The persistence of a fixed relationship between the two fetuses (e.g., face-to-face) over a period of time should suggest the possibility of conjoined twins.

d. Management

The presence of multiple fetuses may be associated with a number of complications, such as preeclampsia, premature rupture of the membranes, premature delivery, hydramnios, and abruptio placentae. Early spontaneous abortion is probably quite common in multiple pregnancies, and in addition, the death and absorption of just one fetus during pregnancy may occur **(i.e., vanishing twin).** In one instance, a patient who passed an intact fetus and placenta at about three months, who had a closed cervix and no further bleeding, was allowed to go to term and delivered a viable second twin. In the rare instance of monoamniotic twinning, as many as 30–50% of cases involve a fetal death due to umbilical cord entanglement. **The overall perinatal mortality rate for twins in the United States is about 10–15%, with the fetal loss being due not only to prematurity, but also to congenital abnormalities, which are doubled in twins.**

1) Premature delivery

Although singleton pregnancies tend to deliver at between 38 and 42 weeks' gestation, twins seem to deliver on the average at about 36.5–37.5 weeks, while triplets seem to deliver at about 35 weeks. However, *premature delivery* may occur at a much earlier time in multiple gestation, unless the patient makes a concerted effort to obtain as much rest as possible. More than 50% of the morbidity and mortality that occurs in twins takes place in the 10% of patients who deliver prior to 30 weeks' gestation. Prolonged bedrest during the third trimester, either at home or in the hospital, has been found to be effective in preventing premature delivery and low–birth weight infants. In addition, bedrest also seems to be effective in preventing *toxemia,* which occurs more frequently in these

patients. The patient should be monitored closely between 20 and 32 weeks' gestation for cervical changes and premature uterine contractions, and the maternal work habits should be carefully evaluated. In addition, the growth rate of the twin fetuses should be evaluated ultrasonically every 2–4 weeks beginning at about the 30th week. Nonstress testing should be carried out weekly from the 32nd week onward. If a nonreactive nonstress test should occur, a biophysical profile may be performed to further assess the fetus.

Premature labor may be treated with tocolytics, however, there is conflicting data in the literature as to the effectiveness of these agents in multiple gestation. Electronic fetal monitoring of both fetuses should be performed during labor by placing a spiral electrode on the first twin and an external Doppler transducer on the second twin.

2) Nutritional needs

Since there are additional nutritional needs in a multiple pregnancy, the mother's diet should be supplemented by 300 Kcal per day over and above the requirements of a normal pregnancy, with an adequate increase in protein. The maternal weight gain should consist of at least enough weight to account for the additional fetal weight, as follows: a normal weight gain to include (1) uterus, 2.5 lbs; (2) blood volume, 3.5 lbs; (3) edema, 3 lbs; (4) breasts, 2 lbs; (5) amniotic fluid, 2 lbs; (6) fetus, 7.5 lbs; and (7) placenta, 1.5 lbs; for a total of 22 lbs. In addition, (8) a second fetus, 7.5 lbs; (9) amniotic fluid, 2 lbs; and (10) placenta, 1.5 lbs; which adds up to a grand total of 33 lbs. Iron supplementation will be necessary, since anemia is more common in patients with multiple fetuses.

3) Labor and delivery

The labor and delivery process poses a number of problems in patients with multiple gestations. The position of the fetuses, uterine dysfunction, cord prolapse, supine hypotensive syndrome, abruptio placentae, premature labor, and postpartum hemorrhage are important considerations. **The fetal mortality rate in twin gestations ranges between 4–33%, with the second twin usually being at a greater risk. The risk of a second twin dying is 1.5–2.5 times greater than the risk to the first twin if the second twin is premature, small for gestational age,**

or has an abnormal presentation. In addition, following the delivery of the first twin, there may be a degree of hypoxia in the second twin secondary to an abnormal presentation, an unrecognized umbilical cord compression, or a minor occult abruptio placentae. In some series, an intracranial hemorrhage may occur in the premature infant due to birth trauma.

If the second twin's position is a complete or footling breech and the head is flexed with intact membranes, then an external cephalic version should be attempted with a subsequent vaginal delivery of a vertex presentation. If the membranes are ruptured, then a complete breech extraction may be effective in delivering the fetus, but this should only be attempted by an experienced physician, since the risk of uterine rupture is high in inexperienced hands. If either of these approaches is unsuccessful or not feasible, then a cesarean section is indicated. Keep in mind that if the second twin's position is breech and the head is hyperextended, then a vaginal delivery is contraindicated and a cesarean section should be performed.

If the second twin is mature, with a fetal weight of at least 2,000 grams, then the risk of perinatal mortality should be the same as for the first twin, and the outcome should not be related to the method of delivery (i.e., vaginal delivery or cesarean section).

In the preparation for the delivery of a patient with twins, 1,000 ml of blood should be typed and crossmatched, a large-bore intravenous catheter should be secured, electronic fetal monitoring should be applied to each twin, and adequate anesthesia support and obstetric attendants should be made available. Since there are two infants in a twin gestation, there should be two physicians available for the delivery and two pediatric attendants available for the possible resuscitation of the infants, especially if they are quite premature.

Each combination of fetal positions in multiple gestations must be evaluated on their own merits in deciding whether a vaginal delivery or a cesarean section will be necessary. A vertex/vertex presentation can usually be delivered vaginally. If the first twin presents as a breech and the second twin as a vertex, the possibility that the chin of the first twin may lock onto the chin of the second twin **(i.e., locked twins)** during delivery must be considered. In some instances, the first twin breech may not fill the pelvis completely (i.e., complete and incomplete breeches), and with the rupture of the membranes, the umbilical cord may prolapse into the vagina. Usually, after the

first twin has been delivered, the second twin will need to be guided into the pelvis before the membranes are ruptured. At times, the membranes will rupture prematurely on the second twin in a transverse lie, requiring that an experienced physician be available to perform an **internal podalic version,** which is performed by grasping the legs of the second twin, and then carrying out a full breech extraction. Adequate anesthesia (i.e., general) should be utilized for such a procedure. In some cases, the first twin may be delivered vaginally, but due to adverse circumstances, fetal distress, or lack of experienced personnel, the second twin may need to be delivered by cesarean section.

Recently, there has been an increase in the use of cesarean section in multiple gestations in which one or both fetuses are not in a vertex position. This approach has been prompted by the need to perform a delivery that is as atraumatic as possible, on a fetus that is generally premature by dates and by size, so as to avoid any unnecessary morbidity and mortality. Due to the increased positional complications that are associated with triplets or quadruplets, cesarean section is often recommended in these cases.

8. Fetal death

The incidence of intrauterine fetal death (i.e., stillbirth) is about 7.9:1,000 live births. The death of a fetus early in pregnancy is usually not too difficult to recognize. Usually, the uterus fails to enlarge appropriately over a period of several weeks. An ultrasonogram may detect a *low-lying distorted gestational sac;* however, this evidence is only suggestive of fetal death. Failure to detect the fetal heart activity by seven weeks' gestation or later will assist in confirming the diagnosis. The presence of human chorionic gonadotropin and a positive pregnancy test will merely confirm the continued functioning of the placenta, which does not require the presence of a living fetus.

Fetal death after the first trimester is usually preceded clinically by a cessation of fetal movements, a slight loss of weight, and a change in the breasts (i.e., decreased volume, and occasionally milk letdown). A real-time ultrasonogram will easily detect the *absence of fetal heart action* and confirm the diagnosis.

Roentgenographic signs of fetal death are: (1) the overlapping of the fetal skull bones (Spalding's sign),

(2) the exaggerated curvature of the fetal spine, or an odd or unnatural position of the fetus, and (3) the presence of intravascular gas in the fetus (Robertson's sign).

The management of a fetal death beyond the first trimester may consist of either watchful expectancy or active intervention. While many patients deliver spontaneously within 2–3 weeks of a fetal death, the active evacuation of the uterus is frequently elected due to the maternal emotional and psychological burden of carrying a dead fetus. About 10–25% of these patients will develop disseminated intravascular coagulation (DIC) about five weeks after the fetal demise, so the blood fibrinogen levels, the prothrombin time, and the partial thromboplastin time should be periodically monitored until delivery.

In many instances, the fetal death is unexplained (50%). In addition to the autopsy findings, total body X-rays of the fetus may provide additional information. *If chromosomal studies are to be performed on the dead fetus, a sample of the fascia lata femoris on the lateral aspect of the thigh should be obtained and placed in either Hanks' solution or in normal saline prior to being transported to the cytogenetics laboratory.*

9. Premature labor

a. Etiology

Premature labor is defined as the onset of labor before 38 weeks' gestation. The cause of premature labor is often unknown; however, the following conditions have been implicated: (1) distension of the uterus by hydramnios or multiple gestation, (2) spontaneous rupture of the membranes, (3) uterine abnormalities, such as a uterine septum or a bicornuate uterus, (4) the presence of severe fetal anomalies, (5) abnormal placentation, such as placenta previa or abruptio placentae, and (6) a history of a previous premature delivery.

b. Diagnosis

Premature labor may be difficult to differentiate from false labor. Since early intervention is necessary if tocolysis is to be effective, treatment should begin when there are moderately strong contractions at less than 10-minute intervals. It is most important to be certain that the labor should be inhibited before this ap-

proach is taken, since in some situations, the intrauterine environment may be so hostile that the extrauterine environment may be infinitely better. On the other hand, in many cases the fetus may benefit much more by remaining in the uterus for an additional amount of time so that it has the opportunity to become more mature.

c. Treatment

There are a number of treatment regimens that have been recommended to inhibit premature labor contractions. *Bedrest,* in the left lateral decubitus position, and *hydration* are commonly utilized.

The use of beta-adrenergic receptor stimulants (or agonists) have been perhaps the most popular labor-inhibiting agents. There are two types of beta-adrenergic receptors: beta-1 and beta-2. The beta-1 receptors are primarily found in the heart and intestines, whereas the beta-2 receptors are found in the blood vessels, bronchioles, and the myometrium.

Compounds similar to epinephrine are therefore often utilized to inhibit myometrial contractions. Ritodrine hydrochloride, terbutaline sulfate, and isoxsuprine hydrochloride have been the most commonly used tocolytic agents in this country. Recently, magnesium sulfate and diazoxide have gained attention as tocolytic agents.

Isoxsuprine hydrochloride was initially used; however, its effectiveness was counterbalanced by the adverse side effects of hypotension and tachycardia. **Terbutaline sulfate** (Brethine) has also been used with some success, but carries a possible side effect of pulmonary edema. It has had the same success rate in stopping contractions as has been reported for ritodrine. **Ritodrine hydrochloride** (Yutopar) has become the most popular tocolytic agent in the United States today (and the only one that is approved by the FDA); however, it carries a risk of several serious side effects, such as hypotension, tachycardia, pulmonary edema, and even death. Hypokalemia, hyperglycemia, and ketoacidosis may also occur. If glucocorticoids are concomitantly administered along with terbutaline or ritodrine to assist in the maturation of the fetal lungs, the occurrence of pulmonary edema seems to be more common.

The use of **magnesium sulfate** as a tocolytic agent has been successful, with the initial results being similar to those that have been obtained with terbutaline or ritodrine therapy. (Note: Magnesium sulfate should not be used in patients with myasthenia gravis). The patient should be placed in a left lateral decubitus position, hydrated (400 ml over 2 hours), and given magnesium sulfate, 6 grams I.V. over 15 minutes, followed by an infusion of magnesium sulfate at 3 grams/hour. Serum magnesium levels should be obtained every six hours and should be maintained at a level between 5.5–7.5 mg/dl. The intravenous fluids should be limited to 3,500 ml/day. This agent has gained considerable popularity because its widespread use as a treatment of PIH has made it a more familiar medication to most physicians.

A recent study has indicated that the use of **diazoxide** at a rate of no more than 5 mg/kg I.V. over 15 minutes will stop uterine contractions in almost all patients. In this study, it was postulated that it is possible to determine whether the underlying stimulus for labor is increasing or decreasing by giving two successive infusions of diazoxide. If the contractions recur and the second dose inhibits the contractions for a longer time than the first dose, then the gestation will be prolonged for over 72 hours in most cases. If the inhibition of contractions on the second infusion is less than that of the first infusion, then 60% of the patients will deliver within 24 hours. The patients in this study were placed in a left lateral decubitus position and were given 500 ml of normal saline or Ringer's lactate. The patients were then given 5 mg/kg of diazoxide, for a total dose of 300 mg delivered over 15–20 minutes in most patients. If the contractions recurred, a second 300-mg dose was administered. The side effects consisted of a transient decrease in both systolic and diastolic pressures and an increase in the heart rate. Dizziness, nausea, and headache may occur with the rapid administration of the drug. This drug has not been approved as a tocolytic agent by the FDA.

A delay in the delivery of the fetus for about 72 hours may be expected to occur in 80% of patients treated with any of these agents. In patients who are at less than 34 weeks' gestation, the administration of **corticoids** has been recommended in an effort to decrease the incidence of the neonatal respiratory distress syndrome (RDS). This regimen may be used in patients who are between 28 and 34 weeks' gestation, since outside of this gestational range, the corticoids have not been shown to be of benefit. **Black** infants and **female** infants apparently receive the less benefit from the use of corticoids. The corticoids that have been most commonly used

are betamethasone, 10 mg, or dexamethasone, 5 mg, once a day for two doses. The pulmonary maturational effect on the surfactant only occurs after about 24 hours and then lasts for only seven days. The fetal hazards of antenatal cortisone administration consist of the possible impairment of the fetus's ability to respond to an immunologic stimulus, and the possible occurrence of growth retardation in the neonatal -period. In view of the fact that cortisone has been administered to many pregnant women for a variety of diseases without any discernable damage to the fetus, it would seem that this therapy should be safe.

Recently, some studies have been published in which patients used a **contraction "guard-ring" monitor** at home, which records up to 200 minutes of uterine activity at a time. This belt-like device weighs less than 4 lbs, and the recording is transmitted via telephone lines to a central monitoring station for data interpretation. High-risk patients for premature labor who have used this device have experienced fewer preterm deliveries than those who did not use the monitor; however, it is uncertain whether it was the use of the monitor, or the extra almost daily patient contact and support by health professionals, that caused the improved results. In view of the high cost of neonatal intensive care, the use of these expensive monitors may eventually turn out to be cost-effective.

10. Premature rupture of the membranes

a. Definitions

Premature rupture of the membranes (PROM) has been defined as the rupture of the membranes at any time prior to the onset of labor; however, there is confusion regarding this definition. Since the time of membrane rupture could be anywhere from one hour prior to labor on up to several weeks or months prior to labor, I would like to suggest that PROM should be renamed **"preterm" rupture of membranes (PTROM)** when it occurs prior to 38 weeks' gestation, and reserve the term **"premature" rupture of membranes (PROM)** for the rupture of the membranes occurring after the 38th week. In addition, the use of "premature rupture of membranes" is often not distinguished from "prolonged rupture of the membranes." If the membranes have been ruptured for more than 24 hours prior to the onset of labor, then it would seem reasonable that we should add the term **"prolonged"** to the type of rupture (i.e., prolonged PTROM or prolonged PROM) to delineate this type of problem.

b. Risks of premature rupture

The primary risks involved in the premature rupture of the membranes are puerperal sepsis with fetal infection or death on the one hand, and prematurity and respiratory distress syndrome in the infant after the delivery on the other hand. It is very important for the first physician who sees the patient to be certain that the membranes are truly ruptured. This confirmation can be accomplished by a *sterile speculum examination* to detect the presence of amniotic fluid, by visualizing the fluid emanating from the cervical os, or by obtaining a positive nitrazine test of the fluid in the posterior vaginal vault. The presence of fetal squames or evidence of ferning in the amniotic fluid is also valuable information (i.e., dried amniotic fluid on a microscopic slide will show a "fern pattern"). An evaluation of the vaginal amniotic fluid for the L/S ratio, or for the presence of phosphatidylglycerol (PG), may be helpful in determining the fetal pulmonary maturity. Vaginal examinations thereafter should be interdicted, in an effort to prevent any further undue contamination.

In all patients who have evidence of premature labor or premature rupture of the membranes, a vaginal Gram stain and vaginal cultures should be obtained in an effort to detect the presence of **group B streptococci and/or Neisseria gonorrhoeae.** Since prematurity is present in more than 90% of the fetal deaths that are due to group B streptococci, ampicillin or erythromycin therapy should be instituted prior to delivery when the membranes are ruptured in an effort to prevent an infection of the fetus (see Chapters 12 and 28). If the labor is stopped by tocolysis in the patient with intact membranes, and one of these organisms is identified, antibiotic treatment should be administered and a repeat culture obtained in two weeks.

c. Management considerations

A knowledge of the fetal salvage statistics in your hospital nursery is essential in the management of cases involving preterm rupture of membranes (PTROM). In some hospitals, infants may have a very good salvage rate at 32 weeks' gesta-

tion with a comparable fetal weight, whereas in other hospitals, a similar salvage rate may not be obtained until 33–34 weeks' gestation. If the fetus is of a gestational age or weight that is not likely to result in a satisfactory outcome, then observation should be carried out until a greater degree of maturity can be obtained or until you are forced to deliver the patient because of chorioamnionitis or spontaneous labor. Close evaluation of the maternal temperature, the white count, and in some instances, an evaluation of the amniotic fluid for the presence of bacteria, should be carried out. **In patients who develop signs of uterine infection, prompt delivery should be performed.**

One study using the **fetal biophysical profile** every 1–2 days to determine the presence of infection after PROM noted that in those patients who had a biophysical profile score of 8 or more, the incidence of infection (maternal/neonatal) was 2.7%. If the score was less than 7, the infection rate was 93.7%. Those patients who had the smallest amount of amniotic fluid (less than 1 cm in a vertical diameter) had the highest incidence of amnionitis (47.3%), suspected neonatal sepsis (26.3%), and proven neonatal sepsis (31.5%). **In those patients who had a reactive NST initially that became nonreactive later, there was a 90% infection rate.** The fetal breathing movements had a negative predictive value for the presence of infection (95.3%).

In one study, in patients who had prolonged PTROM prior to 26 weeks' gestation that lasted for more than 5 weeks, 46% of the fetuses developed pulmonary hypoplasia and/or skeletal anomalies. In those who had prolonged PTROM between 26 and 32 weeks' gestation, only 10% of the fetuses were affected. If prolonged PTROM occurred after 32 weeks' gestation, then there was no risk for the development of either of these entities.

In one recent study of 70 singleton pregnancies with preterm rupture of the membranes between weeks 20 and 27, who were followed conservatively, 58.6% developed chorioamnionitis and 33.6% of the mothers had other postpartum complications. **Of 17 infants in this study who were included in long-term follow-up observations, only 5 (29.4%) were physically and mentally normal at six months of age.** While there have been some dramatic changes in the intensive care of immature and premature infants in recent years, the results have often been disappointing, as was shown in this study.

d. Delivery

If the patient's gestation is sufficiently mature to warrant delivery, and if the infant is in the vertex position, then an oxytocin induction of labor should be performed. If the fetus is in a footling breech presentation or in a transverse lie, cesarean section should be performed. In some studies, it has been shown that if the membranes have been ruptured for more than 24 hours, the incidence of fetal respiratory distress syndrome appears to be much less common than if the fetus delivers before 24 hours. **A similar acceleration of surfactant production has been demonstrated in patients who have pregnancy-induced hypertension (PIH), heroin addiction, sickle cell anemia, hyperthyroidism, and amnionitis.**

11. Premature delivery

A premature fetus is one that has been delivered before 38 weeks' gestation. The majority of fetal problems occur in the premature infant secondary to the immaturity of one or more organ systems. Brown fat accumulates during the last few weeks of pregnancy; since the premature infant lacks this type of adipose tissue, it consequently is more susceptible to *cold stress*. Due to the immaturity of the gastrointestinal tract in the premature infant, additional supplementation of calories and nutrients is often needed. The excretion of bilirubin is hindered by the lack of maturity in the liver enzymes, and the resulting jaundice in the neonatal period may cause damage to the infant's brain if this problem goes untreated.

Great care should be exercised during the labor of a premature infant to avoid excessive sedation or hypotensive episodes due to regional anesthesia. The delivery should be as atraumatic as possible, with the careful, slow delivery of the fetal head across an adequate episiotomy so as to minimize any rapid expansion of the fetal skull. The infant should be handled gently, suctioned carefully, and prevented from developing undue hypothermia. If possible, pediatric assistance should be present in the delivery room.

a. Respiratory distress syndrome

Probably the most common and perhaps the most dreaded immediate complication that the premature infant must face is the respiratory distress syndrome (RDS). While extrauterine survival is possible at 25 weeks' gestation when the lung tissue becomes anatomically mature, it is only after **26–28 weeks** that the pulmonary vascular network becomes sufficiently mature to support adequate extrauterine respiration.

The biochemical functioning of the lung involves the development of **type II pneumocytes,** which secrete surfactant material that assists in maintaining the surface tension of the alveoli during respiration. Some of these cells are present as early as 20 weeks' gestation. Minimal to moderate secretion is present after 28 weeks; however, at about 34–35 weeks' gestation, there is a dramatic increase in the active secretion of surfactant.

About 85% of the surfactant is phospholipid, with lecithin (phosphatidylcholine) being the principal type. Its function is to prevent the collapse of the alveolar sac with each expiration. In its absence, the alveoli will collapse with each breath, making reexpansion difficult with each succeeding respiration. As a consequence, atelectasis occurs with poor gas exchange, leading to a progressive asphyxia and the development of respiratory distress syndrome.

The lecithin that is secreted by the type II pneumocytes is released into the alveolar sacs of the in-utero fetal lung and is carried into the amniotic fluid. The classic studies of **Dr. L. Gluck and colleagues** in 1971 described for the first time the relationship of the amniotic fluid lecithin:sphingomyelin ratio to the amount of fetal surfactant present and the risk of developing the respiratory distress syndrome (RDS). The lecithin can be measured against another rather constant phospholipid, sphingomyelin, which serves as a baseline reference. The value of the lecithin:sphingomyelin (L/S) ratio is generally greater than 2:1 when the fetus is mature. Another phospholipid, phosphatidylglycerol (PG), in the amniotic fluid is quite significant, since its presence signifies that the lecithin has been stabilized and that RDS is unlikely to occur.

There are a number of factors that may stimulate or inhibit the secretion of lecithin, which influences the functional maturity of the fetal lungs. **Those factors that seem to accelerate lung maturity and surfactant production include heroin addiction, prolonged rupture of the membranes, labor, and placental insufficiency. Those that inhibit lung maturation include fetal distress, acidosis, twinning, hemorrhagic accidents of pregnancy, and uncontrolled diabetes mellitus.** It is important that the fetus be delivered with a minimum of birth trauma, asphyxia, or cold stress, since these conditions may result in a loss of surfactant production.

b. Hazards of prematurity

A number of other complications may occur in the premature fetus in association with RDS. **They include pneumothorax, pneumomediastinum, pneumopericardium, and bronchopulmonary dysplasia.** These problems stem from pulmonary air leaks, which often occur as a result of the resuscitative efforts at the time of delivery and may lead to fetal death.

The initial breaths by the infant cause an increase in the pO_2, which, along with the loss of the prostaglandin effect, will result in the functional closure of the ductus arteriosus. Blood is thereby diverted to the rapidly expanding low resistance pulmonary circuit, which has also responded to the elevated oxygen tension by decreasing the pulmonary vascular resistance. With the clamping of the umbilical cord, the peripheral systemic vascular resistance increases and the foramen ovale between the two atria functionally closes, which then allows each of the two ventricles to pump equal amounts of blood. If all of the above events occur in an appropriate manner, then there is an orderly transition between the in-utero *placental* respiratory system to that of the neonatal *pulmonary* respiratory system.

In the premature infant who has RDS, asphyxia, or meconium aspiration, **pulmonary hypertension** may develop, in which case the blood will be diverted away from the pulmonary circuit. **Due to the low pO_2, the ductus arteriosus again opens up and begins to shunt blood away from the pulmonary circuit.** This process leads to even greater hypoxia and even more pulmonary hypertension, resulting in a vicious circle of "hypoxia—decreased pulmonary blood flow—further hypoxia—," which has been called the **"persistent fetal circulation" syndrome, or the "pulmonary hypertension syndrome."** Furthermore, this shift in the volume of blood into the systemic circulation may lead to cardiac failure. Persistent pulmonary hypertension may be due to: (1) hypoxia, (2) excessive muscularization of the pulmonary vessels, secondary to congenital heart defects, and (3) the underdevelopment of the pulmonary vascular bed, due to pulmonary hypoplasia.

Prematurity also poses **growth and developmental** hazards to the infant. These infants are subject to chronic interrelated disorders of the central nervous system, including cerebral palsy, mental retardation, sensory loss (e.g., hearing and sight), cerebral dysfunction (e.g., learning and language disorders), hyperactivity, and behavioral problems.

Cerebral palsy is a disorder that involves the movement and the posture of the individual resulting from damage to the basal ganglia (extrapyramidal system) in the deeper portion of the cerebrum. Severe hypoxia in the *term infant* (at more than 35 weeks' gestation) affects primarily the superficial areas of the cerebral cortex and may result in mental retardation, but it does not usually involve the basal ganglia. In the premature infant, however, severe hypoxic damage may extend from the cerebral cortex to the deeper basal ganglia and cause cerebral palsy with superimposed cortical manifestations of mental retardation, epilepsy, and psychopathy. Therefore, according to one study, the occurrence of cerebral palsy in a *term infant* should not be attributed to the hypoxic events that occurred at the time of labor and delivery, but rather, should be assigned to events that occurred weeks or months before the onset of labor.

The most common type of cerebral palsy is that of **spastic diplegia,** which involves primarily the lower extremities; however, it may consist of spastic quadriplegia and athetosis. Cerebral palsy occurs in 6–24% of infants who have a birth weight of 750–800 grams, and is primarily a disease of prematurity.

Mental retardation (i.e., I.Q. of less than 70) may occur in premature children, and as many as 13–28% of these children have a borderline intelligence (i.e., I.Q. between 70 and 80). The various degrees of mental retardation below an I.Q. of 70 are: 55–70 (mild), 40–55 (moderate), 25–40 (severe), and less than 25 (profound). In one study, 50–70% of the children who weighed less than 1,500 grams at birth had behavioral problems. The children in this weight group also have a 20–36% chance of having a learning disability as well. Retrolental fibroplasia is common in premature infants. Chronic lung disease can also occur in the premature infant (e.g., bronchopulmonary dysplasia).

c. Central nervous system hemorrhage

Intracranial bleeding occurs in 30–45% of the infants who are delivered prior to 35 weeks' gestation. The more premature the infant, the greater the risk that an intracranial hemorrhage may occur. There are generally four locations that hemorrhage may occur in the fetal central nervous system (CNS): **(1) subdural, (2) subarachnoid, (3) intracerebral, and (4) intracerebellar.** Recent studies have indicated that fetal hypoxia is infrequently associated with intracranial hemorrhage in the mature infant. Intracranial hemorrhage in **premature infants** may be due to the head compression that occurs during the delivery process. Neonatal respiratory complications presumably may lead to **hypoxia** in infants weighing less than 1,500 grams at birth. The use of maternally administered phenobarbital prior to a premature delivery has been reported to have a salutary effect in decreasing the incidence and severity of fetal intracerebral hemorrhage. Phenobarbital also seems to be helpful in maturing the liver enzymes and in preventing hyperbilirubinemia, and perhaps in preventing the respiratory distress syndrome in premature infants.

1) Subdural hematoma

Lacerations of the tentorium or of the falx cerebri due to trauma often involves the veins. Any hemorrhage from these vessels may form a subdural hematoma that will usually be unilateral. These infants may have focal seizures and may show a dilated pupil on one side; most of these infants die. A hemorrhage from the superficial veins over the cerebral convexity is relatively common, and usually involves only one side. About 50–80% of these infants will end up with no residual problems; however, a small number may develop hydrocephalus or focal neurological signs.

2) Subarachnoid hemorrhage

A subarachnoid hemorrhage is the most common form of CNS bleeding in the neonate, and nearly 75% of all cases occur in premature infants. While such a hemorrhage can be rapidly fatal, even those infants who have seizures may eventually do quite well. Some premature infants will manifest significant neurological sequelae from severe hemorrhage secondary to hypoxia. The most common end result, however, is hydrocephalus.

3) Intracerebral hemorrhage

A hemorrhage into the substance of the brain (germinal matrix) may remain within the parenchymal tissue (40%) or may rupture through the ependyma into the lateral ventricles. **Hypoxia** seems to be the major cause of the vascular congestion and endothelial damage that leads to such a hemorrhage. Due to the silent nature of many of these lesions, this type of hemorrhage is now thought to be more common than previously believed. **The incidence of this lesion may approach 50% in infants who weigh less than 1,500 grams at birth.**

In cases in which there has been a severe hypoxic insult, the infant may become comatose, flaccid, apneic, and develop seizure activity. The infant's vital signs will then rapidly deteriorate, with death occurring within 24 hours. In lesser degrees of hypoxia involving intracerebral hemorrhage into the ventricles, hydrocephalus may result due to the development of arachnoiditis and the blockage of the posterior fossa, which stops the flow of cerebral spinal fluid from the fourth ventricle.

4) Intracerebellar hemorrhage

A hypoxic insult in the very premature fetus may also cause hemorrhage into the cerebellum. This condition may be associated with intraventricular hemorrhage as well.

d. Necrotizing enterocolitis

Many premature infants develop necrotizing enterocolitis during the first month of life. **About 70% of these cases occur in infants who weigh less than 1,500 grams.** The infant may manifest symptoms of lethargy, poor feeding, apnea, abdominal swelling, and tenderness, and may have blood in their stools. The cause of this condition is apparently due to an ischemic insult to the intestinal wall, which, in the presence of gas-forming enteric bacteria, causes necrosis and ulceration of the bowel. The glucose that is present in the initial feedings is converted to gas, which leads to ileus, intestinal distension, and increased intraluminal pressure. Perforation of the intestine may occur. Early recognition of this condition has lowered the mortality rate; however, in cases in which there has been a rupture of the bowel with peritonitis and sepsis, the mortality rate may be as high as 80%. The treatment consists of fluid replacement, antibiotics, oxygen, and intestinal decompression.

12. Teenage pregnancy

a. Incidence

Premarital sexual activity has continued to increase over the last 20 years, especially in girls under the age of 16. Initially, sexual activity in the 1960s and 1970s occurred more frequently in women aged 18–19 years. In the late 1970s, about 65% of white women and 88% of black women in this age group were sexually active. The increase in sexual activity in the younger age groups (i.e., ages 13–15) rose from 0.2–2.0% (whites) and 1.4–6.9% (blacks) in the 1950s to 1.0–7.6% (whites) and 3.0–15.3% (blacks) in the same age group in the 1970s. The risk of pregnancy is increased in this younger group (under 15 years) since they are less likely to use contraception with the first coitus (23%) as compared to the 18–19 age group (53%). It has been reported that nearly 60% of American teenagers are sexually active, with over 1.2 million becoming pregnant each year. Approximately 14% of all pregnancies occur in teenagers. Teenagers account for 37% of all births out of wedlock. Abortion is more prevalent in teenagers, with 15% of those aged 14–19 years having had at least one abortion.

b. Risks in pregnancy

It would appear that teenagers are at a greater risk for a number of pregnancy complications, such as pregnancy-induced hypertension (PIH), abruptio placentae, and urinary tract infections. The poor eating habits of the adolescent leads to anemia and poor nutrition, with a resultant intrauterine growth retardation of the fetus. Prematurity is also common. Maternal death may be 60% higher in adolescents under 15 years of age than in women in their twenties. Due to the poor life-style of the teenager, sexually transmitted diseases (e.g., herpes, gonorrhea, syphilis, chlamydia, hepatitis) are more common. Furthermore, the involvement of the adolescent with illicit drugs and alcohol may produce adverse effects on the fetus.

c. Emotional factors

The pregnant adolescent may have a long history of a poor adaptation to her environment. Her home life may be chaotic and stress-producing enough to force her to seek a means of "getting back" at her parents (i.e., by dumping a baby on them) or to "produce someone" (i.e., the baby) who will love her and need her. The family dynamics may be confusing, with the attitudes of the mother, the father, and the girl often being at variance. The parents may even give tacit approval to the child to have sexual relations. Often these girls do not do well in school and they do not

compete well. They may be in constant conflict with the authorities, the school officials, and sometimes with the law. They fall in with a disenchanted crowd of teenagers who have the same types of problems, and who frequently do not finish school. The girl may succumb to sex through peer pressure, and then may use her body to be socially accepted by a boyfriend, to be part of a peer group of friends, or to proclaim to the world that she is an adult and sexually mature. One investigator has described the teenage pregnant girl as being a **syndrome of failure.** The girl fails to fulfill the functions of adolescence, to remain in school, to limit her family size, to establish a stable family, to find a vocation and become self-supporting, to have healthy infants, and to have children who will reach their full potential in life.

The pregnant adolescent is usually unmarried, and her partner usually does not want any responsibility or commitment. The girl's family often provides little support for the girl, or for the couple if they get married. In addition, there are few community services available to assist such young people, although about 60% of unwed adolescents in one study were on welfare. Of those who got married, 80% were divorced within five years. Most of these girls have almost no marketable skills by which to obtain a job and support themselves.

Finally, it should be remembered that the children of teenagers are at greater risk of being victims of child abuse and neglect. These adolescents do not learn effective parenting skills, and their children have a poor prognosis in terms of both physical growth and in cognitive development.

d. Nutritional requirements

It is important in the management of the pregnant teenager that an attempt be made to reverse some of the adverse factors that are present in their lives. In addition to the usual nutritional requirements, an additional 30 grams of protein per day and an extra 300–350 calories per day should be added to their diet. You should try to convince the patient to stop smoking and using alcohol or drugs, and to obtain plenty of rest. The Special Supplemental Food Program for Women, Infants and Children (WIC) should be available in the community if financial problems interfere with her nutrition. Psychological support and encouragement of the couple by a concerned and caring physician may be very beneficial.

CHAPTER 38

Abnormal labor

. . . .

As one watches a man handle a patient it is easy to tell whether or not he has had a proper training, and for this purpose fifteen minutes at the bedside are worth three hours at the desk.

—*Sir William Osler**

. . . .

1. Dystocia due to fetal position

Dystocia, or difficult labor, may be due to: (1) an abnormal fetal position or fetal size, (2) abnormalities of the bony pelvis, (3) the presence of abnormal uterine contractions due to either hypotonia or hypertonia, or (4) soft tissue obstruction.

a. Abnormal fetal positions

1) Breech

The breech position may be present quite often in the late second trimester; however, by term, only about 3% of the fetuses still remain in the breech position. Some of the factors that may predispose the fetus to assume this position include: (1) prematurity, (2) a lax abdominal musculature, (3) high parity with a relaxed uterus, (4) hydramnios, (5) oligohydramnios, (6) the presence of multiple fetuses, (7) fetal hydrocephalus, (8) placenta previa, (9) a cornual-fundal placental implantation, (10) uterine tumors, or (11) uterine abnormalities. *The incidence*

of congenital anomalies in breech infants is increased more than twofold over nonbreech infants. **The breech position exposes the infant to certain problems, such as umbilical cord prolapse, possible traumatic delivery, and/or the necessity for a cesarean section.**

a) Types

The types of breech position are: (1) the complete breech, (2) the incomplete breech, and (3) the frank breech (Fig. 38-1). The **complete breech** position is said to be present when the legs are flexed at the hips and one or both knees are flexed. The **incomplete breech** occurs when one or both hips are unflexed and one or both feet or knees lie below the breech. If one foot is down, it is referred to as a **single footling presentation,** whereas if both feet are down, then it is called a **double footling presentation.** The **frank breech position** is said to be present when the hips are flexed and the knees are extended, so that the legs come to lie alongside the fetal head. This position is the most common breech presentation and the one that is safest if a vaginal delivery is to be performed, since the fetal buttocks will fill the pelvic inlet completely and prevent the prolapse of the umbilical cord.

b) External cephalic version (ECV)

The performance of an external cephalic version (ECV) of the fetus, from the breech to the vertex position, in the last trimester of pregnancy, has been advocated by some authors in an attempt to prevent a breech presentation from occurring at term (Fig. 38-2). The risks involved are abruptio placentae (3%), premature labor (1.2%), fetal death (0.9%), and premature rupture of the membranes (0.6%). However,

---

*Reprinted with permission from Robert Bennett Bean, *Sir William Osler: Aphorisms from His Bedside Teachings and Writings,* William Bennett Bean, ed. Springfield, Ill.: Charles C Thomas, Publisher, 1968, p. 49.

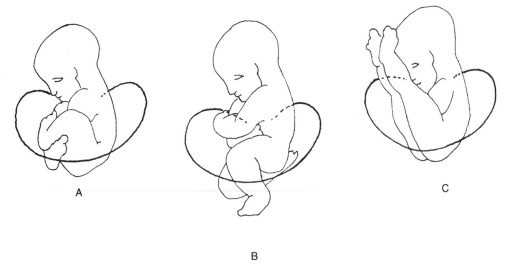

FIGURE 38-1. Types of breech presentation. (A) Complete or full breech. (B) Incomplete breech, or single footling. (C) Frank breech.

when the version is successful, prematurity and the risk of a vaginal breech delivery or a cesarean section may be prevented. On rare occasions, the uterus may be ruptured during the performance of this procedure. In one study, it was shown that when an external cephalic version was utilized, only 27.4% of the patients had to be delivered by cesarean section because of a recurrent and persistent breech presentation, whereas in those patients in which the external cephalic version had failed, 87.5% required a cesarean section because of a persistent breech presentation. It has been recommended that an ECV should be accomplished while the patient is under beta-mimetic tocolysis (e.g., ritodrine), after verification by both an ultrasonogram and a nonstress test that the fetus is completely normal and in good condition. Following the ECV, a Kleihauer-Betke stain of a maternal peripheral bood smear should be performed to detect any evidence of a significant fetomaternal hemorrhage secondary to the procedure.

c) Diagnosis

The diagnosis of a breech position can be accomplished by performing **Leopold's maneuvers.** The position can easily be confirmed during a vaginal examination by the identification of the fetal anus and the ischial tuberosities, which may be found to lie in the same plane with each other, through the dilated cervix. Ultrasonography will further confirm the fetal position. It is important to be certain that the fetal head is not **hyperextended** if vaginal delivery is being considered, since this complication is a contraindication to performing a vaginal delivery of an infant in the breech position (Fig. 38-3).

d) Management

The overall fetal mortality rate for breech deliveries in one study was about 8.5%, as compared to the rate of 2.2% for vertex presentations. In another study, the perinatal mortality rate of vaginal breech deliveries was reported to be five times greater than vertex presentations. The vaginal delivery of a breech may result in undue trauma to the fetus, since the brain, the spinal cord, the liver, the adrenal glands, and the spleen, as well as the brachial plexus, may be injured. In addition, fractures of the lower jaw, clavicle, humerus, and femur may occur during a breech extraction. The presence of prematurity, especially with a fetal weight below 1,500 grams, may predispose the infant to additional trauma and fetal distress, which may result in intracranial hemorrhage, asphyxia, and death.

In order to vaginally deliver a breech infant safely, it is essential that the fetus be of average

Text continues on p. 512

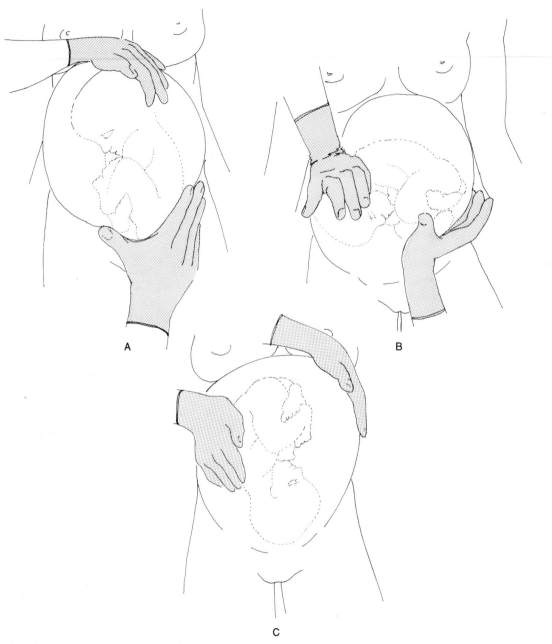

FIGURE 38-2. External cephalic version. (A) The breech is in a left sacrum transverse position. The fetus is grasped at each pole and gradually maneuvered with short adjustments of position in whichever direction the fetus will move easily (i.e., backward or forward somersault). (B) The fetus is now in a transverse lie. The fetal heart rate should be checked periodically as the fetus is maneuvered into position. (C) Frequently, the fetus may slowly struggle its way into the vertex position. If not, then gentle maneuvering will assist it to do so. Excessive force should not be used to perform this maneuver.

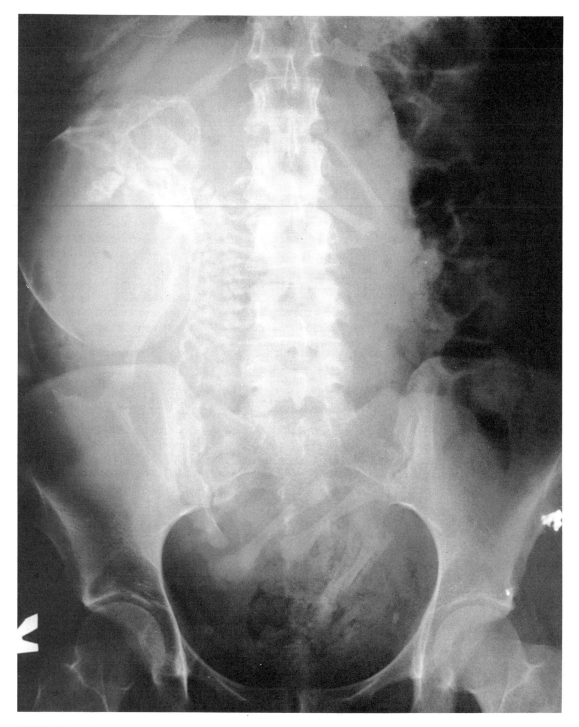

FIGURE 38-3. Hyperextended head in breech presentation.

size and that the mother have an adequate pelvic capacity. The labor should be completely normal with a good progression in the cervical dilatation and in the fetal descent, and a physician who is experienced in breech delivery should be in attendance. In a **spontaneous breech delivery,** the infant delivers without any assistance, except for the support of the fetal body as it delivers. In a **partial breech extraction,** the infant should be allowed to deliver spontaneously to the level of the umbilicus before the obstetric attendant intervenes and assists in the remaining part of the delivery. In a **total breech extraction,** the feet are grasped by the physician and the total body of the fetus is delivered. This procedure has been replaced by cesarean section in most cases.

The aftercoming head should be delivered by means of **Piper forceps** whenever possible. Any variation from an absolutely "normal" labor in a breech presentation should be viewed with suspicion and a cesarean section should be considered. Even with "perfectly normal conditions," a breech delivery may end up with a less than satisfactory result in regard to fetal morbidity.

In view of the three- to five-fold overall increase in the fetal mortality rate associated with vaginal deliveries of breech infants, it is difficult to ever recommend vaginal delivery in these cases; however, the fact remains that in **well-selected cases,** the risk of a vaginal delivery probably approaches that of a vertex delivery. It has been suggested that vaginal delivery should be considered in patients with a breech presentation who have an adequate pelvis on X-ray pelvimetry along with: (1) a transverse diameter of the inlet of at least 11.5 cm, (2) an anteroposterior (AP) diameter of the inlet of 10.5 cm, (3) a midpelvis transverse diameter of 10 cm, and (4) an AP diameter of the midpelvis of 11.5 cm. In addition, these patients should have a *frank* breech presentation, with a gestational age of at least 36 weeks, and a fetal weight estimation of between 2,500 and 3,800 grams. In such patients, the labor may be allowed to proceed and a vaginal delivery accomplished. Some investigators have even suggested that the judicious use of oxytocin may be allowed in these patients, if there is only minimal uterine contraction dysfunction. Failure to progress normally, however, is usually an indication of cephalopelvic disproportion and the need to perform a cesarean section.

In one study, the incidence of birth injuries in **spontaneous** vaginal breech deliveries was 3%, whereas in **partial breech extractions** it was 5%, and for **total breech extractions** it was 20%. Most of these injuries involved lesions of the brachial plexus (e.g., Erb's palsy and Klumpke's paralysis), damage to the fetal soft tissues, and fractures of the long bones.

It would appear from the evidence in the literature that there is little doubt that a cesarean section (C/S) should be performed for the **premature breech.** It has been shown that breech infants with birth weights between 1,000 and 2,500 grams have a significantly lower perinatal mortality rate when delivered by cesarean section. In infants who are less than 1,000 grams, however, there does not seem to be any particular benefit in delivering by cesarean section, perhaps because of the already poor salvage rate in this weight group. Infants in excess of 3,800 grams should also be delivered by C/S, because of the increased risk of fetal damage secondary to the increased size of the fetus.

Since prolapse of the umbilical cord may occur with complete breeches (5%) or footling breeches (15%), these infants should be delivered by cesarean section. When prolapse of the umbilical cord occurs, the presenting part may be manually held up off of the umbilical cord until a cesarean section can be performed, or the bladder may be filled with 500–700 ml of saline, and the patient treated with ritodrine, to accomplish the same goal, while preparations are being made to deliver the patient by cesarean section. Some of the other indications for a cesarean section delivery in a term breech presentation include a borderline or small pelvis, a bad obstetric history, dysfunctional uterine contractions with poor labor progress, and the primigravida breech.

2) Persistent occiput posterior presentation

More than 90% of infants with a persistent occiput posterior (OP) presentation will spontaneously rotate in the second stage of labor and deliver in the occiput anterior (OA) position. As the labor progresses, the fetal head will undergo the cardinal movements of labor, which, in the occiput posterior position, are: engagement, descent, **extension,** internal rotation, **flexion,** external restitution, and expulsion. While the deceleration phase of labor may be prolonged somewhat (about two hours), vaginal delivery can usually be anticipated without difficulty in most cases.

a) Management

In those instances in which the occiput posterior fetal head position has reached the perineum and is without caput formation or molding, delivery may be accomplished by: (1) the manual rotation of the fetal head to the occiput anterior position, followed by spontaneous delivery, (2) the rotation of the fetal head with Kielland forceps (or a Scanzoni maneuver using outlet forceps) to the occiput anterior position and then delivery by forceps, or (3) a low forceps delivery of the persistent occiput posterior position without cephalic rotation. The delivery of a persistent occiput posterior presentation without rotation is associated with an increase in perineal lacerations because of the need for additional room to deliver the head in this position.

b) Caput formation

It is important to determine the presence of caput formation and fetal head molding in an occiput posterior presentation. Although the leading portion of the fetal head may be almost on the perineal floor, if there is excessive molding and caput formation, then the fetal head may be elongated sufficiently so that it may still be unengaged. Your failure to recognize this fact might lead you to attempt to use forceps to effect delivery in this situation inappropriately. A cesarean section would be the procedure of choice in this situation.

c) Etiology

The occiput transverse position (OT) is the initial and transitory position of the fetal head as it enters the pelvis. The factors that allow the head to rotate into the **occiput posterior (OP)** position, instead of the occiput anterior position (OA), are: (1) a large anteroposterior diameter of the inlet, such as may be found in the anthropoid pelvis, and (2) a more posterior lie of the fetal body [i.e., right occiput posterior position (ROP)], such as may be found in a right-sided presentation with the fetus lying over on its back in the right paracolic gutter. Due to the more solid stool on the left side, and its frequent evacuation through the descending colon, the infant in the left occiput anterior position (LOA) is usually unable to roll over onto its back in the left gutter. As a consequence, a left-sided fetal lie is rarely associated with an occiput posterior presentation. **In contrast, a right-sided fetal lie, in an anthropoid pelvis, is much more prone than a left-sided fetal lie to have a persistent right occiput posterior presentation (ROP) during the course of labor (perhaps as high as 30%).**

3) Persistent occiput transverse presentation

In patients who have either a platypelloid or an android pelvic configuration, a persistent occiput transverse arrest may occur with the fetal head being arrested at or above the spines. If there is an arrest of the descent for over one hour in the occiput transverse position (OT), then an *occiput transverse arrest* may be diagnosed. Often, the occiput transverse position develops because there has been a failure of the head to flex appropriately, with the consequence being that the **occipitofrontal diameter (about 11 cm)** is the presenting area (see Chapter 2). If there is enough room in the midplane of the platypelloid pelvis (i.e., with the sacrum being slightly curved and posterior, instead of being flattened and anteriorly displaced), the head may rotate as it descends further into the birth canal and a vaginal delivery may be anticipated. In contrast, since the android pelvis funnels and becomes even more narrow in the midplane, the fetal head usually cannot descend appropriately and a deep occiput transverse arrest will result, necessitating the performance of a cesarean section to effect delivery.

In early labor, the fetal head enters the pelvis in an oblique or occiput transverse position. A persistent occiput transverse presentation should alert you to the possibility that there may be some cephalopelvic disproportion (CPD) present. If CPD is present, labor usually slows, the patient no longer makes adequate progress in cervical dilatation, and the presenting part fails to descend, so that the head remains high in the pelvis (i.e., zero station or above). **If there is fetal head molding (i.e., overriding of the fetal skull sutures on vaginal examination), and/or caput formation, then the probability that there is cephalopelvic disproportion is very high and cesarean section should be strongly considered.** If molding and caput formation are not present, then judicious oxytocin augmentation of the labor may be carried out if it is judged that ineffective uterine contractions are the problem. If the labor does not progress normally after effective uterine contractions have been reestablished, then cesarean section should be performed. The use of **Kielland forceps** to effect the rotation of the fetal head from the occiput transverse position to the occiput anterior position should only be attempted by a physician who is trained in forceps procedures, and only if there is no cephalopelvic disproportion present. In this situation, the fetal head should be below the spines (+ 1 station or more) before the forceps are applied. A gentle "jockeying" motion of the forceps (i.e., **Stillman's maneuver**) is used to effect the rotation, with the head being slightly elevated up into the pelvis and rotated 15–30 degrees. This allows the head to settle again into the pelvis, followed by a repetition of the maneuver until the head has been rotated into the desired position.

4) Face presentation

Face presentations occur in about 1:300–1:600 deliveries. Leopold's maneuvers may suggest the diagnosis; however, a vaginal examination should be carried out to confirm it. The bony features of the mouth in particular may help to differentiate it from the anus of a breech presentation. *The fact that the mouth lies at the apex of a triangle, in relation to the malar bones, will serve to differentiate it from the anus, which lies more in a line with the ischial tuberosities.* Furthermore, meconium staining of the examining finger will occur if the anus is entered.

The hyperextension of the fetal head that produces a face presentation may be caused by such factors as an inlet pelvic contraction, a lax maternal abdominal wall, fetal neck muscle contraction, a short nuchal cord, prematurity, hydramnios, uterine anomalies, and the presence of anencephaly. As the fetal head descends into the inlet of the pelvis, the brow initially presents, which is then followed by the face as the head further extends with descent. The submentobregmatic diameter (9.5 cm) presents, but since it is about the same size as the normal suboccipitobregmatic diameter of the vertex presentation, there is no prolongation of early labor (see Chapter 2).

If the face presents in a mentum posterior position, delivery becomes impossible because the head cannot extend any further in its attempt to extend over the perineum at the point of delivery. **It is only when the face presents with the chin beneath the pubis that the head may deliver by flexion, rather than by extension, over the perineum.** Usually, when the fetus is small and the pelvis is adequate, a mentum anterior position will progress to delivery without difficulty. If the descent of the face is slow, or if the mentum is posterior, cesarean section should be considered.

5) Brow presentation

The brow presentation is an unstable fetal head position that occurs in 1:1,000–1:3,000 deliveries. With the descent of the fetal head, the brow presentation usually converts either to a face or to an occiput presentation. If cephalopelvic disproportion is present, the brow presentation may persist. If this occurs, then the largest diameter, the occipitomental diameter (13.5 cm), will present (see Chapter 2). Considerable molding would be necessary for the head in this position to pass the inlet and descend into the birth canal. As a consequence, the presence of a brow presentation is an indication for cesarean section, unless the infant is quite small or the pelvis is very large.

6) Shoulder presentation (transverse lie)

An acromion presentation (i.e., shoulder) occurs whenever the long axes of the fetus and the mother are at right angles to each other (i.e., transverse lie). The incidence of this presentation is about 1:500 deliveries. This position may occur in association with a placenta previa, a multiple pregnancy, hydramnios, uterine anomalies, or a contracted pelvis. The position is described in relationship to the position of the shoulder (i.e., left or right) and the back (i.e., anterior or posterior, and superior or inferior). **A transverse lie in labor is an indication for cesarean section.** If labor is allowed to progress with a transverse lie, there is a great risk of uterine rupture with possible maternal death.

In very rare instances, when the fetus is very small and the pelvis is very large, delivery may occur by the folding of the infant upon itself *(conduplicato corporis)*, in which case both the head and the thorax pass through the birth canal simultaneously.

7) Compound presentation

A compound presentation is said to be present when one or more limbs prolapse alongside of the presenting part. Upper extremity prolapse occurs in about 1:700 deliveries, whereas lower extremity prolapse is less frequent, occurring in about

1:1,600 deliveries. **An associated prolapse of the umbilical cord occurs in 15–20% of the cases.** Prematurity is perhaps the most common finding, and is perhaps the cause for the incomplete occlusion of the pelvic inlet, which allows for the prolapse of the limb or umbilical cord to occur in the first place. The perinatal mortality rate in these cases varies between about 4.8 and 25%. While the replacement of the prolapsed limb may be attempted, overzealous attempts at replacement have been found to lead to high fetal and maternal death rates. Therefore, nonmanipulation of the fetus is the procedure of choice in a compound presentation. As the labor progresses, the extremity may gradually retract back into the uterine cavity as the vertex descends into the vaginal canal, after which the delivery may then become uneventful. In some instances, the prolapsed extremity prevents the descent of the fetal head, and cesarean section becomes necessary. A cesarean section is usually necessary in a fetus of normal or of large size with a compound presentation.

b. Fetal macrosomia

1) Incidence

While the position of the fetus may result in a *relative* cephalopelvic disproportion, the size of the infant may be such that an *absolute* cephalopelvic disproportion may exist. Infants who attain the weight of 4,000 grams or greater are considered to be macrosomic. **The incidence of infants who weigh more than 4,000 grams is about 5%, with about 0.5–1% weighing 4,500 grams or more.** The infant size may be increased when: (1) the parents are large, especially the mother, (2) the mother is a multipara, (3) the mother has delivered large infants in the past, (4) the mother is diabetic, (5) the mother is obese, and (6) the pregnancy is post-term.

2) Diagnosis

A large infant may be suspected when the maternal height and the fundal measurement are taken into account. A fundal measurement of 36–38 cm in an average-sized woman is usually indicative of a moderately sized infant (i.e., 7–8 lbs), whereas a fundal measurement of 40 cm or more in a singleton pregnancy is almost always indicative of an infant that weighs 9 lbs or greater, unless hydramnios or twins are present. In patients in one study who had fundal measurements at term that were above the 90th percentile (in

which the relationship between the maternal height and the symphysis-fundal height were adjusted), there was a higher incidence of abnormal labor and operative delivery (Fig. 38-4). These patients and fetuses experienced an increased amount of shoulder dystocia, meconium aspiration, birth asphyxia, brachial plexus injuries, and midforceps deliveries.

3) Treatment

The perinatal mortality rate in macrosomic infants is about 7%; these deaths are most often due to cephalopelvic disproportion, shoulder dystocia, respiratory depression, and neurologic damage. The mother will often have a severe postpartum hemorrhage resulting from the excessive distention of the uterus by the macrosomic infant, which results in uterine atony in the immediate postpartum period. Some authors have suggested that women who have delivered a macrosomic infant previously can probably deliver another one vaginally, whereas those women who have not previously delivered large babies should probably be delivered by cesarean section.

c. Shoulder dystocia

1) Incidence

In general, the incidence of shoulder dystocia is of the order of 0.15–0.20%; however, in infants of more than 4,000 grams, the incidence is about 1.6%. A prolonged second stage of labor (longer than one hour) may be associated with shoulder dystocia in 35% of cases with a fetal mortality rate of 50%. The finding of a fundal measurement of more than 38–40 cm, associated with a prolonged second stage of labor, should alert you to this possibility; however, in many instances there are no warning signs to indicate that a shoulder dystocia may occur. If, on an ultrasonogram, the fetal head circumference is subtracted from the chest circumference and the resulting value is greater than 1.6 cm, then it has been suggested that there will be a greater risk of shoulder dystocia occurring at the time of delivery. Furthermore, if the shoulder-to-head circumference difference exceeds 4.8 cm, then there may also be an increased risk of shoulder dystocia. In another study, the shoulder width was measured by computerized tomography (CT) scan in an effort to determine the presence of a macrosomic baby, which might also indicate the possibility of shoulder dystocia. A CT shoulder measurement of

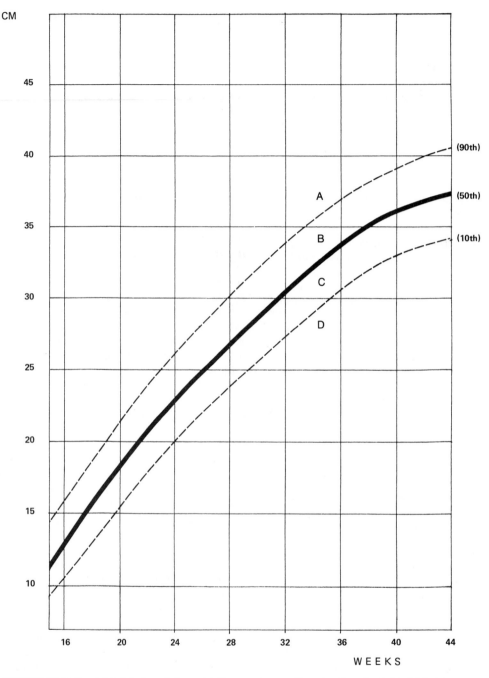

FIGURE 38-4. Fundal height in relation to delivery outcome. Zone A—Symphysis-fundal height above 90th percentile line. Zone B—Symphysis-fundal height between 50th and 90th percentile lines. Zone C—Symphysis-fundal height between 10th and 50th percentile lines. Zone D—Symphysis-fundal height below 10th percentile line. Group A women constitute a high-risk population for abnormal labor and operative delivery due to increased fetal size. (Redrawn with permission from A. B. Hughes, D. A. Jenkins, R. G. Newcombe, and J. F. Pearson, "Symphysis Fundal Height, Maternal Height, Labor Pattern, and Mode of Delivery," *American Journal of Obstetrics and Gynecology* 156 (1987), p. 644.)

more than 14 cm had a sensitivity of 100%, a specificity of 87%, a positive predictive value of 78%, and a negative predictive value of 100% in predicting that the weight of the infant would exceed 4,200 grams.

The definitive cure for bad fetal outcomes associated with shoulder dystocia would be to perform ι prophylactic cesarean section in those cases in which this diagnosis is considered. In one study, it was estimated from the data collected that if a cesarean section had been performed on all patients with fetuses weighing more than 4,000 grams, their primary cesarean section rate would have increased from 9.3% to 13.3%. This would have entailed the performance of an additional six cesarean sections for every case of shoulder dystocia that would have been prevented. Understandably, it was decided that this was too high a price to pay to prevent this condition and its consequences. A further projection of the data, however, to determine the effect of delivering all patients with infants that weighed more than 4,500 grams (10 pounds) by cesarean section showed that this approach indeed might be effective, in that it did not appreciably increase the number of unnecessary sections but did prevent the problems of shoulder dystocia. At the present time, there is no way to accurately predict the occurrence of shoulder dystocia.

2) Precautions

There are several techniques that may be utilized to effect the delivery of the infant with shoulder dystocia. **It is very important to avoid any flexion of the neck on the shoulders or any twisting motions of the head during attempts at delivery, since brachial plexus injuries may occur.** Such stretching of the infant's neck may result in damage to the upper nerve roots of the brachial plexus and cause **Erb-Duchenne paralysis.** This condition involves the flexor muscles of the forearm, the deltoid, and the infraspinous muscles. The arm will lie close to the side of the body with the forearm extended and internally rotated. If the lower roots of the brachial plexus are torn or injured, with paralysis of the hand, then **Klumpke's paralysis** is present.

3) Management

Hyperflexion of the maternal thighs upon the hips will often provide sufficient room to release a shoulder dystocia **(McRobert's maneuver).** This underlies the fact that even in a routine delivery, it is important

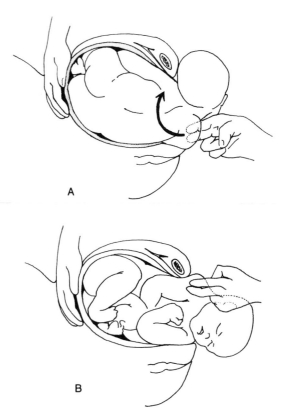

FIGURE 38-5. Wood's maneuver for shoulder dystocia. (A) Rotation of the posterior shoulder toward the pubis. (B) Delivery of the now anterior shoulder as it rotates outside of the pubic bone.

to have the patient's buttocks slightly over the edge of the delivery table in order to produce **hyperflexion of the thighs** with an opening of the pelvic outlet. The technique of **rotating the fetal shoulders into an oblique or horizontal position,** with the pressure on the back of the baby being directed posteriorly, will also sometimes allow the shoulder to deliver, if a **Kristeller maneuver** is used judiciously (i.e., broad fundal pressure on the uterus by the nurse in an attempt to push the baby out). If the shoulder rotation is then continued from the oblique or horizontal shoulder position on around in a "screwing" motion to allow the anterior shoulder to become the posterior shoulder, the posterior shoulder may rotate anteriorly and deliver, after which the posterior shoulder can then be delivered **(Wood's maneuver)** (Fig. 38-5). In some instances, the delivery of the posterior arm across the chest may provide sufficient room to

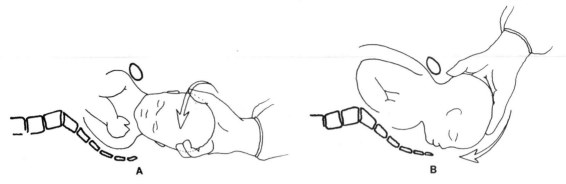

FIGURE 38-6. The Zavanelli maneuver. (A) Diagram of first part of the Zavanelli maneuver. If restitution has occurred following expulsion of the head, as in this case, the head is first manually returned to its prerestitution position, full extension in a direct occipital anterior position. (B) Diagram of second part of the Zavanelli maneuver. The head is manually flexed, recapitulating, in reverse, the birth of the head by extension. Upward pressure to recapitulate expulsion, in reverse, was not required in this instance. (Adapted from E. C. Sandberg, "The Zavanelli Maneuver: A Potentially Revolutionary Method for the Resolution of Shoulder Dystocia," *American Journal of Obstetrics and Gynecology* 152 (1985), pp. 479–484.)

then deliver the anterior arm and then the infant in a shoulder dystocia situation. Finally, often as a last resort, it has been recommended that a deliberate **fracture of the clavicle** of the impacted shoulder should be performed, which will usually cause a sufficient reduction of the shoulder width to effect the delivery.

A maneuver that has recently been developed, called the **cephalic replacement maneuver** (i.e., the Zavanelli maneuver, or the O'Leary maneuver), relies upon the fact that the umbilical cord is pulled into the pelvis when the head delivers and is thus compressed within the birth canal (Fig. 38-6). This umbilical cord compression may eventually cause the death of the infant if delivery is not carried out promptly. If the fetus *does not breathe* when the shoulder dystocia occurs (with the head recoiled into the perineum), it is possible to reposition the head in the predelivery position (i.e., the position of the chin on one shoulder that existed prior to external restitution) and push the fetal head back up into the birth canal. By so doing, the umbilical cord is automatically replaced into the uterine cavity and is no longer compressed. A cesarean section can then be carried out at your leisure, if the fetal heart tones remain good.

d. Fetal anomalies

Any abnormal enlargement of the fetal structures may cause dystocia due to obstruction of the birth canal.

Internal hydrocephalus with an accumulation of a large amount of spinal fluid may preclude vaginal delivery until decompression drainage has been carried out. The fetal head may be tapped, either transvaginally or transabdominally, just prior to delivery in order to decrease the cranial size. A greatly distended fetal abdomen secondary to ascites or a greatly distended bladder may be decompressed by needle aspiration in some instances. Moreover, a large sacrococcygeal teratoma may prevent vaginal delivery and necessitate a cesarean section. About 25% of these tumors are malignant.

2. Dystocia due to cephalopelvic disproportion (CPD)

a. Pelvic contraction

Classically, pelvic girdle contraction has been classified with regard to the specific portion of the pelvis in which the major contraction occurs. Thus, the contraction might be at the *pelvic inlet,* at the *midpelvis,* at the *pelvic outlet,* or at a combination of all three places (*i.e., generalized pelvic contraction*). Since the biparietal diameter of the fetal head at term is about 9.5 cm, it would seem that the inlet anteroposterior diameter should be at least 10 cm and the transverse diameter should be at least 12 cm. Of even more importance, however, is the configuration of the pelvis, as outlined in the Caldwell-Moloy classification system.

1) Inlet contraction

In patients who have a contracted inlet, the incidence of face, brow, or shoulder presentations may be increased, as is the incidence of cord prolapse and compound presentations. During labor, the cervix may dilate slowly up to 7–8 cm, but due to the high station of the presenting part and its inability to descend into the pelvis, there may be no pressure against the cervix for further dilatation. Since the cervix does not continue to dilate effectively, and the presenting part does not descend below the spines, an obstructed labor results. A persistent obstructed labor that lasts two hours beyond complete cervical dilatation may result in the development of a **pathologic retraction ring (Bandl's ring)** with the subsequent rupture of the uterus. The excessive pressure of the fetus upon the bladder and other pelvic structures in such prolonged obstructed labors may result in necrosis of the maternal soft tissues and the formation of fistulas between the bladder and vagina (vesicovaginal fistula), or between the cervix and the vagina (cervicovaginal fistula). Prolonged labors with ruptured membranes also frequently lead to an ascending infection of the uterus (chorioamnionitis), which may be accentuated by frequent vaginal examinations. Fetal bacteremia and aspiration pneumonia may occur as the result of the amnionitis.

An obstructed labor results in the development of a caput succedaneum, which consists of edema of the scalp in the most dependent portion of the fetal head. Fetal head molding also occurs in obstructed labors, as the bones of the fetal skull overlap each other in an attempt to compress enough to pass through the narrow pelvis. Localized compression of the fetal skull by the spines may be so severe in some instances that indentations and fractures of the fetal skull may occur.

A significant obstructed labor, such as may occur with an inlet contraction, can easily be diagnosed in modern obstetrics before the mother and the fetus become jeopardized. **Such a problem can be identified early in the course of labor if you pay close attention to the time sequences and the progression of labor and are aware of any failure of the fetal presenting part to descend ap-** propriately. **Finally, the development of a caput and fetal head molding will confirm the diagnosis of cephalopelvic disproportion.** The treatment of a cephalopelvic disproportion that is sufficient to produce a significant caput and fetal head molding is to perform a cesarean section.

2) Midpelvic contraction

The midpelvis consists of a plane from the lower border of the symphysis pubis through the ischial spines to the junction of the 4th and 5th sacral vertebrae. The anteroposterior measurement is about 11.5 cm, with the transverse diameter being about 10.5 cm. While these measurements cannot be obtained clinically with any degree of accuracy, an appreciation of the midpelvis dimensions may be detected by manual pelvimetry. If the spines are prominent, the side walls of the pelvis converge, there is a narrowing of the sacrosciatic notch, and the sacrosciatic ligament measurement is less than 2.5 cm (i.e., android pelvis), then a midpelvic contraction is probably present. **If a vaginal examination shows that the fetal presenting part does not descend well with Valsalva's maneuver or with a contraction (i.e., Müller-Hillis' maneuver), especially when the presenting part is below the zero station, then there is a good possibility that there is cephalopelvic disproportion present.** Confirmation of these findings may be obtained by noting whether the biischial diameter of the outlet is less than 8.5 cm, with a pubic angle of less than 90 degrees (i.e., android pelvis). If a midpelvic contraction is present, it is important not to employ a forceps delivery, unless the fetal head is bulging on the perineum (without caput), since only then can it be assumed that the obstruction has been passed. Midforceps are thus contraindicated in patients who have a midpelvic contraction.

3) Pelvic outlet contraction

If the biischial diameter is less than 8.5 cm and the pubic angle is less than 90 degrees, then an outlet contraction is present. This type of contraction, as with the midpelvis contraction, occurs in the **android pelvis,** since the passageway funnels from the inlet through the midplane to the outlet. Thus, the fetal presenting part only descends part of the way down the birth canal, where it then arrests (deep occiput transverse arrest). In general, if an outlet contraction is present, then a midpelvis contraction will

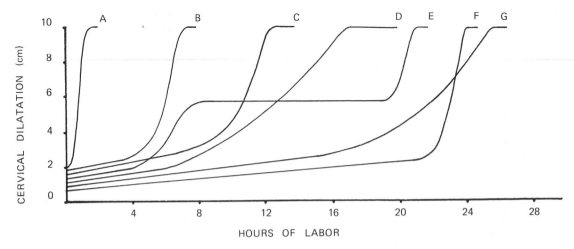

FIGURE 38-7. The major types of deviation from normal labor progress may be noted by observing the dilatation of cervix at various intervals after labor begins. (A) Precipitate labor. (B) Multiparous labor. (C) Primigravida labor. (D) Prolongation of active phase of labor and of the second phase. (E) Labor with a secondary arrest of dilatation. (F) Labor with a prolonged latent phase. (G) Prolonged latent phase and active phase of labor. (Adapted from M. L. Pernoll and R. C. Benson, *Current Obstetric and Gynecologic Diagnosis and Treatment.* Norwalk, Conn.: Appleton & Lange, 1987, p. 189.)

also be present. The treatment for a patient with a pelvic outlet contraction is a cesarean section.

b. General pelvic contraction

The normal gynecoid pelvic configuration is small enough in some patients to preclude normal vaginal delivery. This problem commonly occurs in patients who are of small stature and are **less than five feet in height.** In a few of these patients, the pelvis may be small because the individual is a true dwarf, a hypoplastic dwarf, or a chondrodystrophic dwarf. There are other patients, however, who have distorted pelves, including those that are seen in patients who have kyphosis, scoliosis, rickets, or a variety of other pelvic deformities that may result from either pelvic disease or fractures. If the fetus is of average size, many of these patients will require a cesarean section to effect delivery.

3. Dystocia due to dysfunctional labor

a. Dysfunctional labor

Uterine dystocia during parturition may be secondary to either weak uterine contractions or due to inadequately coordinated contractions. In either case, a lack of progress in the labor will result. Often, weak contractions accompany cephalopelvic disproportion; thus, it is essential to assess all four of the factors that may impede the progress of labor (i.e., the passenger, the passage, the powers, and the patient). **Dr. E. A. Friedman** in 1978 noted that the incidence of abnormal labor was about 8%. He identified nine different types of dysfunctional labor: (1) prolonged latent phase, (2) protracted active phase dilatation, (3) protracted active phase descent, (4) prolonged deceleration phase, (5) a secondary arrest of dilatation, (6) an arrest of descent, (7) a failure of descent, (8) precipitate dilatation, and (9) precipitate descent. Some of these patterns are more common than others (Fig. 38-7).

1) Prolonged latent phase

About one-half of the cases of dysfunctional labor may be ascribed to a prolonged latent phase. **A prolonged latent phase is one that lasts for longer than 20 hours in the primigravida and for more than 14 hours in the multiparous patient.** The incidence of this entity in a primigravida patient may be as high as 30%. The causes of a prolonged latent phase are: (1) the patient may have only been in false labor, or (2) the patient is in the early latent stages of labor but has been given an excessive amount of sedation too early (75%). This problem does not presage other abnormal labor patterns, and rest for 6–10 hours is usually all that is needed to effect the onset of good labor. The administration of subcutaneous morphine sulfate will allow the patient to rest. Upon awakening, about 85% of these patients will develop a good labor pattern, and 5% will continue to have ineffective contractions; however, they may then respond to oxytocin stimulation. About 10% of these patients will not be in labor.

2) Protraction disorders

A protracted descent of the fetus or a protracted active phase of labor may be due to excessive sedation, regional anesthesia, or a minor degree of cephalopelvic disproportion. Continued close observation of these patients should be carried out with attention being paid to the progress of the cervical dilatation and of the fetal descent. A failure of the presenting part to descend should strongly suggest that a significant cephalopelvic disproportion might be present that may require a cesarean section. The judicious use of oxytocin in this situation may be of value, but only if the contractions are weak. **The active phase of labor is said to be protracted when the cervical dilatation is less than 1.2 cm per hour in the primigravida, or less than 1.5 cm per hour in the multigravida. Furthermore, if the descent advances less than 1.0 cm per hour in the primigravida, or less than 2.0 cm per hour in the multigravida, then a protracted descent phase is said to be present.** While the fetal descent below the zero station may occur somewhat later in the course of the cervical dilatation (i.e., at about 6–7 cm), it is important to note the time when the presenting part drops below the level of the spines without caput formation or molding. **In summary, as the cervix dilates from 3 cm to 10 cm (i.e., complete dilatation), the time elapsed in a normal labor should not exceed 5.8 hours (i.e., 5 hours and 48 minutes) in the primigravida and 4.6 hours (i.e., 4 hours and 36 minutes) in the multigravida.** It is very important to keep these times in mind when managing a woman in labor; otherwise, uterine dysfunction may be missed and further procrastination may jeopardize both the fetus and the mother. It is equally important for you to recognize that these time limits are not absolute and that you do not need to rush into doing a cesarean section when they are exceeded. However, if you use these limits as an **early warning system,** then you will be able to manage the patient in a more intelligent manner.

3) Arrest disorders

If two hours elapse without any change in the cervical dilatation, then an arrest of dilatation has occurred; however, a minimum time period of only one hour is all that is necessary to make this diagnosis. About 5% of primigravidas will have a secondary arrest of dilatation during labor. The incidence of cephalopelvic disproportion (CPD) in primigravidas with a secondary arrest of labor may be as high as 50%, whereas it is only about 20% in multigravidas. If CPD is not the cause of the arrest, then oxytocin augmentation of the uterine contractions should be effective in 90% of the remaining cases within four hours. In these cases, excessive sedation, regional anesthesia, and mild fetal malposition may be the cause of the secondary arrest of labor.

4) Hypotonic labor

Two forms of uterine dysfunction have been described: hypotonic and hypertonic. The most common form of dysfunction is the **hypotonic type,** in which the contractions, although well coordinated, are not strong enough to produce adequate progress in cervical dilatation. *While cephalopelvic disproportion may accompany hypotonic uterine dysfunction, in the absence of fetal head molding and/or caput formation, the judicious use of oxytocin stimulation of labor should be attempted.* If such augmentation of the labor does not immediately restore the labor to normal (i.e., within 60 minutes after adequate contractions are reestablished), with the resumption of adequate progress in cervical dilatation and in the descent of the fetal head, then cesarean section should be strongly considered. **When augmentation of the labor is utilized, the oxytocin should be administered by a constant flow infusion pump at an initial rate of no more than 1 mU/minute. The flow rate should be increased by 1 mU/minute at intervals of at least 30–40 minutes until adequate contractions occur.** The previous teaching that the oxytocin dosage could be increased every 15 minutes is incorrect and may lead to hyperstimulation (i.e., tetanic contractions) and fetal dis-

TABLE 38-1. Bishop scoring index

Factor	Rating			
	0	1	2	3
Dilatation	Closed	1 cm–2 cm	3 cm–4 cm	5 cm+
Effacement	0–30%	40–50%	60–70%	80% +
Station	−3	−1, −2	11	+1, +2
Consistency	Firm	Medium	Soft	
Position	Posterior	Middle	Anterior	

Range of scores: 0–13

Prerequisites: Multiparity, gestation at least 36 weeks, and vertex presentation with a normal past and present obstetric history.

Predictions: Patients with a score of 9 or more will have a safe, successful induction with an average length of labor of less than 4 hours.

Reprinted with permission from The American College of Obstetricians and Gynecologists, E. H. Bishop, "Pelvic Scoring for Elective Induction," *Obstetrics and Gynecology* 24 (1964), p. 266.

tress. Indeed, it has been found that the length of the augmented labor-to-delivery time seems to be less when the dosage is increased only every 30–40 minutes as opposed to every 15–20 minutes. Good contractions should occur at a dosage level of about 4–7 mU/minute; however, about 15–20% of the patients will respond to as little as 1 mU/minute. Dosages of oxytocin of more than 8 mU/minute should be used with caution, and the presence of cephalopelvic disproportion should be considered in these patients if there is not adequate progress. At levels of 20–40 mU/minute or greater, a strong antidiuretic effect is produced.

a) Induction and augmentation of labor

It is important to recognize that the term **induction** of labor consists of the use of oxytocin stimulation *prior* to the onset of labor, or at a cervical dilatation of less than 3–4 cm. In contrast, the **augmentation** of labor consists of the use of oxytocin stimulation *after* the onset of labor, or beyond 3–4 cm of cervical dilatation. Hypotonic labor occurs after the labor has been established (i.e., beyond 3–4 cm of cervical dilatation). Artificial rupture of the membranes is often helpful in stimulating labor. *It has been stated that the prolonged labor that occurs in the primigravida is commonly due to poor uterine contractions, whereas the prolongation of labor seen in the multigravida is usually considered to be evidence of cephalopelvic disproportion.*

Endogenous **oxytocin** is an octapeptide that is produced in the paraventricular and supraoptic nuclei of the hypothalamus. Oxytocin is packaged with a neurophysin in a secretory granule that is transported down the hypothalamic neurohypophyseal tract to the posterior lobe of the pituitary gland. The oxytocin then stimulates the uterine muscular activity by its interaction with the calcium ion transport system in the myometrium. Oxytocin has a half-life of about 3–6 minutes. Commercial oxytocin has the same pharmacologic properties as the naturally occurring oxytocin. Oxytocin will stimulate rhythmic uterine contractions, especially in the third trimester, and should only be administered by an intravenous infusion pump.

The **Bishop scoring system of the status of the cervix** has frequently been used to determine whether the cervix is favorable for induction (Table 38-1). The sum of the five factor scores equals the total score. A low score of less than 4 is indicative of about a 20% failure rate if labor induction is carried out, whereas a score of between 9 and 13 has been associated with a high incidence of successful inductions.

In making the decision to induce labor for medical reasons, the decision should be based upon the concept that **"the medical indications are such that the patient must be delivered."** This statement implies that the patient's condition requires delivery within 24 hours. Too often, if the induction fails and labor does not develop, then the physician will agonize over whether to perform a cesarean section to effect delivery, since this is a more dangerous procedure. If the reasons for the induction were valid initially, then there is no question as to whether to perform a cesarean section or not—it should be done. If the indications were not logical or medically acceptable initially, then the physician has probably used bad judgment and could be accused of practicing meddlesome obstetrics.

The use of oxytocin for the induction or augmentation of labor requires that there be no evidence of known relative or absolute cephalopelvic disproportion, nor of a previous scar of the uterus (e.g., previous cesarean section). The presence of a breech presentation, grand multiparity, or a multiple pregnancy are relative contraindications for the use of oxytocin; however, clinical judgment should be exercised with each individual patient.

There are a number of side effects that have been associated with the use of oxytocin. Oxytocin has an **antidiuretic effect** that results in the retention of water by renal tubular reabsorption. Large amounts of I.V. fluids should not be administered to the patient who is receiving high doses of oxytocin, due to the risk of **water intoxication and pulmonary edema.** Oxytocin may also produce **severe tetanic contractions** of the uterus, which may result in abruptio placentae or a rutpure of the uterus.

5) Hypertonic labor

Hypertonic labor is characterized by very painful contractions that do not prove to be effective in dilating the cervix. It generally occurs early in latent labor before the cervix has dilated to 3–4 cm. It would appear that these contractions are probably uncoordinated, with an asynchrony of the electrical impulses and the pressure gradients. Oxytocin is not indicated in these patients. Maternal rest with morphine or meperidine will usually relieve the pain for a short period of time, after which the patient may then resume spontaneous normal labor contractions.

6) Poor voluntary expulsive forces

In patients who have been heavily sedated or who have received conduction anesthesia, the voluntary expulsive forces in the second stage of labor may be blunted or absent. A lack of adequate maternal "pushing" may lead to the use of midforceps for delivery.

7) Precipitate delivery

A labor that is more rapid than normal may lead to a **precipitate delivery. Precipitate dilatation** refers to progress in the accelerated phase of labor of 5 cm per hour in a primigravida or 10 cm or more per hour in the multipara. **Precipitate descent** has been defined as a descent of the fetal head at a rate of 5 cm per hour in the accelerated phase of labor in the primigravida or 10 cm per hour in the multipara. **Thus, the delivery of a primigravida within about two hours, or of the multigravida within one hour of the onset of the accelerated phase of labor, would be classified as precipitate labor.** Another author has defined precipitate labor as a labor of less than 3 hours. This is in contrast to a prolonged labor, which is one that lasts for more than 18 hours. Usually, precipitate labor is of no concern as long as the uterine contractions have not been too close together (tachysystole), which prohibits the uterine muscle from relaxing appropriately, in which case it is possible that the fetal oxygenation may have been compromised. Furthermore, precipitate expulsion of the fetus at delivery may result in intracranial hemorrhage and trauma, especially if the delivery was unattended. Postpartum hemorrhage secondary to uterine atony may also occur.

b. Uterine contraction bands

In prolonged, obstructed labors, especially when the cervix has been dilated completely for more than two hours, a pathologic contraction ring, or Bandl's ring, may occur. This ring demarcates the thinned-out lower uterine segment from the thickened upper uterine fundus, and will gradually migrate superiorly over a short period of time as the upper segment continues to retract. **In so doing, the lower uterine segment becomes progressively thinned out until it eventually ruptures.**

In contrast, the **physiologic retraction ring** that is seen after the delivery of one twin is usually benign, unless it impedes the delivery of the second fetus by contracting about the fetal body.

4. Dystocia due to soft tissue obstruction

Soft tissue obstruction is a rare cause of dystocia in labor. Vulvar hematomas or massive edema may cause obstruction of the birth canal, as may extensive condylomatous lesions of the vulva and vagina.

a. Vaginal conditions

Thick vaginal septa, either longitudinal or transverse, may become an obstructive problem at the time of delivery and may also be associated with other urologic abnormalities. These septa are often stretched to the point that they are torn during delivery by the descending fetal presenting part. On occasion, it may be necessary to incise these bands or transverse septa in order to relieve the obstruction. Rarely, strictures of the vagina or severe scarring from previous inflammatory disease, corrosive abortifacient agents, or trauma may all but obliterate the vaginal canal. In such situations, a cesarean section may be necessary to effect the delivery of the infant.

b. Cervical conditions

Cervical cicatrical stenosis may occur following cervical conization, cryosurgery, traumatic injuries, or chemical damage to the cervical os. During normal labor, the softening of the cervix, plus effacement, may gradually allow the cervical os to dilate. At times, *conglutination of the cervical os* prevents its dilatation. The insertion of a fingertip into the cervical os will frequently result in a dramatic and almost instantaneous dilatation of the cervical os in these cases.

c. Abdominal conditions

In the presence of a diastasis recti abdominis and a pendulous abdomen, the direction of the uterine contractile forces may be distorted sufficiently that the engagement of the fetal presenting part cannot occur. The use of an abdominal binder may result in a better positioning of the uterus and may redirect the uterine contractile forces more effectively on the fetal body to allow for a normal progression of labor.

d. Tumors

During pregnancy, *leiomyomas* of the lower uterine segment or of the cervix may occupy the pelvis and prevent the fetal presenting part from descending into the pelvis for delivery. Cesarean section should be performed in this situation.

Cystic or solid ovarian masses may also at times occupy the pelvis and prevent the descent of the fetus. A cesarean section should be carried out whenever this type of obstruction occurs. On rare occasions, a cystic mass (e.g., dermoid cyst) may rupture and produce a chemical peritonitis. Furthermore, an obstructing mass may develop torsion and become infarcted and necrotic. Most of these conditions may be managed at the time of the cesarean section.

Other pelvic masses, such as a **congenital pelvic horseshoe kidney,** or a kidney transplant, may not only obstruct labor but also may be traumatized and damaged during labor and delivery.

CHAPTER 39

Puerperal complications

. . . .

Half of us are blind, few of us feel, and we are all deaf.
—*Sir William Osler**

. . . .

1. Postpartum hemorrhage

a. Hemorrhagic conditions

Postpartum hemorrhage is defined as the loss of 500 ml or more of blood within the first 24 hours postpartum. Since the average patient with an episiotomy probably loses this much blood (i.e., 500–600 ml), this definition should be abandoned. It has been suggested that the definition should more properly be based upon a loss of 1,000 ml or more, since only about 5–8% of patients would qualify for the diagnosis of postpartum hemorrhage under such a definition. The usual blood loss following a cesarean section is of the order of 1,100–1,200 ml.

The treatment of hemorrhage basically consists of the replacement of the blood. While intravenous fluids (e.g., lactated Ringer's solution) may assist in replacing the fluid volume in the intravascular compartment, it should not be forgotten that the red blood cells themselves are necessary in order to provide for an adequate perfusion of the vital organs and to avoid organ hypoxia. *The hematocrit should be maintained at about 30% and the urine output should be kept at least at 30–60 ml per hour.* The blood loss may be replaced with packed red blood cells. Coagulation

problems may be corrected with cryoprecipitate, platelet concentrate, and fresh frozen plasma.

Postpartum hemorrhage may be further divided into "early" hemorrhage (i.e., during the first 24 hours postpartum) and "late" hemorrhage, which occurs after the first 24 hours and up to six weeks' postpartum.

1) Early postpartum hemorrhage

Hemorrhage during delivery and in the immediate postpartum period may be due to: (1) atony of the uterus, (2) lacerations of the genital tract, (3) retention of placental tissue, or rarely (4) coagulation disorders.

a) Uterine atony

In many instances, a potential postpartum hemorrhage may be predicted prior to delivery. Patients who have hydramnios or a multiple gestation will have an **overly distended uterus** that will frequently result in uterine atony postpartum. Those patients who have had either **precipitate labor or prolonged labor** may have postpartum uterine atony, as will many patients who have had **oxytocin stimulation** of their labor. In patients who have had a number of **previous pregnancies (e.g., grand multipara),** the uterus may be "flabby," which may also result in uterine atony. **Amnionitis** will not only interfere with good labor contractions but may also result in postpartum uterine atony. Those patients who have had a **previous episode of postpartum uterine atony** may often have another episode of hemorrhage due to uterine atony in subsequent pregnancies. The use of **general anesthesia for delivery,** especially halothane anesthesia relaxes the uterus sufficiently to cause excessive blood loss in many patients.

---

*Reprinted with permission from Robert Bennett Bean, *Sir William Osler: Aphorisms from His Bedside Teachings and Writings,* William Bennett Bean, ed. Springfield, Ill.: Charles C Thomas, Publisher, 1968, p. 37.

b) Genital lacerations

Difficult deliveries and those involving episiotomies, rotating forceps, or manipulative procedures may cause lacerations of the genital tract. **Lacerations** may be easily visualized postdelivery by the use of a speculum and sponge forceps to inspect the vagina and cervix. **Uterine rupture** is more difficult to diagnose, even with manual exploration of the uterus. If, however, significant uterine bleeding persists immediately after delivery in the absence of uterine atony or lacerations, then a uterine rupture should be strongly suspected.

c) Retention of placental fragments

The retention of small placental fragments or of a succenturiate lobe may result in postpartum hemorrhage. The placenta should always be carefully inspected at the time of delivery to detect any missing cotyledons or vessels that may extend from the edge of the placental disk. Should a cotyledonary fragment be missing, the uterine cavity should be explored manually under adequate anesthesia. You should insert your hand into the uterine cavity and curette the walls from the fundus to the cervix in a "scraping" motion with closed fingers to avoid the perforation of the uterine wall by any individual finger. Any fragments will usually scrape off of the uterine wall easily.

The placenta will usually separate within 30 minutes of delivery. This step is heralded by a lengthening of the umbilical cord, a gush of blood from the vagina, and an elevation anteriorly of the uterine fundus. A cessation of the umbilical cord pulsations will also occur at this time. If the placenta does not deliver within 30–60 minutes, or if severe bleeding should occur, then a manual removal of the placenta should be performed (Fig. 39-1). In rare instances, the placenta may be attached to the myometrium of the uterus **(placenta accreta).** This condition is due to a defective decidua basalis, which normally underlies the placental implantation site. Usually in such cases, **Nitabuch's layer** is absent also. Placenta accreta may occur as a result of a previous D&C of the uterus or from scars of the uterus resulting from a previous cesarean section. If the placenta actually invades deeply into the myometrium, a **placenta increta** is said to be present, whereas if the placenta penetrates all the way through the myometrium to the peritoneal surface of the

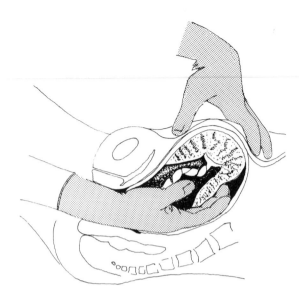

FIGURE 39-1. Manual removal of the placenta. Develop a cleavage plane between the uterine wall and the base of the placenta, while the other hand steadies the uterus.

uterus, then it is called a **placenta percreta.** Only rarely can a placenta accreta be manually removed, much less the other invasive placentas, so a hysterectomy is usually required to treat these entities. If there is only a small amount of invasion of the placenta into the myometrium in a focal area, the main body of the placenta may be manually removed, leaving only a small placental remnant (i.e., placental polyp).

An **inversion of the uterus** occurs in about 1:2,000 cases if undue traction is placed upon the umbilical cord during the delivery of the placenta, especially if the placenta has not yet detached itself from the uterine wall, or if a placenta accreta is present. The excessive uterine relaxation that occurs with halothane anesthesia also in rare cases may result in a spontaneous uterine inversion during the delivery of the placenta. *These patients have shock that is thought to be disproportionate to the amount of blood loss; however, the bleeding can be considerable and at times may be life threatening.* The treatment in these cases consists of the immediate manual replacement of the uterus under halothane anesthesia or under magnesium sulfate tocolysis treatment, and the restoration of the blood volume with packed red cells and intravenous fluids. In almost all cases, the uterus may be reinverted into its normal position without difficulty. In the rare instances where this approach is not successful, laparotomy may be necessary. If surgery becomes necessary, the anterior cervical constriction ring should be incised through an abdominal excision and a tenaculum placed on the uterine fundus to restore the uterus to its normal position, after which the cervical incision may then be closed. Oxytocin or prostaglandins, e.g., carboprost tromethamine (Hemabate) should be administered to decrease the uterine bleeding after the uterus has been replaced in its normal position.

d) Coagulation disorders

The coagulation disorders that may be seen in pregnancy consist of consumptive coagulopathy, or disseminated intravascular coagulation (DIC); hemophilia A (Factor VIII deficiency); hemophilia B (Factor IX deficiency); and von Willebrand's disease. Since hemophilia A and B are X-linked recessive diseases, the female carrier is not affected clinically. Von Willebrand's disease may cause hemorrhage in the pregnant patient (see Chapter 35). Abruptio placentae, toxemia (PIH), and amniotic fluid embolism may be associated with DIC. The supportive treatment of these conditions consists of the administration of packed red blood cells, fresh frozen plasma, and/or cryoprecipitate.

e) Management of early postpartum hemorrhage

The most common cause of early postpartum hemorrhage is uterine atony. If the uterine fundus is held tightly between the hands (with one hand positioned in the vagina and the other on top of the abdomen) for 20–30 minutes, most patients will cease bleeding (Fig. 39-2). Initially, oxytocin or Methergine may be utilized to assist in causing a contraction of the uterus. If the bleeding persists in spite of these measures, then the administration of carboprost tromethamine (Hemabate) will almost always control the bleeding. If clotting is present, then a coagulation defect is not a factor in the bleeding problem.

In rare instances, a hypogastric artery ligation or a uterine artery ligation may become necessary in a serious postpartum hemorrhage (Fig. 39-3, Fig. 39-4). Recently, interest has been directed toward the use of **bilateral selective embolization** of the internal iliac arteries with Gelfoam. If these

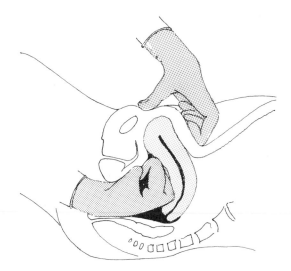

FIGURE 39-2. Bimanual compression of the uterus.

procedures do not control the blood loss, then it may be necessary to perform a hysterectomy in order to control the hemorrhage. The pneumatic anti-shock trousers, or Military Anti-Shock Trousers (MAST), may be used to temporarily control serious hemorrhage until surgery can be carried out.

2) Late postpartum hemorrhage

Postpartum hemorrhage that occurs after the first 24 hours following delivery and up to six weeks' postpartum is usually due to **subinvolution** of the placental site, although occasionally it may be due to retained secundines. Although curettage usually removes any fragments of secundines that are present, minimal tissue may be returned and the hemorrhaging may actually increase. This complication may become severe enough to require a uterine or a hypogastric artery ligation and/or a hysterectomy. The treatment of subinvolution usually consists of the administration of methylergonovine maleate (Methergine) 0.2 mg p.o. q4h for 24–48 hours. If an endometritis proves to be the cause of the subinvolution, then antibiotic therapy should also be administered.

3) Postpartum pelvic hematomas

Hematomas of the pelvic area may occur as the result of: (1) accidental trauma (i.e., car accidents), (2) pelvic surgery, or (3) obstetric trauma. The most

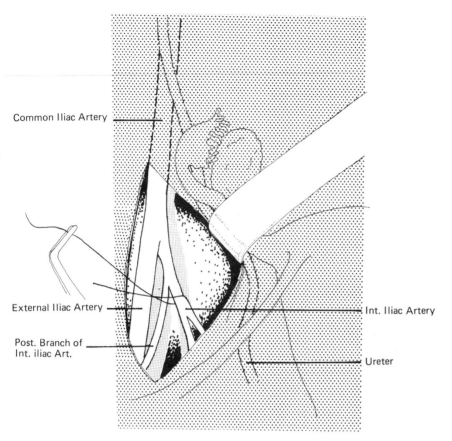

FIGURE 39-3. Ligation of the right internal iliac (hypogastric) artery. The anterior division of the internal iliac artery should be ligated with two silk ligatures. Note the retraction of the ureter, which normally overlies the bifurcation of the iliac artery into the external and internal iliac branches.

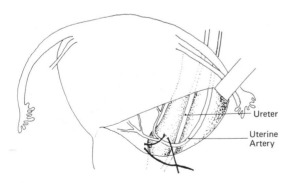

FIGURE 39-4. Uterine artery ligation.

common causes of pelvic hematomas are vaginal deliveries involving obstetric manipulation, large lacerations or episiotomies, or the injection of local, pudendal, and paracervical block anesthesia. In the case of a laceration or an episiotomy incision, the development of a hematoma can be perhaps prevented by placing the first suture in the repair above the apex to include any retracted blood vessels. If a hematoma is identified in the absence of an incision or laceration, the placement of a relatively deep suture above the hematoma may stop its further growth; however, care must be exercised in order to prevent injury to the underlying structures. In some cases, the development of a pelvic hematoma may be very insidious and may take several hours to manifest itself. **Patients**

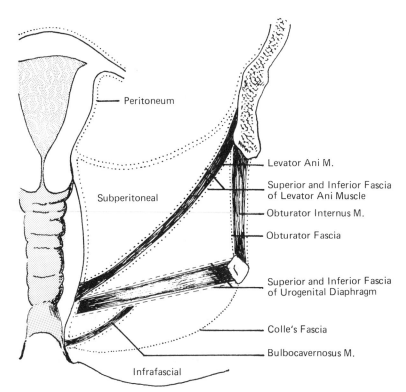

Peritoneum

Subperitoneal

Levator Ani M.

Superior and Inferior Fascia
of Levator Ani Muscle

Obturator Internus M.

Obturator Fascia

Superior and Inferior Fascia
of Urogenital Diaphragm

Colle's Fascia

Bulbocavernosus M.

Infrafascial

FIGURE 39-5. Pelvic fascial planes involved in postpartum hematomas.

who complain of undue perineal pain in the postpartum period should have a sterile pelvic examination performed to determine if a pelvic hematoma is present.

If on pelvic examination there appears to be a small **vulvar hematoma,** cold compresses and pressure over the vulva may limit its spread. The endopelvic fascial planes will define the development of a hematoma (Fig. 39-5). If the hematoma is obviously enlarging over the next 30–60 minutes of observation, then the area should be opened, the hematoma evacuated, and the bleeding vessels ligated.

If a **vaginal hematoma** is found, then it should be opened and any bleeding vessels ligated. When hemostasis has been achieved, a vaginal pack may provide additional pressure on any oozing from the incision. A Foley catheter should be placed in the bladder. Both the pack and the catheter may be removed in 24 hours.

If the pelvic examination reveals a **retroperitoneal hematoma** in the adnexal area, then the evaluation of serial hematocrits may be of value. An ultrasonogram, especially with a vaginal transducer, may

help to delineate the problem. Blood transfusions should be administered if there has been a significant loss of blood, and the patient may require a laparotomy. Rarely is it possible to identify the bleeding vessels in such a hematoma in order to ligate them. As a consequence, the hypogastric artery on the affected side may be ligated. If the hematoma appears to be due to a laceration of the uterine artery on one side, then the ligation of the ascending uterine artery along the side of the uterus and/or the ovarian artery on the affected side may control the bleeding.

b. Sheehan's syndrome

Severe intrapartum or postpartum hemorrhage with hypotension in an obstetric patient may result in necrosis of the anterior pituitary gland. This event will in turn cause the development of panhypopituitarism (i.e., Sheehan's syndrome), in which **postpartum milk letdown will not occur, due to the failure of the lactation process.** It has been recommended that the patients who experience hypotensive episodes during parturition should not receive lactation suppression drugs postpartum, since such agents may mask this failure of lactation.

2. Postpartum infection

a. Endometritis

1) Historical aspects

In 1843, **Oliver Wendell Holmes** wrote about the "Contagiousness of Puerperal Fever." During the next 20 years, another pioneering physician, **Ignaz Semmelweis** (1818–1865) in Vienna, contributed significantly to the understanding and prevention of **puerperal sepsis,** or "childbed fever." He attracted considerable attention from such medical luminaries of his day as Gustav Michaelis and Alfred Hegar of Germany and James Simpson of Scotland, who were ardent supporters of his concepts of asepsis in the management of patients in labor. Another man, who became famous for his forceps rotation maneuver, Friedrich Scanzoni, was bitterly opposed to this doctrine of the contagiousness of puerperal sepsis. Charles D. Meigs, an American obstetrician, was also strongly against the theory of Holmes and Semmelweis.

2) Organisms involved

Although group A beta-hemolytic streptococci were the most common pathogens in the puerperal infections of the past, recent studies have implicated many other organisms, such as Escherichia coli, the Klebsiella species, Peptococci, Peptostreptococci, the Bacteroides species, and group B streptococci. It is well known that all of these organisms are common inhabitants of the vagina and the rectum and that, in the presence of tissue damage, they become opportunistic invaders. Group B streptococci will commonly cause a postpartum fever within the first 24 hours.

Following vaginal delivery or cesarean section, the conditions within the vagina (i.e., possible lacerations) and the uterus (i.e., the placental bed, with its thrombosed decidual vessels, and the raw decidual surface and possible retained fragments of the placenta) form an excellent culture media for infective bacteria to produce puerperal sepsis. The fact that all patients do not develop such infections is perhaps

due to a number of factors involved in the labor and delivery process, and to the **patient's inherent host resistance to infection.** The incidence of endometritis after a vaginal delivery is about 3%, whereas the incidence following a cesarean section has been reported to be between 12 and 85%. The incidence of endometritis varies with the socioeconomic class of the patient, with the lower socioeconomic levels having a higher infection rate. Infectious complications are also usually more severe following a cesarean section, with an abscess or pelvic thrombophlebitis occurring in as many as 2–4% of patients who develop puerperal endometritis.

3) Factors involved

Some of the factors that have been implicated in the development of postpartum endometritis are: (1) the amount of trauma to the genital tract, (2) the presence of retained secundines, (3) the length of labor, (4) the length of time that the membranes have been ruptured, (5) the number of vaginal examinations during labor, and (6) the socioeconomic status of the patient. The amount of the bacterial inoculum involved is also of paramount importance, but this factor is difficult to define in a given case.

Febrile morbidity has been defined as a temperature of 38° C (100.4° F) on two or more days of the first 10 days' postpartum, excluding the first 24 hours. The temperature should be taken by mouth at least four times daily. Due to the fact that many patients are discharged within 48 hours of delivery, this definition should probably be modified. The presence of an abnormal temperature on either of the first 2 days should be considered an indication of possible infection sufficient to delay the patient's discharge until the problem is resolved.

The initial manifestations of postpartum endometritis include fever in association with a tender uterus. Upon examination, a *Gram-stained smear* of the cervix and the uterus should be obtained in order to determine the predominant organism involved. *Cultures for aerobic and anaerobic bacteria* should be obtained for confirmation; however, these cultures are frequently not helpful, due to the polymicrobial flora that is normally present in the vagina. If a cesarean section was performed prior to complete cervical dilatation, it is especially important to be certain that there is not a blockage of the cervical os with blood clots and lochia **(i.e., lochial block).** *The choice of antibiotic therapy should be such that broad-spectrum coverage is provided.*

The persistence of a fever in a postpartum or postoperative patient with a pelvic infection in spite of the administration of appropriate broad-spectrum antibiotics over the course of 4–5 days should alert you to the possibility of a **septic pelvic thrombophlebitis.** This entity occurs in 2–4% of patients with pelvic infections. The pelvic infection involves the pelvic and ovarian vessels and entails the development of thrombosis and pulmonary embolism. The use of the **heparin sodium test** in these patients will cause a lysis of the patient's fever within 48–72 hours after it has been initiated. The heparin should be administered intravenously in full therapeutic dosage so as to prolong the activated partial thromboplastin time to two times the normal value. If the patient responds and becomes afebrile, then the heparin sodium should be continued for seven days. If the activated partial thromboplastin time exceeds the recommended range of twice normal (i.e., 55 seconds), protamine sulfate, 1 mg of a 1% solution, may be administered for every 100 units of heparin sodium in the patient's body to reverse the heparinization.

b. Episiotomy infection

An infection in an episiotomy incision is uncommon because of the excellent blood supply that is present in the perineal region. When it does occur, it usually follows the development of an incisional seroma or hematoma. The treatment consists of the evacuation of the infected hematoma and the establishment of adequate drainage, so that the episiotomy can heal by second intention. The use of hot sitz baths, with detergent soap added to the water, is beneficial and soothing. Systemic broad-spectrum antibiotics should also be administered.

There have been 14 cases of **clostridial myonecrosis** of the episiotomy incision reported. These patients have myonecrosis associated with positive cultures for clostridial species; however, in other respects these infections are similar to a necrotizing fasciitis. Aggressive debridement is indicated until free bleeding is encountered. High-dose wide-spectrum antibiotic therapy should be administered.

Another rare infection that occasionally occurs in an episiotomy incision, or more commonly in an abdominal incision, is that of a **"synergistic bacterial gangrene,"** or **"necrotizing fasciitis."** This infection presents with rapidly progressive edema, necrosis, and gangrene of the skin and the underlying fascia. Extensive debridement must be carried out with the excision of all nonbleeding tissues. Broad-spectrum antibiotics must be utilized and should be administered in high dosage. Skin grafts are generally needed after the infection has been cured.

3. Amniotic fluid embolism

Amniotic fluid embolism is fortunately quite rare (1:20,000 to 1:80,000 deliveries), but when it occurs, it is a catastrophic event, with the death of the patient in 86% of the cases. The delivery is often complicated by a large fetus (sometimes dead), a rapid and explosive labor with strong, "tetanic" contractions, and occasionally a ruptured uterus or an abruptio placentae. **Disseminated intravascular coagulation (DIC) is almost always present in these cases, and a severe hemorrhage ensues. The development of DIC is due to the entrance of the thromboplastin-rich amniotic fluid into the maternal bloodstream. The amniotic fluid embolism results from intravascular particulate matter (i.e., meconium, fetal squames) that rapidly travels to the lungs to produce a vascular embolism.** If the woman survives, these vessels will recannulate after about two weeks and leave the patient with no residual symptoms. Right heart blood that is obtained at autopsy, or via a central venous catheter or a pulmonary artery monitoring catheter, will demonstrate upon centrifugation three fluid zones, with the top one being the amniotic fluid. The site of entry for the amniotic fluid is unknown, but it is probably at the cervix, which ruptures in 54–60% of these cases. It may also gain entry through the open sinuses beneath the placental site, secondary to placental abruption, which occurs in 45% of the cases.

The cardiorespiratory response to the amniotic fluid embolism is perhaps due to several hemodynamic factors. The obstruction of the microvasculature of the lung results in **systemic hypotension (shock), pulmonary hypertension,** and **acute cor pulmonale.** The lack of adequate ventilation and perfusion in the lungs results in **hypoxia, cyanosis,** and **dyspnea.** As a consequence, there is a general systemic **cardiovascular collapse,** with pulmonary edema (which may progress to the adult respiratory distress syndrome if the patient survives) and left ventricular failure.

The treatment of amniotic fluid embolism primarily consists of supportive management of the cardiovascular and respiratory systems. A **Swan-Ganz catheter** is essential to monitor these parameters. **Fluids and blood replacement should be judiciously administered to maintain the blood pressure.** The treatment of the patient with dopamine hydrochloride and digoxin may be necessary. **While endotracheal intubation and positive end-expiratory pressure (PEEP) ventilation with oxygen will relieve some of the hypoxia, the administration of corticosteroids has been of variable benefit. They may be of value in aborting the develop-ment of the adult respiratory distress syndrome.** DIC should be treated by the administration of cryoprecipitate and fresh frozen plasma.

Amniotic fluid embolism has occurred so infrequently that little is actually known as to the full pathophysiological events involved, except by conjecture. During the management of the patient, the events that occur are so rapid and catastrophic that little information has been developed as to the interplay of the various local and systemic responses of the organ systems in this condition. It would seem from animal experiments that the particulate matter itself plays a major role; however, the presence of vasoactive substances such as prostaglandins or other agents in the amniotic fluid, and their role in the production of the symptomatology of the amniotic fluid embolism syndrome, have not as yet been fully defined.

PART V

Reproductive endocrinology and fertility control

CHAPTER 40

Amenorrhea

1. Primary and secondary amenorrhea

a. Definitions

Amenorrhea (G., *a*, "without," + *men*, "month," +
rein, "to flow") is defined as an absence or cessation
of menstruation. **Primary amenorrhea** refers to an
absence of menses in a woman who is past the age of
14–16 years, who has never had a menstrual period,
and who has not developed secondary sexual characteristics. If secondary sexual development has occurred but there has been no menses by the age of 16,
then the patient should undergo investigation. **Secondary amenorrhea** has been defined as the absence of menses for either a period of 3 of the previous cycle lengths or 6 months. Thus, any woman with
a usual menstrual interval of 28 days duration may be
a candidate for investigation after 3 months of
amenorrhea. The designations of primary and secondary amenorrhea are no longer utilized in clinical practice, however, since such categorization of these patients has proven to be of only limited value.

*Reprinted with permission from Robert Bennett Bean, *Sir
William Osler: Aphorisms from His Bedside Teachings and
Writings,* William Bennett Bean, ed. Springfield, Ill.: Charles
C Thomas, Publisher, 1968, p. 37.

b. Diagnostic workup

The evaluation of either primary or secondary
amenorrhea requires a *systematic approach* to the hypothalamic-pituitary-ovarian axis and the uterine and
vaginal outflow tract. An interruption in the functioning of any one of the organ systems involved in the
cyclic hormonal control of the menstrual cycle may
result in amenorrhea. Furthermore, the presence of
certain congenital abnormalities of gonadal differentiation or function may be the underlying reason
for a primary amenorrhea.

*There are four times in a woman's life when
amenorrhea is considered to be "physiologic": (1)
prior to puberty, (2) during pregnancy, (3) during
lactation, and (4) after the menopause.*

The principles underlying the initial diagnostic
workup of the patient with amenorrhea involve the
interpretation of the history, the physical examination,
and some of the basic tests of genital system function.
**The organ systems that may be involved in the
development of amenorrhea are: (1) the uterus
and vagina, or the outflow tract** (e.g., imperforate
hymen; developmental abnormalities of the vagina,
cervix, or uterus; Asherman's syndrome; cervical stenosis), **(2) the ovary** (e.g., insensitive ovocytes, premature ovarian failure, hormone-producing tumors of
the ovary), **(3) the adrenal gland** (e.g., adrenal hyperplasia, adrenal tumors), **(4) the pituitary gland**
(e.g., pituitary insufficiency, pituitary tumors), **(5) the
thyroid gland** (e.g., hypothyroidism, hyperthyroidism), and **(6) the hypothalamus** (e.g., hypothalamic
dysfunction). In addition, **drugs** (e.g., oral contraceptives, phenothiazines), **psychological disorders**
(e.g., anxiety, stress, emotional shock, psychosis,
pseudocyesis), and **chromosomal abnormalities**
(e.g., testicular feminization syndrome, gonadal dysgenesis, Turner's syndrome) may cause amenorrhea.

535

2. Secondary sex characteristics not present

In patients who have not developed their secondary sex characteristics, a **gonadal abnormality** should be strongly suspected, since about 40% of these individuals will have a congenital abnormality involving the gonadal tissues. A buccal smear may be obtained to detect the presence of Barr bodies or the fluorescent Y chromosome. A more accurate determination of genetic sex may be obtained from a *karyotypic analysis using leukocytes.*

a. Turner's syndrome (45,X)

Turner's syndrome (45,X) may be obvious in patients who have no secondary sexual development and who present with the classic stigmata of the disease. These patients are usually short (less than 63 inches or 150–160 cm), have a webbed neck, high arched palate, low-set ears, shield chest, increased carrying angle at the elbow, short fourth metacarpal, coarctation of the aorta, and abnormalities of the genital system (streak gonads). In some cases of Turner's syndrome, mosaicism (XX/XO) may be present or there may be structurally abnormal X-chromosome problems (e.g., deletions, isochromosome formation, or a ring chromosome) that may allow the patient not only to menstruate, but even to bear children. In addition, these patients may have none of the stigmata of Turner's syndrome and may be of normal height. In some patients who have a mosaicism, there may be a silent Y chromosome present in the gonads, which should be removed prior to puberty. Probably all of the patients who have elevated levels of follicle-stimulating hormone (FSH) and luteinizing hormone (LH) should have a **karyotype** performed to rule out the diagnosis of Turner's syndrome. Patients with Turner's syndrome are said to have *gonadal dysgenesis.*

b. Swyer's syndrome (46,XY)

Another primary cause of amenorrhea is *Swyer's syndrome,* in which the patient has an **XY karyotype,** a palpable uterus, normal female testosterone values, and no secondary sexual development. The gonads, which consist of fibrous bands, should be removed as soon as the diagnosis is made, because of the presence of the Y chromosome and the risk of tumor formation.

3. Secondary sex characteristics present

In patients with amenorrhea who have already developed secondary sex characteristics, the evaluation should proceed in an orderly fashion. Any woman in the reproductive age group who has amenorrhea **must be considered to be pregnant until proven otherwise,** and a **pregnancy test** should be performed prior to the institution of the diagnostic workup and the administration of progesterone. **Initially, the thyroid-stimulating hormone (TSH) and prolactin levels should be determined and a progesterone challenge test should be performed.** ↳ what is this?

The **TSH value** will quickly allow you to determine whether the thyroid function is normal. If **hypothyroidism** is found, it may be easily corrected and normal menses restored with the administration of thyroxine. The **prolactin level** will occasionally also be elevated in hypothyroidism, but will almost always be below 100 ng/ml.

a. Abnormal outflow tract

Initially, it is important to define the presence of a functioning vagina, uterus, and ovaries in the patient who has developed secondary sexual characteristics. If you find an absent vagina on pelvic examination, then you should consider such syndromes as the Rokitansky-Kuster-Hauser syndrome and the testicular feminization syndrome.

In addition, some patients will develop intrauterine synechiae following a D&C after a pregnancy or an abortion and will cease to menstruate (Asherman's syndrome).

1) Gonadal organ absence/abnormality

During the physical examination, it is possible to detect such abnormalities of the genitalia as an imperforate hymen, a transverse vaginal septum, or the absence of either the uterus and/or the vagina. Rarely, the endometrial lining of the uterus will be missing.

A congenital absence of the vagina, the **Rokitan-**

sky-Kuster-Hauser syndrome (RKH), is usually associated with a rudimentary functioning uterus, cryptomenorrhea, and cyclic abdominal pain. Since this syndrome may be confused with the testicular feminization syndrome (TF), the finding of a testosterone level in the "female range" and a female **karyotype** will define the RKH syndrome. The testicular feminization syndrome patient will have an elevation of the **testosterone levels** to the normal "male range" of values and a male karyotype, in addition to the absence of the vagina. About one-third of these patients will have a renal tract abnormality, such as a horseshoe kidney or an abnormal collecting system. The treatment of the RKH patients consists of the creation of an artificial vagina by means of gradual dilatation with a vaginal dilator, or if there is a functioning uterus, then it must be determined whether a functioning uterus, vagina, and cervix can be surgically developed.

Those patients who have the **testicular feminization syndrome** or the complete androgen insensitivity syndrome clinically present as a phenotypic female; however, they are genetic males with a 46,XY karyotype (i.e., male pseudohermaphrodite). The testicular feminization syndrome is transmitted as an *X-linked recessive gene* that is responsible for the defective or abnormal intracellular androgen receptor. These individuals may be suspected because of their well-developed secondary sex characteristics *(i.e., breast growth)* and their *complete or partial lack of pubic and axillary hair* (due to their androgen insensitivity). The renal anomalies occur in both the RKH and TF syndromes. Usually in patients in whom the gonadal tissues contain a Y chromosome, the gonads should be removed prior to puberty to prevent undue masculinization and possible tumor formation. However, since patients with the testicular feminization syndrome have target cell receptors that are insensitive to androgens, the gonads should not be removed until after the individual has gained her full sexual development at puberty.

True hermaphroditism patients have both testicular and ovarian tissue present. They may present with either a male phenotype or as a female in appearance, even to the point of having menses. The gonads of these patients should be removed, since the incidence of gonadal tumors (i.e., gonadoblastoma, dysgerminoma, embryonal carcinoma, or choriocarcinoma) is about 25%. A malignancy due to the Y

chromosome has not been reported in these patients under the age of 20 years.

2) Test of the outflow tract

The progesterone challenge test assesses the outflow tract and the ovary. It determines the presence of: (1) adequate amounts of endogenous estrogen from the ovary, (2) the physical integrity of the uterine endometrium, and (3) the ability of the endometrium to be sloughed from the uterus through the cervix and vagina to the outside (i.e., the outflow tract). Progesterone (100–200 mg) should be administered intramuscularly, or it may be given orally as medroxyprogesterone acetate (Provera), 10 mg/day for seven days. Within 3–5 days after receiving the progesterone, the patient will withdraw from the hormone and manifest uterine bleeding, but only if there has been an adequate amount of endogenous estrogen stimulation present and if the uterus and the vagina are intact. Patients who respond with withdrawal bleeding and who do not have elevated prolactin levels may be considered to be *anovulatory, with a normal outflow tract.* Furthermore, patients who have normal prolactin levels, normal withdrawal bleeding, and no galactorrhea do not have a prolactin-secreting pituitary tumor.

Those patients who fail to bleed after a progesterone challenge test either do not have a sufficient amount of endogenous estrogen present to prime the uterus or do not have a functioning endometrium. In order to correct for this possible lack of estrogen, they should have **estrogen administered to them and then they should again be challenged with progesterone.** The administration of conjugated estrogens (Premarin), 2.5 mg/day for 21 days, plus medroxyprogesterone acetate (Provera), 10 mg/day from day 16–21, should result in withdrawal bleeding. This therapy should be repeated for one additional month if no bleeding occurs, in order to be certain that the test has been completely accurate and that the endometrium has been sufficiently stimulated by the estrogens to be able to respond to the progesterone administration.

If bleeding does occur after the administration of both estrogen and progesterone, then this indicates that the ovaries have failed, in which case the FSH and LH levels should be elevated. The finding of **elevated values of the gonadotropins (FSH and LH)** signifies ovarian failure or premature menopause in almost all cases. Exceptions to this are: (1) gonadotropin-producing carcinomas of the lung, (2) single gonadotropin deficiency, (3) early normal elevation of FSH in the perimenopausal period, (4) the resistant ovary syndrome (Savage syndrome), in which there are ovarian follicles present, but they are unresponsive to hormonal stimulation, and (5) a 17-hydroxylase deficiency, in which case there would be no secondary sexual characteristics present, due to the lack of the sex steroids.

Finally, the failure of the patient to bleed following the administration of both estrogen and progesterone may indicate that there is an end organ failure and that the endometrium is not functioning (e.g., Asherman's syndrome or congenital absence of the endometrium).

b. Ovary

Anovulation, with oligomenorrhea or amenorrhea, may occur whenever there is interference with the normal ovulatory process. When this condition persists for a period of time, the characteristic **polycystic ovary syndrome (PCO)** results (see Chapter 15). In contrast to the normal variations in the hormonal components of the normal menstrual cycle, during prolonged anovulation the LH levels become elevated and both LH and FSH assume a "steady state" level that does not fluctuate in the normal manner. **The LH will usually be more than 30 mIU/ml, whereas FSH will be normal or low. The elevated LH level stimulates the ovarian stroma to produce androstenedione and testosterone.** The androstenedione is converted by the extraglandular tissues to estrone, resulting in elevated estrone levels in the blood. These patients are therefore exposed to **unopposed estrogenic stimulation** of the endometrium and are at risk for abnormal endometrial changes (e.g., adenomatous hyperplasia or adenocarcinoma of the endometrium). In addition, due to the suppression of the sex hormone binding globulin (SHBG), there is an increase in the free testosterone levels. Normally, 80% of the circulating testosterone will be tightly bound to β-globulin, or SHBG, 19% will be loosely bound to albumin, and 1% will be free. Since hirsutism is due to the free fraction, this value may be increased up to 2% in hirsute women. **The increased circulating free testosterone levels that are seen in PCO syndrome result in clinical hirsutism.** The normal free testosterone level will be about 20–80 ng/dl. The treatment of hirsutism in this condition consists of the administration of birth control pills to suppress the secretion of LH and FSH, which will eliminate the ovarian stromal stimulation and decrease the secretion of the androgens. The hirsutism can also be treated by the administration of spironolactone (Aldactone), which effectively competes with testosterone for the androgen receptors at the hair follicle level.

c. Hirsutism

Excess androgen secretion may be produced by either the ovary or the adrenal glands (Fig. 40-1). Patients who have **hirsutism** or virilization will present with **oligomenorrhea/amenorrhea,** due to the effects of the elevated androgens. Whenever there is a significant amount of hirsutism to cause amenorrhea, then the patient should be evaluated thoroughly. *Patients with severe virilization or masculinization will usually show the advanced effects of androgens, such as hirsutism, increased muscle mass, deepening of the voice, clitoral enlargement, acne, and a male hair pattern with temporal balding.*

1) Cushing's syndrome

Cushing's syndrome, or hyperadrenocorticism, may occur as a result of an overproduction of ACTH (Cushing's disease), as an ectopic ACTH tumor, as an autonomous adrenal tumor (Cushing's syndrome), or with the exogenous administration of corticosteroids. The overnight dexamethasone test consists of the administration of dexamethasone, 1 mg administered at bedtime, followed by a **plasma cortisol** at 8:00 A.M. The normal value should be less than 5–6 μg/dl. When a 2-mg low-dose suppression test is administered for two days in these patients after two days of baseline urinary 17-hydroxysteroid measurements, those patients who have Cushing's syndrome will not suppress their urinary 17-hydroxysteroids below 4 mg per day.

If the 8-mg high-dose dexamethasone suppression test is carried out for two days along with a comparison of the basal levels of the blood ACTH and the urinary 17-hydroxysteroids, then the following findings may be noted: (1) if the basal ACTH is not detectable and there is not a decrease in the urinary 17-hydroxysteroid levels by a minimum of 40%, then

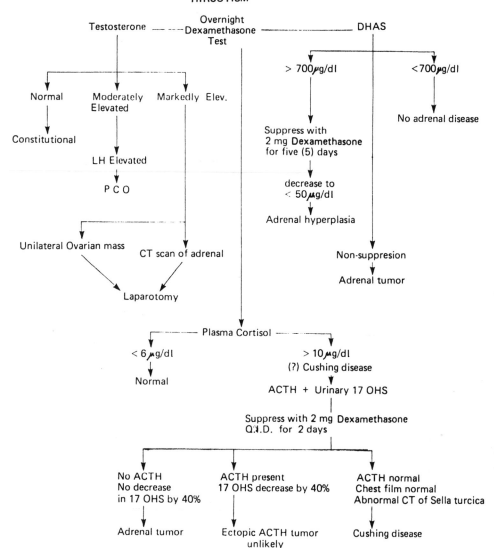

FIGURE 40-1. Suggested flow chart for the diagnosis of hirsutism.

the diagnosis is an adrenal tumor; (2) if the 17-hydroxysteroids decrease by at least 40% and the blood levels of ACTH can be detected, then an ectopic ACTH tumor is probably not present; and (3) if the following findings, such as an abnormal sella turcica on CT scanning, a normal chest film, and a normal ACTH blood level is found, then Cushing's disease is present.

Dehydroisoandrosterone sulfate (DHAS) is derived almost exclusively from the adrenal gland. The normal level (upper limit) is 250 μg/dl. It may be elevated in association with an elevated prolactin level for unknown reasons. If it is normal in the face of a clinical androgen excess, then the androgens that are causing the hirsutism are originating from the ovary. **If the androgens are produced by the**

adrenal gland, then the DHAS will be elevated. Levels of up to 700 μg/dl may be found in cases of polycystic ovary syndrome (PCO), and these patients apparently do not need any further evaluation, according to some experts. If the DHAS levels are over 800 μg/ml, an adrenal tumor should be suspected and an intravenous pyelogram (IVP) and a computerized tomography (CT) scan of the adrenal gland should be obtained. If the DHAS is suppressed by dexamethasone (2 mg q.i.d. for five days) and a DHAS value is obtained on the fourth day, then with these results the following diagnoses may be entertained: (1) if there is no decrease in DHAS, then the diagnosis is an autonomous adrenal tumor, and (2) if the DHAS decreases to less than 50 μg/dl, then the diagnosis is adrenal hyperplasia.

2) Adrenal hyperplasia

Patients with **adrenal hyperplasia** (i.e., 21-hydroxylase, or 11-β-hydroxylase deficiency) should have elevated blood levels of 17-hydroxyprogesterone. Adrenal hyperplasia, adenomas, or carcinoma may cause hirsutism and amenorrhea.

3) Androgenic tumors of the ovary

Androgen-producing tumors of the ovary are usually palpable, but not always (see Chapter 15). They include the arrhenoblastoma (the Sertoli-Leydig cell tumor), the hilar cell tumor, and the adrenal rest cell tumor. Other tumors that *stimulate the stroma of the ovary* to produce androgens are Krukenberg tumors and mucinous cystadenomas. The ingestion of exogenous androgens can cause drug-induced hirsutism in female patients who practice muscle building and power lifting. **Testosterone levels** in ovarian lesions are usually over 200 ng/ml, if the DHAS levels are normal.

d. Pituitary lesions and galactorrhea syndromes

Certain nonneoplastic lesions of the pituitary gland may result in amenorrhea. When there has been destruction of the pituitary gland due to postpartum hypoxia, thrombosis, or hemorrhage **(Sheehan's syndrome)** or by infectious process **(Simmonds' disease),** panhypopituitarism may occur, which will result in amenorrhea.

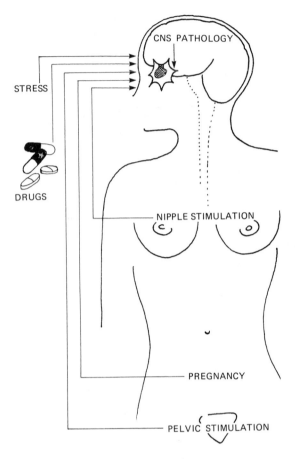

FIGURE 40-2. Causes of hyperprolactinemia.

Tumors of the pituitary gland, such as a chromophobe adenoma, a basophilic tumor (Cushing's disease), or acidophilic tumors (acromegaly or giantism) may also cause amenorrhea. These patients usually do not respond to a progesterone challenge because they have low gonadotropin levels. The **sella turcica** will usually be enlarged on X-ray films whenever there is a pituitary tumor present.

Pituitary tumors are often associated with **galactorrhea** and have **elevated levels of prolactin** present (Fig. 40-2). These tumors may be microadenomas (less than 1 cm in diameter) or macroadenomas (more than 1 cm in diameter). Due to the small size of the microadenomas, a **CT scan** is required to detect these lesions. The old eponyms of the Chiari-Frommel syndrome (galactorrhea and amenorrhea following a pregnancy), Ahumada-del Castillo syndrome (galactorrhea and amenorrhea unrelated to pregnancy), and the Forbes-Albright syndrome (galactorrhea and amenorrhea associated with a pituitary tumor) are no longer used, since they all appear to be due to either micro or macroadenomas of the pituitary gland. **It should be remembered that breast suckling, surgical trauma or stress, hypothyroidism, and drug ingestion may also cause hyperprolactinemia, galactorrhea, and oligomenorrhea.**

The treatment of patients with microprolactinomas may take either a medical or a surgical approach. *Transsphenoidal hypophysectomy* is the most common surgical approach, whereas the use of *bromocriptine mesylate* (Parlodel), 5–10 mg per day, has been an effective medical treatment. Usually, the lowest possible dose of bromocriptine is utilized to suppress the prolactin levels. A prolactin determination and a visual field examination should be obtained every 6–12 months, as well as a magnetic resonance image (MRI) scanning of the pituitary every 1–2 years in these patients. Due to the normalization of the prolactin levels with the bromocriptine treatment, pregnancy may occur in these women.

e. Hypothalamic amenorrhea

1) Anorexia nervosa

Low gonadotropin levels may be seen in patients who have a tumor of the pituitary or who have hypothalamic amenorrhea secondary to the suppression of the pulsatile gonadotropin releasing hormone (GnRH) below a critical level (e.g., due to anorexia and/or weight loss). **Anorexia nervosa occurs in young women who have a distortion of their body image and can result in a weight loss of up to 25%.** The patient may experience episodes of overeating (binge eating), followed by self-induced vomiting (purge-gorge syndrome, or bulimia). Some authors separate anorexia nervosa from bulimia and classify the anorexic patient who also has bulimia as a "bulimia nervosa," or a "bulimorexic."

The young anorexia nervosa patient will have a strong desire to be thin and may be very achievement oriented. Amenorrhea, constipation, hypotension, hyperactivity, bradycardia, edema, hypercarotenemia, and a mild partial diabetes insipidus may be present in these patients. There is a decreased release of the gonadotropin releasing factor (GnRH), and a resultant decrease in the secretion of FSH and LH, which causes a decrease in estrogen production in the ovary. Due to the low estrogen levels, these patients will generally not respond to a progesterone challenge test, in contrast to the anovulatory patient with simple weight loss, who will experience withdrawal bleeding after progesterone administration. A reversal of the hypogonadotropic hypogonadism with a return of the menses may occur if the dietary carotene is lowered in the hypercarotenemic patient. A gain in body weight will also assist in reestablishing a normal menstrual pattern. Estrogen replacement therapy (ERT) and intermittent progesterone therapy should be administered to hypoestrogenic patients in an effort to prevent osteoporosis. Birth control pills may accomplish this replacement and also may prevent the occurrence of an unwanted pregnancy. Nutritional and psychiatric counseling should be carried out in these patients.

2) Exercise amenorrhea

Recently, a new form of amenorrhea has been identified in women who exercise, especially in marathon runners and in ballet dancers. Often these women fall below a "critical weight," which in terms of body fat seems to be about the 10th percentile. A loss of body weight of about 10–15% of the normal weight for height will result in a loss of one-third of the body fat, which will be less than the 22% value which seems to be necessary to maintain normal menstruation. Competitive female athletes may fall even further below the 10th percentile, or the 22% body fat line, and develop secondary amenorrhea. It has been thought that the release of the endogenous opioid **beta-endorphin** by the exercise activity may suppress the GnRH pulsatile secretion at the arcuate nucleus. It has been shown that the administration of naloxone hydrochloride (Narcan), an opioid inhibitor, will restore the pulsatile pattern of secretion. **It also increases the levels of prolactin, by suppressing hypothalamic dopamine secretion.** The treatment of these patients consists of decreasing the amount of exercise and promoting weight gain. If the patient will not decrease her exercise level, then hormone replacement therapy will be necessary to prevent osteoporosis.

3) Kallmann's syndrome

A rare congenital syndrome of **hypogonadotropic hypogonadism** that is associated with **anosmia**

(Kallmann's syndrome) is characterized by primary amenorrhea, sexual infantilism, low gonadotropins, a normal female karyotype, and an inability to smell strong odors. These patients will not respond to clomiphene citrate (Clomid) ovulation induction, but may respond to exogenous gonadotropin stimulation. The use of priming doses of luteinizing hormone releasing hormone (LHRH), a hypothalamic decapeptide, has demonstrated a normal LH response in these patients.

4) Drug ingestion

An elevated prolactin level (i.e., higher than 20 ng/ml) may occur in association with the administration of phenothiazines, birth control pills, or in the presence of a pituitary microadenoma or macroadenoma. If the patient has **galactorrhea** (even without amenorrhea), a coned down view of the sella turcica should be ordered. These patients may bleed after a progesterone challenge.

CHAPTER 41

Abnormal uterine bleeding

. . . .

Patients should have rest, food, fresh air, and exercise—the quadrangle of health.

—*Sir William Osler**

. . . .

1. Dysfunctional uterine bleeding

a. Definition

Dysfunctional uterine bleeding (DUB) may be defined as uterine bleeding that occurs due to variations in the secretion of estrogen and progesterone and/or abnormalities of hormone receptor interaction. This is in contrast to **uterine bleeding due to organic disease,** such as occurs as a result of neoplasms, infection, pregnancy, or other pathologic conditions that affect the uterus.

About 10% of dysfunctional bleeding occurs as a result of defective ovulation, such as: (1) a shortening of either the proliferative or the secretory phase of the cycle (e.g., a corpus luteum deficiency or luteal phase defect), or (2) a prolongation of the corpus luteum activity (i.e., persistent corpus luteum). Polymenorrhea and oligomenorrhea are common in these patients.

b. Corpus luteum problems

The presence of a corpus luteum insufficiency (i.e., luteal phase defect) occurs in about 3.5%

*Reprinted with permission from Robert Bennett Bean, *Sir William Osler: Aphorisms from His Bedside Teachings and Writings,* William Bennett Bean, ed. Springfield, Ill.: Charles C Thomas, Publisher, 1968, p. 98.

of infertility patients and in perhaps 35% of patients who have a history of habitual abortion. The patient may give a history of a bleeding pattern that may include intermenstrual spotting, menorrhagia, or polymenorrhea. An endometrial biopsy during the latter half of the cycle will show that the endometrium is out of phase with the chronological date by at least two days on two consecutive cycles.

On occasion, the function of the corpus luteum may be prolonged with a persistent or prolonged secretion of progesterone (i.e., Halban's disease, or persistent corpus luteum). The histologic picture is one of a decidua-like transformation of the endometrium, which is due to the persistent progesterone influence. Clinically, the patient presents with 6–8 weeks of amenorrhea followed by spotting and the finding of an ovarian corpus luteum cyst on the pelvic examination. The differential diagnosis of the patient's problem must include the diagnosis of an ectopic pregnancy, which may present with similar findings. An ultrasonic evaluation and a specific pregnancy test may differentiate the two syndromes (see Chapter 27).

c. Anovulation

About 90% of dysfunctional uterine bleeding occurs as a result of anovulation. It occurs most commonly in patients who are at the extremes of the reproductive life—the teenage years and the perimenopausal years. During these times, the menstrual periods may become irregular in interval, duration, and flow. It was demonstrated in one study that the menstrual periods in these patients may be of normal length (50%), associated with oligomenorrhea (28%) or with polymenorrhea (22%). It is then evident that the menstrual pattern in patients who

menorrhagia - excessive uterine bleed

have anovulation may be quite variable. Due to the unopposed estrogen stimulation that occurs with anovulation, breakthrough bleeding may often occur intermenstrually. **If an anovulatory pattern persists, the unopposed estrogenic stimulation of the endometrial lining of the uterus is thought to produce adenomatous hyperplasia initially, then atypical hyperplasia, and then finally adenocarcinoma of the endometrium.** Menorrhagia is more commonly found in association with hyperplasia, whereas menometrorrhagia may occur with carcinoma. *excessive bleeding during menses & irreg intervals*

Psychological stress has been shown to be associated with an elevation of neurotransmitters, such as norepinephrine and serotonin, and with a decreased excretion of dopamine. Norepinephrine also may have an effect on LH secretion. **It has been suggested that the polycystic ovary syndrome in certain patients may be related to an imbalance in these hormones secondary to psychological stress.** Women who were captured during World War II developed amenorrhea **(i.e., "war amenorrhea")** long before the effects of malnutrition could produce such an effect. Recently, it has been noted that women who **exercise excessively** (i.e., marathon runners, ballet dancers) may experience amenorrhea secondary to perhaps an increased opioid activity **(i.e., endorphin secretion)** (see Chapters 4 and 40). Certainly, the central nervous system has some degree of control over the menstrual cycle, since traumatic events in the patient's life may often precipitate amenorrhea or irregular menstruation.

d. Treatment

The treatment of dysfunctional uterine bleeding should be individualized according to the age of the patient, her desire for fertility, and other factors.

1) Adolescent age group

In the first few years after menarche, about 50% of a woman's menstrual cycles are anovulatory, probably secondary to the immaturity of the hypothalamic-pituitary-ovarian axis. You should keep in mind that a pregnancy may be present in sexually active adolescents as the reason for amenorrhea or irregular bleeding. Generally, menstrual irregularities are not considered to be significant in this age group, as long as they do not lead to a severe anemia, and as long as the pelvic examination is entirely normal. Young girls with **leukemia,** however, will occasionally present with menorrhagia. A peripheral blood smear should show the early blast forms in these patients. The influence of *emotional or psychological factors* on the menstrual cycle is well known. Young women will often have a disruption of their menstrual cycles when: (1) they first go away to school or college, (2) they have their first sexual experience, (3) they get married, divorced, or widowed, and in other stressful situations.

The treatment of menstrual irregularity in the adolescent usually consists of *observation* in most cases, with the patient using a **menstrual calendar** to document her periods. The hemoglobin and hematocrit levels should be monitored and oral iron therapy should be utilized as necessary. The use of medroxyprogesterone acetate (Provera), 10 mg per day from day 13 to day 25, will frequently serve to regulate the menstrual cycles. In some instances, especially if the woman is sexually active, *birth control pills* will serve to not only regulate the cycles, but will also provide protection against an unwanted pregnancy.

In some patients with heavy bleeding who are severely anemic (e.g., hemoglobin of less than 6 grams/100 ml), hospitalization should be considered. You should be certain that there are no coagulation defects in the patient and that she does not have hypothyroidism.

2) Reproductive age group

During the reproductive years, conditions other than dysfunctional bleeding may be present to account for a history of irregular vaginal bleeding. **Pregnancy must always be ruled out,** since both a threatened abortion or an ectopic pregnancy may present in this manner. Blood dyscrasia or uterine and cervical pathology may also be present and must be eliminated as a consideration before therapy for DUB can be instituted.

In the absence of pregnancy, *acute severe bleeding* may require the use of intravenous conjugated estrogens (Premarin), 25 mg q4h, for three doses or until the bleeding decreases. At the same time that the I.V. Premarin is started, the oral estrogen (Premarin) should be begun, using 2.5–7.5 mg per day for 21 days, with the addition of medroxyprogesterone acetate (Provera), 10 mg per day, for the last 10 days (i.e., day 15–25). Alternately, if the bleeding is not so profuse, the administration of combination birth control pills, 1 tablet 3–4 times per day, should cause a cessation of the blood flow within 12–24 hours in a majority of patients.

In patients who have irregular menses only, with no acute hemorrhaging, the administration of *birth control pills* for about three months will usually regulate the menstrual cycles.

3) Perimenopausal age group

The occurrence of abnormal vaginal bleeding in a patient who is beyond the age of 40 years has a greater likelihood of being due to neoplastic causes than in the younger age groups. It is especially important in these women to be certain that a genital neoplasia is not involved. *As a consequence, it is mandatory that the endometrium be evaluated by either a thorough endometrial biopsy (multiple sampling technique) or, better still, by a fractional dilatation and curettage (D&C), prior to the initiation of therapy.* **If endometrial adenomatous hyperplasia is found, then a total abdominal (or vaginal) hysterectomy should be considered, since this is a premalignant lesion.** The finding of a proliferative endometrium or a cystic hyperplasia of the endometrium on the biopsy is indicative of an anovulatory menstrual pattern. *In perimenopausal patients with anovulatory bleeding, the use of medroxyprogesterone acetate (Provera), 10 mg per day from day 13 to day 25 of each menstrual cycle, will provide an effective withdrawal of the endometrium on a regular continuing basis.* **Such therapy is currently thought to be protective in preventing adenocarcinoma of the endometrium, and perhaps also may be protective in preventing breast carcinoma.** As long as the patient has enough endogenous estrogen to prime her endometrium, the progesterone therapy will be effective and will result in an orderly monthly menstruation. **If at any time during therapy the bleeding should again become irregular, then organic causes must be considered and appropriate steps taken to identify the cause of the bleeding (e.g., fractional D&C).** If the patient has repeated attacks of irregular bleeding in spite of hormonal treatment, or

if she has had repeated D&C's, then definitive therapy is indicated in the perimenopausal patient. A hysterectomy should be performed in such patients, after first being certain that a carcinoma of the endometrium is not present.

Recently, an alternative to hysterectomy for **severe menorrhagia** has been recommended. This technique involves the use of the **laser** to ablate the endometrium. It has been shown to be safe and has about a 97% success rate. About 50% of these patients will not have any further menses, while the other half will have only slight spotting at the time of their menses. This procedure would be quite valuable in the treatment of some high-risk patients for hysterectomy; however, either a general or spinal anesthetic may still be required. This technique should not be utilized in patients in whom there is a history of pelvic inflammatory disease or in whom a premalignant endometrial lesion has been identified. The uterus must be sounded one month postoperatively to prevent the development of a hematometra or a pyometra due to cervical stenosis.

2. Menorrhagia

The loss of more than 80 ml of blood during menstruation has been defined as primary **menorrhagia.** While this may occur in as many as 2–10% of women, its etiology often remains obscure. Recently, the prostaglandin cascade has been implicated in the etiology of this condition.

The endometrium and myometrium are capable of producing both prostacyclin and thromboxane A_2. **Prostacyclin, a potent vasodilator,** originates primarily in the endothelial cells in the vessel wall. Prostacyclin *inhibits* platelet aggregation and in addition produces tachycardia, flushing, hypotension, and the stimulation of the renin-angiotensin-aldosterone system. It also causes an increase in the blood levels of glucose, glucagon, prolactin, and cortisol.

Thromboxane A_2 is produced from cyclic peroxides through the action of thromboxane synthetase in various tissues, such as the platelets, the vascular walls, and the endometrium or myometrium. Thromboxane A_2 is a potent vasoconstrictor and *can cause platelet aggregation.*

It has been noted that there is often an increase in the level of prostaglandin E in the en-

dometrium of women who have menorrhagia. Furthermore, it has been shown that **prostacyclin will promote menorrhagia** and that this agent may be produced by the cooperation of both the endometrium and the myometrium. The balance between prostacyclin and thromboxane A_2 in the uterine tissues therefore may be important in the etiology of menorrhagia. **If there is a dominance of prostacyclin, then the patient may experience primary menorrhagia, whereas if the F series of the prostaglandins are predominately present in the uterine tissues, then dysmenorrhea may be produced instead of menorrhagia.**

CHAPTER 42

Menstrual problems

Consider the virtues of taciturnity. Speak only when you
have something to say.

—*Sir William Osler**

1. Dysmenorrhea

a. Incidence

Painful menstruation (i.e., dysmenorrhea) may be
found in more than 50% of all women, and in about
10% of these patients the pain will be severe enough
to cause incapacitation for 1–3 days each month. In
the United States alone, the absenteeism of adolescents from school because of this entity approaches
25%. Furthermore, in some studies it has been found
that those adolescents who had dysmenorrhea also
had lower grades in their school work and had a
poorer adjustment to the school environment.

b. Symptoms

The symptoms of dysmenorrhea may be characterized
by the presence of cramping pains in the lower abdomen that may be associated with nausea and vomiting
(89%), fatigue (85%), diarrhea (60%), lower backache
(60%), headache (45%), dizziness, and various degrees of nervousness. The initial onset of dysmenorrhea usually occurs within two years of menarche
in 88% of the patients. These symptoms generally last

*Reprinted with permission from Robert Bennett Bean, *Sir
William Osler: Aphorisms from His Bedside Teachings and
Writings,* William Bennett Bean, ed. Springfield, Ill.: Charles
C Thomas, Publisher, 1968, p. 89.

for about 2–3 days each month; however, they may
seriously interfere with the patient's activities and life-
style.

c. Etiology

Clinically, dysmenorrhea has been divided into primary and secondary dysmenorrhea. Primary dysmenorrhea is not associated with any significant pathology, whereas secondary dysmenorrhea may often be
associated with pathologic conditions such as endometriosis or pelvic inflammatory disease.

1) Primary dysmenorrhea

The etiology of primary dysmenorrhea has been attributed to such conditions as psychological factors,
cervical stenosis, uterine ischemia, an increase in
prostaglandin release, and an increase in the vasopressin levels. It has been noted that **ovulatory cycles** are almost always associated with mild dysmenorrhea. The presence of **cervical stenosis** also
seems to be associated with dysmenorrhea, since dysmenorrhea usually disappears after the first vaginal
delivery, when the cervix has been dilated with the
delivery of the fetus.

2) Secondary dysmenorrhea

Since **endometriosis** may occasionally occur in
young girls, this diagnosis must always be kept in
mind. Typically, pelvic adhesions due to endometriosis usually occur at a later time. **Adenomyosis** is
also associated with dysmenorrhea. Some of the other
causes of dysmenorrhea include such conditions as
pelvic inflammatory disease or the use of an **intrauterine contraceptive device (IUD).** Those patients who have **chronic pelvic pain,** which may be

due to a variety of different causes, may also have dysmenorrhea as part of the clinical picture.

d. Treatment

There is some evidence to indicate that abnormal uterine contractions are caused by an increased production and release of prostaglandins. The muscular contractions that are produced by these agents result in ischemia and hypoxia of the uterus. The use of **prostaglandin (PGF$_{2\alpha}$)** for the induction of labor produces symptoms similar to those that occur with primary dysmenorrhea. In addition, since there is a higher concentration of prostaglandins present in the secretory endometrium, the presence of uterine cramps with ovulation (and their absence with anovulation) would further support the role of prostaglandins in the production of dysmenorrhea. Finally, those medications that are prostaglandin synthetase inhibitors are highly effective in the treatment of dysmenorrhea, indicating again that the basic mechanism for the development of dysmenorrhea is most likely due to the presence of the prostaglandins.

The various treatment regimens that have been suggested become more sensible in light of this concept of the etiology of dysmenorrhea. Although analgesics may be used in mild cases, **oral contraceptive pills** will decrease the level of prostaglandins present in the endometrium by suppressing endometrial growth and ovulation, and thus dysmenorrhea will not occur. In addition, **prostaglandin synthetase inhibitors,** such as ibuprofen, naproxen sodium, and ketoprofen (type I inhibitors), interfere with the production of prostaglandins between the arachidonic acid metabolic step and the production of cyclic endoperoxides, whereas agents such as phenylbutazone (type II inhibitors) interfere with the further conversion of the endoperoxides to PGE or PGF$_{2\alpha}$. **In either case, the prostaglandin cascade is blocked at various levels and the dysmenorrhea is relieved.** The type I inhibitors appear to be more effective than the type II ones due to their inhibition of the endoperoxides, which are potent uterotonic agents.

In most instances, medical therapy utilizing the prostaglandin synthetase inhibitors will effectively relieve the symptoms of dysmenorrhea. *In addition, agents such as mefenamic acid may also reduce the amount of menstrual flow in those individuals who have menorrhagia.*

Those patients who do not obtain relief from their symptoms with an adequate trial of medical therapy should be investigated further to determine the possible presence of other pathologic conditions. Dilatation of the cervix is indicated if cervical stenosis is suspected. The removal of an intrauterine device (IUD) may be necessary, since the IUD causes a leukocytic infiltration and an increased prostaglandin production in the endometrium; however, the administration of a prostaglandin synthetase inhibitor usually relieves the dysmenorrhea without requiring the removal of the IUD. **The presence of persistent dysmenorrhea that is unresponsive to medical therapy may require a diagnostic hysteroscopy or a laparoscopy to determine the exact diagnosis.**

2. Premenstrual syndrome (PMS)

a. Incidence

The premenstrual syndrome (PMS) was first described by **H. T. Frank** in 1931. This syndrome has drawn increasing attention over the past few years, because there are perhaps as many as 10 to 12 million women in the United States who suffer from this condition. With more than 50% of the women in the work force having this syndrome, the loss of time from work and the loss of efficiency in the workplace have important economic implications. In addition, there have been legal ramifications with regard to the personal accountability of women who have PMS and who commit criminal acts during the period of time just prior to the onset of their menses.

b. Symptoms

The patient with premenstrual syndrome may experience irritability, tension, combativeness, mastodynia, fluid retention, bloating, constipation, insomnia, fatigue, emotional lability, alterations in libido, and changes in her appetite. In addition, she may have a desire for sweets and salty foods, an inability to concentrate, poor judgment, motor incoordination, and a desire to withdraw from the company of others. *These symptoms begin at about 7–14 days prior to the onset of menses and generally resolve at the beginning of menstruation.* It has been shown that women who have shorter cycles (i.e., 20–24 days) have more autonomic and physical symptoms than those who have cycles of a normal length (i.e., 25–30 days).

Some authors have described four types of premenstrual syndrome: (1) **PMS-A** (80–90%), which consists of anxiety, nervousness, and irritability, (2) **PMS-H** (60–65%), which consists of edema, abdominal bloating, weight gain, and breast tenderness, (3) **PMS-C** (40%), which consists of an abnormal craving for sweets associated with fatigue, palpitation, syncope, and headaches, and (4) **PMS-D** (less than 3%), which consists of symptoms of an affective disorder, such as depression and withdrawal.

c. Etiology
1) Progesterone deficiency

While the cause of PMS is unknown, a number of investigators have suggested that the symptoms of PMS may be due to a relative **lack of progesterone** that occurs in the luteal phase of the menstrual cycle (PMS-A), which results in a relative estrogen excess. Controlled studies do not support this theory, however.

2) Hypoglycemia

Previous studies have reported that there may be an increased carbohydrate intolerance in patients with PMS. This increased hypoglycemia during the luteal phase supposedly resulted in symptoms of hunger, fatigue, and nervousness (PMS-C). Recently, this theory has been refuted.

3) Vitamin B_6 deficiency

Vitamin B_6 (pyridoxine) deficiency has also been proposed as a possible cause of the headaches, breast changes, emotional lability, and tension in PMS. In one placebo-controlled study, however, pyridoxine treatment was found to be effective only in reducing tension, anxiety, and irritability.

4) Fluid retention

The symptoms of fluid retention have been recognized as being part of the PMS syndrome for many years and have resulted in the widespread use of diuretics to treat this condition in clinical practice. The edema and abdominal bloating of PMS has also been attributed to aldosteronism (PMS-H); however,

the serum aldosterone has not been found to be significantly increased in PMS in controlled studies.

5) Psychosomatic dysfunction

While psychosomatic dysfunction has been implicated in PMS, there has been limited evidence to support this etiology.

6) Endogenous hormone allergy

An allergic reaction by the patient to the endogenous progesterone hormone has been suggested as a possible etiology for PMS; however, there has been little evidence to support such a contention.

7) Psychiatric disease

When the symptoms of an affective disorder are mimicked by depression and withdrawal symptoms (PMS-D) in the patient, psychiatric referral should be considered, since suicide may be a real risk; however, most investigators do not consider PMS to be a psychiatric disease. Recently, the American Psychiatric Association has suggested that this disease may be a psychiatric disease and has termed it the **"premenstrual dysphoric disorder" (PDD), or the "late luteal phase dysphoric disorder." PDD has been defined as a disorder that has at least four of the following symptoms present during the week prior to menses:** (1) affective lability, (2) persistent and marked anger or irritability, (3) anxiety and tenseness, (4) depression, (5) decreased interest in friends, hobbies, etc., (6) easy fatiguability and a lack of energy, (7) difficulty in concentrating, (8) changes in appetite, with special food craving, (9) insomnia or hypersomnia, and (10) other symptoms such as breast swelling or tenderness, bloating, and weight gain. This disorder may be severe enough to interfere with the patient's work and other activities. It is not, however, considered to be a continuation of other disorders, such as panic disorders, dysthymic disorders, or personality disorders. The above information may be obtained by daily self-ratings by the patient over the course of two menstrual cycles.

There has been considerable controversy concerning the labeling of the 10–12 million women in the population who have this disorder as having a "psychiatric disease." The effects of this kind of "psychiatric" diagnosis on the social, psychological, emotional, and business aspects of a woman's life could be catastrophic.

8) Endogenous opiate peptides (EOP)

Recently, it has been suggested that the etiology of PMS may be related to changes in the **endogenous opiate peptide (EOP)** activity during the menstrual cycle. There has been increasing evidence that the EOPs function as neurotransmitters and that they may have an influence on the individual's mood and behavior. The levels of EOPs are apparently influenced centrally by progesterone alone or in combination with estrogen, both of which are present in the luteal phase. With the abrupt withdrawal of the EOPs as the progesterone/estrogen levels fall just prior to menstruation, it is thought that the clinical manifestations of PMS may be triggered. It has been shown that there are lower levels of EOPs in patients who have symptoms of PMS during the luteal phase. Indeed, the use of high doses of naloxone hydrochloride (an opiate receptor antagonist) in normal women has been shown to produce a variety of symptoms identical to those of PMS.

Decreased levels of EOPs during the mid-luteal phase may account for the binge eating due to stimulation of the appetite in some PMS patients. The decreased release of norepinephrine or dopamine, due to the inhibition of the biogenic amines by the EOPs, might also account for the fatigue and depression that is seen in PMS patients. The withdrawal of the EOPs might result in a rebound hyperactivity in the nervous system, which might result in aggression, irritability, anxiety, and tension. It has been postulated that the effect of the EOPs on inhibiting the prostaglandin E_1-stimulated fluid secretion and its effect on the bowel (i.e., decreased peristalsis) may be responsible for the bloating and constipation that are seen in the luteal phase, and also for the diarrhea that occurs in some women just prior to menstruation as the EOPs fall and the effects of prostaglandin are again exerted on the bowel.

d. Treatment

The treatment of PMS in the past has consisted of many different approaches, none of which have been successful in all patients. The use of *birth control pills* in the younger patient, who may also have concomitant dysmenorrhea, has usually been effective. While the use of *diuretics* has been widespread, their effect on PMS symptoms has not been well documented. In those patients who show clear evidence of recurrent weight gain and edema in the luteal phase, the judicious use of diuretics may be of some value. A decrease in the intake of salt by the patient may also be of benefit. The use of spironolactone, 25 mg p.o., q.i.d., for 7 days just prior to menses, has also been advocated to decrease the amount of water retention. *Bromocriptine (2.5 mg b.i.d., p.o. for 10 days)* and *Danocrine (200 mg b.i.d. p.o.) have also been successfully used in the treatment of mastodynia.*

The regulation of the patient's diet by the reduction of carbohydrates and the elimination of chocolate and caffeine has been suggested and seems to be somewhat effective in the treatment of some of these patients. Supplementation with vitamin B_6, 25–100 mg b.i.d., has also been used; however, its effectiveness has not been well documented and doses of more than 2 grams per day may be associated with the development of neurological symptoms. Oil of evening primrose (linoleic acid), calcium, zinc, and tryptophan, which can be obtained over the counter, have been used in PMS, but there is no documented evidence of any benefit in the administration of most of these agents.

Tranquilizers have been used to alter the mood of patients with PMS; however, the use of these drugs in these patients has not been researched adequately. Stress reduction and counseling have a strong placebo effect and have also been advocated. The administration of progesterone, 200–800 mg/day by vaginal suppository, from the onset of symptoms to the beginning of the menses, has been suggested by some authors as definitive treatment. Prostaglandin synthetase inhibitors, such as mefenamic acid have been found to be effective in the treatment of dysmenorrhea but have generally been thought to be ineffective in the treatment of patients with premenstrual syndrome. Psychotherapy and the use of tricyclic antidepressants have not been found to be effective in the treatment of PMS, although patients with manic behavior or severe depressive symptoms probably should have a psychiatric evaluation. Most PMS patients are normal, healthy individuals the majority of the time, and the traditional psychiatric therapeutic approach may be inappropriate in these patients. Lithium carbonate (600–1,800 mg/day p.o.) has been used with some success in patients who have cyclothymic behavior; however, this agent is not generally indicated in PMS.

3. Mastalgia

Some women experience a cyclic discomfort in their breasts in association with their menstrual periods. This condition has been termed **mastalgia.** The use of diuretics in these patients has been strongly advocated in the past; however, these drugs have proved to be of little benefit. The treatment of the patient with testosterone in small doses (5 mg methyltestosterone every other day) has been advocated, but care should be taken that virilization of the patient does not occur. *Recently, danazol (100–400 mg/day) has been found to be effective in decreasing the breast discomfort in these patients.* The use of vitamin E (600 units/day of tocopherol acetate) has also been found to be effective.

CHAPTER 43

Menopause

. . . .

Never let your tongue say a slighting word of a colleague.

—Sir William Osler*

1. Perimenopause

a. Symptoms

As the ovarian function begins to wane during the perimenopausal years, estrogen deprivation will be manifested clinically by the onset of **vasomotor instability (hot flushes), insomnia, irritability, fatigue, headaches, depression, loss of libido, loss of concentrating ability, poor mental performance, nervousness, and mood changes.** The **hot flushes,** which may occur at any time during the day or night, are present in 85% of women in the perimenopausal years. They last on an average of about 2.0–4.7 minutes and are associated with a slight elevation in the heart rate. There is an increased amount of heat and redness to the skin of the face, the neck, and the upper anterior chest during the hot flush. These vasomotor episodes often occur at night and produce profuse **sweating,** which may interfere with the patient's sleep. The hot flush is associated with a surge of circulating LH, and the patient will usually have a prodromal awareness of the impending flush.

The **skin changes** of wrinkling, thinning, and a loss of elasticity have been attributed to the lack of

estrogen. There has been little evidence presented to substantiate this claim, although there are estrogen receptors present in the skin.

During the perimenopausal years (i.e., 40–55), the number of primordial ovarian follicles gradually decreases. The serum estrogen levels also decrease as fewer and fewer follicles remain. **The serum FSH levels at this time may increase in an effort to stimulate the remaining follicles, which may be less sensitive to the usual FSH output.** As a consequence, more cycles become anovulatory and **menstrual irregularities** begin to develop. Eventually, the serum estrogen levels fall to low enough values that the endometrium is no longer stimulated, and menstruation then ceases. During the first one to three years after the cessation of the menses, the serum FSH and LH levels increase to reach their maximal values. **The elevated LH levels stimulate the stroma of the ovary to produce testosterone and androstenedione, which accounts for the mild degree of hirsutism that is observed in some women in the postmenopausal period.**

b. Concerns during the perimenopausal period

During the perimenopausal years, a number of clinical problems may occur. **The increasing number of anovulatory cycles leads to irregularities in the interval, duration, and the amount of flow of the menses. Such altered bleeding patterns in this age group raise questions concerning the possibility of the presence of a neoplastic lesion.** Indeed, persistent unopposed estrogen has been thought to lead to adenomatous hyperplasia or even to adenocarcinoma of the endometrium. Thus, it is important that a **fractional D&C** be performed

---

*Reprinted with permission from Robert Bennett Bean, *Sir William Osler: Aphorisms from His Bedside Teachings and Writings,* William Bennett Bean, ed. Springfield, Ill.: Charles C Thomas, Publisher, 1968, p. 89.

before any treatment regimen is instituted. If there is no evidence of cancer on the pathology report, then the patient should be placed on medroxyprogesterone acetate (Provera), 10 mg/day from day 13 to day 25 of each cycle, which is continued until the patient has failed to menstruate for at least three to six months (i.e., menopause). **As long as there is no bleeding at any other times than during the normal withdrawal time (i.e., three to five days after the cessation of the pills), you can be relatively confident that the patient does not have an adenocarcinoma of the endometrium; however, good clinical judgment should be utilized in the individual patient.** It is interesting that the degree of protection against endometrial hyperplasia seems to be related to the duration of the medroxyprogesterone acetate (Provera) treatment. If unopposed estrogens are administered, then the incidence of endometrial adenomatous hyperplasia has been noted to be as high as 10%. If the medroxyprogesterone acetate (Provera) is administered for seven days, then the incidence decreases to about 4%. Treatment regimens of ten days will not completely protect against the development of endometrial hyperplasia (i.e., incidence of 2%), whereas treatment with 13 days of medroxyprogesterone acetate (Provera) virtually eliminates the risk of developing endometrial cancer.

2. Menopause

a. General considerations

The menopause was known even in ancient times. In the sixth century A.D., it was noted that menopause occurred between the ages of 35 and 50. **Menopause in the United States occurs at a median age of 51.4 years (range 43.8 to 59).** With the current female life expectancy, a woman may expect to live nearly one-third of her life after the ovaries have stopped functioning.

At about 20 weeks' gestation, the fetal ovary contains 6–7 million germ cells; however, this number will decrease to about 1–2 million at the time of birth. By the onset of puberty, the number of ovocytes will have been further depleted by atresia to about 300,000. During the reproductive life of the female, assuming 100% ovulation, only about 400 follicles could possibly be ovulated. Obviously, not every cycle is ovulatory, so even fewer follicles will eventually

reach ovulation. Since **almost all of the follicles will be gone by the time of menopause,** it would appear that at least 1,000 follicles are lost by atresia each month.

There is a decrease in the estradiol production in menopause. As a consequence, the predominant estrogen now becomes estrone, which is derived from the peripheral conversion of androstenedione in the adipose tissues. This decreased level of estradiol affects all of the tissues that have estrogen receptors (e.g., genital tissues, urinary tract, breasts, and the central nervous system). There is an increase first in the FSH levels and then in the LH levels as the ovarian follicles fail to respond. This LH stimulation of the ovarian stroma causes an increased amount of androstenedione and testosterone to be produced.

The cessation of menses for at least 12 months constitutes the menopause. Any bleeding beyond this point requires that a fractional D&C be performed in order to rule out cancer (i.e., the diagnosis being **postmenopausal bleeding**).

The adrenal gland produces almost all of the androstenedione that is present in the postmenopausal woman (85%). **Androstenedione is then converted by the peripheral adipose stromal tissue into estrone, which is the principal estrogen in the postmenopausal patient.** Although this extraglandular conversion of androstenedione to estrone is normally only slightly more than about 1% (i.e., 45 μg/24 hours), the percentage of this conversion may increase proportionally with an increase in the patient's body weight. Obesity also decreases the sex hormone binding globulin (SHBG) levels, which allows for an increase in the circulating levels of the free sex steroid hormones. Thus, in the postmenopausal period, the obese woman will have significantly higher circulating levels of estrone than will be found in the thin patient. In some cases, the level of estrone produced may be sufficient to support some of the estrogen-dependent tissues, such as the urethra and the vagina.

As the estrogen loss becomes even more marked after the menopause has taken place, the thin patient may complain of **dyspareunia,** which is due to the thinning and atrophy of the vaginal mucous membrane. **Urinary frequency, dysuria, urgency, and even incontinence** may occur, since the mucous membranes of the bladder and urethra also have estrogen receptors. These patients also have an increased incidence of urinary tract infections, which may be prevented by the administration of estrogen (see Chapter 12).

After about 10–15 years, the continued gradual loss of calcium from the bones due to the decreased level of estrogens may result in **osteoporosis.** This loss of bone mass may be diagnosed with either single- or dual-photon absorptiometry, as well as by a quantitative CAT scan. If the bone density values fall to less than 80% of young normal values, then they are considered to be abnormal. This much bone loss and more may be sufficient to result in fractures. Classically, the **dowager syndrome** occurs as the vertebrae fracture and condense upon themselves to produce a shrinkage in the patient's height and the development of a dorsal hump. As much as 2.5 inches of loss in the height of white women may occur. Normally, there is no more than a 1-inch difference between the crown-to-pubis measurement and the pubis-to-heel measurement. The crown-to-pubis measurement will be 1.5 inches less than the pubis-to-heel measurement in patients who have lost bone in the upper spinal column. It has been reported that about 26% of white women will have vertebral fractures by age 60, and 50% will have them by age 75. Both hip and long bone fractures are also common in these women. A hip fracture in a 90-year-old woman is tantamount to a death sentence, since 15–20% of these patients will die within three to six months of the injury. There are about 200,000 hip fractures and 100,000 forearm fractures in the United States each year.

Since only about 20–25% of white women will develop osteoporosis in the postmenopausal period, it has been suggested that only women with certain characteristics are at risk for the disease. These characteristics are: (1) a lack of body fat, (2) a sedentary life-style, (3) an inadequate diet, (4) smoking, and (5) excessive alcohol consumption.

3. Treatment concerns

The treatment of the postmenopausal woman with **estrogen replacement therapy (ERT)** has been controversial for a number of years. While estrogen administration may correct the patient's symptoms of hot flushes and vaginal atrophy, and also will decrease the risk of osteoporosis, its possible adverse effects on other organ systems have been the cause of some concern.

a. Cardiovascular system

The effect of estrogen therapy on the cardiovascular system has always been thought to be protective for women, since there seems to be an apparent sex difference in the incidence of coronary artery disease and stroke in women as opposed to men. Current evidence has indicated that estrogen is also cardioprotective on the basis of its salutary effect on high-density lipoproteins (HDL) (i.e., high levels of HDL are cardioprotective). The addition of a progestogen to the estrogen treatment has caused some concern from a cardiovascular standpoint because of its adverse changes in lowering the HDL levels. This still needs to be evaluated by controlled studies.

Some of the complications, such as thromboembolism, that have been attributed to estrogen in the higher dose birth control pills have not been seen in postmenopausal patients who have been treated with lower and more physiological regimens of estrogen. High-dose estrogen therapy may be relatively contraindicated in patients with hypertension, familial hyperlipidemia, epilepsy, or migraine headaches. Patients with thromboembolic problems, cerebrovascular disease, myocardial infarction, or severe liver disease should also not receive high-dose estrogens. There is an increased incidence of gall bladder disease in these patients taking high-dose estrogens. The side effects of low-dose estrogens and progestogens, however, seem to be much less or even absent, so that some of these contraindications may no longer be valid, both in the use of 30–35 mcg oral contraceptive pills in the younger patient and also in the postmenopausal patient who is receiving low-dose estrogens and progesterone.

b. Breast carcinoma

About 1:11 women in the United States eventually develops breast cancer. The mortality rate for this disease has been nearly constant for 45 years at 23:100,000. While there appears to be an association of breast cancer and estrogens, the exact relationship is unknown. Certainly, the dramatic increase in estrogen usage over the past 30 years has not resulted in an overall increased incidence of breast carcinoma. In one study conducted at the Wilford Hall USAF Medical Center, the incidence of carcinoma of the breast in **estrogen only** users was 142.3:100,000. Additional evidence from this study has shown that, in women who received both **estrogen and progesterone** in the postmenopausal period, the incidence of breast cancer was only 66.8:100,000.

c. Uterine cancer

Endometrial hyperplasia and endometrial adenocarcinoma have both occurred in relation to unopposed estrogen administration and have raised the question of a cause-and-effect relationship. Indeed, studies have shown that there is a four- to eight-fold increase in the risk of adenocarcinoma in those patients who take estrogens orally. Furthermore, 25–30% of patients who have adenocarcinoma of the endometrium have had a previous diagnosis of adenomatous hyperplasia. In patients with adenomatous hyperplasia of the endometrium, about 10% have been found to later progress to obvious cancer. In one study, it was demonstrated that the incidence of endometrial carcinoma was 390.6:100,000 in patients who received **estrogen alone** in the postmenopausal period. In those patients who received **no hormones** in the postmenopausal period, the incidence of adenocarcinoma of the endometrium was 245.5:100,000. In contrast, the incidence of adenocarcinoma in those patients who received both **estrogen and progesterone** in the postmenopausal period was 49:100,000. It should be noted that in all of these latter patients, estrogens had been administered alone from 2.5–8 years before the progesterone was added to their regimen.

4. Management

The decision to treat the patient with progesterone during the **perimenopausal period** is often not a difficult one. If there is no evidence of adenomatous hyperplasia or endometrial cancer on a multiple sampling biopsy of the endometrium (or a fractional D&C), then the patient should be placed on medroxyprogesterone acetate (Provera), 10 mg/day from day 13 to day 25 of each cycle, which is continued until the patient has not menstruated for at least 3–6 months. The patient's bleeding episodes should be monitored with a menstrual calendar. This therapy will serve to regulate the menses and remove the concerns about the development of endometrial cancer. Regular withdrawal menses 3–5 days after the cessation of treatment should be expected each month. If endometrial hyperplasia is found initially on the fractional D&C, then a hysterectomy should be considered.

The selection of the postmenopausal patient for estrogen replacement therapy (ERT) should take into consideration the presence of any medical risk factors that may be involved, the patient's symptomatology, and the risk of developing osteoporosis (20–25%). If the patient's symptoms are severe, then estrogen administration may be beneficial in improving the quality of life. To be really effective in retarding the bone loss, the estrogen should be administered within the first three years of the onset of the menopause; however, some investigators believe that a retardation of bone loss can be obtained whenever estrogens are administered.

Estrogens should not be administered alone, however, due to their growth stimulating propensity. **The minimal dose of conjugated estrogens that will inhibit bone resorption and the development of osteoporosis is 0.625 mg/day × 25 days/ month.** Most authorities recommend using the lowest possible dose and that the minimal dose of 0.625 mg/day for 25 days each month should probably not be exceeded if at all possible. Medroxyprogesterone acetate (Provera), 10 mg/day from day 13 to day 25, should be administered to any patient who receives estrogens in the postmenopausal period. Recently, some authorities have recommended continuous estrogen therapy with the addition of continuous medroxyprogesterone acetate therapy (i.e., Provera, 2.5 mg or 5.0 mg) daily throughout the month. Progestins inhibit the growth of endometrial cells and decrease the numbers of cytoplasmic estrogen receptors, thereby counteracting the effects of the estrogen.

Equivalent dosages of other estrogens as compared to 0.625 mg of conjugated equine estrogens are as follows: (1) Ogen (a derivative of estrone), 1.25 mg; (2) Estrace (micronized estradiol), 1 mg; (3) ethinyl estradiol, 20 μg; (4) estradiol valerate, 1 mg; and (5) transdermal patches of estradiol, 0.05 mg. The patches are changed twice each week on days 1 through 25.

In addition to hormone replacement therapy, postmenopausal patients should also receive 1.0 gram of calcium each day. Those patients in the postmenopausal period who are not receiving estrogen should be given about 1.5 grams of calcium per day.

CHAPTER 44

Infertility

The young physician should be careful what and how he writes.

—*Sir William Osler**

1. Infertility

If a pregnancy cannot be achieved after 12 months of unprotected intercourse, then the diagnosis of infertility may be made, since the chance for conception in a fertile couple should be about 90% during this period of time. It has been estimated that 10–15% of American couples are infertile. An infertility workup carried out in these cases should involve an investigation of both partners whenever possible.

Such a workup should proceed in a systematic and orderly fashion. An initial **history and physical examination** should be performed, followed by a **semen analysis** on the male and **basal body temperature** charting on the female. A **postcoital test** should be scheduled at the time of the next ovulation to detect the presence of a hostile cervical mucus, and a **repeat three-day abstinence sperm analysis** should be obtained during the same cycle. On the next appointment after the postcoital test, an **endometrial biopsy** should be obtained in the **midluteal phase** to detect ovulation and the possibility of a luteal phase defect. A serum progesterone obtained at the same time may confirm ovulation. A **hysterosal-**

*Reprinted with permission from Robert Bennett Bean, *Sir William Osler: Aphorisms from His Bedside Teachings and Writings,* William Bennett Bean, ed. Springfield, Ill.: Charles C Thomas, Publisher, 1968, p. 61.

pingogram should then be performed between two and six days after the menses have ceased in order to detect or rule out the presence of tubal defect. This simple infertility evaluation may be accomplished in about 2–3 months. Between 6 and 42% of the couples who undergo investigation, however, will remain infertile with no explanation provided by these studies.

It is important to recognize that the infertile couple is emotionally involved with their problem. Their inability to conceive may bring on feelings of anger, disbelief, and denial. They may grieve for the child that was never conceived. Their self-image may be damaged by their reproductive inadequacy, and their sex lives may suffer. If the couple is forced to make a choice concerning artificial insemination or other techniques for correcting the infertility, it may be difficult for them to make a rational decision. Many couples will change physicians or will fail to follow through with the infertility workup for long periods. The workup itself may be stressful to either or both of the marital partners. You should be aware of these feelings and allow the couple to express their concerns and help them to emotionally work through their problems.

2. Screen of the infertile couple

A thorough **history and a complete physical examination** should be performed on the female, and if possible, on the male as well. A history of any previous pregnancies and their outcome should be obtained if the patient is a secondary infertility patient. You should attempt to determine the **patient's general health status,** her menstrual history, and the other pertinent details of her **social and economic life.** You should investigate the couple's use of medications, tobacco, alcohol, and drugs of abuse, as well as the their general life-style. A detailed **sexual history** should be evaluated with regard to the frequency of intercourse, the use of douches or lubricants, and whether the woman goes to the bathroom immediately following intercourse, since in the upright position the bulk of the semen may leak out of the vagina and reduce the chances of conception. *Sexual factors account for perhaps 5% of infertility problems.*

If the male uses sauna baths or wears jockey shorts, this may produce sufficient heat to the testicles to further reduce the sperm count in men who already have low sperm counts. **Men who are under legitimate drug therapy for various conditions may also have a problem, since about 15% of the commonly used medicinal drugs may interfere with reproductive performance.** A decrease in the libido in the male may occur if **sedatives, tranquilizers, or hypnotics** are used, except in rare instances in which there is a high degree of anxiety present. Other agents, such as **tricyclic antidepressants** (amitriptyline hydrochloride, doxepin hydrochloride, impramine hydrochloride, and cyclobenzaprine hydrochloride) may alter the libido and cause testicular swelling. **Methyldopa hydrochloride,** a medication that is used for hypertension, may reduce libido in a dose-related manner and may also inhibit ejaculation. **Other ejaculation inhibitors include monoamine oxidase inhibitors and guanethidine. Antiandrogenic drugs** (medroxyprogesterone acetate and spironolactone) will decrease the libido. Clonidine may cause impotence in as many as 20% of these patients. The use of one of the **phenothiazines** (chlorpromazine and trifluoperazine hydrochloride) has been associated with an inability to ejaculate in some men.

Centrally acting drugs that affect men will also affect the woman's reproductive performance. **Spironolactone** may alter the menstrual periods. **Methyldopa hydrochloride** may result in anorgasmia in women, and the libido may be decreased with **reserpine and prazosin hydrochloride. Barbiturates** affect both the libido and the orgasmic response of the woman, as well as the menstrual regularity.

3. Male infertility factors

The male is responsible for infertility in about 40% of the cases. **Male infertility factors involve: (1)** spermatozoa production, (2) obstruction of the ducts, (3) ejaculation disturbances, and (4) abnormal semen.

a. Spermatozoa production

Spermatozoa production may be affected by: (1) the presence of a varicocele, (2) testicular failure, (3) cryptorchidism, (4) endocrine diseases, and (5) heat, smoking, stress, and systemic infections. Those individuals who have sperm counts in the range of 10–19 million/ml, who have over 50% abnormal forms, or a motility of less than 35% should have a thorough evaluation. **Spermatozoan motility is directly correlated with fertility.** Couples in whom the male has severe oligospermia, azospermia, or other severe seminal defects may be candidates for alternative procedures of assisted reproductive technology (ART), such as artificial insemination or in-vitro fertilization.

The male should be evaluated by a **semen analysis** to detect any abnormalities of the sperm number, morphology, and the volume of the ejaculate (Table 44-1). A semen analysis should be performed initially and then again after a few weeks to get a good idea of the range of values. The specimen should be obtained by masturbation into a clean jar after a three-day period of abstinence. The liquefaction of the semen will usually occur within about 20–45 minutes. *The volume should be about 2.0–6.0 ml. The sperm count should be above 20 million per ml, with at least 50–60% motility, and with 50–60% forward progression. The morphology should be normal in at least 60% of the sperm* (Fig. 44-1). Some authors have suggested that these values can be more easily recalled as the "rule of sixties" (Table 44-1). The presence of white blood cells in the semen requires further evaluation.

In order for the sperm to have the capacity to fertilize the ovum, **capacitation** must also take place. This process usually occurs in the female generative tract, but it may also occur in a defined media during the process of in-vitro fertilization. The reaction during capacitation involves the acrosome, the cap of lysosome overlying the head of the sperm. Once the sperm is capacitated, it is capable of penetrating the ovum and causing fertilization. After one spermatozoon has entered the ovum, usually no other sperm can penetrate the membrane. The sperm then loses its tail and becomes the male pronucleus that fuses with the female pronucleus to form the zygote. The female

TABLE 44-1. Standard semen analysis

Parameter	Average values
Consistency	Fluid (after liquefaction)
Color	Opaque
Liquefaction time	<20 min
pH	7.2–7.8
Volume	2–6 ml
Motility (grade 0–4)	>50%
Count (millions/ml)	20–100
Viability (eosin)	>50%
Morphology (cytology) cell types	>60% normal oval
Cells (white blood cells, others)	None to occasional
Agglutination	None
Biochemical studies (e.g., fructose, prostaglandins, zinc), if desired	

Reprinted with permission from D. N. Danforth and J. R. Scott, eds., *Obstetrics and Gynecology,* 5th ed. Philadelphia: J. B. Lippincott Company, 1986, p. 933.

has thus provided not only her haploid number of the chromosomes to the new zygote with her pronucleus, but has also provided all of the cytoplasm with its cytoplasmic chromosome (see Chapter 22).

1) Varicocele

A varicocele is the cause of infertility in 40% of infertile men. This condition causes changes in the sperm analysis that have been called a **"stress" pattern,** which consists of oligospermia, with decreased sperm motility and the appearance of "tapered" forms of sperm. It is thought that this pattern results from the increased local testicular heat, which is due to the varices. With the surgical correction of the varicocele, there will be an improvement in the sperm in about 70–80% of patients, and in about 22–68% of these men, a pregnancy with their mate may be achieved.

2) Testicular failure

Individuals who have severe seminal problems with unexplained oligospermia or azospermia should be suspected of having testicular failure, which is a cause of infertility in 14% of the cases. Germinal aplasia is the most common reason for testicular failure, and it can be differentiated from maturational arrest by a testicular biopsy. A serum FSH to document failure

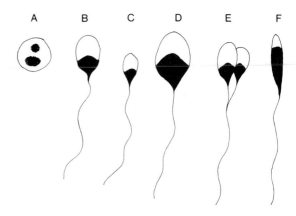

FIGURE 44-1. Morphologic variations of spermatozoa. (A) Immature cell. (B) Oval sperm (normal). (C) Small (microcytic) sperm. (D) Large (macrocytic) sperm. (E) Double-headed (bicephalic) sperm. (F) Tapering form.

and a chromosomal analysis should be obtained, since patients with Klinefelter's syndrome (47,XXY) or a variant of this condition may have gynecomastia and small testes.

3) Endocrine diseases

The adrenogenital syndrome, hypopituitarism, or hypothyroidism may cause difficulties with spermatozoa production in about 8% of infertility patients. A "stress" spermatozoan pattern may be seen in the adrenogenital syndrome. Hypothyroidism is a rare cause of problems (2%). While hypogonadotropic patients have low gonadotropins, they will respond to human menopausal gonadotropins (hMG), or to clomiphene citrate (Clomid).

4) Cryptorchidism

It is essential that the testicles be placed in the scrotum by the age of six years, since if they remain intraabdominally after puberty, they will become sterile. This is a cause of azospermia in 4% of infertile men.

5) Stress, smoking, heat, work, infections

Cigarettes, alcohol, and long working hours often affect the sperm count. Nicotine inhibits both the quality and the quantity of the spermatozoa. Alcohol ingestion decreases the circulating levels of testosterone, and heat has an adverse effect upon spermatogenesis. **Since spermatogenesis requires 74 days for completion, any effects of these agents on the sperm count will not be observable until 2.5 months later.** Infections, both viral and bacterial, may also have a deleterious effect on spermatogenesis. The use of drugs such as nitrofurantoin, sulfasalazine, or chemotherapeutic agents have also been implicated in the production of low sperm counts. Frequent coitus may reduce the sperm count in men with borderline counts, just as abstinence beyond seven days may also cause a reduction of the sperm count to levels that are similar to those found immediately after coitus. The optimum time between coital acts is about 36–48 hours.

b. Obstruction of the ducts

If the male has a history of an infection involving the testicles (i.e., epididymitis), an enlarged, obstructed epididymis may be found on examination. The obstruction of the vas deferens is the cause of azoospermia in 7% of infertile men. A congenital absence of the vas deferens is associated with a low semen volume. The ducts will be blocked after a vasectomy, but a surgical reanastomosis results in the return of testicular function with an adequate sperm count in 40–80% of cases.

c. Ejaculatory disturbances

Marked hypospadia results in retrograde ejaculation into the bladder in about 2% of infertile men. Retrograde ejaculation may also occur following prostatic surgery, or if there is an obstruction of the ejaculatory duct.

d. Abnormal semen

Abnormal semen problems are the cause of infertility in 12% of infertile men. The normal ejaculatory volume is about 2.0–6.0 ml. A low volume is considered to be present when the volume is less than 1 ml. The use of homologous intracervical or intrauterine insemination may be successful in these patients, since the low volume of the ejaculate may preclude the proper deposition of the semen at the cervical os. If the volume is too large (i.e., more than 6 ml), a split ejaculate using the half with the most spermatozoa may be of value. While the bulk of the sperm is in the first half of the ejaculate in most men, this should be checked, since on occasion it is in the other half.

When the ejaculate is too viscous, a poor postcoital test may result. If there is agglutination of the sperm, then an autoimmune reaction or an infection should be considered as the cause. The presence of white blood cells in the ejaculate may point to a low-grade infection.

4. Evaluation of the male

The **Sims' test (or Huhner test)** evaluates the compatibility of the sperm with the cervical mucus. This test consists of having the woman have intercourse about 2–8 hours prior to her visit at the time in her cycle when she is ovulating (i.e., midcycle). A specimen of the cervical mucus is then obtained and the number of sperm that are present is noted. *If there are five or more actively motile sperm present per high power field, then the test is considered to be normal.* If there are no sperm present in the analysis of the ejaculated specimen, then the male may have a **poor delivery of the sperm into the vagina,** due to a possible **retrograde ejaculation into the bladder,** in which case the sperm may be recovered from the bladder. If the cervical mucus is hostile and the sperm are dead, and the postcoital test is persistently abnormal, then the presence of sperm-agglutinating or sperm-immobilizing antibodies should be sought.

5. Treatment of male factors

The male infertility factors may be difficult to treat. Azospermia precludes pregnancy; in these cases, **artificial donor insemination (AID)** should be considered. If a very low sperm count, a low volume, or a sperm delivery problem is present, then **artificial insemination (AIH)** using the husband's sperm from a split ejaculate may be successful in producing a pregnancy in 4–12% of cases where this is tried. The use of a cervical cap may increase this success rate to 27% by concentrating the sperm at the cervical os.

The zona-free hamster egg penetration test, the bovine cervical mucus migrating capacity of the sperm, and the acrosin assay test are some of the experimental tests that have been used in evaluating the spermatozoa. Since one of the most common causes of a low sperm count is a varicocele, the surgical correction of this problem may improve the quality of the spermatozoa and result in a pregnancy. Usually, ductal obstruction, retrograde ejaculation, cryptorchidism, and the variety of endocrine problems that affect fertility require the expertise of specially trained physicians. Interestingly, the recovery of spermatozoa from the cul-de-sac via a laparoscope following coitus, or after AIH, has been strongly correlated with the eventual successful establishment of a pregnancy.

6. Female factors

Female infertility factors include: (1) ovulation failure, (2) tubal obstruction, (3) cervical and uterine factors, (4) vaginal factors, (5) immunologic incompatibility, and (6) nutritional and metabolic factors.

a. Ovulation factors

Usually, chronic **anovulation** is associated with irregular menstrual cycles or oligomenorrhea (see Chapter 40). The menstrual bleeding associated with an anovulatory cycle may be light or heavy and is generally not associated with cramps. Ovulation failure accounts for 15% of the cases of infertility in women. An inadequate corpus luteum (i.e., luteal phase defect) may also result in shortened menstrual cycles.

Recently, it has been recognized that ovulation may occur without the release of the ovum; this condition is called **the luteinized unruptured follicle syndrome (LUF).** For unknown reasons, there is a failure of the follicle to rupture, causing entrapment of the ovum. The basal body temperature, the serum progesterone, and the endometrium, however, all undergo changes that are indicative of normal ovulation. This problem occurred in about 10% of infertile women in one study.

Another phenomenon has recently been described as a cause of infertility where the follicle ruptures appropriately, but **the ovum is retained in the follicle.**

1) Basal body temperature chart

The woman should be evaluated by a **basal body temperature chart (BBT)**, an **endometrial bi-**opsy, and/or a **midluteal serum progesterone level test** to determine if ovulation is occurring with her cycles. The **basal body temperature chart** is a daily measure of the patient's temperature, which should be taken upon arising in the morning and recorded to the nearest tenth of a degree. *If ovulation occurs in a particular menstrual cycle, then the increased levels of progesterone cause an increase in the body temperature of 0.8–1.0° F that persists throughout the last half of the cycle* (Fig. 44-2).

2) Endometrial biopsy

An **endometrial biopsy** taken in the latter half of the menstrual cycle (e.g., day 24–26) or on the first day of the menses will show a *secretory endometrium,* if ovulation has occurred. If there is at least a two-day lag in the maturation of the endometrium on two separate cycles, then a luteal phase defect may be said to be present.

3) Serum progesterone

There is an elevation of the serum progesterone level, due to the corpus luteum formation, if ovulation occurs. A **serum progesterone** value of greater than 10 ng/ml in the latter part of the menstrual cycle when the progesterone level has peaked is indicative of ovulation.

4) Treatment

In anovulatory patients, ovulation may be induced by treating the patient with **ovulation-inducing agents,** such as **clomiphene citrate (Clomid)** or **human gonadotropins (Pergonal).** This latter compound contains 75 IU of FSH and 75 IU of LH per ampule. One of the serious side effects of these agents, especially with human gonadotropins, is the hyperstimulation of the ovaries, which may result in a massive enlargement of the ovaries with the development of ascites. The dosage of these medications is critical in preventing this problem. In addition, the occurrence of twins is more common with clomiphene citrate, and multiple fetuses are more common with the gonadotropin therapy.

Clomiphene citrate (Clomid) is an anti-estrogen that acts by binding with the estrogen receptors of the uterus, ovaries, breasts, vagina, pituitary gland, and the hypothalamus. Clomiphene citrate should be adminis-

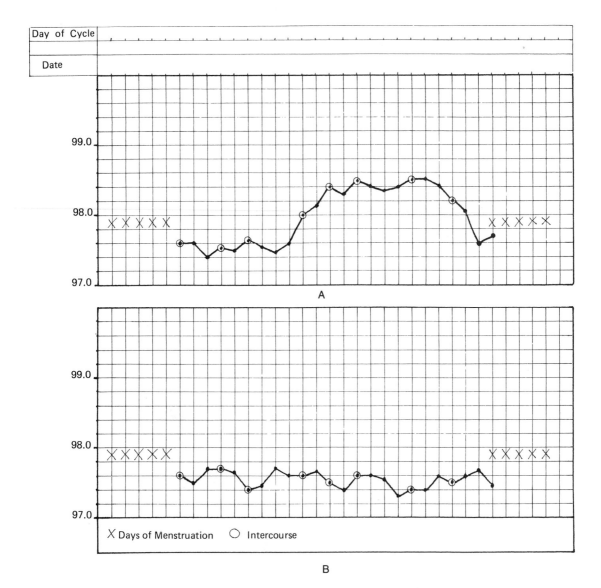

FIGURE 44-2. Basal body temperature records suggesting (A) ovulatory and (B) anovulatory cycles. The increase in the temperature on the 15th day of the ovulatory cycle is consistent with ovulation on day 14. Intercourse on the 16th day should result in a pregnancy; however, this is not always the case. (Adapted from D. N. Danforth and J. R. Scott, eds., *Obstetrics and Gynecology,* 5th ed. Philadelphia: J. B. Lippincott Company, 1986, p. 939.)

tered in doses of 50–200 mg daily for 5 days beginning on day 3 to 5 of the menstrual cycle. Ovulation will occur about 7–10 days after the cessation of the treatment. Tamoxifen citrate has also been used in *experimental* situations to induce ovulation; however, its primary use has been in patients with breast cancer as an antitumor agent. As an anti-estrogenic agent, it can affect the same receptors as the clomiphene citrate.

b. Tubal obstruction

Obstruction of the fallopian tubes may involve: (1) the cornual region, (2) the isthmus, (3) the fimbria, or (4) the peritubal areas (i.e., adhesions). Infections with Neisseria gonorrhoeae or Chlamydia trachomatis will produce intraluminal adhesions, as well as peritubal adhesions, which may cause blockage of the tubes (see Chapter 14). Tuberculosis and other pelvic infections also generally involve the ovaries and the fallopian tubes. Appendicitis, pelvic surgery, or endometriosis usually involves the cul-de-sac and may produce dense adhesions involving the tubes and ovaries. Tubal obstructions account for about 20% of the cases of infertility in females.

1) Rubin test

An **obstruction of the fallopian tubes** may be clinically demonstrated by passing CO_2 into the uterus and the tubes and listening with a stethoscope over the lower abdomen to hear the passage of the gas through the ends of the tubes **(Rubin's test).** The patient will often complain of transient shoulder pain upon sitting up due to the intraperitoneal gas and the irritation of the diaphragm.

2) Hysterosalpingogram

A technique that will demonstrate tubal patency much more easily than the Rubin's test is the **hysterosalpingogram.** In this procedure, radiopaque dye is injected through a cervical cannula into the uterus and the tubes (Fig. 44-3). The configuration of the uterine cavity can be determined by this technique, and it frequently provides a much more definite demonstration of the tubal patency on X-ray than the use of the Rubin's procedure. Tubal spasm may be present in as many as 50% of patients who appear to have tubal occlusion on a hysterosalpingogram. **Both of these tests should be performed after menstruation** **has ceased and before ovulation could take place (i.e., usually between day 6 to day 9).**

3) Laparoscopy

In some cases, a **laparoscopy** will be needed to determine the extent of the pelvic pathology that may be interfering with tubal patency. An injection of a solution of indigo carmine or methylene blue dye into the uterus and out the tubes at the time of the laparoscopy may provide visual evidence of the level of the tubal blockage or provide definitive evidence of patency by the free flow of the dye out the ends of the tubes **(i.e., chromotubation).**

4) Treatment

The main tubal problem involved in infertility is tubal obstruction; restoring the patency of the tube frequently requires plastic reconstruction. Due to the delicacy of the surgical technique, these procedures should be performed by physicians who are specially trained in microsurgical techniques. If peritubal adhesions are involved, a laparotomy should be performed and a lysis of the adhesions carried out. It is important in pelvic surgery, and especially in infertility surgery, to handle the tissues gently in an attempt to avoid the development of postoperative adhesions. In those patients who have a sterilization reversal (i.e., midsegment tubal anastomosis), about 75% will conceive during the first 18 months following surgery.

c. Cervical and uterine factors

Endocervical polyps, cervical leiomyomas, or other space-occupying lesions may **obstruct the cervical os.** A history of cervical tuberculosis, endometriosis, cauterization, conization, or dilatation and curettage in a patient might explain a **stenosis** of the cervix. The cervical os should be probed to be certain that there is no obstruction. If there are endocervical polyps present, then they should be removed.

The presence of uterine abnormalities, such as the "T-shaped" uterine cavity that has been described in those patients who were exposed in utero to diethylstilbestrol (DES), has been implicated in reproductive wastage in some reports. Other congenital uterine abnormalities may occur and these are usually due to either an abnormal fusion or an incomplete resorption of the müllerian duct septa. Endometrial polyps and leiomyomas may also distort the uterine cavity and interfere with implantation of the zygote. Intra-

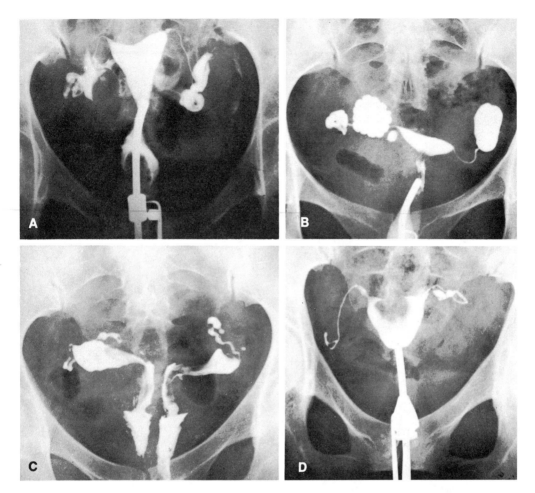

FIGURE 44-3. Hysterosalpingograms. (A) Normal uterus and fallopian tubes with peritoneal spill. Note outline of ovarian beds and leakage into proximal part of vagina. (B) Loculation of contrast material in inflammatory pockets at distal ends of tubes. (C) Didelphic uterus with double vagina. (D) Large filling defect in uterine cavity due to submucous myoma. Note incomplete tubal filling and absence of peritoneal spill. (Reprinted with permission from D. N. Danforth and J. R. Scott, eds., *Obstetrics and Gynecology,* 5th ed. Philadelphia: J. B. Lippincott Company, 1986, p. 935.)

uterine synechiae may be found at times to almost obliterate the endometrial cavity (i.e., Asherman's syndrome). Cervical and uterine problems have been implicated in as many as 10% of the cases of infertility. The presence of a hypoplastic uterus is very rare.

1) Hysteroscopy

The use of a 7-mm panoramic hysteroscope, with dextran 70 (Hyskon) or carbon dioxide distending media, provides an excellent evaluation of the uterine cavity.

Intrauterine polyps and submucosal leiomyomas can be removed via hysteroscopy.

2) Vaginitis/cervicitis

An evaluation of vaginal secretions may detect a **vaginitis or a cervicitis.** An infection of the cervix (e.g., chlamydial) may alter the cervical mucus and make it hostile for the sperm. The specific treatment of a cervical erosion due to chlamydia should be carried out using tetracycline or erythromycin.

3) Treatment

Uterine synechiae may be corrected by hysteroscopy or by a D&C followed by several months of high-dose hormone therapy. Uterine polyps should also be removed, and if the leiomyomas are large enough to significantly encroach upon the intrauterine cavity, then these should probably be removed in selected cases.

d. Vaginal factors

The congenital absence of the vagina may be easily found upon examination (see Chapter 40). An imperforate hymen may also be discovered in a woman who complains of infertility, attesting to the fact that the marriage has never really been consummated. The presence of vaginismus may prevent intercourse and could also lead to infertility in rare instances. Severe vaginitis may affect the survival of the sperm in the vagina and could contribute to infertility. Such problems as these have been thought to be the cause of infertility in less than 5% of infertility cases.

e. Immunologic incompatibility

In order to detect antispermatozoa antibodies it is necessary to do serial postcoital tests. The finding of less than five motile spermatozoa per high power field, in an otherwise normal semen analysis and in the presence of a well-estrogenized cervical mucus, may point to an immunologic problem. Often on the postcoital test, **a "shaking" movement of the spermatozoa** may be seen. The degree of spermatozoal survival, and their ability to penetrate the cervical mucus, is an important factor. Immunologic incompatibility occurs in less than 10% of infertility patients.

The immunologic mechanism may be tested by means of the sperm immobilization test or the sperm agglutination test. The Franklin-Dukes, Friberg, and Kibrick agglutination tests are well known. The presence of **agglutinating activity** may be a normal finding, however, in that there is normally a tendency for the sperm to spontaneously form a "head-to-head agglutination." It is necessary to separate this normal activity from that of an agglutinating antibody activity by using very careful test conditions. The spermatozoa should be mixed with fresh gelatin and serum in various dilutions, incubated, and then observed for the agglutination phenomenon. The ag-

glutinin apparently resides in the immunoglobulin G (IgG) fraction.

The **immobilizing antibody** appears to be the antibody associated most commonly with problems of infertility. The Isojima sperm immobilization test has been used effectively to test for this type of problem. In this test, the sperm is incubated with complement and inactivated patient's serum for one hour at 37° C. The motility level of the sperm is then compared with that of a control specimen that utilizes inactivated normal serum instead of the patient's serum. The immobilizing factor is present in the immunoglobulin G (IgG) and immunoglobulin M (IgM) fractions.

Recently, radiolabeled antiglobulin tests have been developed that are highly specific for the detection of spermatozoan antibodies. The **immunobead binding** technique is another test that detects antibodies on the surface of the living spermatozoa. An enzyme-linked immunosorbent assay (ELISA) test has also recently become available.

1) Treatment

Immunologic incompatibility problems are usually lessened by the use of a condom for several months, which allows the antibody titer in the woman to decrease considerably.

f. Nutritional/metabolic factors

Thyroid disease is rarely a cause of infertility. Other conditions, such as diabetes, hyperprolactinemia, and severe nutritional disorders, result in infertility in less than 5% of infertility patients.

7. In-vitro fertilization and embryo transfer

More than 50 clinics have performed in-vitro fertilization (IVF) and embryo transfer in the United States in the past few years. In perhaps as many as one-half of these clinics, no successful pregnancies have yet been obtained. **The pregnancy rate per treatment cycle in the other half of the clinics has been of the order of about 20–30%.**

Those couples who have had considerable difficulty in achieving a pregnancy over the course of about 18 months are potential candidates for **in-vitro fertilization and embryo transfer (IVF/ET).** Many of these couples are infertile because of female organic pelvic disease, male subfertility, or cervical mucus insufficiency. The criteria that have been used in some clinics to select a couple for in-vitro fertilization and embryo transfer have included the following questions: (1) Is the couple psychologically stable? (2) Does the female have an ectocervix-to-uterine-fundus measurement of more than 70 mm? (3) Does she have at least one functioning ovary? and (4) Does the male partner have at least 5×10^6 motile sperm per milliliter of ejaculate? If the answer is yes to all four questions, then the couple may be considered possible candidates for the in-vitro fertilization and embryo transfer procedures.

The patient who has been selected for these procedures is initially stimulated with *human menopausal gonadotropin (hMG)*. The objective of this procedure is to achieve a plasma estradiol level of greater than 700 pg/ml by the ninth day in the woman who has two ovaries, or 500 pg/ml in the patient who has only one ovary. Excessive stimulation of the ovaries by hMG may result in the *ovarian hyperstimulation syndrome*, which involves the development of massive ovarian cysts and ascites and can be very dangerous for the patient. As a consequence, the close monitoring of the estradiol levels is quite important. A determination of the ovarian follicular size by ultrasound is then carried out to detect a follicular size of at least 15 mm prior to attempting a laparoscopic ovocyte retrieval. At about 24–48 hours prior to stopping the hMG treatment, 10,000 U of *human chorionic gonadotropin* (hCG) are administered to the patient intramuscularly, with the laparoscopic ovocyte retrieval being planned for 34 hours later. The administration of hCG allows for the augmentation of the corpus luteum function.

Ovulation may be detected ultrasonically by: (1) the disappearance of the follicle, (2) the loss of the circular shape of the follicle, (3) the thickening of the follicular wall, (4) the loss of the clear sonolucent follicle, and (5) the detection of fluid in the cul-de-sac. The ovocyte is then retrieved via laparoscopic technique and placed in special media, where the fertilization can be carried out with prepared sperm. The subsequent fertilized ova (usually four cleaved embryos) are then transferred into the uterine cavity in a special transfer media. Daily intramuscular injections of progesterone are then administered for at least eight days. If the beta-hCG test becomes positive, indicating that implantation and a possible viable preg-nancy has taken place, the quantitative hCG assays may be followed to determine the levels and their trend. An ultrasound evaluation allows for the confirmation of the pregnancy after about six weeks. If the pregnancy does not take, then the patient should skip a menstrual cycle before attempting another in-vitro fertilization procedure. Multiple gestations (20%) as well as ectopic pregnancies (1–2%) may occur in these patients.

In couples in which there seems to be either a male factor or unexplained infertility, **gamete intrafallopian transfer (GIFT)** has been used. After the patient has been hyperstimulated, monitored, and the eggs retrieved at laparoscopy, the washed sperm and ovocytes may be placed in the ampulla of a normal fallopian tube by a plastic cannula. The success rate of such procedures is about 25%.

In those patients who do not have a uterus or accessible ovaries, who have genetic diseases or medical contraindications to having a pregnancy, or who have a poor obstetric history, a **surrogate mother** may be used. In this case, the parent's gametes or embryo may be placed into the surrogate mother's uterus.

These new techniques have stimulated considerable controversy within the medical community as to the **ethics** involved in modern clinical medicine. Is it ethical, for example, to create embryos in a dish? What are the rights and responsibilities of the surrogate mother? What are the risks to the mother or to the fetus in the use of these various techniques? What are the rights of the fetus? In short, such issues have forced the physician to look at many of the new technological advances in medicine with a different perspective. There are four possible issues of **ethical/medical decision making** that should be considered, namely: (1) What are the indications for medical intervention in the first place? (2) What are the patient's goals and preferences? (3) What is the quality of life that can reasonably be expected to occur with or without the intervention? and finally, (4) What is the influence of the cost factors and other societal concerns upon the decision? While these issues have been raised primarily in regard to infertility procedures, similar ethical concerns have also been raised in other areas of obstetrics. For example, should the mother be held liable for in-utero damage to her baby due to alcoholism or drug abuse during pregnancy? Should she be held liable for the intrauterine fetal growth retardation that results from poor eating habits or smoking? Whose rights take precedence when the mother refuses a cesarean section and there are late decelerations present on the electronic fetal monitor—the mother's or the fetus's? Furthermore, what are the obligations and responsibilities of the physician in these situations? Under current laws in many states, the physician is caught in the middle and stands to be in violation of the rights of either the mother or the baby regardless of the final clinical decision. In the future, guidelines will have to be formulated to protect everyone's rights in a moral, ethical, and legal sense. **The broadly trained physician who has been well-grounded in philosophy, ethics, literature, history, and psychology will be more properly equipped to make such decisions in the future.**

CHAPTER 45

Fertility control

The master word in medicine is work—Though a little one, it looms large in meaning. It is the open sesame to every portal, the great equalizer in the world, the true philosopher's stone which transmutes all the base metal of humanity into gold.

—*Sir William Osler**

1. Contraception

a. Historical aspects

Since ancient times, men and women have attempted to control fertility and to limit the size of their families. Such contraceptive measures have included various potions, procedures, and techniques as well as abortion. **Coitus interruptus,** which consists of the early withdrawal of the penis prior to ejaculation, has been commonly employed for fertility control. Douches, the vaginal insertion of animal excreta, and the use of vaginal sponges are only a few of the contraceptive practices that have been utilized.

In 1350 B.C., the Egyptians used decorated covers for their penises. These **penile sheaths** were still in use in 1504. The famous Italian anatomist Gabriele Fallopius (1523–1562) also described penile sheaths made of linen. With the introduction of the vulcanization of rubber in the middle of the 19th century, the modern rubber condom became widely available by 1870.

*Reprinted with permission from Robert Bennett Bean, *Sir William Osler: Aphorisms from His Bedside Teachings and Writings,* William Bennett Bean, ed. Springfield, Ill.: Charles C Thomas, Publisher, 1968, p. 74.

Following condoms, diaphragms and cervical caps were introduced; by 1915, there were 16 different sizes of diaphragms available. By 1923, a couple of intrauterine devices had been developed, most notably the **Grafenberg ring.**

Near the turn of the century, **Margaret Sanger** (1879–1965) of the United States and **Marie Stopes** (1880–1958) of England began their lifelong careers of educating the population about contraception and family planning. In the 1950s, **Dr. John A. Rock,** of Johns Hopkins University School of Medicine, was able to develop contraceptive hormones from the wild Mexican yam. He has since been called **the father of the pill.** By 1956, the first research studies, by **Dr. Gregory Pincus,** and **Dr. Min Chueh-Chang,** on the contraceptive pills appeared. The first clinical studies were performed by **Dr. Celso Ramon Garcia,** and **Dr. Edris Rice-Way,** in Puerto Rico in 1956. In 1960, the "pill" was approved by the U.S. Food and Drug Administration, and the Searle Pharmaceutical Company then began to market the first **birth control pill.**

2. Current birth control methods

a. Types

Birth control methods may be classified as: (1) physiologic, (2) chemical barrier, (3) mechanical barrier, (4) combined chemical and mechanical barrier, (5) intrauterine devices, and (6) systemic hormonal control. The failure rate of these various methods of birth control in many instances is often more dependent upon the patient's failure to use them correctly, rather than being a failure of the method itself.

The **physiologic fertility control method** (i.e., natural family planning, rhythm method, fertility awareness) consists of identifying the time of ovulation so that coitus can be avoided during the fertile portion of the menstrual cycle. This technique is utilized by about 1% of women. The **chemical methods** of birth control consist of the use of foams, creams, jellies, or suppositories that contain spermicidal agents. About 4% of women use this technique of birth control. **The mechanial barrier methods** interpose a membrane (e.g., a condom, diaphragm, or sponge) between the penis and the uterine cervix. Condoms are used by 8% and diaphragms by 3% of couples. **In practice, a combination of both a mechanical barrier (e.g., diaphragm) and a spermicidal cream, foam, or jelly is usually used.** Vaginal sponges have also been used in conjunction with spermicidal agents. **Intrauterine devices (IUDs)** consist of coils, loops, or other shapes of plastic that are inserted into the uterine cavity for extended periods of time. Some of the IUDs release progesterone gradually over time. Other IUDs are partially encased in copper wire that slowly dissolves over several years. IUDs until recently were used by 4% of patients. The **systemic hormonal** control of fertility involves the use of birth control pills or medroxyprogesterone acetate (Depo-Provera) to suppress ovulation. The birth control pills are the most popular form of contraception and are used by 12–18% of women.

b. Physiologic fertility control

The basic premise involved in utilizing physiologic fertility control, or the rhythm method, is that the day of ovulation must be accurately identified so that coitus may be avoided during the fertile part of the cycle. Some women will note the time of ovulation by becoming aware of an increased amount of a *clear vaginal mucoid discharge, lower pelvic heaviness and discomfort, and some lower quadrant pain* (i.e., **mittelschmerz**) that occurs for 2–3 days at about midcycle. In other women, these symptoms may be minimal or absent. When ovulation does occur, the next menstrual period is usually associated with lower abdominal cramps, indicating that ovulation has taken place during that cycle.

In using this technique of fertility control, certain assumptions must be made regarding ovulation. They are: (1) that ovulation will oc- cur on or about the **14th day ± 2 days before the next menses, (2) that the spermatozoa will survive for 2–3 days, and finally, (3) that the ovum will survive for only about 1 day.**

1) Calculating the safe period

A patient's previous 9–12 months of menstrual cycles should be evaluated to determine the shortest and the longest cycles. In calculating the **earliest time that ovulation might occur during a menstrual cycle,** you should take the ovulation time (i.e., 14 days plus 2 days) and add it to the 3 days that the sperm may live, to give a total of 19 days. If this factor is then subtracted from the **shortest menstrual cycle** (e.g., 26 days), the value becomes 26 − 19 = 7. Thus, assuming that the first day of the menses is day number one, then the **earliest** time that ovulation could occur would be on day 7.

To calculate the **latest day that ovulation might occur during a menstrual cycle,** you should take the time of ovulation, minus 2 days, (14 − 2 = 12) and then subtract from it the one day that the ovum may live, to give a total of 11 days. This is then subtracted from the **longest menstrual cycle** (e.g., 32 days) to give the 21st day. Thus, the last day that ovulation could take place would be day 21. **Therefore, between day 7 and day 21 (in this example) intercourse should be avoided, since this would seem to be the possible fertile range for this patient.** Each month, this calculation should be redone using the most recent 9–12 cycles for the calculation. This method allows for a correction of any subtle changes in the cycle length that may have occurred over this period of time.

2) Basal body temperature chart

To further refine this approach to fertility control, it is necessary to more accurately define the time of ovulation. **This may be accomplished by using the basal body temperature (BBT) chart.** The patient should obtain a large, easy-to-read BBT thermometer and should take her temperature orally each morning upon awakening "for 5 minutes by the clock." This should be done before drinking, smoking, or any other activity is carried out. The temperature will be found to dip slightly just before ovulation at midcycle, and then after ovulation, the temperature will increase from 0.8 to 1.0° F, where it will remain for the rest of the cycle.

3) Cervical mucus changes

The last aspect of physiologic fertility control that should be considered involves a confirmation of the time of ovulation by the evaluation of the character of the cervical mucus. The cervical mucus is thick and cloudy and does not have much "stickiness" prior to or after ovulation. *During the 2–3 days that encompass the time of ovulation, the mucus becomes thin and clear (i.e., like egg white), and becomes sticky so that when it is stretched between the fingers, it will produce a thin strand of mucus that exceeds 2.5 inches (6 cm or greater). This mucus-stretching technique has been called spinnbarkeit.* In order to more clearly define the differences in the vaginal discharge during (1) the pre- and postovulatory period, (2) following sexual excitement, (3) in the presence of semen, and perhaps (4) with a vaginal infection, from that of the mucus that occurs at the time of ovulation, it has been suggested that the patient should chart the characteristics of the mucus throughout one month of abstinence in an effort to observe these differences.

4) Effectiveness

The failure rate of the physiologic fertility control method is quite high (2–20%*). The average typical users' failure rate, however, is about 24%.** Accurate data concerning the success or failure of this method of fertility control are difficult to obtain since many individuals have difficulty in following the three parameters. In addition, the technique is often mixed partially with chemical or barrier methods during the fertile period of the cycle.

An additional consideration in the use of a contraceptive approach involves the type of pregnancy that might occur when the technique fails. In the physiologic fertility control method, the fertilization of an *over-ripe egg* may result in fetal abnormalities and in an increased fetal wastage in some animals. This may be true in humans as well.

---

*The **lowest observed failure rate** in 100 users who use the method correctly for one year.
The **average typical users' failure rate in 100 users who use the method correctly and consistently for one year.

c. Condom

The modern condom, otherwise known as a rubber, a prophylactic, a safety, a skin, or a sheath, is a latex rubber sheath-like cover for the penis that contains the ejaculate and thus prevents conception. Initially, sheep intestine (i.e., cecum) was used for the making of condoms; however, with the availability of vulcanized rubber in the 1840s, most of them were then made of rubber. Since 1930, when the latex rubber process became established, thin, strong condoms that were superior to the previous types became possible. Currently, condoms are the second most popular contraceptive after oral contraceptives in the United States, and they are becoming even more popular with the current problems associated with the transmission of sexually transmitted diseases (e.g., AIDS, Chlamydia trachomatis, etc.).

The condom is a thin cylindrical sheath that can be rolled up and easily packaged. They come in different colors, with or without ridges, and with or without lubrication. The shelf life of the condom is more than two years. They are available from a wide variety of business establishments with public restrooms, such as restaurants, gas stations, and bars, as well as drugstores and grocery stores, and thus can be easily obtained. A couple of the common brand names of condoms are Trojan and Ramses. The condom is an excellent birth control method because it affords protection against venereal disease in addition to its contraceptive benefits. **When using a condom, the man should be instructed to allow for adequate room beyond the end of the penis so that the condom can accommodate the ejaculate.** A spermicidal cream or jelly is often used with a condom as an additional chemical barrier. The Ramses Extra type has 0.5 gram of nonoxynol-9 spermicidal cream on both the inner and outer surfaces of the sheath, which apparently has been shown to reduce the motility of the sperm inside the condom to less than 2% within two minutes.

While the **condom may reduce the sensation** somewhat for the male partner, it is a valuable form of contraception that places the responsibility for conception control upon the man rather than on the woman. The condom, if used appropriately and correctly, may approach the effectiveness of the oral contraceptives, with the **lowest observed failure rate** being of the order of 2% (*), and with the **average typical users' failure rate** being about 10% (**).

d. Spermicidal agents

The use of spermicidal agents to prevent pregnancy dates back to ancient times. These agents may act by damaging the cell membrane of the spermatozoa or by interfering with specific essential cellular ezyme systems.

Numerous chemicals have been used as spermicidal agents, including surface-acting chemicals, hypertonic solutions, alkylating compounds, oxidizing agents, and many more. *One chemical that is commonly used as a spermicidal agent is nonoxynol-9.*

Chemical spermicidal agents are usually combined with a vehicle or a base that allows the agent to be delivered to the cervix and the vagina. *These delivery systems consist of foams, creams, jellies, or suppositories.* Of these, the foams are usually the least messy after coitus, and are therefore more acceptable to the patient than are the jellies or creams.

These chemical barrier agents should be placed in the vagina for up to 20 minutes prior to having intercourse. Following coitus, there is no need for the patient to douche; however, if douching is desired, it should not be done for at least four hours. The **lowest observed failure rate** of these chemical agents is of the order of 3–5% (*), with the **average typical users' failure rate** being about 18% (**).

Although there have been essentially no contraindications to the use of the chemical barrier methods, there has been some recent concern regarding the systemic blood levels of these chemicals that may occur in the patient secondary to their absorption from the vaginal mucosa. Furthermore, if a pregnancy should occur, there is some evidence that congenital anomalies, especially limb-reduction defects, may be slightly increased.

e. Diaphragm

The original vaginal diaphragm was designed in 1838, and its construction has not changed appreciably in the past 150 years. The modern diaphragm is a round latex rubber cup-like structure that has a metal rim about its periphery. The rim may be made of: (1) a flat

---

* The **lowest observed failure rate** in 100 users who use the method correctly for one year.
** The **average typical users' failure rate** in 100 users who use the method correctly and consistently for one year.

spring steel band, (2) a coiled spring, (3) an arcing steel band that bends in one direction (i.e., arcing type), (4) a flexible steel band, that is inside of a coiled spring, or (5) a type with a wide seal rim that contains a flexible 1.5-cm flange along the inner edge. This latter type is a more recent innovation (1983), and consists of the addition of a rubber lip that extends out from the rim of the diaphragm and aids in "sealing" the edge of the diaphragm to the vaginal walls. These changes from the original diaphragm have allowed for additional flexibility in the use of the diaphragm and have provided for a more effective shape that fits the vaginal and cervical contours more effectively.

Although **the diaphragm is a mechanical barrier for contraception, a chemical barrier in the form of a spermicidal agent is almost always used in conjunction with it.** The diaphragm must be fitted by the physician initially, and the patient must be carefully instructed on how to insert it and check its position once it is in place. **The largest diaphragm that can be fitted with comfort to the patient should be used, since with sexual excitement the vagina elongates as the uterus rises up out of the pelvis.** The diaphragm comes in a number of sizes to accommodate the range of vaginal depths that may be encountered. *It should be replaced once a year, or whenever there has been a significant change in the patient's body weight (e.g., over 10 lbs).* The anterior rim of the diaphragm should fit snugly behind the symphysis pubis, while the posterior rim lies in the posterior vaginal fornix. The cup of the diaphragm covers the cervix and contains a spoonful of spermicidal jelly or cream. Occasionally, some women will not be able to master the procedure of insertion, or may be so fastidious that they will not touch their genitals in order to check the position of the diaphragm, in which case this method of fertility control cannot be used.

The patient should be able to insert and remove the diaphragm and to also palpate the cervix through the membrane so as to be certain that the posterior rim is in the fornix and that the cervix is covered by the diaphragm. **The diaphragm should be left in place for eight hours following coitus, after which it should be removed, cleaned, and dried.** Cleaning the diaphragm consists of washing it in soap and water, followed by immersing it in 70% alcohol for at least 20 minutes, in order to sterilize any potential sexually transmitted diseases. No powder or lubricants should be used on the diaphragm, except for perhaps cornstarch. The diaphragm should be inspected periodically to be certain that there are no holes present.

The diaphragm has a **lowest observable failure rate** of about 2% (*), and a **typical users' rate of failure** of about 19% (**). The need to insert the diaphragm into the vagina prior to coitus may be aesthetically unsatisfactory for some couples. There are other hazards as well to the patient who uses a diaphragm, although they are rare. These risks include toxic shock syndrome, vaginal ulcerations, allergic responses to the latex rubber or the spermicidal creams, and a putrid vaginal odor if the diaphragm is forgotten and retained for a long period of time. The additional benefits of using the diaphragm are that it conveys a degree of protection against gonorrhea, and perhaps some of the other sexually transmitted diseases as well, when the spermicidal cream or jelly is also used.

f. Cervical cap

The cervical cap is a miniature diaphragm that is placed over the cervix and held in place by suction. While individually molded cervical caps have been used in Europe for contraception with good results, their use in the United States has been limited. Vaginal odor and vaginal ulcerations have been identified as potential problems with this method, which may also pose a risk for the development of the toxic shock syndrome.

A spermicidal cream is placed within the cervical cap in the same manner as with the diaphragm. The continued use of the cervical cap was low in one study, with less than 30% of the patients continuing to use the method after one year. The **lowest observable failure rate** would appear to be about 2% (*), or the **typical users' failure rate** of about 13% (**); however, there is limited information as to its effectiveness at the present time. Some of the caps that are available in Europe are Prentif Cavity-Rim Cervical Cap, Dumas Vault Cap, and the Vimule Cap.

---

*The **lowest observed failure rate** in 100 users who use the method correctly for one year.
The **average typical users' failure rate in 100 users who use the method correctly and consistently for one year.

g. Vaginal sponge

The use of vaginal sponges for contraception is quite ancient, having been used by the Jewish people as long ago as 300 B.C. While sea sponges or balls of cloth were initially favored, the recent development of the collagen protein sponges that contain bacteriostatic and fungicidal agents in association with spermicidal agents has resulted in a contraceptive device that may be a valuable addition to conception control methods. At this time, however, this technique has resulted in an unacceptably high failure rate with the **lowest observed failure rate** of 9–11% (*), or an **average typical users' failure rate** of about 10–20% (**). The only contraceptive techniques that exceed this level of failure are coitus interruptus, with 23% (**); the physiologic fertility methods (i.e., "rhythm"), with 24% (**); douching, with 40% (**); and no method of fertility control at all, at 90% (**).

h. Intrauterine devices

It has been estimated that, in the 1980s, more than 60 million women in the world were using intrauterine devices (IUDs) for contraception. Many of these women resided in China or in Third World countries. Over the past several years there has been considerable concern expressed about the safety of these devices. Recently, due to the excessive litigation surrounding IUDs, almost all of them have been removed from the market in the United States. The progesterone-containing IUD is still available, however, and another copper-containing IUD will be placed on the market again in the near future (i.e., Copper-T 380A).

1) Mechanism of action

The **mechanism of action** of the IUD is supposedly due in part to the local inflammation that is produced in the underlying endometrium, which causes lysis of the blastocyst and sperm. There is an increase in prostaglandins also, which apparently interferes with the implantation of the fertilized ovum. Enzyme interference has been noted in the endometrium when the copper-containing IUDs have been used. The thickened cervical mucus, and the endometrial changes that are produced by the progesterone-containing IUDs, has been cited as the cause for the failure of the zygote to implant in the endometrium with these devices.

2) Failure rate and complications

The **lowest observable failure rate** of the IUD is about 1.5% (*); however, other studies have shown a **typical users' failure rate** of 5% (**). About 15% of patients will have enough difficulty with an IUD that it will have to be removed. Some of the minor problems that have been associated with the use of the IUDs have involved excessive or persistent bleeding, cramping, and expulsion of the IUD (10%). In general, nulliparous women should not be fitted with an IUD because of the risk of infection and possible subsequent infertility, especially in the first few months of use. One of the major complications that have been seen is the **perforation of the uterus.** The perforation may occur during the initial insertion (with an incidence of 1:1,000 to 1:2,000) or it may occur because of the shape and rigidity of the IUD, which allows the IUD to work its way through the uterine wall into the peritoneal cavity. **Another significant complication that has been noted is the increased incidence of pelvic inflammatory disease (PID), although this increase was associated mostly with the shield type of IUD.** There has been a slight increase in the incidence of PID in patients who used the Cu-7 and the loop type of devices, especially during the first four months of use. These infections have occurred more commonly in women who have had many different sexual partners or in women who have had previous episodes of PID. As a consequence, the IUD should not be used in this type of patient. The type of PID that occurs in association with the IUD may be unilateral in some patients, and unusual organisms, such as **actinomycetes, may be involved in perhaps as many as 20% of these cases.**

An increase in the incidence of **ectopic pregnancy** in patients wearing IUDs was initially thought to be due to the device; however, this theory has been revised. Since the IUD is more successful in preventing an intrauterine pregnancy (99.5%) than it is in preventing a tubal pregnancy (95%), there is a 5- to 10-fold increased chance that if a pregnancy does occur in a patient with an IUD, then it will be an ectopic pregnancy.

---

*The **lowest observed failure rate** in 100 users who use the method correctly for one year.
The **average typical users' failure rate in 100 users who use the method correctly and consistently for one year.

i. Oral contraceptives

1) Historical aspects

The oral birth control pills came on the market in 1960 and were widely used in the United States. During the next 15 years, this usage increased to the point that 35.4% of married women, and almost 50% of the unmarried women were "on the pill." With the subsequent adverse publicity over the past few years, the usage of birth control pills has decreased to about 12% of all women in the childbearing age groups (i.e., 9–10 million women). Perhaps as many as 50 million women in the United States have used this form of contraception.

2) Composition of birth control pills

There are more than 30 types of oral contraceptives available in the United States today that contain an estrogen and/or a progestin component. The estrogenic component has consisted of either ethinyl estradiol, 20–50 μg, or mestranol, 50–150 μg. The higher dose oral contraceptives (i.e., 75–150 μg of estrogen) that contain mestranol are generally not advocated, due to the higher incidence of complications reported with these pills, and they have recently been taken off the market. Since the progestin norethynodrel was also used in some of these higher dose preparations, it also is no longer used. The six progestins are: (1) norgestrel, 0.075–0.5 mg, (2) levonorgestrel, 0.15 mg, (3) norethindrone, 0.35–2.0 mg, (4) norethindrone acetate, 1.0–2.5 mg, and (5) ethynodiol diacetate, 1 mg (Table 45-1).

3) Cardiovascular complications

In 1975, a few British studies began to appear linking the "pill" to an increased risk of death from cardiovascular diseases. The reports began to show that women over 40 years of age who were using birth control pills had a three-fold increase in heart attacks. Since 1975, further evidence has accumulated to indicate that the risk of cardiovascular disease is minimal in women taking birth control pills under the age of 30, unless other factors are present, such as hypertension or diabetes. Smoking was also cited as an adverse factor in women who were beyond the age of 35. Estrogens usually cause an increase in high-density lipoproteins (HDL) and a decrease in the

TABLE 45-1. Composition of oral contraceptives currently marketed in the United States

Product	Type	Progestin content	Estrogen content	Manufacturer
Brevicon	Combination	0.5 mg norethindrone	35 µg ethinyl estradiol	Syntex
Norinyl 1 + 35	Combination	1 mg norethindrone	35 µg ethinyl estradiol	Syntex
Norinyl 1 + 50	Combination	1 mg norethindrone	50 µg mestranol	Syntex
NOR-Q.D.	Progestin only	0.35 mg norethindrone		Syntex
Tri-Norinyl 7/	Combination triphasic	0.5 mg norethindrone	35 µ ethinyl estradiol	Syntex
9/		1 mg norethindrone	35 µg ethinyl estradiol	Syntex
5/		0.5 mg norethindrone	35 µg ethinyl estradiol	Syntex
Demulen 1/35	Combination	1 mg ethynodiol diacetate	35 µg ethinyl estradiol	Searle
Demulen 1/50	Combination	1 mg ethynodiol diacetate	50 µg ethinyl estradiol	Searle
Loestrin 1/20	Combination	1 mg norethindrone acetate	20 µg ethinyl estradiol	Parke-Davis
Loestrin 1.5/30	Combination	1.5 mg norethindrone acetate	30 µg ethinyl estradiol	Parke-Davis
Norlestrin 2.5/50	Combination	2.5 mg norethindrone acetate	50 µg ethinyl estradiol	Parke-Davis
Norlestrin 1/50	Combination	1 mg norethindrone acetate	50 µg ethinyl estradiol	Parke-Davis
Lo/Ovral	Combination	0.3 mg norgestrel	30 µg ethinyl estradiol	Wyeth
Nordette	Combination	0.15 mg levonorgestrel	30 µg ethinyl estradiol	Wyeth
Ovral	Combination	0.5 mg norgestrel	50 µg ethinyl estradiol	Wyeth
Ovrette	Progestin only	75 µg norgestrel		Wyeth
Tri-Phasil 6/	Combination triphasic	50 µg levonorgestrel	30 µg ethinyl estradiol	Wyeth
5/		75 µg levonorgestrel	40 µg ethinyl estradiol	Wyeth
10/		125 µg levonorgestrel	30 µg ethinyl estradiol	Wyeth
Ovcon-35	Combination	0.4 mg norethindrone	35 µg ethinyl estradiol	Mead Johnson
Ovcon-50	Combination	1 mg norethindrone	50 µg ethinyl estradiol	Mead Johnson
Modicon	Combination	0.5 mg norethindrone	35 µg ethinyl estradiol	Ortho
Ortho-Novum 1/35	Combination	1 mg norethindrone	35 µg ethinyl estradiol	Ortho
Ortho-Novum 1/50	Combination	1 mg norethindrone	50 µg mestranol	Ortho
Ortho-Novum 1/80	Combination	1 mg norethindrone	80 µg mestranol	Ortho
Ortho-Novum 10/	Combination biphasic	0.5 mg norethindrone	35 µg ethinyl estradiol	Ortho
11/		1 mg norethindrone	35 µg ethinyl estradiol	Ortho
Micronor	Progestin only	0.35 mg norethindrone		Ortho
Ortho-Novum 7/	Combination triphasic	0.5 mg norethindrone	35 µg ethinyl estradiol	Ortho
7/		0.75 mg norethindrone	35 µg ethinyl estradiol	Ortho
7/		1 mg norethindrone	35 µg ethinyl estradiol	Ortho

Adapted from D. N. Danforth and J. R. Scott, eds., *Obstetrics and Gynecology,* 5th ed. Philadelphia: J. B. Lippincott Company, 1986, p. 237.

low-density lipoproteins (LDL). The progestins have an opposite effect on the lipoprotein profile. High-density lipoprotein (HDL) cholesterol has been thought to be antiatherogenic (i.e., high levels are protective; low levels are not protective). Low-density lipoproteins (LDL) and very-low-density lipoproteins (VLDL), on the other hand, have a high triglyceride content and may deliver cholesterol to the walls of the arteries. Estrogens and progestins also have an effect on the coagulation cascade system. A delicate balance exists between thromboxane and prostacyclin at the level of the platelet and vascular epithelium, since the former increases platelet aggregation and arterial va-

sospasm, whereas the latter has just the opposite effect.

In view of these concerns, the amount of estrogen that was present in the original birth control pills was first reduced from 100 µg to 80 µg, then from 80 µg to 50 µg, and finally from 50 µg to 30–35 µg. In doing so, there was a dramatic reduction in the risk of cardiovascular complications that were associated with the birth control pills. **The risk of thromboembolism in association with birth control pills that contain 35 µg of estrogen is about 3:100,000 women per year.** To place this in proper perspective, however, the risk of death from pregnancy is about 25:100,000. Because of this possible risk of thromboembolism, it has been suggested that oral contraceptives should be discontinued about one month prior to elective surgery. Of interest is the fact that the oral contraceptives are somewhat protective against both gonococcal and chlamydial pelvic inflammatory disease. There is recent evidence that women up to the age of 45 who use low-dose pills (i.e., 35 μg of estrogen) are not at an increased risk for fatal heart attacks, provided that they do not smoke and do not have any preexisting cardiovascular disease (hypertension, diabetes, hypercholesterolemia). **Currently, however, the recommendation of the American College of Obstetricians and Gynecologists is that in women over 40 years of age, the use of birth control pills is potentially more of a risk, and that they are relatively contraindicated.**

In a woman who is nursing, the earliest reported time of ovulation is 10 weeks postpartum; therefore, contraception is usually not needed until after this time. **If the woman is not nursing, then the earliest reported time of ovulation is about 4 weeks postpartum, with about 5% of women ovulating by this time.** If bromocriptine is utilized for milk suppression, ovulation may occur as early as the **2nd week** postpartum. The use of oral contraceptives in nursing patients will cause a decrease in the amount of milk that is produced; however, this does not seem to affect the infant's weight gain if the low-dose pills are used. The administration of birth control pills during the first six weeks' postpartum in patients who have received bromocriptine or in those who are not nursing carries the potential risk of thromboembolism. Some authors have found no evidence of adverse effects if the birth control pills are started during the 3rd week postpartum.

4) Contraindications

The **contraindications to the use of the higher dose birth control pills** include a previous history of vascular disease, such as thromboembolism, thrombophlebitis, atherosclerosis, stroke, lupus erythematosus, and sickle cell anemia. Further, diabetes mellitus, familial hyperlipidemia, hypertension, cardiac disease, liver disease, undiagnosed genital bleeding, and breast and endometrial cancer may also be listed. In addition, some of the relative contraindications to the use of birth control pills would include severe

migraine headaches, asthma, heavy cigarette smoking, amenorrhea of unknown origin, depression, varicose veins, and uterine leiomyomas. All of these contraindications are currently being reevaluated in light of the fact that the high-dose birth control pills are no longer administered. Many of these contraindications may no longer apply to the oral contraceptives at the lower dosage levels.

5) Benefits

It has been noted in some studies that women who have used birth control pills seem to have an incidence of ovarian cancer that is about 60% of that of non-pill users. A similar protection has been noted with regard to the development of endometrial carcinoma. In this instance the risk appears to be about 50% of that of non-pill users and is therefore comparable to that of ovarian cancer.

The fact that the ovary is "put to rest" by the use of oral contraceptives probably also decreases the incidence of ovarian inclusion cysts and the later development of other benign ovarian tumors. Birth control pills have virtually eliminated the occurrence of ectopic pregnancy because of their effectiveness as a contraceptive. By regulating the menstrual cycle and therefore the amount of menstrual discharge in most patients, birth control pills have reduced the amount of blood loss each month and therefore the incidence of iron deficiency anemia. The protective action of birth control pills in reducing the incidence of pelvic inflammatory disease has been widely recognized.

There are subtle benefits as well to the patient who uses birth control pills. The decreased incidence of dysmenorrhea is of benefit to many patients. In addition, the patient can plan her activities around the time of her menstrual period without fear of an unplanned menses occurring. Furthermore, the maintenance of estrogen and progestin throughout the month protects against the eventual development of osteoporosis. A contraceptive that suppressed the ovarian function without providing such protection would not be acceptable. Finally, the decrease in the number of hospitalizations secondary to the decreased incidence of pelvic inflammatory disease, benign ovarian tumors, and ovarian and uterine malignancies results in a considerable saving in health-care expenses. In sum, the use of birth control pills has many benefits in addition to the excellent protection it provides against an unplanned pregnancy.

6) Initiation of treatment

Any sexually active woman between puberty and 35 years of age is a candidate for oral contraception, assuming that there are no medical contraindications to their use. Women who have irregular menses prior to using birth control pills will usually continue to have a similar menstrual pattern after they stop the pill. Ideally, teenagers should have had at least 6–12 periods before starting birth control pills; however, the need to protect against an unwanted pregnancy may take precedence over this approach.

The patient should be counseled as to the risks and benefits of the pill, and as to the other alternative forms of contraception, prior to the initiation of the treatment. The birth control pills (BCPs) that contain 30–35 μg of estinyl estradiol are preferred over the higher dosage forms because of safety reasons, since higher doses carry a higher risk of complications. The **lowest observed failure rate** of the combined birth control pills is about 0.5% (*), with an **average typical users' failure rate** of 2% (**).

The selection of a specific formulation for each patient is otherwise dependent upon the patient's ability to tolerate the possible side effects. The side effects are secondary to the relative strengths and the amounts of the estrogenic and the progestationl components of the pill. The incidence of postpill amenorrhea has been reported to be 0.2–0.8%; however, this rate may be higher in those patients who had irregular menses prior to taking birth control pills. The patient on birth control pills should be evaluated closely during the first six months of treatment for evidence of symptomatic side effects, breakthrough bleeding, and an elevation of the blood pressure. If hypertension occurs, the patient may need to be switched to a pill with less estrogen or a progestin-only pill. Spotting and breakthrough bleeding can be watched for three months, and they will usually disap-

---

*The **lowest observed failure rate** in 100 users who use the method correctly for one year.
The **average typical users' failure rate in 100 users who use the method correctly and consistently for one year.

pear as the woman becomes adjusted to the birth control pill. The least androgenic pill is Ovcon-35. A low androgen pill such as this will also prevent the onset of weight gain during the use of the pill. Ovcon-35 has the lowest progestin activity, and Brevicon and Modicon are the next lowest progestin-activity pills.

j. Other hormonal contraceptives
1) Contraceptive intrauterine devices

The only intrauterine device that was still available in the United States until recently was the progesterone-containing intrauterine device, since all of the other IUDs have been removed from the market. This IUD releases a progestin slowly over a period of time. Recently, a new copper IUD is being reintroduced in the United States (i.e., Copper-T 380A).

2) Contraceptive vaginal rings

A vaginal ring that contains a progestin may be inserted into the vagina postmenses for 21 days in a manner similar to the use of a diaphragm. The ring may be temporarily removed for intercourse and then replaced. Vaginal erosion has been a problem in these patients due to the length of time that the ring remains in the vagina. Such erosions could lead to the development of the toxic shock syndrome. Currently, both a three-month and a six-month trial using the vaginal insert are being studied to determine if it has a place among the options of fertility control methods.

3) Contraceptive implants

Hormonal implants have been utilized in Great Britain, China, Finland, Sweden, and Thailand for some time. **The hormone, usually a progestin, is placed in a biodegradable Silastic capsule which can then be inserted under the skin, where it gradually releases the hormone over about a 5-year period.** The Norplant contraceptive implant contains levonorgestrel (i.e., 6 Silastic subdermal implants containing a total of 36 (±) mg of levonorgestrel). The **advantages** of these implants are that they provide effective birth control that is not dependent upon patient compliance. The menstrual blood loss is usually less with the progestin, which allows for the maintenance of a higher hemoglobin level in the patient, and in addition they relieve dysmenorrhea in almost 100% of women. There have been only two ectopic pregnancies reported in 5,000 woman-years of use. It has been estimated that about 20 mcg of levonorgestrel are released each day over the course of the 5-year period. The **disadvantage** involved in the use of these implants is that they must be surgically implanted, and thus there is a minor risk of pain and infection. **The pregnancy rate of the hormone implant varies between about 0.5 to 13.2 pregnancies per 100 woman-years of use, although one recent report lists a 5-year net pregnancy rate of only 0.4.**

k. Postcoital contraception

1) Morning-after pill

It has been noted that an unprotected coitus that occurs at midcycle carries about a 1–17% risk of conception; however, according to some authorities this risk may be as high as 15–30%. Pregnancy may occur when a barrier contraception technique fails (i.e., condom break, diaphragmatic or cervical cap dislodgement). Unprotected coitus may also cause pregnancy in cases of rape.

Currently, the U.S. Food and Drug Administration (FDA) has not approved any contraceptive agent to be used following coitus; however, in the treatment of rape victims, such therapy has been carried out for a number of years in an attempt to protect the patient from an unwanted pregnancy.

The current most popular "morning-after" pill is Ovral (0.05 mg of ethinyl estradiol and 0.5 mg of norgestrel), two tablets within 72 hours of coitus, with two more tablets being taken 12 hours later. The failure rate of this regimen in two reported studies was 0.16% and 1.6%, respectively. Bleeding occurred within 21–30 days in almost all patients.

2) Estrogens in high dose

The use of either diethylstilbestrol (DES), 25–50 mg, or ethinyl estradiol 0.5–2.0 mg daily for five days, has been used for pregnancy contravention in the past. The use of DES, however, is no longer recommended as a method for postcoital contraception.

3) IUD insertion

The insertion of a Copper-T or a Copper-7 IUD might be effective as a postcoital contraceptive, but there is no information on this approach as yet. Since most of the IUD devices have been removed from the market, there will probably be few studies performed in this regard; however, the recent reintroduction of a new copper IUD may rekindle interest in IUDs for this purpose.

4) Menstrual extraction

A suction curettage may be performed during the first six weeks of amenorrhea to interrupt any possible pregnancy that may have occurred. While this procedure may be performed on an outpatient basis, it would probably not be a popular option in most cases of accidental failure of a contraceptive technique, since it consists basically of a D&C for an elective abortion.

5) The future of fertility control

Over the next 50 years, we might anticipate the development of male and female antifertility compounds and vaccines, improved sperm and ovulation suppression techniques, and reversible male and female sterilization procedures. A recently developed once-a-month contraceptive compound, anordrin, is undergoing trials as an ovulation inhibitor. When given within the first six days of the menstrual cycle, anordrin suppresses the maturation of the ovum and the development of the follicle, with a significant decrease in estrogen and progesterone.

As the world population increases, there will be an even greater research thrust in these areas than in the past. Indeed, we may see governments becoming more interested in this area as the world's resources become more limited. Governmental control of the population may be instituted as in China, where a couple must seek the authorization of the government to have a child. The failure of a couple to abide by such laws may result in punitive measures, with a "loss of income" instead of an increase in financial aid. Certainly, governmental policies, medical care concerns, and human ethics will become more tightly intertwined over the next 50 years in the field of fertility control.

I. Induced abortion

1) General considerations

The performance of an abortion is not a very cost-effective form of population control, aside from the moral and ethical considerations. **As a surgical procedure, the maternal mortality rate is of the order of 0.5 deaths:100,000 abortions in the first trimester and 10:100,000 abortions in the late second trimester.** Surgical techniques have been shown to be somewhat safer than medical procedures up to 20 weeks' gestation. Most women who have abortions are single (78%), under the age of 25 (63%), and white (70%). **A first-trimester abortion is one in which the abortion occurs within the first 13 weeks, whereas a second-trimester abortion occurs between 14 and 24 weeks' gestation.**

2) Workup

Patients who wish to undergo abortion should have the pregnancy confirmed by a β-hCG pregnancy test and the gestational age should be estimated by an ultrasonogram. The Rh factor and the routine blood studies, including the hemoglobin and hematocrit, should be obtained. A routine history and physical examination should be performed to determine the presence of any medical complications, allergies, or other medical problems.

3) Surgical evacuation

The use of a Laminaria tent (or synthetic cervical dilator) to gently dilate the cervix over the course of 6–24 hours prior to the performance of the dilatation and evacuation (D&E) is of great value in preventing unnecessary trauma to the cervix. Prostaglandin gels, hydrophilic resins, and magnesium sulfate sponges have also been used with success to dilate the cervix.

A dilatation and curettage should be performed in abortion patients whose pregnancy is at less than 13 weeks' gestation. A vacuum curettage may be utilized up to 16 weeks' gestation. In patients who are in the second trimester (i.e., weeks 13–24), a dilatation and evacuation should be performed. While the techniques of hysterotomy and hysterectomy may be used in rare situations, they are usually not performed due to the associated higher morbidity and mortality rates. It is important for the patient to be closely followed

postoperatively to avoid complications. You should also provide emotional support for the patient during this psychologically and emotionally trying experience.

4) Medical evacuation

There are three medical techniques that may be used to evacuate the uterus between 13 and 24 weeks. These approaches utilize the instillation of intra-amniotic agents, such as (1) prostaglandins, (2) hypertonic saline, or (3) hypertonic urea.

Prostaglandin F_{2_α} (about 40 mg) may be instilled into the amniotic fluid; however, the primary problem with this technique when it is performed between weeks 20 and 24 is the risk of delivering a live infant. In addition, there are a number of uncomfortable side effects associated with the prostaglandins. Although the use of 20 mg vaginal suppositories of prostaglandin E_2 to instigate labor has been recommended by some authors in early abortions, the side effects may be quite uncomfortable and consist of fever and gastrointestinal complaints.

The use of hypertonic saline solution has the benefit of being fetocidal. About 200 ml of a 20–25% saline solution may be instilled into the amniotic cavity, after the removal of an equal amount of amniotic fluid. This method will result in the development of uterine contractions and the expulsion of the fetus over the course of 18–24 hours. The use of urea, 80 mg in 200 ml of sterile water, will accomplish this same purpose.

The above techniques should be combined with the use of Laminaria tents (Laminaria japonica or Laminaria digitata) to dilate the cervix in a nontraumatic manner. A synthetic polymer **(Dilapan)** may also be used to dilate the cervix. Another synthetic osmotic dilator made of polyvinyl alcohol surgical sponge with magnesium sulfate impregnation **(Lamicel)** has also been used to rapidly and atraumatically dilate the cervix in pregnancies that are at 14–16 weeks' gestation. In addition, oxytocin may be added to facilitate the uterine contractions and the ultimate expulsion of the products of conception.

5) Maternal mortality

The maternal mortality rates of the above procedures vary depending upon the length of gestation and the type of procedure used. The mortality rate of legal abortions in the United States from 1977–1981, as related to the number of weeks of gestation, was: (1) 0.5:100,000 at less than 8 weeks' gestation, (2) 0.8:100,000 at 9–10 weeks, (3) 1.1:100,000 at 11–12 weeks, (4) 1.5:100,000 at 13–15 weeks, (5) 7.8:100,000 at 16–20 weeks, and (6) 3.6:100,000 at more than 21 weeks.

When the maternal mortality rate was evaluated according to the type of evacuation procedure used, the following death rates were noted: (1) instrumental evacuation, 0.8:100,000, (2) intra-amniotic fluid instillation, 4.9:100,000, and (3) hysterotomy/hysterectomy, 58.9:100,000. The maternal morbidity includes infection, hemorrhage, cervical or uterine trauma, retained secundines, and the continuation of the pregnancy.

m. Sterilization

1) Female

a) General considerations

During the past 10 years it has been estimated that 800,000 to 1 million or more women have been sterilized annually in this country. Both laparoscopy and minilaparotomy procedures have been the most common techniques employed, and they have comparable failure rates. Sterilization should not be viewed as a temporary procedure to control childbearing. When it is performed, it should be considered to be a permanent operation. **About 1–3% of sterilized women request a reanastomosis of their tubes; however, depending upon the amount of tissue damage and the type of sterilization procedure, probably only 50% of these patients will ultimately have a subsequent pregnancy.**

It is important to thoroughly evaluate the patient and her motives for wishing to be sterilized. This is especially true for women in their early twenties or who only have 1–2 children. Later marital instability or divorce may cause many of these patients to eventually regret having undergone a sterilization procedure. The risks and benefits of sterilization should be thoroughly explained. Often it is worthwhile to ask the patient if she would like to have more children in the following circumstances: (1) if her husband died and she remarried, or (2) if she lost all of her children. A "yes" answer to either of these questions should alert you to the fact that this patient may have some ambivalent feelings about being sterilized and therefore may not be a good candidate for this procedure.

It is often good advice to encourage the woman who is between 20 and 30 years of age to utilize the nonpermanent forms of birth control until she is over the age of 30, after which a permanent sterilization procedure could be carried out if she so desires. Unfortunately, a large number of these young women are unable or unwilling to utilize temporary forms of contraception and will demand a permanent sterilization procedure.

b) Minilaparotomy sterilization procedures

A tubal ligation sterilization procedure may be carried out either as an outpatient or an inpatient procedure. The ligation of the fallopian tubes by the **Pomeroy technique, which consists of the ligation of a knuckle of the fallopian tube with plain catgut and the excision of a loop of the tube,** is perhaps the most common sterilization procedure that is performed when a **minilaparotomy** is utilized (Fig. 45-1). Other tubal sterilization procedures, which may require a larger abdominal incision, include: (1) the **Irving technique** (i.e., removal of a 1–2 cm segment of tube with ligation of each tubal end and the burial of the proximal tubal end into the posterior peritoneum of the uterus) (Fig. 45-2); (2) the **Kroener fimbriectomy technique** (i.e., the removal of the distal fimbriated portion of the fallopian tube) (Fig. 45-3); (3) the **Madlener technique** (i.e., the ligation of a knuckle of fallopian tube with nonabsorbable suture without resection of the tube) (Fig. 45-4); or a modification of this procedure by doubly ligating each limb of the loop; (4) the **Parkland technique** (i.e., the tube is ligated in 2 places about 2 cm apart and the intervening segment is excised) (Fig. 45-5), (5) the **Uchida technique** (Fig. 45-6), and (6) the **St. Louis Maternity Hospital (Barnes Hospital) technique,** which is similar to the Uchida technique, where the proximal end of the fallopian tube is buried between the leaves of the broad ligament (Fig. 45-7). The St. Louis Maternity Hospital, or Barnes Hospital, technique was being utilized from at least 1947 onwards. This technique was thought to be highly successful in preventing any further pregnancies, and yet

Text continues on p. 582

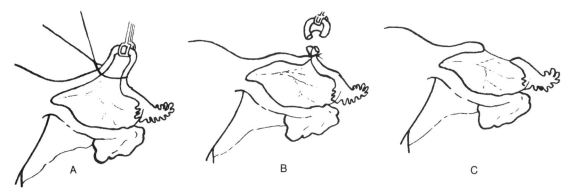

FIGURE 45-1. The Pomeroy technique of sterilization. (A) The tie should be of no. 1 plain gut with no previous crushing of the tube. (B) The loop of tube is removed. (C) The end result shows the separation of the tubal stumps.

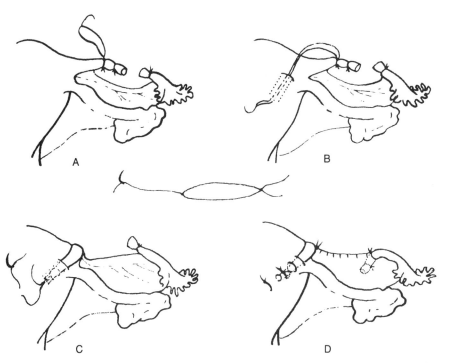

FIGURE 45-2. The Irving technique of sterilization. (A) The cut proximal tube is doubly ligated with catgut with one tie left long. The proximal mesosalpinx is cut back toward the uterus. (B) The long suture is threaded through a tunnel in the uterine peritoneum. (C) The end of the proximal tube is buried. (D) The distal end of the tube is ligated and buried between the leaves of the broad ligament, which is also closed with interrupted sutures. A special traction suture is demonstrated between the drawings.

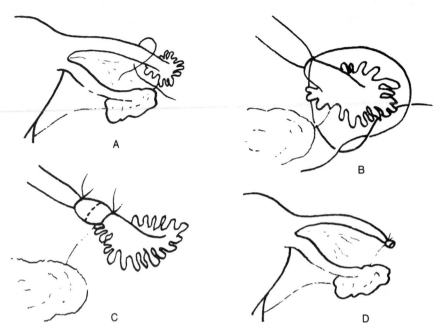

FIGURE 45-3. The Kroener technique of sterilization. (A) The fallopian tube is ligated at the ampulla. (B) A second ligature is placed. (C) The dotted line shows the placement of the division of the distal tube. (D) The ampulla with all of the fimbria is resected.

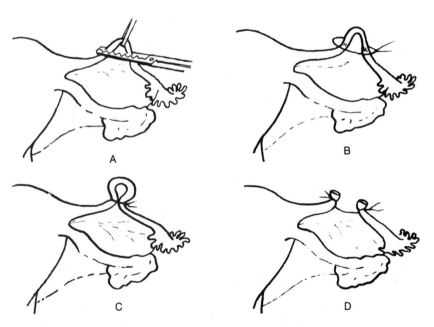

FIGURE 45-4. The Madlener technique of sterilization (modified). (A) While the tube is held up with an Allis clamp, the base of each limb of the tube is crushed with another clamp. (B) Nonabsorbable suture material is used to tie the base of the tubes. (C) The suture is tied. (D) The loop of tube is excised and the tubal stumps are doubly tied with a nonabsorbable suture. In the original Madlener technique only (A), (B), and (C) were carried out and the loop was not excised.

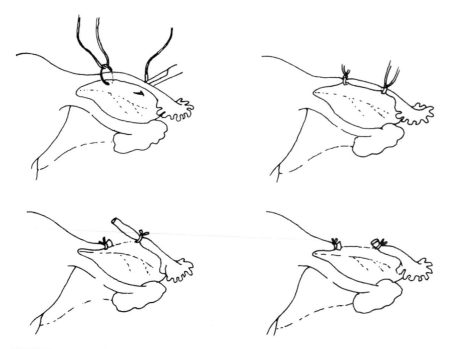

FIGURE 45-5. Parkland technique. The tube is ligated in two places and the intervening segment removed.

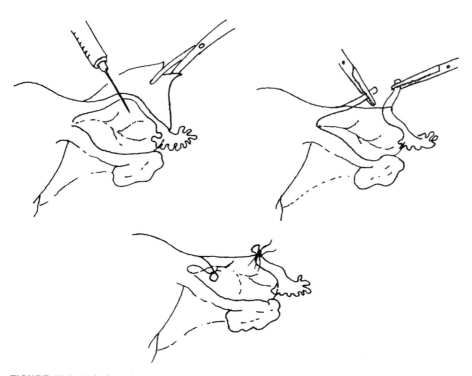

FIGURE 45-6. Uchida technique.

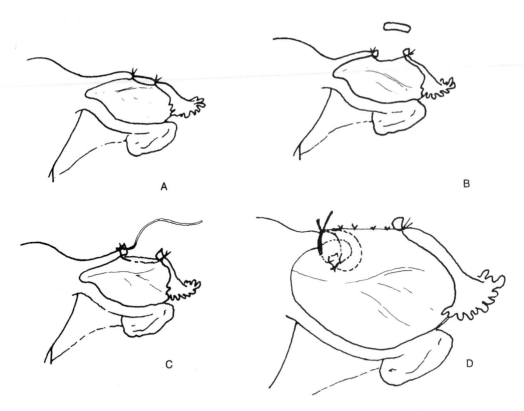

FIGURE 45-7. St. Louis Maternity Hospital (Barnes Hospital) technique of tubal sterilization. (A) The fallopian tube is ligated. (B) A 1-cm segment of the tube is removed. (C) The leaves of the broad ligament are opened. (D) The proximal portion of the fallopian tube is tunneled into the broad ligament and the suture ends brought back through the broad ligament and ligated on top of the proximal portion of the tube. The broad ligament is closed with interrupted sutures.

is easy to repair if a reanastomosis is needed. The Pomeroy technique has a failure rate that is slightly higher than some of the other procedures, especially when it is performed in the immediate postpartum period. The Madlener technique also has a high failure rate and is mentioned only to be condemned. **The Irving technique, the Parkland technique, the St. Louis Maternity Hospital (Barnes Hospital) technique, and the Uchida technique are probably the best laparotomy tubal sterilization procedures.**

c) Laparoscopy sterilization procedures

If a **laparoscopic** procedure is employed, the fallopian tubes may be fulgurated in 1–2 locations along the length of the tube through a very small periumbilical incision. A **bipolar coagulation** instrument is safer than a unipolar laparoscope and is more effective in performing a sterilization. **The complication rate of this procedure is about 1.7:100 laparoscopic procedures, and the complications consist mainly of hemorrhage and injuries to the abdominal organs (e.g., bowel and blood vessel puncture, bowel burns). The failure rate of laparoscopic fulguration of the fallopian tubes is about 1:1,000.** Some other laparoscopic procedures utilize metallic spring-loaded Lexan clips (Hulka-Clemens clip), bands, or rings (Falope ring), or a titanium device that is lined with silicon rubber (Filshie clip) to occlude the fallopian tubes. These procedures have a failure rate of about 2:1,000.

2) Male

A vasectomy is a simple office procedure that may be performed in the male in about 15–20 minutes under local anesthesia. The scrotum is opened and the vas deferens is identified, cut, ligated, and replaced into the scrotal sac. **Hemorrhagic complications occur in perhaps 1.6% of vasectomies, infection in 1.5%, epididymitis in 1.4%, and granuloma formation in 0.3%.** Several semen analyses should be performed for 1–2 months after the procedure to be certain that there are no more sperm present. It requires about 10–15 ejaculations to eliminate all of the sperm after the vas has been ligated to produce a negative sperm analysis. When two negative sperm analyses have been obtained, the man may be considered to be sterile. **The failure rate of a vas ligation is about 0.4%.** The anatomic reversibility of this procedure is of the order of 40–90%; however, only about 18–60% of the reversals will result in a pregnancy.

Index of Names

Index

The letter *f* following a page number indicates a figure; *t* indicates tabular material.